# Ultrastructural Appearances of Tumours

# Ultrastructural Appearances of Tumours

## DIAGNOSIS AND CLASSIFICATION OF HUMAN NEOPLASIA BY ELECTRON MICROSCOPY

**Douglas W. Henderson** MB, BS, FRCPA

Director of Electron Microscopy, Department of Histopathology, Flinders Medical Centre, Adelaide, South Australia; Honorary Consultant in Ultrastructural Pathology, The Queen Elizabeth Hospital, Woodville, South Australia; Senior Lecturer in Pathology, The Flinders University of South Australia

**John M. Papadimitriou** BA, MD, PhD, MRCPath, FRCPA

Associate Professor of Pathology, The University of Western Australia; Consultant in Pathology, Royal Perth Hospital and Queen Elizabeth II Medical Centre, Perth, Western Australia

**Mark Coleman** MB, BS, FRCPA

Senior Staff Specialist in Pathology, Flinders Medical Centre, Adelaide, South Australia; Lecturer in Pathology, The Flinders University of South Australia

And with the technical assistance of

*Peter J. Leppard and Terry A. Robertson*

Electron Microscopy Units, Departments of Pathology, Flinders Medical Centre and The University of Western Australia

SECOND EDITION

CHURCHILL LIVINGSTONE

EDINBURGH LONDON MELBOURNE AND NEW YORK 1986

CHURCHILL LIVINGSTONE
Medical Division of Longman Group Limited

Distributed in the United States of America by Churchill
Livingstone Inc., 1560 Broadway, New York, N.Y. 10036 and by
associated companies, branches and representatives throughout the
world.

First edition 1982
Second edition 1986

ISBN 0 443 03111 8

**British Library Cataloguing in Publication Data**
Henderson, Douglas W.
    Ultrastructural appearances of tumours :
    diagnosis and classification of human neoplasia
    by electron microscopy.——2nd ed.
    1. Tumors——Diagnosis  2. Diagnosis, Electron
    microscopic
    I. Title  II. Papadimitriou, John M.
    III. Coleman, Mark
    616.99′20758    RC255

**Library of Congress Cataloging in Publication Data**
Henderson, Douglas W.
    Ultrastructural appearances of tumours.
    Bibliography: p.
    Includes index.
    1. Tumors——Diagnosis.  2. Diagnosis, Electron
    microscopic.  3. Oncology——Classification.  4. Ultra-
    structure (Biology)  I. Papadimitriou, John M.
    II. Coleman, Mark.  III. Title.  [DNLM: 1. Microscopy,
    Electron——atlases.  2. Neoplasms——diagnosis——atlases.
    3. Neoplasms——ultrastructure——atlases.  QZ 17 H452u]
    RC270.H45  1985    616.99′20758    84–23760

Printed and bound in Great Britain by
William Clowes Limited, Beccles and London

# Preface to the Second Edition

The favourable reception accorded the first edition of this book and recent advances in our knowledge of tumour ultrastructure have necessitated preparation of a second edition after an interval of less than four years. The acceleration of information in this field can be gauged to some extent from the fact that most of the 1867 reference citations in the first edition appeared over a decade, whereas the updated bibliography contains approximately 1400 new references — most accessioned between July 1980 and 31 December 1983 — which could be accommodated only by deletion of many older and less important entries. As remarked by one reviewer, the writing of books on ultrastructure can be a truly Sisyphean task!

The basic objectives of *Ultrastructural Appearances of Tumours* remain unchanged, yet the entire text has been extensively revised, with the addition of three new chapters and many new tables. Although diagnostic features are still emphasized, the expanded text discusses issues of differential diagnosis and tumour classification in greater detail; the distinction between *differentiation* and *histogenesis* is stressed throughout, and we also attempt to define minimal criteria for the diagnosis of a number of tumours. Once again, we have adopted both a 'tumour-type' and 'organ-based' orientation, in the belief that this avoids repetition and partly conforms to a 'decision-tree' approach complementary to light microscopy. The reference numbers in the text have been deliberately restricted in an attempt to preserve the cadence for the reader; more exhaustive listings are appended to the tables and appropriate captions.

Almost half the illustrations in the first edition have been modified or replaced, with a wider spectrum of neoplasms being covered. As a matter of policy we have again decided to exclude light micrographs from the illustrations. The reasons for this decision are two-fold:

1. Ultrastructural *diagnosis* cannot be carried out meaningfully in isolation from pathological expertise; in such circumstances the interpretations are likely to be irrelevant or spurious. Light microscopy (LM) is a prerequisite for *diagnostic* electron microscopy (EM); we believe that the best results are likely to be achieved by surgical pathologists skilled in EM,[85,127] by electron microscopists with experience in surgical pathology, or by close collaboration of pathologist and electron microscopist. In all of these situations, background expertise in LM will be available, rendering it unnecessary to include a series of light micrographs, which, in the available space, could only be a token collection.

2. In any case, the histological appearances of tumours are depicted in a plethora of standard pathology texts and atlases; the interested reader is advised to consult these for LM descriptions of the tumours considered in this work.

Once again, we hope that this book will stimulate interest in the fine structure of pathological processes and, above all, that it will prove useful to everyone engaged in diagnostic electron microscopy.

Adelaide and Perth
1986

D.W.H.
J.M.P.
M.C.

# Preface to the First Edition

In reviewing the history of the light microscope in pathology, Majno & Joris[1] commented on a curious gap of some 250 years between its discovery and its introduction into surgical pathology.[2] The reasons given to explain this delay included 'secrecy of the art, high cost of the apparatus, technical difficulty, the notion that the microscope was a toy, lack of new ideas, neglect by Universities' and poor resolution of early instruments. Many of these observations could equally have been applied to electron microscopy; yet in the comparatively short space of about four decades, the electron microscope has come to occupy a well established role in diagnostic tissue pathology, haematology, and virology.

Over the past few decades, ultrastructural information on known neoplasms has accumulated to the point at which the data can be used for the diagnosis of tumours which are poorly differentiated or atypical by routine optical techniques. It is with this exercise that this atlas is primarily concerned. The lack of specificity of many architectural features is emphasized, and we have concentrated on the important differential ultrastructural features of the following groups of tumours:

1. Neoplasms such as the small round cell tumours, in which the fine-structural appearances are characteristic and often decisive in diagnosis.
2. Neoplasms with distinctive fine-structural appearances, which, although generally less crucial in diagnosis, may nevertheless contribute to the final pathological classification.
3. Neoplasms such as malignant fibrous histiocytoma, in which electron microscopy is ordinarily of limited or little diagnostic value, but which nevertheless enter into the differential light-microscopic and/or ultrastructural diagnosis of tumours in the first two groups.
4. Neoplasms not included in the above three groups, with unusual or interesting fine-structural features, illuminating the light-microscopic appearances wherever possible.

This volume is therefore primarily intended for the practising surgical pathologist, and not the research-orientated oncologist or cell biologist. Its purpose is to outline and illustrate the oncological problems encountered by surgical pathologists which can be solved by electron microscopy. It is hoped, however, that both the electron micrographs and the accompanying bibliography will also be useful to oncologists whose interest focuses on cell biology; the fine structure of various neoplasms must surely contribute to an understanding of the neoplastic process. Moreover, the tumours illustrated may aid researchers employing various experimental models, by providing information on the ultrastructural appearances of human neoplasms.

No attempt has been made to give an encyclopaedic description of the detailed ultrastructural appearances of human neoplasia. The text has been deliberately kept brief and only major diagnostic features have been emphasized; we have also made liberal use of tabular summaries to facilitate comparative ultrastructural recognition. In compiling many of the tables (such as the occurrence of fibrous long-spacing collagen in tumours) it has again not been our intention to be exhaustive, but to emphasize non-specificity by listing a range of tumours in which a particular structure may be found. The descriptions and illustrations are intended to facilitate problem-solving in surgical oncopathology by a process of major pattern recognition; if more detail is needed, relevant references should be sought in the bibliography.

Major categories of neoplasms have been grouped and their fine structure is illustrated in descending orders of differentiation with ascending sequences of magnification. In compiling the electron micrographs we have tried to illustrate a spectrum of appearances ranging from the representative to the unusual wherever applicable. Restrictions on space have precluded inclusion of light micrographs, but we have attempted to compensate for this by extensive use of low power electron-micrographic illustrations. Generally, special features have been grouped in one section while non-specific characteristics have been collected in another. The selection of material was governed by the principle that it was representative and/or that it possessed unique diagnostic features. Constraints of space and avoidance of unnecessary repetition have, however, influenced our choice, and to some extent selection of material was determined by our own practice.

An extensive bibliography was thought essential for deeper knowledge of the fine structure of particular neoplasms. Much of the material published in the last ten years is included, and most human neoplasms are listed. The references are predominantly grouped according to organ or tissue systems, or characteristic tumours, to help search and retrieval. Important references have been listed beneath the tables and many of the captions (particularly those at the beginning of various topics). It is hoped that this atlas will prove useful to the surgical pathologist in everyday practice and that it will generally stimulate interest in the fine structure of pathological processes.

Adelaide and Perth                              D.W.H.
1982                                            J.M.P.

# Acknowledgements

Production of the second edition of this work would have been impossible without the continuing support and enthusiasm of Prof. M. N-I. Walters (Perth) and Prof. R. Whitehead (Adelaide); we also owe a special debt of gratitude to Drs A. E. Seymour (Adelaide) and J. M. Skinner (Adelaide) for reading and criticizing the manuscript.

The clinicians, pathologists and haematologists who secured biopsy material for our evaluation are now too numerous to be listed in full. However, we pay particular tribute to the following colleagues, many of whose contributions are also acknowledged elsewhere, in the captions: Dr J. Armstrong (Perth): Dr D. K. Burns (Dallas, Texas); Prof. B. Corrin (London, England); Dr T. O. Ekfors (Turku, Finland); Dr C. M. Fenoglio (Albuquerque, New Mexico); Prof. R. L. Kempson (Stanford, California); Prof. J. F. R. Kerr (Brisbane, Queensland); Dr Li Ling (Beijing, People's Republic of China) — who participated actively in the diagnostic EM workload during his stay at the Flinders Medical Centre as a visiting scholar; Dr T. M. Mukherjee (Adelaide); Dr A. E. Seymour (Adelaide); Dr F. G. Silva (Dallas, Texas); and Dr E. J. Wills (Sydney, New South Wales).

The technical staff who processed the tissues for electron microscopy are again too many to list individually, but we must express our profound gratitude to Mr P. J. Leppard (Adelaide) who singlehandedly prepared all the new illustrations.

For secretarial help we thank Ms M. A. Seats, and in particular Miss C. McCaw, who spent many long hours processing the manuscript; her ability to convert seemingly illegible and disorganized handwriting into accurate typescript raised decipherment to new levels of sophistication. Assembly of the bibliography was facilitated by Mr D. Gardner who devised a computer programme to carry out this task.

We are also indebted to the following authors, editors and publishers for permission to modify and reproduce several of the tables and figures in this atlas: Dr F. W. Gunz, editor of *Pathology*, for Table 9.1 and Figs. 18.6–18.8; Dr P. B. Marcus and the editor of the *Journal of Submicroscopic Cytology*, for Table 5.2; Dr P. B. Marcus and the editor of *Ultrastructural Pathology*, and Hemisphere Publishing Corp. for Table 2.6; Prof. J. F. R. Kerr, Dr J. W. Searle, Dr A. H. Wyllie and the editors of *Pathology Annual* and *International Review of Cytology*, and the respective publishers (Appleton-Century-Crofts and Academic Press) for Table 1.3; Dr E. Solcia and the editor of *Gut Hormones*, and Churchill Livingstone for Table 14.1.

We are no less grateful to our publishers, Churchill Livingstone, for their continuing forebearance, patience and co-operation in the face of our many questions and requests.

Any success which this edition enjoys will be in large measure due to the co-operation and enthusiasm of our colleagues listed above. Once again, its deficiencies are ours and ours alone.

Adelaide and Perth                        D.W.H.
1986                                  J.M.P.
                                      M.C.

# Contents

# List of Tables

To our families, and to the memory of Rolf E. J. ten Seldam (1906–1982), Foundation Professor of Pathology in The University of Western Australia.

'At the beginning it was confined to very few; who, making a Secret of it, endeavoured all they could to keep it to themselves; and, when it became a little more publick, the Price was fixt so high, that the most Curious and Industrious, who have not always the greatest Share on Money, could not conveniently get at it. Of late Years, indeed, the Expence has been much less; but then new Discouragements have started up from Mistake and Prejudice.

'For Many have been frighted from the Use of it, imagining it required great Skill in Optics, and abundance of other Learning . . . whereas nothing is really needful but good Glasses, good Eyes, a little Practice, and a common Understanding, to distinguish what is seen; . . .'

Baker, H. (1744) *The Microscope Made Easy*[1]

# Introduction

Electron microscopy (EM) has contributed enormously to an understanding of the structural intricacies of normal and disordered cells and tissues. It is also an important and sometimes indispensable technique in the investigation and diagnosis of disease. Although most pathological diagnoses in surgical oncology can be made by light microscopy (LM), a minority of tumours — perhaps 1 to 8 per cent in selected series[55,91,126,139,149,158] — resists exact classification. In such circumstances, EM can often contribute to the diagnosis by demonstrating structures beyond the resolution of the light microscope (Table 0.1).[39,45,64,85,109]

In experienced hands, ultrastructural examination is

**Table 0.1 Stages in the ultrastructural assessment of tumours**

| Feature | Comments |
|---|---|
| *Topographic cellular relationships* | See Introduction |
| *External lamina* | See Chapters 3, 4, 18, 19 and 21 |
| *Cell contours* | See Chapters 5, 9, 18, 27 and 28 |
| *Intercellular junctions* | See Chapters 4, 5, 21 and 27 |
| *Cytoplasmic granules* | See Table 2.5 and Chapter 2 |
| *Cytoplasmic filaments* | See Tables 2.7–2.9 and Chapters 2, 4, 21 and 22 |
| *Cytoplasmic vacuoles and vesicles* | See Introduction and Chapters 2, 5, 11, 13 and 27 |
| *Organellar patterns* | See Introduction, Table 2.1 and Chapters 2, 10, 11 and 13 |
| *Nuclear and nucleolar morphology* | See Chapters 1, 20, 27 and 28 |
| *Stroma* | See Chapter 3 and Tables 3.2 and 3.3 |

remarkably effective in resolving difficulties in diagnostic tumour pathology; of 1030 problem cases examined by Erlandson,[39] only 120 defied an accurate diagnosis. The improved diagnosis so achieved often has clinical and therapeutic importance. In an evaluation of 49 tumours submitted over a 12-month period, Kuzela et al[78] found that EM confirmed the LM diagnosis in 40 cases, leading to more exact typing in 11; EM corrected the original LM interpretation in three instances, but did not solve two problems. The tissue submitted for EM was judged to be technically inadequate in the remaining four cases, because of either unrepresentative sampling or poor fixation. The precise tumour typing facilitated by EM was considered clinically helpful in up to 25 of 45 cases (56 per cent) by way of influencing patient management. There are indications that in some tumours the more precise classification achieved by EM has prognostic significance (see Chapters 6 and 7).

Diagnostic electron microscopy of tissues can be regarded as an extension of routine optical techniques, in the same category as any other specialized cytomorphological procedure. Although EM may be definitive occasionally in tumour diagnosis, ultrastructural examination is often most effective when LM has restricted the diagnostic possibilities to only a few. In some circumstances, negative ultrastructural information may still be of value in excluding certain possibilities, even when an exact diagnosis is not feasible. However, because of the considerable time and costs associated with the technique, judgement and selectivity should be used whenever fine-structural examination is contemplated.

## GENERAL PRINCIPLES AND THE APPLICATION OF DIAGNOSTIC ELECTRON MICROSCOPY IN ONCOLOGY; CONCEPTS OF DIFFERENTIATION AND HISTOGENESIS CONTRASTED

**1.** Light microscopy is an indispensable prelude to ultrastructural examination of tumours, and the best results are achieved by correlation of these techniques, using specialized LM procedures such as histochemistry and immunocytochemistry whenever appropriate. An apparent conflict between the LM and EM findings is an indication for a careful re-evaluation of both; if the conflict still cannot be resolved, we believe that precedence should generally be accorded to the light microscopy, because of the far greater area of tissue examined. This type of disagreement is most

1

likely to result from the vagaries of tissue sampling, one example being the ultrastructural identification of mesenchymal cells in a neoplasm which is clearly epithelial by LM. These remarks do not, of course, preclude the ultrastructural demonstration of a distinctive pattern of differentiation which may be far less obvious by LM; for example, in one of our referred cases, EM conclusively demonstrated neuritic differentiation in a cerebral tumour resembling an oligodendroglioma by LM, thereby yielding a diagnosis of neuroblastoma. Indeed, EM has helped to establish some neoplasms as distinct entities (for example, neuroendocrine carcinoma of skin, also known as Merkel cell carcinoma; see Chapter 6), and is of value as a form of quality control in surgical pathology;[46] in fulfilling these roles it has also clarified and refined the LM criteria for the diagnosis of some tumours.

**2.** As demonstrated by many investigators[39,45,63,119,126] and emphasized in the general section of this atlas, there are no consistent or specific fine-structural indicators of malignancy, or of neoplasia itself; electron microscopy has little, if any, place in these evaluations which are far more effectively made by light microscopy.

**3.** The fundamental role of EM in tumour diagnosis is the assessment of differentiation within cells and tissues as expressed by cytoplasmic characteristics and cell relationships; when applied to the diagnosis of neoplasms, the exercise is essentially one of detecting and evaluating aberrant submicroscopic morphology. The concept of *differentiation* should be sharply distinguished from that of *histogenesis*, the latter being an hypothesis as to the cell of origin, based on an assessment of differentiation. For example, rhabdomyoblastic differentiation cannot be equated with an origin from striated muscle. On the contrary, rhabdomyoblasts may be encountered in tumours apparently unrelated to striated muscle and which sometimes show pluripotential differentiation (see Table 22.1); it has been recognized for decades that many pure embryonal rhabdomyosarcomas develop in sites ordinarily devoid of striated muscle. Thus a rhabdomyosarcoma — whether it arises in the urinary bladder,[2407] prostate,[2445] lower oesophagus,[2456] biliary tract[2434] or brain[2437,2444] — is so designated, not because of any putative origin from striated muscle, but because of *unidirectional rhabdomyoblastic differentiation*.

This issue is further highlighted by the phenomenon of composite differentiation in carcinomas, exemplified by the presence of neuroendocrine cells in some adenocarcinomas (see Chapter 7). Such mixed cell patterns — and even the presence of both mucous and neurosecretory granules within single cells — call into question the postulated neural crest derivation of enterochromaffin cells,[28] and the hypothesis is further undermined by heterotransplantation experiments. Thus Cox & Pierce[28] transplanted single cells from a colonic adeno-carcinoma of the rat which contained mucous, columnar, endocrine and undifferentiated cells; the resultant tumours reproduced all four cell lines, albeit in varying proportions. Similarly, Goldenburg & Fisher[847] transferred a human

carcinoid tumour to immunosuppressed rodents, with subsequent growth as a signet-ring cell carcinoma.

The situation has been lucidly summarized by Gould et al:[52]
  *'. . . certain patterns of differentiation are shared by many different groups of cells . . . and these groups of cells may be of diverse histogenesis and may cut across the boundaries of the three primitive embryonic layers. These observations have resulted in more fluid notions of differentiation, and have served to underline the importance of local (micro-environmental) and regional influences on its development. Thus, histogenesis and differentiation though intimately related are nonetheless distinct concepts. Transfer of these concepts from embryology to pathology, and particularly to diagnostic pathology, has been very useful but, perhaps inevitably, it has also resulted in certain confusion. This confusion has been most pronounced when pathologists have rigidly persisted in equating certain neoplastic cellular structures and functions with a given histogenetic derivation.'*

Taxy & Battifora[2229] have also emphasized the practical importance of the distinction between differentiation and histogenesis:
  *'. . . the identification of the predominant tumor cell type is the major diagnostic point; . . . the extent that this identification reflects the cell of origin cannot truly be ascertained. Histogenesis is, after all, a conclusion arrived at by inference and not by direct observation of the original cell or cell clone. In many instances, histogenesis remains controversial, perhaps unresolvable, and of questionable clinical importance.'*

Finally, Shikary and associates[1339] have reached similar conclusions:
  *'. . . the classification of tumors in general cannot . . . rely on the cell of origin, but rather should be based on the tissues actually being produced. 'Differentiating (as)' may be substituted for 'arising from' with more objectivity, and without loss of descriptive or prognostic information.'*

These observations are not intended to decry the value of histogenetic concepts, which are widely regarded as indispensable to an understanding of the development of neoplasms; they simply emphasize that speculation about histogenesis is an exercise distinct from diagnosis in surgical pathology. At the same time, it should be acknowledged that some of the most significant errors in EM have involved overinterpretation of non-specific features to satisfy pre-existing concepts of histogenesis, exemplified by 'synovial histogenesis' — a will-o'-the-wisp adduced to explain a variety of non-specific ultrastructural findings in mesenchymal tumours, such as microvillous processes, intermediate junctions and external lamina (see Chapter 24).

It is likely that histogenetic concepts will be further de-emphasized as a result of progress in cell biology. There are indications that patterns of normal and presumably neoplastic cell differentiation can be modulated by components of the extracellular matrix (ECM; see Chapter 3), some of which are instrumental in cell-substratum adherence. Such micro-environmental influences of ECM include the following:

1. The in vitro stimulation of smooth muscle differentiation by collagen.[339]
2. Inhibition of smooth muscle growth resulting from heparin production by endothelial cells.[339]
3. The role of collagen in promoting the fusion of myoblasts to form multinucleated myotubes.[346]
4. The apparently greater influence of type II than type I collagen in the development of cartilage.[338,339]
5. The conversion of normally non-chondrogenic cells into cartilage by components of collagenous bone matrix.[338,339]
6. Loss of fibronectin/chondronectin during both chondrogenic and myogenic differentiation, and myoblast fusion in myogenesis.[342]
7. The requirement for ECM in the development of corneal epithelium.[338,339]
8. The influence of glycosaminoglycans in the development and branching of salivary gland epithelium in the mouse.[374]
9. The role of collagen in promoting the polarity of thyroid follicular epithelium.[338]
10. Prolonged in vitro retention of hepatocyte characteristics resulting from cell attachment to components of the biomatrix.[352]
11. Maintenance of neuritic properties in neuroblastoma cells in vitro by components of ECM, preventing an overgrowth of fibroblasts.[352]
12. The depletion and reduced binding of cell surface-related fibronectin during oncogenesis.[342]
13. Ingber et al[343] investigated a transplantable carcinoma of rat exocrine pancreas in which the viable neoplastic cells had lost both epithelial polarity and the capacity to form a complete external lamina. However, in areas of contact with microvascular adventitia the cells produced, and were orientated along, a linear basal lamina. Immunocytochemistry demonstrated a linear distribution of type IV collagen and laminin in the areas of reorientation, whereas in the disorganized tissue type IV collagen was undetectable and laminin had a punctate distribution. The authors suggested that failure of the neoplastic cells to maintain an external lamina resulted in their disorganization. Repolarization of tumour cells also occurred in relation to the connective tissue capsule of the tumour, suggesting that the regional differences were not attributable to nutritional influences of the microvasculature.
14. In a tissue culture study of glioblastoma cells, we have observed a loss of glial fibrillary acidic protein and the acquisition of striated muscle differentiation, presumably influenced by the altered microenvironment (Jacobsen & Papadimitriou, unpublished observations).
15. Plasma membrane-attached glycoproteins known as cell-adhesion molecules (CAMs) have been identified in embryonic tissues.[3147] The molecular structure of the CAMs present at different stages of development and in different regions of the embryo is known to vary; for example, the N–CAM found in neural tissue contains large amounts of polymerized sialic acid, whereas the L–CAM originally isolated from liver lacks polysialic acid and only mediates cell adhesion in the presence of calcium ions.[3147] CAMs are distributed on a regional basis in the embryo; the central N–CAM regions are destined to give rise to the neural plate among other tissues, and are surrounded by a ring of tissue expressing L–CAM. Moreover, in renal tissues originating from mesoderm, L–CAM and N–CAM appear, disappear and reappear in sequence. Evidence indicates that CAMs are instrumental in the development and differentiation of embryonic tissues (see the review by Edelman[3147]); for example, anti-N–CAM antibody disrupts the orderly development of chick embryo retina in tissue culture, while the conversion of epithelia into mesenchyme is accompanied by deletion of CAMs from the cell surface. It is also possible that CAMs interact with components of the ECM; changes in CAM expression during neural crest cell migration are inversely related to the fibronectin content. One can therefore speculate that impaired and even aberrant differentiation in some neoplastic tissues — which are generally characterized by cell incohesiveness — may be at least partly influenced by disturbances in CAM expression, perhaps involving an interaction with components of the ECM.

The possible role of the cellular environment in modulating both differentiation and malignant behaviour is even more dramatically illustrated by transplantation experiments with so-called teratocarcinomas. Transplantation of these tumours to syngeneic mice results in progressive anaplastic tumour growth leading to death of the host; however, small numbers of such cells introduced into normal mouse blastocysts fail to develop as malignant cells. Instead, they differentiate as normal blastocyst cells, producing a variety of normally functioning cells (such as spermatozoa and ova) in the mice developing from the blastocysts.[94]

Nevertheless, the histogenesis of many neoplasms is well established. For example, there is little doubt that adenocarcinomas of the colon originate from colonic epithelium, and a strong body of evidence links testicular embryonal and teratoid tumours with a germ cell precursor.[1128] The concepts of histogenesis and differentiation are to some extent reconcilable by the following epigenetic microenvironmental 'drive' hypothesis:

1. *By synthesizing various components of the ECM, cells are at least partly responsible for their own microenvironment and hence pattern of differentiation.*
2. *Components of the ECM may function as gene amplifiers or repressors by as yet obscure mechanisms; it is conceivable that these mechanisms involve an initial interaction between the ECM and the cytoskeleton, mediated via receptors for ECM molecules on the plasmalemma,[338,339,376] the cytoskeletal components then affecting the distribution of messenger RNA.*
3. *As long as the microenvironment and genetic profile are appropriate for a particular cell line, persistence of clonal properties is to be expected, and under these circumstances the pattern of differentiation will accurately reflect the cell of origin (parallel differentiation-histogenesis).*
4. *If somatic mutation-gene deregulation accompanying neoplasia renders the microenvironment inappropriate for the normally differentiated cell type, aberrant patterns of differentiation may result, making it impossible to determine the cell of origin (divergent differentiation-histogenesis).*

Finally, it is notable that the histogenesis and even the pattern of differentiation of some tumours (such as alveolar soft part sarcoma and Ewing's sarcoma) are obscure or controversial (see Chapters 24 and 25), but EM may still contribute to their diagnosis.

**4.** Clearly, familiarity with normal ultrastructure is essential before abnormal fine structure can be interpreted. Numerous texts and atlases of normal ultrastructure are available[176–191,1988,2883] and we make no attempt to supplant them. Instead, this atlas deals with the submicroscopic morphology of human neoplasia, emphasizing those areas in which light microscopy may fail to identify differentiation precisely.

**5.** The approach adopted is to group the non-specific features found in a variety of different neoplasms and then to review the major groups of tumours, including epithelial, mesenchymal, lymphoid, and mixed types. The distinction between these groups is usually obvious by LM but it is sometimes difficult to determine whether a given neoplasm represents a carcinoma, sarcoma, or lymphoma, and EM may facilitate this assessment, as discussed in Table 0.2.

**Table 0.2  Comparative ultrastructure of major tumour types***

| | Carcinoma | Sarcoma | Lymphoma |
|---|---|---|---|
| Cell shape | Often rounded to polygonal | Often elongated and bipolar | Rounded |
| Disposition of cells | Arranged in groups or sheets | Dispersed singly, with intervening extracellular matrix | Form sheets |
| External lamina (EL) | Present. Amount variable | Variable. Absent from purely fibroblastic tumours. Varying amounts of EL occur adjacent to myofibroblasts, smooth muscle cells and occasionally rhabdomyoblasts. EL is also seen next to endothelial cells, pericytes and nerve sheath cells. When present, EL is usually fragmentary | Absent |
| Distribution of EL | Invests cell groups or individual cells | If present, surrounds individual cells | Absent |
| Intercellular junctions | *Present between neoplastic cells* Number and type vary greatly with tumour type and degree of differentiation. Desmosomes are highly characteristic of epithelial/epithelioid neoplasms. Intermediate junctions often present. Tight junctions occur as a component of junctional complexes of glandular tumours. Melanocytic cells possess few junctions | Variable. Absent from purely fibroblastic neoplasms. Intermediate-type junctions present between myofibroblasts, smooth muscle cells, pericytes and occasionally rhabdomyoblasts. Tight junctions occur between endothelial cells, but are often poorly developed ('leaky') in tumours. Desmosomes absent | Not present between lymphocytoid cells* Junctions may be seen between stromal endothelial cells, but these have no diagnostic significance. Desmosomes may be found occasionally between dendritic cells of follicular centre cell lymphomas |
| Cell processes | Variable. Processes with desmosome-tonofilament complexes characterize squamous tumours. Microvilli are a major feature of glandular epithelial tumours | Cytoplasmic extensions may be present, for example in fibroblastic cells. Cytoplasmic flaps characterise histiocytes | Lymphocytoid cells usually have only poorly developed processes, but elaborate intertwining cytoplasmic extensions occur in follicular centre cell lymphomas. Although recorded, microvillous processes are rare |
| Terminal filamentous web | Often present beneath microvilli in glandular tumours, especially intestinal adenomas and adenocarcinomas | Absent | Absent |
| Filaments† | Present. Number varies with tumour type and degree of differentiation. Tonofilaments (cytokeratin filaments) are a major feature of epithelial neoplasms, especially squamous tumours. Peripheral microfilaments may also be present | Tonofilaments typically absent. Intermediate and micro-filaments often present. Myosin filaments typify striated muscle tumours | Usually absent or inconspicuous, but intermediate filaments are found occasionally and presumably correspond to the presence of vimentin |
| Cytoplasmic granules | Various types of granule (see Table 2.5) ± lysosomes. Granule morphology may be characteristic of a particular type of epithelial tumour; see Figs. 5.8–5.14 | Lysosomes, especially in histiocytic cells | Few lysosomes occasionally present, ± immunoglobulin granules |
| Remarks | Cell disposition and shape, together with desmosomes, cytoplasmic tonofilaments and granules are the principal diagnostic features of epithelial neoplasms by electron microscopy. The markers of particular subtypes are also of general diagnostic value | Cell disposition and shape, together with cytoplasmic filaments and absence of true desmosomes are principal diagnostic features | Cell disposition and shape, as well as nondescript and often sparse organelles, in the absence of intercellular junctions and cytoplasmic filaments, are principal diagnostic markers |

*This table is intended only as an introductory guide to the differential diagnosis of broad categories of tumours and as such embodies a number of oversimplifications. At the same time, it is meant to be reasonably comprehensive, in the belief that identification of the major tumour type (e.g. carcinoma) is often inseparable from more specific subtyping (e.g. adeno- or squamous carcinoma). Absence of junctions between neoplastic cells is a useful guide to the ultrastructural diagnosis of lymphoma, but we have once observed convincing intermediate-type junctions between a small group of 3–4 immunoblasts in an undoubted immunoblastic lymphoma; Perez-Atayde et al[2787] have also described similar junctions in a retroperitoneal lymphoma

†See Tables 2.7, 2.8 and 21.1

References: 14, 39, 45, 48, 55, 63, 64, 70, 86, 97, 109, 119, 126, 2787

**6.** Although a few subcellular structures (such as Weibel-Palade bodies and Langerhans' cell granules) appear to be specific for certain cell lines (see Chapters 3, 23 and 28), there is probably no single structure pathognomonic of a particular tumour when taken in isolation. Most findings assume discriminant value only in the appropriate cellular environment. What is ultimately important is the sum total of the appearances, as emphasized by Schlote:[2001]

> *'Like light microscopy, electron microscopic findings are relevant only in the context of the clinical symptoms and the tentative diagnosis; the typical, characteristic picture therefore may support the tentative diagnosis or an incompatible observation suggest another diagnosis. The individual structural deviations should not be overevaluated; ultrastructural details are not diagnostically important until they are considered in the context of the other alterations present in the tissue.'*

**7.** Any poorly differentiated malignancy is likely to consist largely of primitive cells devoid of distinctive features. Prolonged scrutiny of multiple tissue blocks may be necessary to identify a definite line of differentiation, but the search is sometimes fruitless. Negative findings are therefore of restricted value in tumour diagnosis and failure to demonstrate a particular pattern of cell differentiation does not necessarily preclude the suspected diagnosis. A positive result is most likely to be obtained when areas of tumour showing a hint of differentiation by LM are selected for examination, rather than totally anaplastic tissue (but see Chapters 6, 7 and 29).

**8.** EM may also indicate the possible source of a metastasis of unknown origin. For example, the cellular organization and/or secretory granules characteristic of some adenocarcinomas developing in particular organ systems may be of value in predicting the source of a corresponding metastasis (see Chapter 5).[37] Thus, the presence of glycocalyceal bodies is an indicator of gastrointestinal adenocarcinoma (see Table 5.2), while frequent cytoplasmic neolumina are typical (but not pathognomonic) of some mammary carcinomas. Metastasizing acinic cell, bronchiolo-alveolar and endocervical adeno-carcinomas may also be recognizable by persistence of their secretory granules; in addition, prostatic carcinomas may be detected by the presence of lysosomal granules and cytoplasmic vacuoles and vesicles (see Fig. 5.19), but the immunocytochemical demonstration of prostatic acid phosphatase and/or prostate-specific antigen by LM offers greater diagnostic accuracy. Finally, the presence of melanosomes should prompt a search for a primary malignant melanoma (see Chapter 8).

## IMMUNOCYTOCHEMISTRY IN TUMOUR DIAGNOSIS

Recent developments in immunohistological techniques have added a new dimension to tumour typing. Whereas conventional light- and electron-optical methods provide a static architectural perspective, the use of peroxidase- and alkaline phosphatase-conjugated antibodies (including hybridoma-generated monoclonal antibodies) constitutes a complementary system of cell identification based on the detection of an increasing variety of both functional and structural antigenic cell components. The most important of these cell markers in tumour diagnosis are:

1. *Cell products* (for example hormones, enzymes and immunoglobulins).
2. *Cytoplasmic filaments* (for example cytokeratins, vimentin and glial fibrillary acidic protein).
3. *Tumour-associated antigens* (for example oncofetal antigens, and tissue-specific and tumour-specific antigens).

Examples are listed in Table 0.3 and elsewhere in the text, but are not intended to be exhaustive, and for further information the interested reader should consult standard references on this subject.[167-175]

Immunocytochemical analysis at the ultrastructural level is primarily a research procedure, but the methods are readily applicable to examination of formalin-fixed, paraffin-embedded tissue sections by LM and are used routinely in this way in our laboratories as part of a tripartite approach to tumour diagnosis, involving LM, EM and immunohistology.

Although justifiably riding a wave of popularity, immunocytochemistry is no panacea for all diagnostic problems in tumour pathology. Positive immunostaining is most likely to be seen with non-problematical highly differentiated tumours, whereas poorly differentiated malignancies may yield negative results for predicted antigenic markers, even when the diagnosis is not in dispute. False positive reactions also occur, some being attributable to cross-reactivity of antisera. It is therefore desirable that the reliability of antisera be tested regularly and that the procedure be monitored by using both positive and negative control sections. Monoclonal antibodies do not necessarily constitute a definitive answer to these problems. As monoclonal antibodies are raised against ever smaller antigenic targets on cell membranes, the probability that the antigens are part and parcel of the functional properties of particular cell lines diminishes, and the likelihood of antibody cross-reactivity with diverse cell types increases.

## SAMPLING, MATERIALS AND TECHNIQUES FOR ELECTRON MICROSCOPY

Transmission electron microscopy has proved to be the most informative ultrastructural technique in tumour diagnosis. Scanning EM has provided diagnostic information only rarely, while electron cytochemistry and immuno-electron microscopy have been used in selected cases. Lastly, X-ray microanalytic techniques may be used occasionally, but their value at present is limited.

For adequate and representative ultrastructural examination of tumours, multiple blocks of tissue from different areas of a given tumour are highly desirable. These ensure that most of the features seen by LM will also be available for EM. Diagnostic ultrastructural detail may not be present uniformly

**Table 0.3    Immunocytochemistry in tumour diagnosis – examples of tumour-associated antigens detectable by immunocytochemical techniques**

| Tumour type | Antigen(s) | Comments |
| --- | --- | --- |
| Bladder (urothelial) carcinoma | Blood group isoantigens | Loss of isoantigens correlates with invasiveness |
| B-cell malignant lymphomas; plasma cell neoplasia | Immunoglobulin components<br>B-cell-surface differentiation antigens<br>J-chain | Monoclonal proliferations typify neoplasia |
| Breast carcinoma | $\alpha$-lactalbumin<br>Casein<br>Pregnancy-specific $\beta_1$-glycoprotein<br>Human chorionic gonadotrophin (HCG)<br>Mammary epithelial membrane antigens<br>Placental lactogen<br>Placental protein 5<br>Oestradiol-oestrogen receptor<br>Carcinoembryonic antigen (CEA)<br>Transferrin<br>Insulin | — |
| Cervical adenocarcinoma | CEA<br>Blood group isoantigens | CEA positive in cervical adenocarcinoma, but negative in endometrial adenocarcinoma |
| Colon carcinoma | CEA<br>Blood group isoantigens | — |
| Endodermal sinus tumour | Yolk sac-specific $\alpha$-fetoprotein<br>Haemoglobin F<br>Laminin | — |
| Epithelial neoplasms | Cytokeratins<br>Epithelial membrane antigen<br>Secretory component | General markers. See Chapter 2 |
| Erythroblastic proliferations | Haemoglobin A<br>Haemoglobin F | — |
| Gastroenteropancreatic endocrine tumours | Insulin<br>Glucagon<br>Somatostatin<br>Gastrin<br>Vasoactive intestinal polypeptide<br>Pancreatic polypeptide<br>Cholecystokinin | See Chapter 14. Neurone-specific enolase and chromogranin are two further markers for neuroendocrine cells, including pancreatic endocrine tumours; chromogranin appears to be localized to the secretory granules of neuroendocrine cells and may represent the site of silver binding in the Grimelius and related stains. |
| Gliomas | Glial fibrillary acidic protein<br>Vimentin | See Chapter 17 |
| Granulocytic leukaemias; granulocytic sarcoma | Granulocyte cell-surface differentiation antigens<br>Lysozyme (muramidase)<br>Lactoferrin | — |
| Hepatocellular carcinoma | $\alpha_1$-antitrypsin ($\alpha_1$-antiprotease)<br>$\alpha$-fetoprotein<br>Hepatitis B virus antigens | — |
| Histiocytic lymphoma (true histiocytic lymphoma; lymphoma of mononuclear phagocytes) | Monocyte-specific cell-surface antigens<br>Lysozyme<br>$\alpha_1$-antitrypsin | — |
| Hodgkin's disease | $\alpha_1$-antichymotrypsin<br>(Nuclear membrane peanut lectin binding) | Positive in Reed-Sternberg cells and mononuclear Hodgkin's cells |
| Lymphoblastic lymphoma; acute lymphoblastic leukaemia | Lymphocyte cell-surface differentiation antigens<br>Terminal deoxynucleotidyl transferase | — |
| Malignant melanoma | Neurone-specific enolase<br>S-100 protein<br>Vimentin | — |
| Mesothelioma | Cytokeratins<br>Mesothelioma antigen | Negative or weak reactions for CEA<br>See Table 9.1 |
| Neuroblastoma | Neurofilaments<br>Neurone-specific enolase<br>S-100 protein | — |
| Ovarian carcinoma | Alkaline phosphatase (placental isoenzyme) | — |
| Ovarian granulosa and theca cell tumours | Oestradiol | — |
| Paneth cells in neoplasms | Lysozyme | See Chapter 7 |
| Parathyroid tumours | Parathormone | — |
| Peripheral nerve sheath cell tumours | S-100 protein<br>Vimentin | S-100 protein often negative in malignant Schwannomas |

**Table 0.3 (continued)** Immunocytochemistry in tumour diagnosis – examples of tumour-associated antigens detectable by immunocytochemical techniques

| Tumour type | Antigen(s) | Comments |
|---|---|---|
| Pituitary (adenohypophyseal) tumours | Adrenocorticotrophic hormone<br>Growth hormone<br>Prolactin<br>Luteinizing hormone<br>Follicle-stimulating hormone<br>Thyroid-stimulating hormone | See Chapter 10 |
| Prostatic carcinoma | Prostate-specific epithelial antigen<br>Prostatic acid phosphatase | — |
| Salivary gland neoplasms | Salivary duct epithelial antigen<br>Lysozyme<br>Lactoferrin<br>Epidermal growth factor | — |
| Small cell neuroendocrine carcinoma of lung | Oat cell carcinoma plasma membrane antigen<br>Neurone-specific enolase<br>Bombesin | — |
| Smooth muscle tumours | Desmin<br>Actin<br>Myosin | See Chapter 21 |
| Soft tissue tumours (non-myoid) | Vimentin | General marker |
| Striated muscle tumours | Myoglobin<br>Desmin<br>Actin<br>Myosin | See Chapter 22 |
| Testicular Sertoli and Leydig cell tumours | Testosterone | — |
| Thyroid follicular epithelial tumours | Thyroglobulin | — |
| Thyroid parafollicular (C) cell tumour (medullary carcinoma) | Calcitonin<br>CEA | — |
| Trophoblastic neoplasia: trophoblastic components in germ cell and other tumours | HCG<br>Placental lactogen<br>$\beta_1$-glycoprotein | — |
| Vasoformative (endothelial) neoplasms | Factor VIII-related antigen (VIII-RAG)<br>Vimentin<br>(*Ulex europaeus* I-lectin binding) | — |

It is emphasized that although some of the markers listed above are highly specific (for example, prostate-specific antigen), many are shared by multiple cell types. Therefore, interpretation of immunocytochemical reactions must be undertaken within the context of an established differential diagnosis, based particularly on light microscopy. An immunocytochemical profile, using several antisera to reveal both positive and negative reactions, will usually be more rewarding than a single examination

References: 167–175, 3148; see also individual text and caption citations

throughout the tumour, and normal or necrotic tissue may be sampled inadvertently. Moreover, atrophic and reactive alterations affecting specialized cells in the vicinity of, or incorporated into, tumours may be a source of error in assessing patterns of neoplastic differentiation. For example, reactive type II pneumocyte hyperplasia and alveolar compression within the lung may simulate glandular epithelial differentiation, including alveolar cell carcinoma (Figs. 0.1–0.4). Similarly, atrophy of myocytes resulting from invasion of striated muscle by non-myoid tumours can be mistaken for rhabdomyoblastic differentiation (Figs. 0.5–0.8).

For optimal ultrastructural preservation, tissues should be fixed within seconds of removal, using an appropriate fixative such as glutaraldehyde. The various fixatives and their uses and limitations are dealt with at length in other texts on methods in electron microscopy,[156,157,162,163] and will not be reiterated here. Even if fixation is suboptimal, enough ultrastructural detail may still be present to be useful (if unaesthetic). Formaldehyde-fixed material is often acceptable[151] and the superiority of buffered formalin as an EM fixative, compared to unbuffered formol-saline, is strongly emphasized. Even material embedded in paraffin can be retrieved and sometimes subjected successfully to ultrastructural analysis,[158] although the poor state of tissue preservation is disappointingly uninformative in most cases. Techniques are also available for the retrieval and examination of routine smears and tissue sections from glass slides.[158]

Fine needle aspiration biopsy specimens represent an expanding proportion of our workload. This 'minibiopsy' technique is now widely used in tumour diagnosis, but problems are sometimes encountered because of the limited volume of tissue sampled. Even in such circumstances, cytological examination greatly restricts the possible diagnoses and EM is often highly effective in distinguishing between these, despite suboptimal cell preservation. Cohesive minibiopsy fragments are sometimes obtained, especially with use of the Nordenström screw needle.

As a matter of policy, we routinely fix tissue for EM from

any unusual or undiagnosed tumour received in the fresh state. On the basis of the frozen or paraffin sections, a decision can then be made to discard the specimen, process and file the tissue for future reference, or to proceed immediately to ultrastructural examination.

The techniques of embedding in epoxy resins and subsequent sectioning are well described in standard texts.[148,156,157,162] One aspect of the procedure which cannot be stressed too strongly is the value of close scrutiny of the semithin (0.5–1 $\mu$m) sections of various blocks from the specimen.[126] These not only provide the link between LM and EM,[147,160] ensuring that the features seen by optical techniques are actually subjected to ultrastructural examination, but also permit a more refined light-microscopic assessment of the neoplastic tissues, because of the improved cytomorphology provided by the semithin sectioning technique. Finally, if an answer is urgently required, there are reliable embedding schedules which allow the preparation of useful sections within a few hours of the sample being obtained.[149,153,164] Infiltration and embedding can be accomplished in about one hour by use of a medium containing vinyl cyclohexane dioxide and cyanoacrylate.[166]

Most of the material illustrated in this atlas is from tissues fixed at the time of biopsy. Glutaraldehyde was the primary fixative in the majority of cases, but sometimes mixtures of glutaraldehyde and paraformaldehyde were used. Less frequently, formaldehyde was employed, with variable delays occurring between biopsy and fixation. Rarely, necropsy material was obtained, or tissue which had been previously frozen or embedded in paraffin. The blocks were post-osmicated and dehydrated in graded ethanol solutions. The tissue was then usually embedded in Araldite, but Spurr's resin or Epon were used occasionally. Sections were cut with LKB or Reichert ultramicrotomes and the sections stained with uranyl acetate and lead hydroxide or citrate. Grids were examined with a Philips 201 or 301, or a Siemens 101 electron microscope.

When scanning electron microscopy was used, specimens were subjected to 'critical point' drying, and then coated with a thin layer of gold-palladium. They were then examined with a Philips PSEM500 scanning electron microscope.

## AN INTRODUCTION TO THE PATHOBIOLOGY OF MALIGNANT CELLS

Before detailing the ultrastructure of a variety of neoplasms (Chapters 1–30), the biological characteristics of malignant cells will be considered briefly. In many instances the functional properties of these cells correlate with their morphological features and account for the behaviour of neoplastic growths. However, no single biological property qualifies as the distinctive trait of all malignant cells and it is very likely that no such unique feature exists.

### Genetic considerations

Genetic transmission of the neoplastic trait from parent cell to progeny characterizes neoplasia. The properties of unrestricted growth, invasion and metastasis appear in all descendants, producing a tissue which is potentially immortal.[17] Despite these anomalies, few if any gene products are found in malignant cells which are not also present in normal cells at some stage of development.[129,131]

The hypothesis that the fundamental abnormality responsible for neoplastic change resides in the genome of malignant cells has stimulated extensive chromosomal analysis of many tumours. Although some malignant neoplasms have normal chromosomes, most display a variety of chromosomal abnormalities, both of number and structure.[60] These have been observed in most solid malignancies, whereas a significant proportion of acute leukaemias have no demonstrable chromosomal lesion. Although the chromosomal alterations are often constant for all cells of a given neoplasm, they are only rarely specific for a particular tumour; usually there is no clear relationship between the type of neoplasm and the chromosomal abnormality.

In chronic myeloid leukaemia, however, a characteristic marker chromsome, the Philadelphia (Ph') chromosome, is found in the majority of cases. The chromosomal abnormality in this disease is the result of a translocation of part of the long arm of chromosome 22 onto another chromosome, most frequently chromosome 9.[21,107,111] Similarly, a translocation from the long arm of chromosome 8 to that of chromosome 14 is found in a large number of Burkitt's lymphomas of both African and non-African origin, irrespective of either positive or negative status for Epstein-Barr virus.[71,144] The 14q+ anomaly of Burkitt's lymphoma is not, however, highly specific and a similar aberration has been observed in other malignant lymphomas and in multiple myeloma.[115] Furthermore, abnormalities of the G group of chromosomes have been reported as a feature of meningiomas.[88]

The possibility of anomalous gene regulation in malignancy has resulted in the comparison of histone and nuclear non-histone proteins (NHP) of neoplastic cells with those of normal cells. Much interest has focussed on NHP because these are thought to exert specific controls on genes compared to the general blocking effects of histones.[17,67] Comparison of histone and NHP profiles of normal and malignant cells has shown both qualitative and quantitative differences but their exact significance is unclear.[17,67,131]

Various differences in the process of transcription have also been detected between normal and cancerous cells,[17,66,124] but it has not been shown that these alterations account for the very efficient protein synthesis of malignant cells. Similarly, the levels of ribosomal precursor molecules and ribosomal RNA products in malignant cells differ from those of normal cells.[17] The significance of these findings and their relationship, if any, to a common nucleolar antigen found in a broad range of human malignant neoplasms,[32] remain to be elucidated.

### The metabolism of malignant cells

Although the basic biochemical lesion underlying neoplastic transformation is still unknown, biochemical investigations of a range of experimental hepatomas have revealed a pattern of enzyme imbalance, affecting a few key enzymes, which suggests a reprogramming of gene expression.[136,137] This imbalance is both qualitative and quantitative, some alterations being associated with transformation (transformation-linked changes), others correlating with the degree of malignancy (progression-linked changes).

An imbalance of the pentose pathway and purine, pyrimidine and DNA metabolism are the major transformation-linked discriminants. There are increased levels of glucose-6-phosphate dehydrogenase and transaldolase of the oxidative and non-oxidative branch of the pentose pathway respectively. Excess ribose pyrophosphate is formed and is shunted towards RNA and DNA synthesis.[136,137]

Imbalance of pyrimidine, DNA, purine and carbohydrate metabolism, as well as alterations in the rate of protein synthesis, the concentration of phosphorylating enzymes and the isoenzyme profile are the major progression-linked discriminants. Generally, there is an increase in the concentration of the enzymes favouring pyrimidine and DNA synthesis and a simultaneous decrease of those involved in catabolism. More than 70 markers have been mooted as correlates of neoplastic progression while the concentration of inosine monophosphate dehydrogenase is directly proportional to the rate of tumour growth.[136,137]

Altered carbohydrate metabolism is reflected by increased activity of key glycolytic enzymes, decreased activity of those involved in gluconeogenesis, and a distinct isoenzyme shift.[129,136,137] The latter is a likely qualitative manifestation of the genetic reprogramming thought to be responsible for the malignant state. It is noteworthy that although hepatomas, fetal and regenerating liver all have similar growth rates, the enzyme profile is different in the neoplastic cells.[136,137]

Neoplastic cells appear to be specialized not only in processes involved in growth and replication, but in addition they are able to survive under relatively adverse conditions.[17] For example, cancer cells are relatively resistant to hypoxia as well as the effects of cyanide ions.

## Properties resembling those of embryonal and fetal cells

Structural and functional similarities between neoplastic cells, and fetal and embryonic cells have often been observed.[129,131] It is noteworthy that invasiveness is also a distinguishing characteristic of normal trophoblast,[76] and a specific protease plasminogen activator — which has been correlated with the ability of cells to invade — has been demonstrated in both trophoblastic and malignant cells.[120,141] Such similarities between neoplastic and embryonal tissue are further reflected in their biochemical and antigenic profiles.

Various isoenzymes, thought previously to be confined mainly to fetal tissues, have been identified in neoplasms.[10,26,29,116,129] Examples of such fetal isoenzymes include glucose-ATP phosphotransferase, pyruvate kinase and alkaline phosphatase. The last of these, known as the Regan isoenzyme of alkaline phosphatase, has been detected in more than 10 per cent of patients with a variety of malignancies.[129]

Similarly, many embryonic and fetal analogues of adult proteins have been observed in neoplasms. For example, chorionic gonadotropin is produced by a variety of malignant neoplasms[54,93] and may be of some significance, since it acts as a lymphocyte suppressor[5] and possibly enhances tumour survival. Other pregnancy-specific and pregnancy-associated proteins have been reported in trophoblastic and non-trophoblastic malignancies.[68]

In addition, an increasing number of embryonic and fetal antigens has been found to be associated with neoplastic tissue.[3,8,23,24,81,129] The most extensively studied is $\alpha$-fetoprotein (AFP) which is produced by hepatocellular carcinomas and embryonal carcinomas of testis and ovary.[53,65,118] AFP binds to oestrogens,[134] providing a possible mechanism for the control of gene expression. Carcinoembryonic antigen (CEA), found in human fetal gut and a high proportion of human colonic carcinomas,[65,100,125] is another oncofetal antigen which has also aroused a great deal of interest, although its precise significance in oncogenesis is unknown.

The expression of such normally repressed genetic information is reflected in the reactivation of the normally condensed X chromosome in cervical and gastric carcinomas of females.[132] Such a process may parallel the embryonic state where both chromosomes must be active for the normal development of a female fetus.[82]

## Cell-surface alterations of malignant cells

It is now evident that the surface of malignant cells is abnormal in many different ways.[138] These anomalies could contribute to the escape of neoplastic cells from the controls and restraints to which normal cells are subject.[104]

Various alterations of surface glycoproteins have been reported. As already mentioned, two fetal glycoproteins — AFP and CEA — may appear on the surface of human malignant cells. In other instances, glycoproteins such as fibronectin are lost or reduced in amount.[90,113,143] Another common finding in malignant cells is increased binding of concanavalin by 100-K glycoproteins.[101,103,143] Concanavalin and other lectins also readily cause the agglutination of neoplastic cells.[101] The effectiveness of this is thought to reflect free diffusion of lectin-binding sites in the cell membrane, forming dense patches of lectin receptors and facilitating cross-linking.

In neoplasms of experimental animals a variety of glycoprotein tumour-associated transplantation antigens are often detected.[49] The available data suggest that there is often an association between these antigens and those controlled by the major histocompatibility complex.[41] It is likely, however, that these antigens are not new entities but reflect a change or re-expression of pre-existing molecules.[49] Such studies can only be performed on syngeneic animals and there is little evidence that similar antigens occur in man. Nevertheless, alterations of blood group substances have been recognized in several human malignancies;[143] these changes include deletion of blood group antigens, accumulation of precursors of blood group structures and the appearance of new blood group determinants.[74]

In addition, changes in the chemical composition of membrane glycosphingolipids occur, probably due to a reduction in the activity of particular glycosyl transferases.[16,59,143] A decrease in the levels of more complex glycolipids may also be present and suggests loss of ability of glycolipid synthesis to respond to stimuli such as cell contact, lectins and enzymes. Sialic acid — an important constituent of both glycosphinglolipids and glycoproteins — is, on the other hand, consistently elevated in malignant cells.[143] This alters the surface charge and may be related to both the invasive properties of malignant cells and their ability to metastasize.

The transmembrane transport of several sugars and certain amino acids is increased in malignant cells,[69,102] and may be related to increased membrane fluidity[123] — a suggestion supported by the observation that antigens on transformed cells are often more mobile than similar antigens on untransformed cells.[38,102] These changes in cell membrane transport are accompanied by increases in the levels of cGMP,[117] while the concentration of cAMP in neoplastic cells is often reduced.[138] The low levels of cAMP may account for the lack of contact inhibition of growth which malignant cells exhibit.[138] (It is thought that in normal cells intercellular contact releases cAMP which then inhibits DNA synthesis and restricts growth).

In addition, neoplastic cells do not display a need for substrate-dependency or attachment in order to initiate cellular proliferation, and have the capacity to grow in suspension in liquid or semisolid media.[121] Such behaviour is likely to involve transmembrane linkages to cytoskeletal components and this is supported by the finding of a reduction in the concentration of membrane-associated microfilaments and microtubules in transformed cells compared to their normal counterparts.[102] On the other hand, the increased numbers of actin microfilaments[42] and increased concentration of myosin[83] in a variety of malignant neoplasms may partly explain the increased mobility and invasiveness of cancer cells. It may also account for the differences in ruffling which have been reported between normal and tumour cells.[135]

Contact inhibition of movement is another surface phenomenon which is defective in neoplastic cells.[4] Neoplastic cells which are not inhibited by each other are, however, inhibited by contact with either normal cells or cells from a different neoplasm, indicating that the phenomenon is highly specific.[130]

## Secretory products

Various materials are secreted by neoplastic cells. Probably one of the most important is the production of 'tumour angiogenesis factor',[40] which is mitogenic for capillary endothelial cells and permits neovascularization and consequent growth of the neoplasm. In addition, hormones and biogenic amines may be produced and secreted.[54] Peptide hormones are the most frequently produced ectopic hormones, while corticosteroids and thyroid hormones are only rarely elaborated, presumably because they require more sophisticated enzyme synthesis.

**Fig. 0.1** *(Top — left)* **Alveolar Remnant: Peripheral pulmonary squamous cell carcinoma**

These illustrations (0.1–0.4) are arranged to demonstrate a sequence of diminishing alveolar compression and type II pneumocyte proliferation. Changes of this type are commonly found at the periphery of pulmonary mass lesions and have contributed to the controversy surrounding alveolar cell carcinoma (see Chapter 5). Alveolar remnants may be found incorporated into infiltrative tumours, inviting misdiagnosis as adenocarcinoma or a mixed tumour such as adenosquamous carcinoma. Sequestered alveolar remnants are also described in metastatic haemangiopericytoma and smooth muscle tumours, accounting for the 'pseudoglandular' spaces sometimes seen by LM.[2367,2495] The problem can be overcome by awareness of these reactive epiphenomena, critical scrutiny of semithin sections by LM, and careful sampling of tissue for examination (utilizing tissues lacking such specialized elements if possible, such as lymph node metastases); in addition, EM reveals a distinct two-cell population in the affected lung tissue.

The compressed alveolus (A) is bordered by microvillous cells probably representing altered type II pneumocytes, although no lamellar inclusions are evident. A squamous cell (S) with numerous tonofibrils lies adjacent to the alveolar remnant. In the lung these appearances might be interpreted as evidence of adenosquamous differentiation, but an apparent progression of alveolar compression and obliteration was found in this case (see also Fig. 0.3), and transitional forms between the squamous and alveolar lining cells could not be identified (×4900)

References: 459, 538, 2367, 2495

**Fig. 0.2** *(Top — right)* **Alveolar remnant: Atypical central bronchial carcinoid tumour**

The narrowed alveolar space (A) is lined by cells with sporadic luminal microvilli, and one contains lamelliform osmiophilic inclusions. Basal lamina surrounds the remnant (arrows). (×6800)

**Fig. 0.3** *(Bottom — left)* **Alveolar remnant: Squamous cell carcinoma of lung**

The alveolus is lined by microvillous epithelial cells containing several lamellar inclusions, consistent with hyperplastic type II pneumocytes. Another cell (S), which intrudes upon the lumen, contains prominent perinuclear tonofibrils, suggesting squamous differentiation. Same case as Fig. 0.1. (×4400)

**Fig. 0.4** *(Bottom — right)* **Hyperplasia of type II pneumocytes adjacent to bronchogenic squamous cell carcinoma**

Hyperplastic type II pneumocytes containing concentric lamelliform inclusions line the alveolar space (A) in which an erythrocyte (E) is apparent. Varying stages of alveolar compression and obliteration with type II pneumocyte proliferation were seen at the periphery of the carcinoma in this case; the regional lymph node metastases were entirely squamous. (×3700)

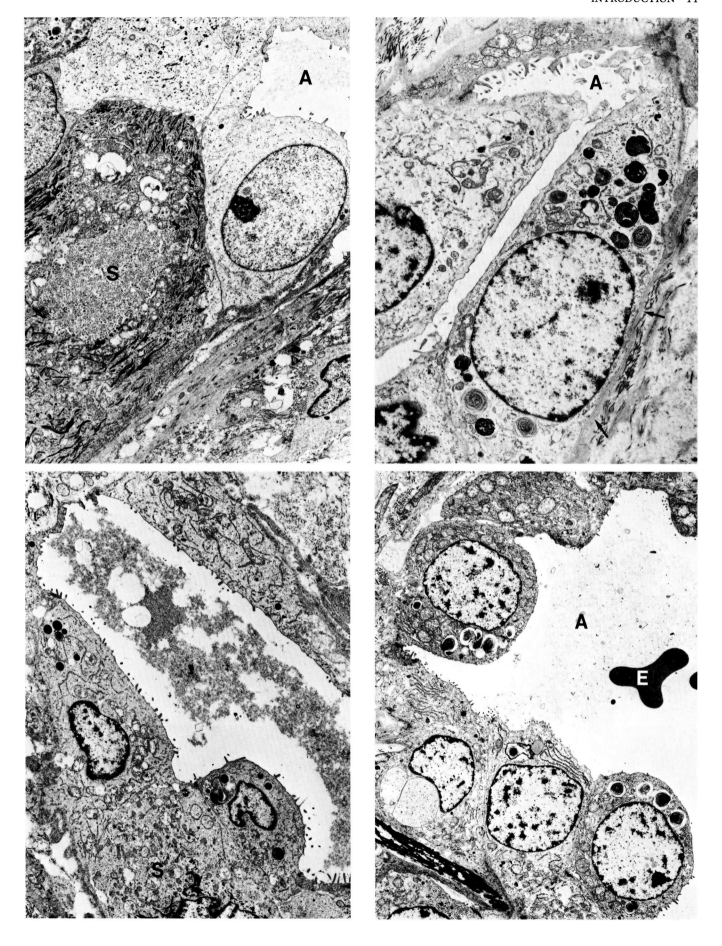

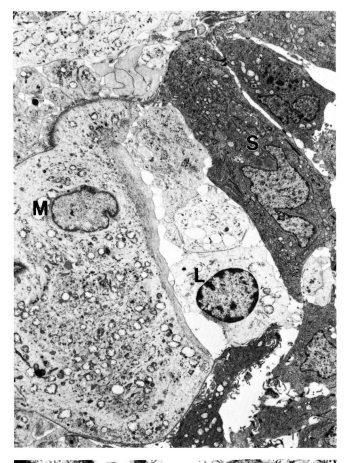

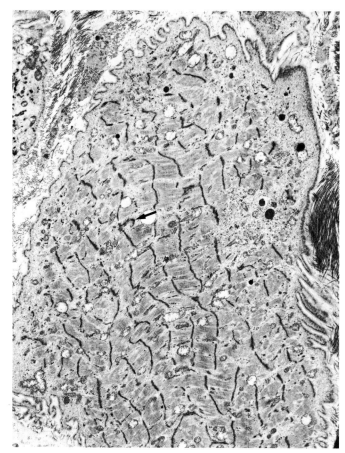

**Fig. 0.5** *(Top — left)* **Squamous cell carcinoma invading striated muscle**

The succeeding Figures (0.5–0.9) are intended to illustrate a progression of myofibrillary disorganization in atrophic myocytes incorporated into carcinomas.

Carcinoma of the floor of mouth. Relatively dark squamous cells (S) lie close to a myocyte (M) which shows marked myofibrillary disorganization. Inflammatory cells, including a lymphocyte (L), separate the squamous cells from the myocyte in one area. (×3000)

References: 44, 45, 2226, 2441

**Fig. 0.6** *(Top — right)* **Myofibrillary degeneration adjacent to squamous carcinoma: I**

The myocyte illustrated displays mild atrophic changes, with malalignment of sarcomeres, early streaming of Z-bands (arrow), and folding of the sarcolemmal membrane. (×4100)

**Fig. 0.7** *(Left)* **Myofibrillary degeneration adjacent to squamous carcinoma: II**

The myocyte shown here exhibits severe sarcomeric atrophy and dissolution. The numerous remaining Z-bands are disorganized and elongated. The sarcolemma and its associated external lamina are focally crenellated. Part of an adjacent activated lymphocyte (L) is also evident. (×11 200)

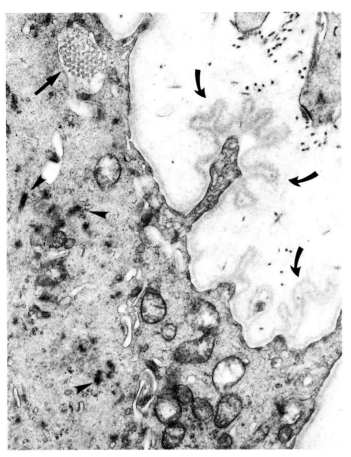

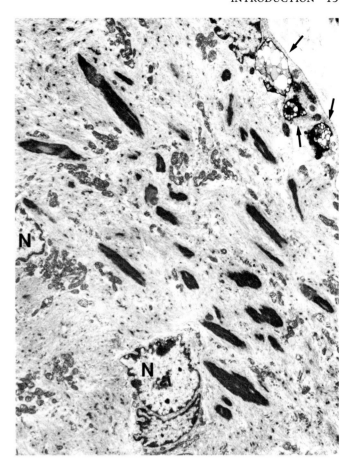

**Fig. 0.8 Myofibrillary degeneration adjacent to metastatic carcinoma: III**

Intramuscular tumour from the vastus intermedius of a 37-year-old woman who presented with multiple lumps in the thigh, buttock and left elbow region. Both LM and EM revealed a large cell carcinoma devoid of further differentiating features. Atrophic myocytes were present, both at the periphery of the tumour and incorporated into the stroma. Autopsy revealed an extremely poorly, but variably, differentiated adenocarcinoma of lung.

One of the atrophic myocytes is depicted. Only a few disorientated myofilaments and Z-lines (arrowheads) remain, but a tubular honeycomb array (straight arrow) is evident (see Fig. 22.1). In some circumstances myofibrillary degeneration may be misinterpreted as evidence of rhabdomyoblastic differentiation in neoplastic cells. However, the atrophic character of the process shown here is indicated by the following observations:

1. The retraction and separation of the sarcolemma from its folded redundant external lamina (curved arrows) in the fashion of a deflated balloon.
2. The wavy sarcolemma associated with a continuous undulant pericellular external lamina in the earlier stages of atrophy, as shown in Fig. 0.7. Compare with Figs. 22.6–22.8.

Atrophic myocytes often contain lipofuscin bodies, and regenerative activity is indicated by nucleolar prominence, and abundant polyribosomes and intermediate filaments.[290] (×18 700)

References: 44, 45, 290

**Fig. 0.9 Myofibrillary degeneration IV: Nemaline body formation**

Atrophic myocyte adjacent to a granulocytic sarcoma of the chest wall. There is marked disorganization of the myofilamentous apparatus, and the cell contains numerous elongated electron-dense nemaline bodies identical to those encountered in so-called nemaline myopathy and adult rhabdomyoma (see Figs. 22.3 and 22.4). Note also apparent displacement of nuclei (N) into the interior of the myocyte, and the peripheral lipofuscin bodies (arrows). (×4400)

# PART ONE

## *The General Fine Structure of Neoplasia*

# 1 The neoplastic cell I: Nuclear ultrastructure

## SUBCELLULAR MARKERS OF NEOPLASIA

The early hopes of electron microscopists of finding subcellular markers specific for neoplasia have not materialized and it is now recognized that neoplastic cells may show no significant structural differences from their normal counterparts.[13,45,58] The criteria for the morphological detection of neoplasia and the prediction of malignant behaviour are therefore still best assessed by light microscopy. Electron microscopy has little to add to this initial phase of evaluation, apart from reflecting the cytological changes which have long been documented by cytopathologists.

To avoid unnecessary repetition in later chapters of this book, some of the ultrastructural features common to neoplasms are briefly outlined. Both nuclear and cytoplasmic aberrations are considered, but the nature of these changes and their possible significance are not discussed in detail; in many instances they are poorly understood.

## THE NUCLEUS

It is ironical that the nucleus, in which the fundamental derangements responsible for the neoplastic process are thought to reside (p. 8), is morphologically perhaps the least informative cell component.[44] Irregularity is probably the only nuclear abnormality which is frequently present in malignant cells,[44,45,58,194] and its severity in a given tumour type may also reflect the degree of malignancy — although a high degree of irregularity may be encountered in some benign tumours (see Fig. 18.11).[45] In addition to complex nuclear contours, heterochromatin projections and bridges may also be present. These irregularities may indicate increased nucleocytoplasmic exchange in parallel with increased nuclear surface area, or even reflect anomalous nucleocytoplasmic interactions ('maturation anarchy'), such as occurs in myelomatosis.[2854]

Nuclear dimensions in malignant cells are often increased,[44,45] largely as a result of euchromatin augmentation. In addition, interchromatin granules and (to a lesser degree) perichromatin granules increase in numbers, although one or the other usually predominates.[44,45] In nasopharyngeal angiofibromas the characteristic intranuclear spheroidal bodies (see Fig. 20.2) may well represent giant perichromatin granules.

Nucleoli are often larger and more frequent than in corresponding normal cells.[45] They may lie at the nuclear periphery (see Figs. 1.6 and 30.8),[44,45,58] and they often have irregular contours or show abnormal arrangements of their major components. Their large size, indicating rapid RNA turnover,[44] perhaps reflects heightened synthetic activity necessary for cell replication.

Various inclusions may be found in the nuclei of malignant cells.[31,44] Some of the most obvious have a fibrillary, crystalline or tubular structure (Tables 1.1 and 1.2), but their significance is obscure. Typically, *convincing* intranuclear virions cannot be demonstrated ultrastructurally in biopsy samples of human malignant neoplasms — one possible exception being rare cases of hepatocellular carcinoma associated with hepatitis B virus[140] — although they are occasionally detectable in cultured material. However, fibrillary and tubular inclusions, and perichromatin and interchromatin granules, may be erroneously identified as viral particles.[44,45,140]

Cytoplasmic (pseudo)inclusions, some of which consist of invaginations of the cytoplasm into the substance of the nucleus, may also be seen.[44,45,291,1745] These can have either regular or irregular contours, but are delineated by the nuclear envelope, and may be another reflection of nuclear irregularity. However, some workers[1727] believe that a proportion of these structures represent sequestered collections of cytoplasm within nuclei (see Fig. 11.3). Rarely, true intranuclear cytoplasmic inclusions lacking a boundary membrane occur, probably resulting from sequestration of cytoplasmic contents within daughter nuclei during mitosis (Fig. 1.15).

Although it is sometimes difficult to distinguish between multinuclearity and the profiles produced by sectioning an extremely irregular nucleus, there is little doubt that multinucleated neoplastic cells are common. Perhaps this indicates an increased tendency of malignant cells to fuse or to undergo nuclear division without cytokinesis.

Metaphase profiles are also seen, but no fine-structural abnormalities have been reported in the chromosomal substructure.[58] Dispersed chromosomal material may be seen within the cytoplasm, despite the presence of a distinct nucleus bounded by a nuclear envelope (Fig. 1.18), possibly reflecting asynchronous nuclear condensation and envelope formation during cell division.

**Table 1.1  Intranuclear fibrillary inclusions**

| Cell type or disorder | Remarks |
|---|---|
| *NON-NEOPLASTIC CELLS* | |
| Circulating lymphocytes | Patients with multiple sclerosis and optic neuritis[232] |
| Neutrophils in renal transplant recipients | — |
| Pulmonary alveolar epithelium | Influenzal pneumonia[231] |
| Endometrial epithelial cells | Massive accumulation of 7–8 nm filaments in the central regions of nuclei with sparing of the periphery corresponds to foci of optically clear nuclei by LM, and may represent a marker for the presence of trophoblast.[207] Identical filaments are also recorded after IM injection of medroxyprogesterone acetate[47,207] |
| Pancreatic B cells | — |
| Neurones | Subacute sclerosing panencephalitis |
| Skeletal muscle | Duchenne muscular dystrophy carriers, and polymyositis with intranuclear inclusions |
| *TUMOURS AND TUMOUR-LIKE CONDITIONS* | |
| Pulmonary hamartoma | In epithelial component[508] |
| Angiomyolipoma of liver* | Formalin-fixed autopsy specimen |
| Infantile haemangiopericytoma | — |
| Proliferating histiocytic lesion | ?Histiocytosis X. Mediastinal and retroperitoneal sclerosing lesion[224] |
| Myoepithelioma of parotid gland | — |
| Pleomorphic salivary adenoma | — |
| Gliomas | Including glioblastoma multiforme |
| Meningioma | In meningiomas these inclusions are sometimes referred to as sphaeridions[2034] |
| Parathyroid adenoma | Intrathyroid tumour associated with hyperparathyroidism[230] |
| Papillary carcinoma of thyroid | — |
| Pancreatic islet tumours | Including B-cell carcinoma[935,976] |
| Adenocarcinoma of lung | Fig. 1.1 |
| Bronchogenic squamous cell carcinoma | Fig. 1.9 |
| So-called Merkel cell carcinoma of skin | — |
| Oesophageal oat cell carcinoma | — |
| Carcinoma of rectum | — |
| Undifferentiated sarcoma | — |
| Malignant lymphoma/lymphocytic leukaemia | In B-lymphocytic lymphomas and adult T-cell leukaemia/lymphoma, and in Sézary cells |
| Acute granulocytic leukaemia | — |
| Acute monocytic leukaemia | — |

*Henderson, Papadimitriou & Coleman, unpublished observation
See also the recent review of this topic by Payne & Nagle[3149]

References: 47, 64, 109, 193, 207, 218, 224, 230-232, 508, 663, 935, 976, 2034

## DEGENERATIVE NUCLEAR CHANGES AND APOPTOSIS

Some nuclear alterations reflect cell injury or the changes which accompany cell death.[44,291] These are indicated by increased amounts of heterochromatin, prominence of perichromatin granules, and, in more severely affected cells, by nuclear fragmentation or dissolution. Such nuclear abnormalities are accompanied by varying degrees of cytoplasmic organellar degradation,[291] sometimes including the changes of apoptosis.[1197]

Apoptosis appears to constitute a mechanism of cell deletion in both normal tissues and a variety of pathological situations, including tumours such as carcinomas of the uterine cervix.[200,212,1197] This phenomenon is characterized by condensation and margination of chromatin, fragmentation of nucleoli, loss of desmosomal attachments, cell retraction, and increased electron-density as a result of dehydration. The cells often undergo phagocytosis at this stage and are then degraded within phagolysosomes, but further extracellular degeneration can occur, such as blebbing and fragmentation of the nucleus and disintegration of the cytoplasm. Affecting individual cells, apoptosis appears to be an active energy-dependent process, different from cell necrosis (Table 1.3).[212] Rapid loss of tadpole tails during amphibian metamorphosis is accomplished by apoptosis; at no stage in this drastic tissue reorganization is the underlying apoptosis especially prominent, suggesting that even small numbers of apoptotic bodies in tissues indicate a high order of cell deletion.[212] Apoptosis is the subject of major recent reviews[200,205,212,219] and is discussed further in Table 1.3.

## NUCLEAR ENVELOPE

No significant abnormality of the nuclear envelope is seen in neoplastic cells.[45] Frequent nuclear pores are found occasionally, perhaps indicating augmented nucleocytoplasmic exchange,[31,194] while in other tumours, such as papillary carcinoma of thyroid, a deficiency of nuclear pores is reported.[1759] Rarely, intranuclear tubular inclusions occur, their morphology suggesting a derivation from the nuclear envelope; these inclusions are encountered especially in type II pneumocytes (Table 1.2). Parallel sets of lamellar structures known as annulate lamellae, resembling and sometimes continuous with the nuclear envelope, may also be seen in the cytoplasm (see Table 2.2). In a few tumours, material may accumulate within the nuclear cisterna, notably immunoglobulin in multiple myeloma.[3109,3121]

**Table 1.2  Intranuclear tubular inclusions: Morphology and comparison with Paramyxovirus nucleocapsids and altered chromatin fibres**

| Conditions associated with intranuclear tubular inclusions | Morphology of component tubules | | | | | Remarks |
|---|---|---|---|---|---|---|
| | Membrane-bound tubular outlines | Branching | Transverse periodicity | Tubular content in transverse section | Diameter of tubules | |
| Alveolar cell carcinoma of lung[472] | + | + | NS | NS | See remarks | Three cases. Inclusions found in type II pneumocytes. Composed of tubules, and granules measuring 35–42.5 nm in diameter |
| Alveolar cell carcinoma of lung[492] | + | + | Periodic striations | Dense core 20 nm in diameter | 60 nm | In neoplastic type II pneumocytes. Corresponded to eosinophilic intranuclear inclusions on LM |
| Bronchiolo-alveolar cell carcinoma[525] | + | + | — | Amorphous, low density | 40-60 nm | Four cases. Tubules seen in tumour cells and hyperplastic type II pneumocytes. Associated lamina fibrosa. Suggested development by invagination of inner nuclear membrane |
| Bronchiolo-alveolar adenocarcinoma* | + | + | — | Some had dense cores | Two distinct forms of tubule noted, one averaging 22 nm, while the larger tubules averaged 45 nm (range 35-95 nm) | Carcinoma with mixed secretory granules (Table 5.3). Tubules found in most neoplastic cells in areas examined and had a bimorphic appearance (Fig. 1.12). The narrow tubules were more uniform and electron-dense than the larger forms. Often closely associated with the nuclear fibrous lamina and envelope (Fig. 1.13), and many inclusions were invested by a scleroprotein-like layer. Nuclei containing the inclusions often appeared degenerate. Corresponding eosinophilic intranuclear inclusions seen by LM |
| Papillary adenocarcinoma of lung[591] | + | + | NS | Central core 18-20 nm in diameter | About 50 nm | Peripheral lung tumours. Inclusions sometimes associated with membranes and chromatin |
| Bronchogenic squamous cell carcinoma[64] | + | + | — | Some had central densities | 30-48 nm, average 37 nm | Within neoplastic cells. Prominent surrounding scleroprotein-like mantle |
| Hyperplastic type II pneumocytes adjacent to mucinous bronchiolar adenocarcinoma[64] | + | + | — | Some had dense cores | 20-53 nm, average 40 nm | Not found in neoplastic cells. Tubular aggregates were sometimes continuous with intranuclear membranes and were surrounded by a layer of scleroprotein-like matter (Fig. 1.11) |
| Hyperplastic type II pneumocytes adjacent to smooth muscle tumour[47] | + | + | — | Some had cores | Approximately 60 nm; range of 30-300 nm mentioned | Narrow electron-dense and larger vesicular tubules illustrated |
| Pulmonary hamartoma[508] | + | + | NS | Tubular, with finely dispersed luminal material | NS | Three cases. Found in approximately 10 per cent of cells in epithelial component. Associated with fibrillary inclusions |
| Alveolar epithelium in fibrotic lung disorders[225] | + | + | — | See remarks | 50-100 nm | Tubules sometimes dilated. Some contained dense matter. Tubules continuous with inner nuclear membrane. No chromatin seen in intertubular spaces. Cases included idiopathic pulmonary fibrosis, sarcoidosis and collagen-vascular disease. In another report, the tubules were 25-50 nm in diameter[222] |

**Table 1.2 (continued)   Intranuclear tubular inclusions: Morphology and comparison with Paramyxovirus nucleocapsids and altered chromatin fibres**

| Conditions associated with intranuclear tubular inclusions | Morphology of component tubules | | | | | |
| --- | --- | --- | --- | --- | --- | --- |
| | Membrane-bound tubular outlines | Branching | Transverse periodicity | Tubular content in transverse section | Diameter of tubules | Remarks |
| Hyperplastic type II pneumocytes in asbestosis* | + | + | — | Cores noted | 20-75 nm, average 45 nm | — |
| Hyperplastic type II pneumocytes in bleomycin- and busulphan-mediated alveolar damage[223] | + | + | — | Cores discernible | 45 nm | Found in 50-80 per cent of type II pneumocytes. Continuity with inner nuclear envelope noted |
| Paramyxovirus nucleocapsids | — | Undulant | Present, 4–7 nm | Hollow | 12–18 nm | Smooth outline. No continuity with membranes. Nucleocapsids may also be present in cytoplasm, with or without viral budding |
| Altered chromatin fibres | — | Coiled | Indistinct | Denser than Paramyxovirus. Tubular configuration rarely apparent | 18–40 nm | Fuzzy outline, more irregular than Paramyxovirus |

+ = present; — = absent; NS = not stated    *Henderson, Papadimitriou & Coleman, unpublished observations
References: 47, 64, 222, 223, 225, 472, 492, 508, 525, 591

**Table 1.3   Comparison of necrosis and apoptosis***

| Feature | Necrosis | Apoptosis |
| --- | --- | --- |
| *LIGHT MICROSCOPY* | | |
| Distribution | Usually involves groups of contiguous cells | Affects single cells scattered through a tissue |
| Associated exudative inflammation with neutrophil infiltration | Usually present | Absent (mononuclear cells may be present if apoptosis is being induced by cell-mediated immunity) |
| Cytology | Cell outlines generally retained, with eosinophilic 'ghosting' of entire cells; nuclei show pyknosis, karyorrhexis or karyolysis† | In transient early stage, nuclear chromatin is marginated. Cellular fragmentation leads to production of round or oval eosinophilic masses, some of which contain basophilic chromatin dots |
| *ULTRASTRUCTURE* | | |
| Chromatin | Marginates in small, loosely textured aggregates; disappears eventually when nuclear membrane destroyed | Marginates in condensed, coarsley granular aggregates abutting on nuclear membrane (Fig. 1.16); in certain planes of section, condensed chromatin may occupy much or all of nucleus |
| Nucleolus | Evident as compact body until cytoplasmic degradation advanced | Disperses to shower of granules while cytoplasm structurally intact |
| Nuclear membrane | Retains pore structures until cytoplasmic degradation advanced; eventually destroyed with other organelles | Progressive convolution; resulting protuberances eventually separate. Pores retained adjacent to euchromatin, but lost next to condensed chromatin. Eventually becomes discontinuous, so that dense chromatin masses lie among cytoplasmic organelles |
| Cytoplasm | Swelling of all compartments followed by rupture of membranes and destruction of organelles. Mitochondrial densities are characteristic | Condensation of cytosol (endoplasmic reticulum may dilate focally); structurally intact mitochondria and other organelles compacted together; cell surface protuberances, developing in association with condensation, separate with sealing of plasma membrane to produce apoptotic bodies |
| *FATE OF CELL REMNANTS* | Ingested and degraded by cells of mononuclear phagocytic system. Duration of persistence of cell remnants in a tissue depends on size of area of necrosis and integrity of microcirculation within the area, for access of phagocytes | Apoptotic bodies are rapidly phagocytosed and degraded by resident cells of a variety of types. The majority of apoptotic cell remnants detected by electron microscopy are intracellular and show evidence of partial degradation |
| *MECHANISM* | Progressive structural and chemical disintegration following irreversible disruption of vital processes maintaining cellular integrity | Apparently active process of cellular self-destruction requiring macromolecular synthesis for its execution |

*The characteristics listed in this table refer to apoptosis occurring within solid tisues and tumours; when the process affects cells in suspension cultures or in ascites tumours, most apoptotic bodies escape phagocytosis and eventually undergo secondary degradation resembling necrosis. Similar degradative alterations are seen in apoptotic bodies extruded into lumina from epithelial surfaces. †The terms 'pyknosis' and 'karyorrhexis' can legitimately be applied to the appearances of chromatin at certain stages of both necrosis and apoptosis.
(Composite table derived from Wyllie et al[219] and Searle et al,[212] and published by permission; modified and prepared in collaboration with Prof. J.F.R. Kerr)
References: 200, 205, 212, 219, 1197

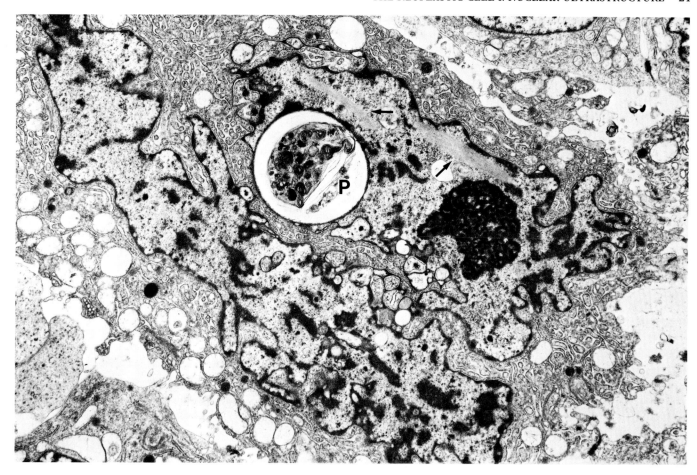

**Fig. 1.1   Nuclear irregularity: Adenocarcinoma**

Extreme nuclear irregularity in a pulmonary adenocarcinoma. Although the two large nuclear lobes are apparently separated by a thin cytoplasmic isthmus, their close proximity suggests that they probably represent profiles of a single highly irregular nucleus (see Fig. 1.2). There are also numerous complex nuclear projections. The nucleolus is prominent, a cytoplasmic (pseudo)inclusion (P) is evident, and there are two intranuclear fibrillary inclusions (arrows). (× 7400)

**Discussion:** Although frequently encountered, highly irregular nuclear profiles are not an invariable component of malignant cells. Conversely, nuclear irregularity is sometimes seen in benign tumours,[45] and in non-neoplastic and even normal tissues.[180] Thus irregular nuclei with protrusions and satellite nuclei are a normal occurrence in polymorphonuclear leukocytes, the epithelium of the human vas deferens and in the epididymis of some species.[180] The nuclei of contractile cells such as smooth muscle, myofibroblasts and cardiac myocytes[31] are often folded due to a 'concertina effect'. Nevertheless, morphometric analysis of the degree of irregularity (nuclear contour index) in T-lymphocytes with cerebriform nuclei *may* be of value in distinguishing mycosis fungoides (MF) from benign cutaneous lymphoid infiltrates, higher orders of irregularity being characteristic of MF (see Table 27.2).

The precise functional significance of nuclear irregularity is uncertain. One obvious consequence is increased nuclear envelope area, and enhanced nucleocytoplasmic exchange has therefore been invoked.[45] Fawcett[180] has argued that if this were so, increased numbers of nuclear pores might also be expected. However, augmented numbers of pores per unit area are not detectable in normal epididymal epithelium; in comparison to other cell types, the level of metabolic-synthetic activity seems insufficient to require such drastic modification of the nuclear surface: volume ratio.[180]

See also Figs. 11.2, 27.1, 27.2 and 27.6–27.9.

References: 13, 31, 44, 45, 47, 58, 180

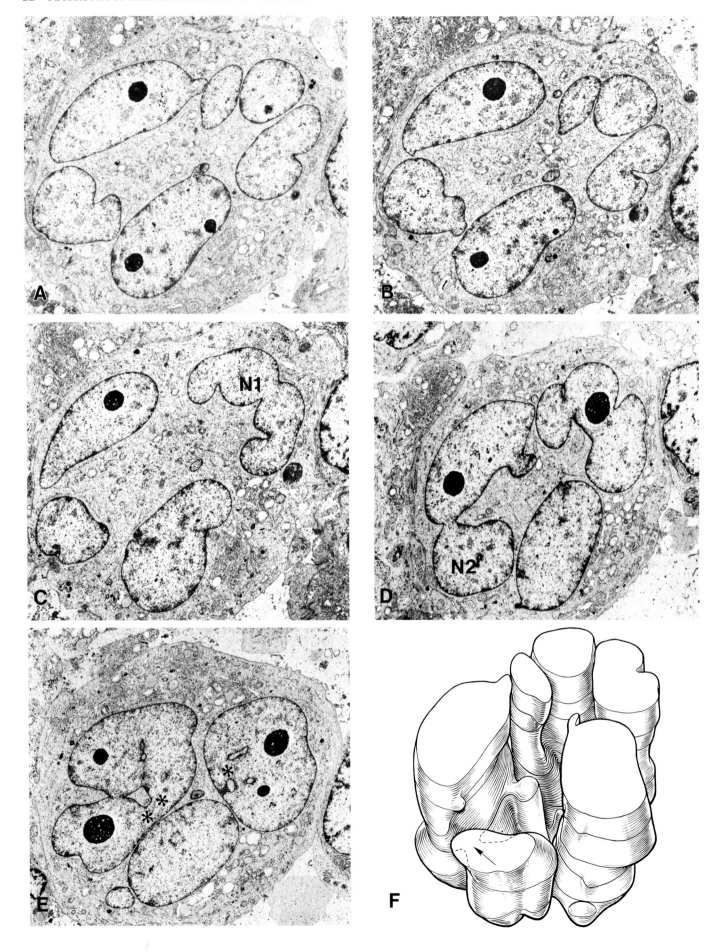

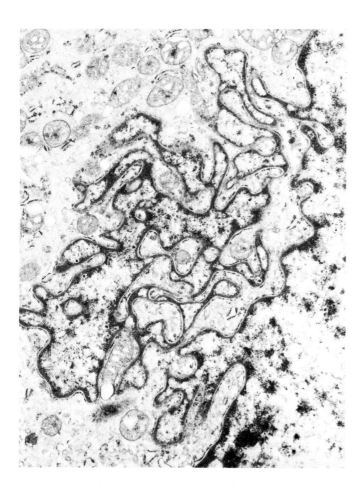

**Fig. 1.3  Nuclear projections: Malignant tumour of undetermined type**

Metastatic neoplasm from the axillary region of a man aged 24 years. An elaborate tangled mass of projections emanates from the nucleus, drastically augmenting nuclear surface area and the potential for nucleocytoplasmic exchange. (Formalin fixation, ×12 100)

**Discussion:** Although occurring in some normal cells, for example polymorphonuclear leukocytes, nuclear projections are frequent in malignant cells, especially in lymphomas, and sometimes achieve extraordinary complexity. They are  also seen in leukaemias, chondroblastoma and medelloblastoma,[39] as well as some cases of the following: leiomyosarcoma, oat cell carcinoma (see Fig. 6.1), malignant melanoma, embryonic neoplasms such as Wilms' tumour, and malignant fibrous histiocytoma (Henderson, Papadimitriou & Coleman, unpublished observations). Satellite nuclei are also said to occur consistently in 'perineurial fibroblasts' in dermatofibrosarcoma protuberans.[39]

The expression 'nucleotesimal' has been used by Elias & Hyde[198] for projections of this type in colonic carcinomas and it has fancifully been claimed that they represent a form of amitotic nuclear division by fragmentation.

References: 31, 39, 44, 47, 192, 198, 213, 216, 217, 291, 2942

**Fig. 1.2** *(Facing page)*  **Multiple nuclear profiles: Large cell undifferentiated carcinoma of lung**

Although multinucleated neoplastic cells are common, caution needs to be exercised in the interpretation of multiple nuclear profiles in electron micrographs, as they can result from ultrathin sectioning of single convoluted nuclei. On the other hand, EM sometimes demonstrates submicroscopic bridges between seemingly separate nuclei, notably in some Reed-Sternberg cells.

**A–E:** Multiple nuclear profiles are evident in these semiserial views of a single neoplastic cell. In successive levels some of the apparently discrete lobes become more closely apposed, eventually fusing to form single lobes (notably N1 in C and N2 in D), while other profiles become more widely separated. (×4200)

**F:** A three-dimensional reconstruction of the profiles is depicted here, suggesting that they represent nuclear hyperlobation within a mononuclear or binuclear cell rather than discrete nuclei in themselves. Beginning at the uppermost plane through the profiles, the continuous lines correspond to each of the sections shown in A–E. One nuclear bridge is indicated by the arrow, but two other areas of fusion (* and ** in E) cannot be visualized in this projection.

Ultrastructural examination of the carcinoma in this case revealed evidence of microacinus formation, indicating a very poorly differentiated adenocarcinoma (see Chapter 5).[468]

References: 44, 468

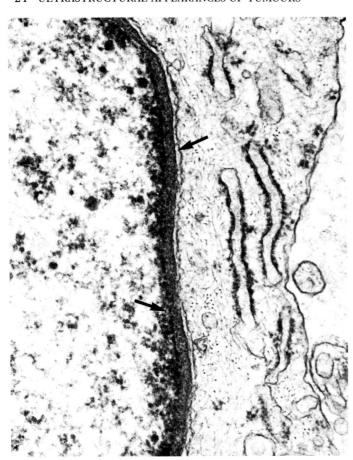

### Fig. 1.4 Nuclear fibrous lamina: Nasopharyngeal angiofibroma

The fibrous lamina in this cell forms a prominent layer of medium density (arrows), situated between the nuclear envelope and the peripheral heterochromatin layer, and measuring 45–60 nm in thickness (see below). The cytoplasm contains RER and intermediate filaments in varying planes of section. (Formalin fixation, × 47 600)

(Case contributed by Dr. A. E. Seymour).

**Discussion:** The nuclear fibrous lamina (FL) represents a layer of medium electron-density between the nuclear envelope and the peripheral heterochromatin masses. In some organisms such as the leech (*Hirudo medicinalis*) the lamina is seen to consist of a network of fine filaments, but this substructure is usually inapparent in the cells of vertebrates. Development of the FL varies greatly among different species, various cell types in an individual, and even within the same cell. Invertebrate cells often have prominent fibrous laminae, measuring up to 200 nm in insects, whereas in vertebrates they are thinner, measuring about 20–80 nm[180] and usually less than 30 nm.[47] In biopsied human tissues the lamina tends to be most prominent in mesenchymal cells; it may be very thin and barely detectable in other cell types,[47] and is deficient in the region of nuclear pores. FL is thought to represent a cytoskeletal polymer, and it is possible that it functions as a peripheral anchoring layer for hypercoiled chromatin fibres; a role in the genesis and maintenance of pore complexes has also been proposed.

The development of the FL is highly variable in tumours and it may apparently be absent, particularly in malignant neoplasms. Inconspicuous laminae are without diagnostic significance, but Ghadially[45] has claimed that a well developed FL in fibroproliferative lesions favours a reparative or benign process. Laminal prominence has previously been reported in elastofibroma,[2286] and mixed salivary tumour, as well as chondroblastoma, chondromyxoid fibroma and highly differentiated chondrosarcoma,[2647] non-ossifying fibroma of bone,[2647] the lymphoid cells in Hodgkin's disease,[47] and in the myofibroblasts of parosteal osteogenic sarcoma[2614] (which has a more favourable prognosis than conventional osteosarcoma). We have also observed prominence of the FL in a case of congenital localized fibromatosis of bone.

References: 45, 47, 180, 2286, 2614, 2647

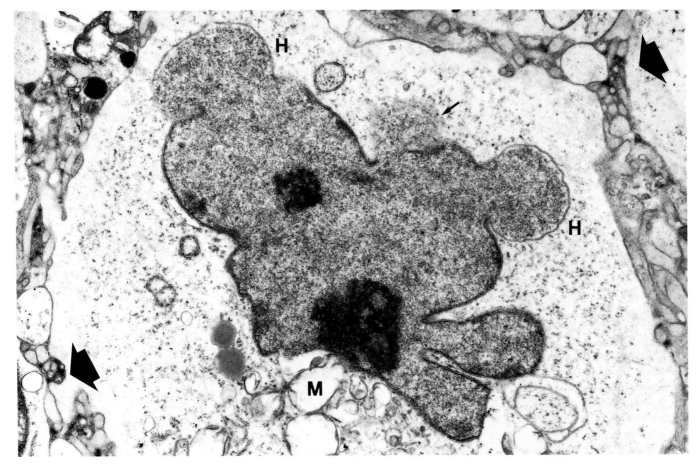

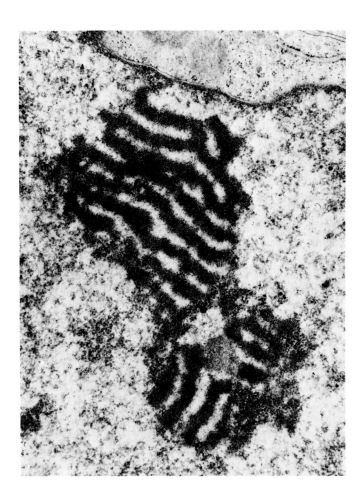

### Fig. 1.6  Nucleolar morphology: Colonic adenocarcinoma

The enlarged nucleolus is marginated at the nuclear envelope and the nucleolonema is arranged in spiremes. ($\times 22\,300$)

Such nucleolar margination in cells, irrespective of their neoplastic status, reflects active protein synthesis and/or heightened cell replication. A fragmented filamentous nucleolonema is usually present in germinomas[70] and is a helpful feature in the differential diagnosis of these tumours (see Table 26.1); however, it lacks specificity and accordingly its significance should be evaluated in conjunction with the other nucleocytoplasmic appearances.

See also Fig. 7.2.

References: 31, 39, 44, 45, 70, 215, 1922

### Fig. 1.7  Nuclear and nucleolar morphology: Malignant fibrous histiocytoma

Of the two cells illustrated, the upper has a prominent nucleolus, with marked elevation of both nucleolar: nuclear and nuclear: cytoplasmic ratios. This large nucleolus consists almost entirely of nucleolonemal material. The upper cell is surrounded by the cytoplasm of another neoplastic cell with less condensation of nuclear chromatin, and a relatively small nucleolus in the plane of section. ($\times 8200$)

Nucleolar prominence is common in poorly differentiated malignancies, but inconspicuous nucleoli characterize others, such as Ewing's sarcoma, neuroblastoma and some non-Hodgkin's lymphomas.

References: 13, 31, 44, 45, 58

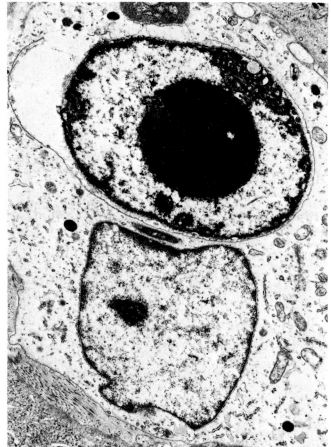

### Fig. 1.5 *(Facing page — bottom)*  Nuclear herniations (evaginations): Follicular centre cell lymphoma (centroblastic lymphoma)

The scleroproteins of the fibrous lamina are deficient in two regions of this hyperlobate nucleus, with associated herniations (H). In another area the nuclear envelope appears to have ruptured, with possible extrusion of chromatin into the cytoplasm (arrow), although this might also be interpreted as a tangential section of a nuclear projection. Cytoplasmic organelles are sparse, and include free ribosomes and swollen mitochondria (M). The surrounding filopodial processes display complex interleaving (bold arrows), but there are no specialized intercellular junctions. The morphology depicted here resembles that of radial segmentation of nuclei. ($\times 13\,100$)

**Discussion:** Nuclear lobulation producing a clover-leaf pattern is sometimes referred to as radial segmentation of nuclei and ultrastructurally characterizes Rieder cells in lymphocytic, granulocytic and myelomonocytic leukaemias (see Table 28.1). Radial nuclear segmentation appears to be a microtubule-dependent phenomenon and is inhibited by microtubule antagonists such as colchicine.[47]

Ruptures of the nuclear envelope resulting in nuclear-cytoplasmic continuity have also been reported in kidney cells of unspecified type in Goodpasture's syndrome.[31] Their role in the transport of nuclear substances is uncertain; nucleocytoplasmic exchange ordinarily takes place by transmembranous transport, and via the endoplasmic reticulum and annulate lamellae, as well as vesicles and blebs.[31]

See also Fig. 20.12.

References: 31, 47, 192, 216, 217

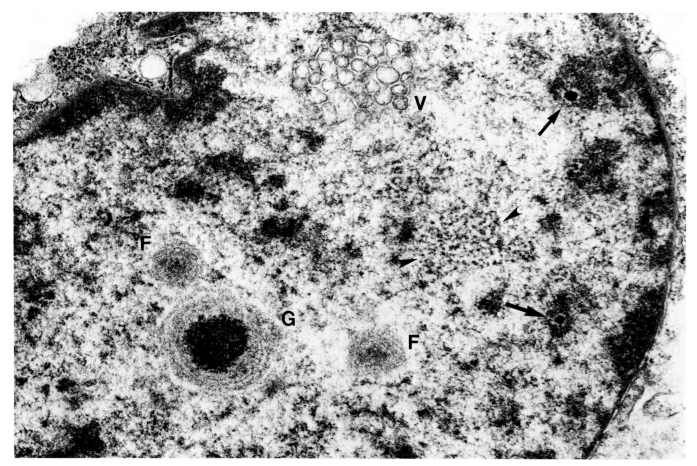

**Fig. 1.8 Nuclear bodies and perichromatin granules: Osteogenic sarcoma**

Several nuclear bodies are apparent in the nucleus, including vesicular (V), small fibrillary (F), and complex granulofibrillary (G) forms. Perichromatin granules are also present (arrows), while the nuclear matrix contains interchromatin granules (arrowheads). (× 38 500)

**Discussion:** The precise nature and significance of nuclear bodies (NB) are uncertain but at least some appear to be proteinaceous and to correlate with the level of cellular metabolic activity. Thus David[31] found that in starved lactating cows the percentage of NB in nuclear sections declined from $13.5 \pm 1.6$ to $2.6 \pm 0.5$! In uterine luminal epithelial cells they are thought to be a structural indicator of oestrogenic stimulation and are related to the duration of localization of the oestrogen receptor complex to the nucleus.[210]

Both complex and simple NB are recognized. The complex forms (G) are composed of a core of ribonucleoprotein granules enclosed by a protein-containing capsule formed by filaments 5–7 nm in diameter, and are included in the extra-nucleolar genome, although some NB may be of nucleolar origin. The simple bodies (F) consist of the filamentous capsular material only, but it is likely that many represent tangential sections of complex NB.

NB are not unexpected in neoplasms, and are recorded in a variety of tumours including prostatic carcinoma, bronchogenic carcinoma, pleomorphic salivary adenoma, thymoma, Hodgkin's disease, smooth muscle and myofibroblastic tumours, gliomas and meningiomas, to mention but a few. Indeed, they are so widely distributed in tissues that they can be considered almost ubiquitous. Perhaps their chief importance is that they may be misinterpreted as viral particles.

Perichromatin and interchromatin granules are abundant in many different tumours (including oestrogen-producing neoplasms and 'scirrhous carcinoma' of the breast),[31] one or the other usually predominating. As their name indicates, perichromatin granules are situated at the periphery of heterochromatin masses; they typically measure 30–35 nm in diameter and are surrounded by a lucent halo 15–50 nm wide. Interchromatin granules are 15–50 nm in diameter and are arranged in clusters. Evidence suggests that perichromatin granules contain messenger RNA, and Ghadially[45,47] regards both types of granules as nuclear ribosomes. Once again, they have sometimes been mistaken for viral particles, particularly the perichromatin granules.

See also Figs. 9.4, 18.10, 20.1, 20.2 and 21.3.

References: 31, 39, 44, 45, 47, 109, 195, 203, 204, 210, 211, 214–217, 1745

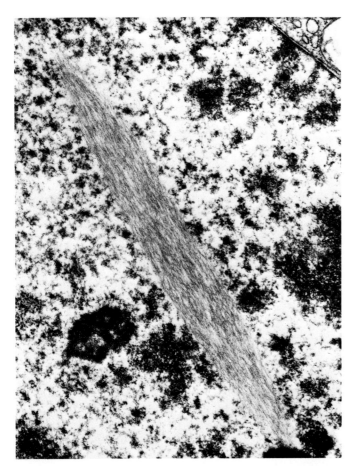

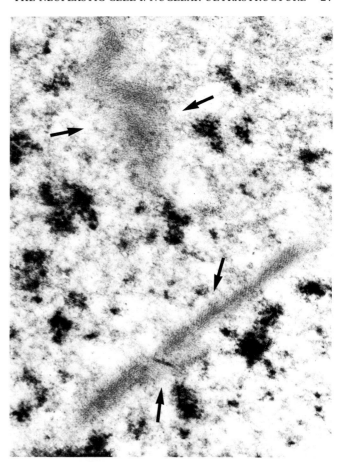

**Fig. 1.9  Intranuclear fibrillary inclusion: Bronchogenic squamous cell carcinoma**

The fibrillary inclusion illustrated here consists of a spindle-shaped sheaf of fine filaments averaging about 7 nm in diameter. (× 18 300)

Intranuclear fibrillary inclusions (intranuclear rodlets[230]) have been reported in many neoplastic and non-neoplastic tissues (Table 1.1), and in normal cells, notably sympathetic neurones in the cat. While they have sometimes been associated with viral infection, their occurrence in such diverse circumstances suggests that they are entirely non-specific, perhaps reflecting altered nucleoprotein.

References: 31, 44, 193, 207, 220, 221, 224, 226–232, 234, 2034, 2484

**Fig. 1.10  Crystalline nuclear inclusions: Anaplastic bronchogenic carcinoma**

A crystalline array of filaments (arrows) is obvious in the euchromatinic regions of this nucleus; a cross-hatched pattern with a periodicity measuring 13–14 nm is present. The nature and significance of such inclusions have not been investigated extensively, but they may represent non-histone DNA envelope protein. (×45 000)

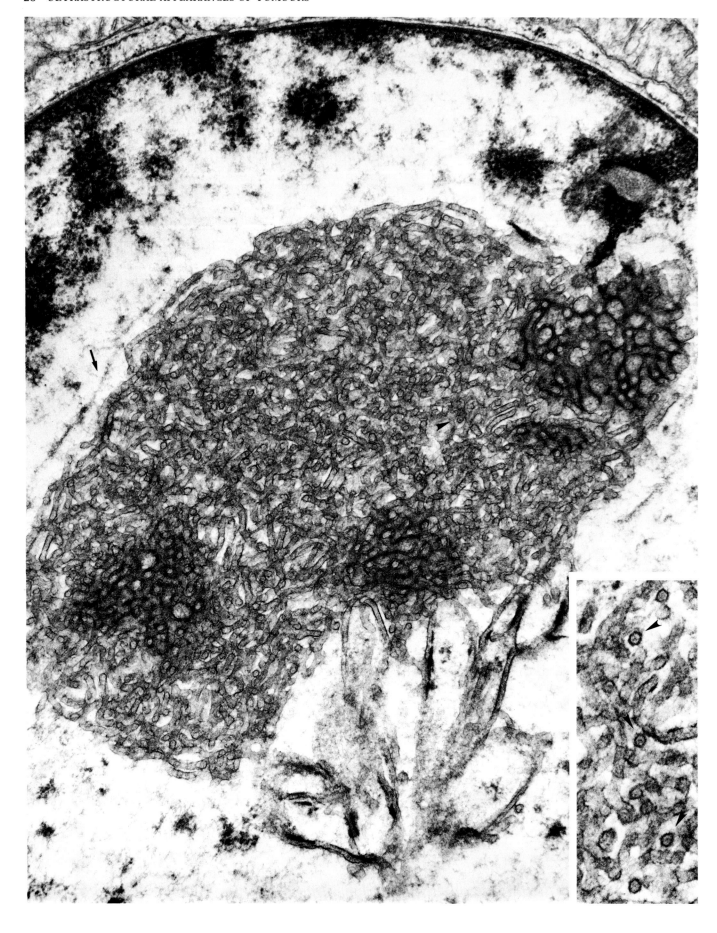

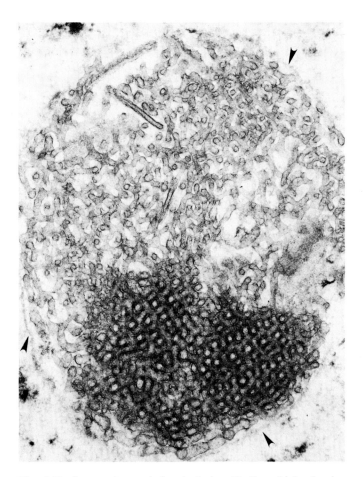

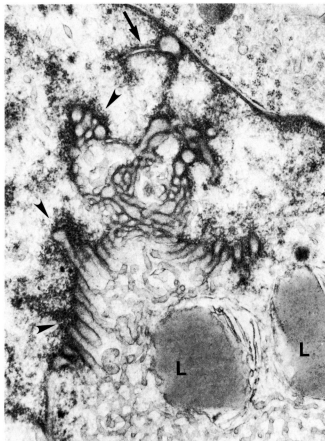

**Fig. 1.12  Intranuclear tubular inclusion II: Bronchiolo-alveolar adenocarcinoma**

In this case the tubules were found in the nuclei of many neoplastic cells; the tumour was a bronchiolo-alveolar carcinoma with a mixed granule population, in a 76-year-old woman. The inclusions were readily apparent by LM as eosinophilic, moderately PAS-positive rounded intranuclear inclusions.

The inclusion illustrated here takes the form of an ovoid mass of tangled and branching smooth tubules with sharp borders. In one area the tubules have a condensed pattern, appearing more electron-dense, regular and narrow than those elsewhere, with the formation of undulant and circular patterns. The narrow tubules have an average diameter of 22 nm; the larger tubules average 45 nm in diameter, with a range of 35–95 nm. Note the thin layer of scleroprotein-like matter partly surrounding the inclusion (arrowheads). (×35 400)

**Fig. 1.11** *(Facing page)* **Intranuclear tubular inclusion I: Hyperplastic type II pneumocytes associated with mucinous bronchiolar adeno-carcinoma**

This inclusion consists of a tightly packed mass of smooth, sharply demarcated branching tubules averaging 38 nm in diameter. A more condensed pattern with narrower tubules is apparent in three areas, and some of the tubules have central cores (inset; arrowheads). The size, branching, sharp demarcation, central cores and absence of transverse periodicity distinguish these tubules from both Paramyxovirus particles and altered chromatin fibres (Table 1.2). Their morphology, occasional continuity with membranous structures, and the presence of a grey surrounding layer resembling scleroprotein (arrow) suggest that they are derived from the nuclear envelope. The nucleolar channel systems occurring in the nuclei of secretory endometrium have morphological similarities to these inclusions and are also thought to originate from the nuclear envelope. (×43 800. Inset ×88 500)

Tubular inclusions of this type have most often been recognized in type II pneumocytes (Table 1.2). We have also found them in a bronchogenic squamous cell carcinoma.

References: 44, 206, 222, 223, 225, 233, 577

**Fig. 1.13  Intranuclear tubular inclusion III: Bronchiolo-alveolar carcinoma**

Here the tubules extend close to the nuclear periphery (arrow), while elsewhere they are intimately related to a layer of heterochromatin (arrowheads), suggesting an origin from interiorized inner nuclear envelope. Two lipid droplets (L) are also present. (×27 100)

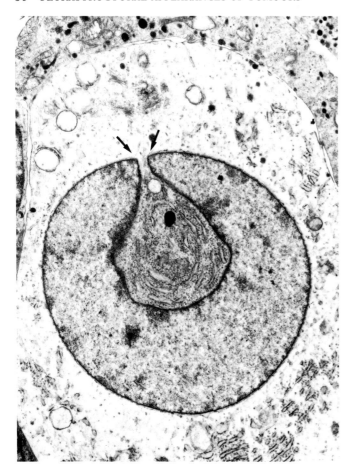

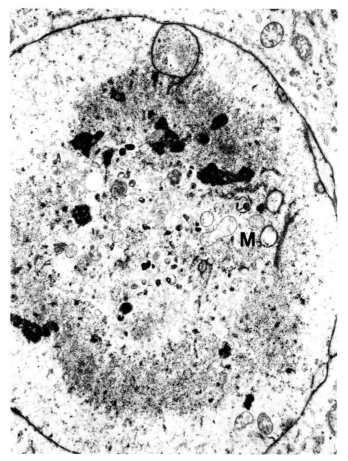

**Fig. 1.14 Intranuclear cytoplasmic pseudoinclusion: Neuro-endocrine carcinoma**

The continuity of the pseudoinclusion with the surrounding paler cytoplasm is clearly shown (arrows). (×7400)

   **Discussion:** Although lacking specificity, these pseudoinclusions are frequently encountered in certain tumour types such as malignant melanoma. They are found in about 90 per cent of papillary carcinomas of thyroid, but only rarely in other thyroid carcinomas and benign diseases.[196] See also discussion to Fig. 11.3.

   References: 44, 47, 196, 291, 1727, 1745, 1766, 2034

**Fig. 1.15** *(Top — right)* **True intranuclear cytoplasmic inclusion: Amelanotic malignant melanoma**

Cerebral metastasis from a 40-year-old man. The nucleus contains a variety of cytoplasmic organelles, including mitochondria (M) and vesicles. The organelles intermingle with the nuclear chromatin, without evidence of a boundary membrane, suggesting that they may have been sequestered during mitosis. Alternatively, this appearance could result from dissolution of the membrane enclosing a pseudoinclusion. (×10 100)

   Concentric laminated (targetoid) inclusions formed by alternating dense and lucent layers have also been described in some animal tumours and in pancreatic acinar cells adjacent to an insulinoma.[47]

**Fig. 1.16** *(Bottom — right)* **Degenerative nuclear changes I: Apoptosis: Large cell lymphocytic (centroblastic) lymphoma**

The chromatin is predominantly arranged as a circumferential layer of heterochromatin, while the central chromatin has a dispersed granular and speckled appearance. These changes conform to an early stage of apoptosis, but as yet there is no increase in electron-density of the cytosol. This morphology is thought to correspond to the doughnut-like pattern of nuclear degeneration seen in lymphomas by LM – especially in Burkitt's lymphoma – in which dense chromatin surrounds a central eosinophilic area. (×13 800)

   References: 200, 205, 212, 219, 1197

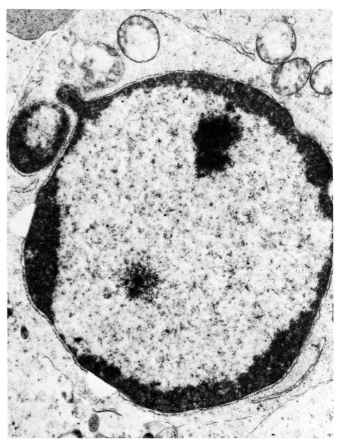

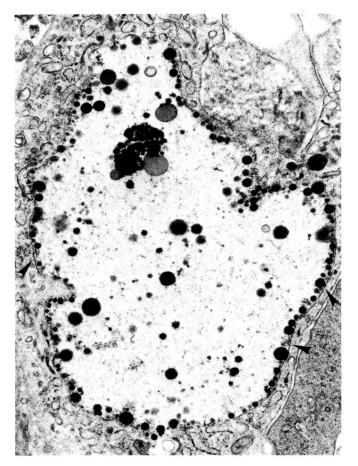

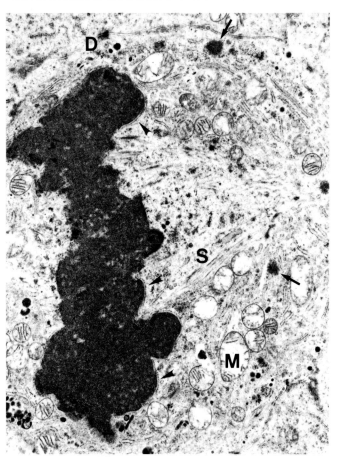

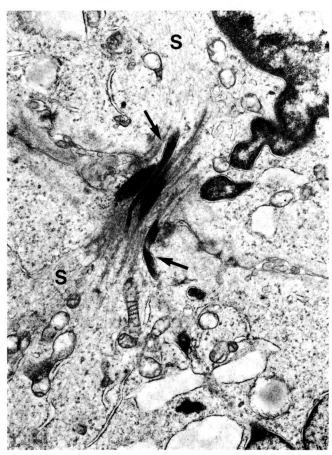

**Fig. 1.17  Degenerative nuclear changes II: Apoptosis: Immuno-blastic lymphadenopathy**

Here the chromatin has fragmented into globules of varying size, some scattered in the lucent matrix but most aligned along the still-intact nuclear envelope (arrowheads). In comparison, the cytoplasmic organelles show little alteration. (×18 400)

**Fig. 1.18** *(Top — right)*  **Mitosis: Large cell undifferentiated carcinoma of lung**

Metaphase mitosis in a malignant cell. Despite dispersal of small chromatinic aggregates (arrows), segments of nuclear membrane border the main chromosomal mass (arrowheads). The microtubular spindle (S) is also evident and some of the mitochondria (M) are swollen. Desmosomal junctions (D) with an adjoining cell are maintained. (×9900)

See also Figs. 6.1 and 20.10.

References: 44, 180, 202

**Fig. 1.19** *(Bottom — right)*  **Late telophase mitosis: Malignant fibrous histiocytoma**

The intermediate body (Fleming's body; *Zwischenkörper*) and the spindle microtubules (S) are shown. Chromatin aggregates (arrows) with surrounding nuclear membrane still extend across the intermediate body. (×13 900)

References: 180, 189, 1131, 2296

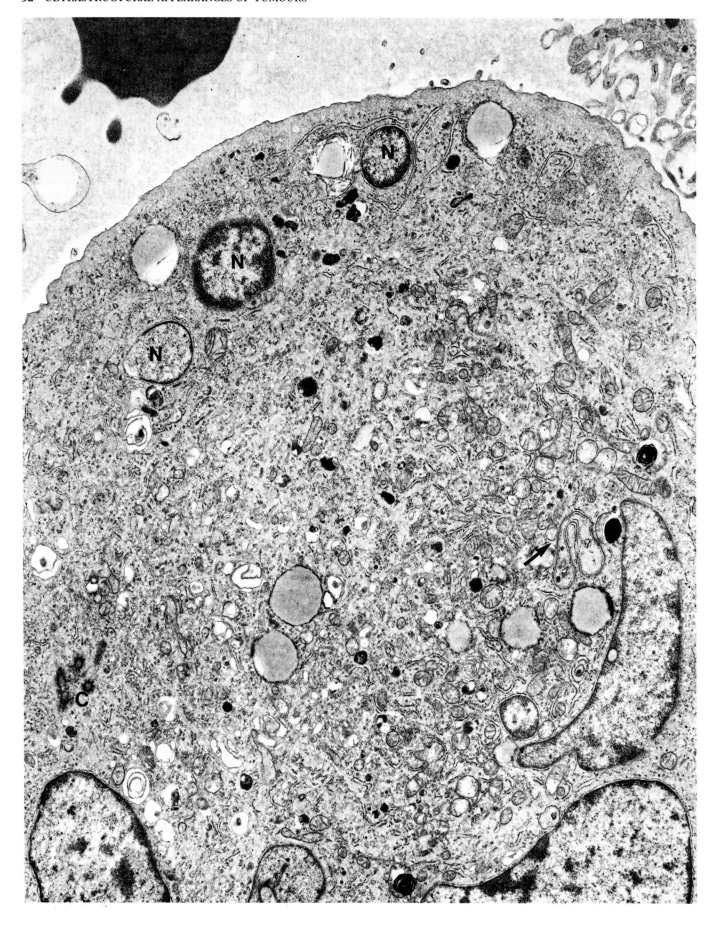

**Fig. 1.20** *(Facing page)* **Multinucleated neoplastic giant cell: Malignant fibrous histiocytoma, giant cell type**

Portions of several widely dispersed nuclei are apparent, including three separate micronuclear profiles (N). The cytoplasm shows considerable organellar disarray, and contains multiple centrioles (C) as well as mitochondria, lysosomes, pale lipid droplets, and confronting cisternae of RER (arrow). (×13 200)

Compare with Figs. 1.1 and 1.2. See also Figs. 20.5, 20.12, 20.13, 27.1 and 27.26.

Reference: 330

# 2 The neoplastic cell II: Cytoplasmic ultrastructure

## MITOCHONDRIA

The mitochondria in malignant cells generally display varying degrees of pleomorphism;[44,58,291] they are often swollen and electron-lucent, but the contents are occasionally electron-dense. Their contours vary from tumour to tumour, in different cells from the same tumour, and even within single cells. Accordingly, mitochondria of unusual shapes and dimensions may be present, and these include branched, crescentic, circular, or giant mitochondria.[44,45] Tubular cristae often characterize cells producing steroid hormones (see Fig. 13.3), and sometimes extreme mitochondrial hyperplasia and hypertrophy saturate the cytoplasm, resulting in a so-called oncocytic appearance (Table 2.1). Tridimensional reconstructions of such mitochondria in oncocytic thyroid adenoma have revealed bipartite and tripartite divisions, thought to reflect rapid mitochondrial replication.[1784]

## ENDOPLASMIC RETICULUM

The amount of rough endoplasmic reticulum (RER) varies according to both the type and degree of neoplastic differentiation;[14] it is generally prominent in highly differentiated cells, especially those engaged in secretion, and is particularly well developed in plasmacytic and fibroblastic cells (see Figs. 27.25–27.27). On the other hand, RER is generally sparse in anaplastic cells. Stacked lamellae of RER are a typical feature of endocrine cells, and are also found in acinic (serous) cells, sometimes forming complex targetoid patterns, while thick branching lamellae are characteristic of fibroblasts. In other situations the cisternae display varying degrees of degranulation. Confronting 'back-to-back' lamellae occur more frequently in neoplastic than normal cells, perhaps due to their predilection for mitotic and post-mitotic cells, while dilatation of RER with accumulation of secretory products suggests secretory asynchrony. So-called micro-sequestration has also been recorded in a pancreatic islet adenoma, but lacks diagnostic significance.[47] Intracisternal tubuloreticular arrays (Fig. 2.11) are seen in a variety of neoplasms, but they are neither confined to neoplastic cells, nor is their significance understood; they should not be confused with intracytoplasmic virions or the products of their replication (Tables 2.3 and 2.4).

Smooth endoplasmic reticulum (SER) is typically abundant in cells producing steroid hormones (see Figs. 30.1 and 30.2).[39] The tubular profiles of SER are best preserved by glutaraldehyde fixation, and they often fragment into a series of vesicles in osmium tetroxide-fixed tissues.[47]

## RIBOSOMAL ROSETTES (POLYRIBOSOMES)

Again, no consistent or specific change is seen in the arrangement and distribution of ribosomal rosettes in the cytoplasm of malignant cells.[44] They usually constitute the predominant cytoplasmic organelle in cells which are poorly differentiated or where cell growth is rapid, and are responsible for the synthesis of endogenous proteins necessary for growth and replication. Generally, the ratio of polyribosomes to the RER is inversely proportional, and is dependent on the degree of differentiation of a particular class of tumour.[47] For example, RER is relatively abundant and polyribosomes are few in highly differentiated fibrosarcomas and osteosarcomas, but in poorly differentiated tumours the reverse applies.

## GOLGI APPARATUS

The degree of development of the Golgi apparatus often reflects the differentiation of the neoplastic cell; the apparatus tends to be well developed in cells actively engaged in secretion and may be accompanied by variable dilatation,[44] whereas it is often poorly developed and may be quite inconspicuous in highly anaplastic tumours. The polarity of the Golgi apparatus relative to other organelles may be disturbed. The Golgi complex is an organelle without diagnostic significance.[39]

## LYSOSOMES AND OTHER SECRETORY GRANULES

There is no consistent pattern in the number and distribution of these organelles within tumour cells. Lysosomes occur in various types of neoplastic cells and profuse autophagosomes are seen occasionally, especially in granular cell tumours (see Table 18.2). Rarely, glycogen accumulates within lysosomes (Fig. 2.16), notably in benign clear cell tumour of lung.[443,570]

In some cases, neoplastic cells contain distinctive granules whose morphology is diagnostic (Table 2.5), and which, in the case of some endocrine tumours, may be equated with a particular secretory product. Secretory granules therefore constitute valuable markers for tumour classification and require careful evaluation. Their dimensions are sometimes of importance, notably in pituitary adenomas, and are usually expressed in the form of either mean or average diameters. For a given population of spheroidal granules, many of the small profiles will result from non-equatorial oblique sectioning, the largest diameters conversely representing equatorial planes of section. The analysis of particle size and shape is a classical and complex stereological problem which is clearly beyond the scope of this work. However, it may be noted that:

1. As with any biological structure, the true granule dimensions will vary, with a normal or skewed distribution.
2. Even in the theoretical case of uniform granule diameters, skewed variability of profiles will result from different planes of section on either side of the equator, the number of intersections depending on granule size and section thickness. The distribution will be skewed in the direction of small profiles.

Throughout this atlas granule dimensions are expressed as either mean diameters with standard deviations, or the size range ± average diameters.

The identification of neurosecretory granules (NSG) is of crucial importance in the ultrastructural diagnosis of neuroendocrine neoplasms such as carcinoid tumours and neuroendocrine carcinomas, and neuroblastoma. In highly differentiated tumours the granules are easily recognized by their morphology, apparent uniformity and profusion. However, they are depleted in poorly differentiated tumours such as small cell neuroendocrine carcinomas, and occasionally it is difficult to decide whether the granules represent NSG or lysosomes. Although the size of NSG may vary according to the site of origin of the neoplasm, the dimensions generally vary only slightly within individual cells; their shape is often round or slightly oval, the electron-dense contents being bounded by a distinct limiting membrane, and they are frequently polarized towards a nearby blood vessel (see Figs. 6.2–6.4, 7.1, 11.5 and 11.6, and Chapter 16). On the other hand, lysosomes are usually larger, more pleomorphic, and are often concentrated in the region of the Golgi complex or near a secretory lumen (see Figs. 16.5 and 30.6). The peripheral submembranous halo is not as clearly demarcated in lysosomes, the contents of which are often less osmiophilic than those of most NSG (see Fig. 20.9). Non-uniform and even apparently extraneous material within granules is characteristic of lysosomal bodies (see Figs. 18.12 and 18.13), while 'zipper-like' junctions between individual lysosomes may be seen on extremely rare occasions (Table 2.12).

## CENTRIOLES AND CILIOGENESIS

Although centriolar abnormalities are rare, multiple centrioles are occasionally found;[44] these may indicate premitosis or cell fusion. The assembly of subcomponents is sometimes aberrant or incomplete in poorly formed centrioles.

Cilia occur in various neoplasms. Although they are most frequently seen in carcinomas, they are not uncommon in sarcomas or neural neoplasms.[39,47] Where multiple cilia are present, various abnormalities of ciliogenesis are more easily detected (see Fig. 5.28). Again, none of these changes is specific for malignancy or neoplasia.

## FILAMENTS

As defined by their diameters, three morphological classes of cytofilaments are found in both normal and neoplastic cells (Table 2.7):

1. Microfilaments (actin-like filaments) 6 nm in diameter.
2. Thick (myosin-like) myofilaments 15 nm in diameter.
3. A heterogeneous class of intermediate filaments approximately 10 nm in diameter.

The intermediate filaments themselves are subdivided into five major types, largely on the basis of immunocytochemical investigations: tonofilaments (cytokeratin filaments), desmin, vimentin, neurofilaments and glial filaments, as discussed in Table 2.8. The individual filaments comprising four of these subtypes lack distinctive appearances, and it is often impossible to distinguish between them on morphology alone. Nevertheless, neurofilaments have a tubular substructure when seen in transverse section at high magnification (such filaments should not be confused with microtubules), and tonofilaments are generally recognizable by their tendency to form electron-dense fibrillary bundles and by their convergence onto desmosomes to produce desmosome-tonofilament complexes (see Chapter 4).

The concentration, arrangement and types of filaments vary with both cell lineage and the degree of differentiation, and they may be sparse or undetectable in some cells, including lymphocytoid and highly anaplastic cells. Immunohistological analysis of various neoplasms suggests that the cytoplasmic actin content is often increased, but there is evidence that this reflects expansion of the polymerized actin fraction rather than true augmentation of the total actin content (see Table 21.1). Microfilaments characterize not only myoid tumours, but also epithelial and other non-myoid neoplasms, and are particularly prominent in myoepithelial cells.[39] On the other hand, elongated thick myosin-like filaments are highly characteristic of striated muscle differentiation, if not entirely diagnostic in the absence of sarcomere formation (see Chapter 22). Aggregates of intermediate filaments (fibrous bodies) with enmeshed secretory granules are sometimes of value in identifying neuroendocrine neoplasms and sparsely granulated growth hormone cell adenomas of the adenohypophysis (Table 2.9 and see Fig. 10.3). Filamentous aggregates indistinguishable from hepatocytic (Mallory's) hyalin are seen occasionally in hepatocellular tumours.

Desmosome-tonofilament complexes are highly characteristic of epithelial differentiation.[39,45] Immunoreactive cytokeratins also represent a valuable marker for epithelial cells; in addition, epithelial cells typically lack vimentin, whereas non-myoid mesenchymal cells generally contain vimentin in the absence of cytokeratins (Table 2.8). Melanocytic cells and renal adenocarcinoma appear to be exceptions to these general rules; thus, Caselitz et al[1560] describe vimentin without detectable cytokeratins in melanocytic cells, while both vimentin and cytokeratins are documented in renal adenocarcinoma,[1009,1011] sometimes coexisting within the same cell.[1009] The simultaneous occurrence of both cytokeratins and vimentin is also recorded in metaplastic myoepithelial cells in pleomorphic salivary adenomas[699,3148] and in spindle cell mesothelioma;[3148] it appears that vimentin is consistently present when two or more intermediate filaments are expressed by single cells.[3148] The relationship of tonofilaments to cytokeratins is discussed in Chapter 4.

## LIPID, GLYCOGEN, AND LIPOFUSCIN

All of these can be found in varying concentrations within neoplastic cells. Lipid material may be abundant in some (Table 2.11),[1030,1031,1509,2328–2348] while large aggregates of glycogen account for the cytoplasmic clarity of most clear cell carcinomas (Table 2.10). Sometimes the accumulation is due to a relative deficiency of one of the enzymes involved in glycogen metabolism, as in some cutaneous tumours.[1461] Autophagosomes, the precursors of lipofuscin, characterize other neoplasms, notably granular cell tumours (see Figs. 18.12 and 18.13); on rare occasions lipofuscin granules are extremely prevalent, imparting the macroscopically visible pigmentation in so-called black adenomas of the adrenal glands.[1827,1831,1838]

## THE DARK CELL-LIGHT CELL PHENOMENON

As the expression implies, the 'dark cell-light cell phenomenon'[47] consitutes variation in the electron-opacity of neighbouring cells of a single type, excluding differences attributable to a mixture of cell lines. Seen in a variety of normal and damaged tissues, this phenomenon is often also encountered in tumours. The dark cells may represent damaged dehydrated cells, the resultant close apposition of organelles producing increased electron-density. The cell 'darkness' may indicate an early stage of apoptosis (see Chapter 1), but dark cells in normal gallbladder have a high enzyme content.[47] However, this observation is not necessarily inconsistent with apoptosis, which appears to be an active process (see Chapter 1), and the dividing line between metabolically active *versus* irreversibly damaged dark cells is not consistently predictable from the morphological appearances alone.

## CELL SURFACE AND INTERCELLULAR JUNCTIONS

Scanning EM studies indicate that the surface of malignant cells is generally more irregular than normal; there is a relative increase in surface microvilli and cytoplasmic flaps, and a loss of microvillous polarity.[36,114,531] Some malignant cells also develop filopodial surface projections which may be implicated in the process of invasion.[401] Occasionally the glycocalyx is thickened, and this may account for the increased negative charge exhibited by some neoplastic cells.[58]

The frequency of junctional specializations between malignant cells is generally reduced in comparison with their normal counterparts.[39,266] The junctions in benign and low-grade malignant tumours are usually highly developed, and may appear normal.[39] However, they are depleted in less differentiated malignancies, and are often poorly formed, being represented merely by sporadic small junctions without diagnostic features. Such vestigial junctions are often designated as intermediate in type, although this tends to relegate intermediate junctions to the status of a wastebasket; nevertheless, we have consistently used this terminology in a morphologically descriptive sense, to emphasize the non-specificity of these junctions and to avoid any assumption that they represent poorly developed desmosomes or tight junctions when interpreted in isolation. Others[39] decline to type them.

Tight, intermediate and desmosomal junctions may be recognizable in mammalian neoplasms (Tables 2.12 and 2.13). The type and configuration of junctional specializations are particularly important in identifying patterns of tumour differentiation. They therefore warrant careful and critical scrutiny in order to detect, for example, unequivocal desmosomes in a background of scattered 'intermediate' junctions, the desmosome being an important, but not exclusive, indicator of epithelial differentiation (see Table 0.2 and Figs. 4.3, 5.3, 6.1 and 9.3). In contrast, subplasmalemmal linear densities with segments of associated external lamina are claimed to represent a useful (but not exclusive) marker for mesenchymal tumours;[2214] these structures are often, but less accurately, referred to as 'hemidesmosomes' (see Table 21.1 and Fig. 20.1). Paired linear densities in areas of close cell apposition may produce the intermediate-type junctions found in some mesenchymal tumours.

Finally, before diagnostic significance is attributed to the presence of junctions in a tumour, care should be taken to ensure that the *junctions are actually present between the neoplastic cells* and not merely between stromal elements such as endothelial cells (see Table 0.2).

## VIRUSES

Virus-like particles are occasionally detected in the cytoplasm of human malignant cells. They may be seen budding from the cell surface, or projecting into the lumina of the lamellae or cisternae of endoplasmic reticulum. They are subdivided into three types (A, B or C) depending on their morphology. Paracrystalline arrays of small particles should be carefully assessed before designating them as viruses.[140] Distinct cores (nucleoids) and capsids must be present, and the dimensions of all similar particles should both be uniform and lie within the range known for viruses replicating in the cytoplasm.

**Table 2.1   Some tumours consistently or occasionally characterized by mitochondrial abundance**

| Tumour | Remarks |
| --- | --- |
| Pituitary adenomas, including:<br>  Pituitary oncocytoma<br>  Acidophilic stem cell adenoma<br>  Corticotroph cell adenoma<br>  Thyrotroph cell adenoma | See Tables 10.2 and 10.3 |
| Oxyphilic (oncocytic) adenoma and carcinoma of thyroid | In typical oncocytic cells the cytoplasm is packed with countless hypertrophied mitochondria in a 'back-to-back' pattern. The mitochondria have clear matrices, stacked lamellar cristae and lack matrical dense granules. Condensed oncocytes with dense cytoplasm and pyknotic nuclei are also seen (apoptosis). See Fig. 11.1 |
| Parathyroid oxyphilic tumours | See Table 12.1 and Figs. 12.3-12.5 |
| Bronchial gland oncocytoma | The bronchial oncocytoma reported by Warter et al[595] had a microcystic and papillary configuration on LM, resembling Warthin's tumour but lacking the lymphoid stroma. On EM the predominant cells were separated by a well defined intercellular space, with plasmalemmal interdigitation (in contrast to the narrow spaces and straight plasma membranes characterizing carcinoid tumours). The cells showed marked mitochondrial hyperplasia and there were occasional intramitochondrial glycogen deposits. The cytoplasm additionally contained serous granules 300–1000 nm in diameter and lipofuscin bodies with diameters up to 2300 nm, as well as fibrillary granules. There were also admixed goblet cells with mucin granules measuring 1200–2300 nm in diameter, and rare suprabasal cells. A single neuroendocrine cell was detected |
| Oncocytic bronchial carcinoid tumour | See Table 16.3 and Fig. 16.8 |
| Warthin's tumour | Epithelial cells are oncocytic |
| Oxyphilic adenoma and carcinoma of salivary glands | Oncocytic change has also been described in a parotid mucoepidermoid carcinoma |
| Proximal tubular adenoma (oncocytoma) of kidney | — |
| Oncocytic breast papilloma | The cells comprising this lesion had smooth plasma membranes, with numerous tightly packed mitochondria; tonofilaments were present, as were secretory granules and other organelles[1420] |
| Fibrolamellar oncocytic hepatoma | — |
| Oncocytic carcinoma of pancreas | — |
| Oncocytic carcinoma of ovary | — |
|  | While the tumours listed above are characteristically oncocytic, those listed below show lesser degrees of mitochondrial hyperplasia and hypertrophy, and usually lack the morphological properties described above, although matrical dense granules are typically absent in hibernomas |
| Hepatocellular tumours | Fig. 5.33 |
| Renal adenocarcinoma | — |
| Adenocarcinoma of lung | Bronchiolo-alveolar and acinar types |
| Apocrine carcinomas | Numberous large mitochondria with incomplete cristae characterize apocrine mammary carcinomas. The mitochondria are usually dispersed in apocrine cells, and secretory granules and other organelles are well represented; plasma membranes are said to be folded. |
| Adrenal cortical tumours | Tubular or vesicular cristae, or both. See Fig. 13.3 |
| Fibroadenoma of breast | — |
| Hibernoma | See text, Chapter 19 |
| Rhabdomyoma | See Figs. 22.2 and 22.3 |
| Alveolar soft part sarcoma | See Fig. 24.1 |

References: 31, 44, 45, 64, 291, 451, 452, 480, 563, 571, 579, 593, 595, 657, 695, 732, 738, 755, 757, 760, 879, 946, 1012, 1014, 1030, 1034, 1038, 1361, 1420, 1432, 1643, 1660, 1681, 1688, 1704, 1739, 1749, 1800, 1805, 1821, 1836, 1872, 2186, 2347

**Table 2.2  Annulate lamellae in human tumours**

| Tumour | Remarks |
|---|---|
| *BENIGN LESIONS* | |
| Parathyroid adenoma | Sporadic annulate lamellae are often present in parathyroid adenomas; they were numerous in one of 16 cases studied by Erlandson[39] |
| Pituitary adenoma | Including sparsely granulated prolactin cell adenoma* |
| Phaeochromocytoma | — |
| Insulinoma | — |
| Warthin's tumour | — |
| Cerebellar haemangioblastoma | — |
| Apocrine hidrocystoma | — |
| Smooth muscle tumour | Fig. 2.8 |
| *MALIGNANT EPITHELIAL/EPITHELIOID TUMOURS* | |
| Parathyroid carcinoma | — |
| Squamous cell carcinoma of lung | Including one glycogen-rich tumour* |
| Pulmonary adenocarcinoma | Fig. 2.9 |
| Large cell carcinoma of lung | — |
| Giant cell carcinoma of lung | EM revealed adenosquamous differentiation* |
| Gastric adenocarcinoma | Found in pulmonary metastasis* |
| Hepatocellular carcinoma* | — |
| Adrenal cortical carcinoma | — |
| Renal adenocarcinoma* | — |
| Adenocarcinoma of prostate | — |
| Adenocarcinoma of rete testis | — |
| Glassy cell carcinoma of uterine cervix | See Table 30.1 |
| Adenocarcinoma of fallopian tube | — |
| Papillary serous cystadenocarcinoma of ovary | — |
| Clear cell carcinoma of ovary | — |
| Endometrioid carcinoma of ovary | In tissue culture |
| Carcinoma of breast | — |
| Malignant melanoma | Including one example in the urinary bladder |
| *EMBRYONAL AND GERM CELL TUMOURS* | |
| Metastatic embryonal carcinoma of testis* | — |
| Yolk sac carcinoma | Annulate lamellae have been found in the neoplastic cells, and in an associated germinomatous component in the suprasellar neoplasm reported by Takei & Pearl[1151] |
| Testicular seminoma | — |
| Ovarian dysgerminoma | — |
| Pulmonary blastoma | — |
| Neuroblastoma | — |
| Retinoblastoma | — |
| Primitive neuroectodermal tumour | In 4 of 5 cases in one series[1930] |
| *SARCOMATOID TUMOURS* | |
| Malignant fibrous mesothelioma | — |
| Malignant fibrous histiocytoma | — |
| Angiosarcoma | — |
| Malignant mesenchymal tumour | Histological type not further classifiable |
| Leiomyosarcoma | Radial cisternae of endoplasmic reticulum |
| Rhabdomyosarcoma | Prostatic tumour |
| *LYMPHOMAS AND LEUKAEMIAS* | |
| Lymphoblastic lymphoma | Both in vivo and in cultured cells |
| Hodgkin's disease | In tissue culture |
| Burkitt's lymphoma | — |
| Multiple myeloma | — |
| Acute lymphoblastic leukaemia | — |
| Chronic lymphocytic leukaemia | Found in 6 of 15 cases, in 0.5–2 per cent of lymphocytes, in one study.[2914] Coexistence with ribosome-lamella complexes in the same cells has been recorded |
| *MISCELLANEOUS TUMOURS* | |
| Metastatic cerebellar tumour | Histological type not further specified |
| Pinealoma | Tumour implantation on cauda equina |

*Henderson, Papadimitriou & Coleman, unpublished observations

References: 39, 44, 47, 55, 64, 313–322, 563, 961, 1118, 1150–1152, 1155, 1188, 1253, 1327, 1551, 1799, 1803, 1811, 1922, 1930, 2003, 2143, 2296, 2914

**Table 2.3    Cytoplasmic tubuloreticular arrays in tumours**

| Tumour | Comments |
|---|---|
| *BENIGN CONDITIONS* | |
| Fibroadenoma of breast | — |
| Subcutaneous myxoma | — |
| *ENDOCRINE TUMOURS* | |
| Pituitary adenomas associated with acromegaly | In endothelial cells, in up to 30 per cent of cases. Identification may require a prolonged search |
| Phaeochromocytoma | — |
| Insulinoma | In stromal endothelium |
| Bronchial carcinoid tumour | In stromal endothelium |
| Medullary carcinoma of thyroid | — |
| *MALIGNANT EPITHELIAL/EPITHELIOID TUMOURS* | |
| Mammary carcinoma | In metastatic carcinoma of breast, tubuloreticular arrays (TRA) have been described in lymphocytes, macrophages and cells designated as reticulum cells |
| Bronchiolo-alveolar cell carcinoma | — |
| Malignant mesothelioma | In neoplastic cells |
| Malignant melanoma | — |
| Hepatoblastoma | — |
| Giant cell tumour of thyroid | — |
| *NEURAL NEOPLASMS* | |
| Gliomas | Fig. 2.11 (glioblastoma multiforme) |
| *SARCOMATOID TUMOURS* | |
| Fibrosarcoma | Identification of TRA in neoplastic cells of sarcomas may require prolonged search |
| Malignant fibrous histiocytoma | — |
| Liposarcoma | — |
| Rhabdomyosarcoma | — |
| Kaposi's sarcoma | — |
| Osteogenic sarcoma | — |
| Chondrosarcoma | In tissue culture |
| *LYMPHOHAEMOPOIETIC PROLIFERATIONS* | |
| Histiocytosis X | So-called Letterer-Siwe syndrome |
| Immunoblastic lymphadenopathy | In endothelial cells of vessels resembling post-capillary venules; coexistence with numerous Weibel-Palade bodies* |
| Hodgkin's disease | TRA may be found in lymphoid cells in a variety of disorders, including both neoplastic and non-neoplastic states, and lymphoproliferative and non-lymphoid diseases |
| Adult T-cell lymphoma and leukaemia | TRA described in both lymphocytic cells and endothelium. In the T-cell lymphoblastic lymphoma reported by Chu et al[2731] the component 40 nm tubules formed complexes measuring 800–1500 nm in diameter; present in more than 80 per cent of cells and often paranuclear in location (?relation to prior chemotherapy) |
| B-lymphocytic lymphoma | In lymphocytic cells and endothelium |
| Burkitt's lymphoma | — |
| Acute lymphoblastic leukaemia | — |
| Acute granulocytic leukaemia | — |

*Henderson, Papadimitriou & Coleman, unpublished observation

References: 44, 64, 303, 304–311, 492, 647, 883, 1743, 2267, 2731

**Table 2.4  Comparison of cytoplasmic tubuloreticular arrays with Paramyxovirus nucleocapsids**

| Feature | Tubuloreticular arrays (TRA) | Paramyxovirus nucleocapsids |
|---|---|---|
| Shape | Tubular, branching and anastomosing | Tubular, undulating |
| Diameter | 20–31 nm | 12–18 nm |
| Transverse periodicity | None | Present, 4–7 nm, related to helical substructure of virus |
| Appearance in transverse section | Rounded, with lucent core. Bounded by membrane approximately 6 nm in thickness | Rounded, with lucent core. Not membrane-bound |
| Site of formation | Within cisternae of rough endoplasmic reticulum (RER) | In cytoplasmic sap, often near cell surface, but not within RER. May be present within nucleus; compare with altered chromatin fibres (Table 1.2) |
| Continuity with membranes | Continuous with membranes of RER | Accumulate at or near membranes, but are not continuous with them |
| Remarks | Widespread occurrence in apparently normal and pathological cells, particularly those of mesodermal derivation. In tumours, TRA may occur in neoplastic cells, endothelium, or other stromal components. See Table 2.3. Contain phospholipid and protein; presence of RNA has not been confirmed. Show high density with permanganate fixation, which may reveal a well defined membrane. Viral cultures of affected tissues are negative, and patients usually show no elevation of titres to a variety of viruses. Compare with glycogen particles (see Figs. 2.16, 2.17 and 25.8). Distinguish from the straight intracisternal tubules (coated parallel tubules) reported in several types of tumours, especially malignant melanoma (see Fig. 8.5) | Marburg virus and certain arboviruses may bud into RER and form tubular structures, but the appearances of the tubules are distinctive, and other spheroidal viral nucleoids may be present. A number of spherical viruses bud into the RER, but once again their appearances are distinctive |

References: 44, 47, 64, 303–311, 492, 647, 883, 1590, 1743, 2267, 2731

**Table 2.5  Distinctive cytoplasmic granules in tumours**

| Type of granule | Representative tumours |
|---|---|
| Mucin granules | Mucin-producing glandular epithelial tumours. See Chapter 5, Figs. 5.8–5.10 |
| Fibrillary mucin granules | Adenocarcinoma of human uterine cervix. See Fig. 5.11 |
| Acinic (serous) granules | Acinic cell neoplasms. Fig. 5.14 |
| Neurosecretory granules | Tumours showing so-called APUD cell differentiation. Figs. 6.2–6.4, 7.1, 11.5, 11.6, 13.7, 16.1, 16.3 and 16.4 |
| Halo (noradrenaline) granules | Noradrenaline-producing phaeochromocytoma. Fig. 13.4 |
| Crystalline (insulin) granules | Insulinoma. Fig. 14.3 |
| Glucagon (double core) granules | Glucagonoma. Fig. 14.4 |
| Gastrin-like granules | Gastrinoma |
| Rhomboidal protogranules | Juxtaglomerular cell tumour. Figs. 15.1 and 15.2 |
| Rhomboidal and elongated crystalloids | Alveolar soft part sarcoma. See Fig. 24.2 |
| Other endocrine granules | Various. See Chapters 10–16 |
| Electron-dense lamelliform granules | Alveolar cell carcinoma of lung. See Table 5.3 and Fig. 5.30 |
| Keratohyaline granules | Well differentiated squamous cell neoplasms. Fig. 4.2 |
| Melanosomes | Melanocytic tumours, including malignant melanoma; Figs. 8.3 and 8.4 Melanotic Schwannoma; Figs. 18.4 and 18.5 Clear cell sarcoma of tendons and aponeuroses; Figs. 24.6 and 24.7 See also Table 8.1 |
| Weibel-Palade bodies | Tumours with endothelial differentiation. Figs. 3.4, 3.5, 23.3 and 23.5 |
| Langerhans' cell granules | Histiocytosis X (Fig. 28.22). See also Table 28.3 |
| Reinke crystals | Interstitial cell tumour of testis (Figs. 30.1 and 30.2) and ovarian analogues |
| So-called Charcot-Böttcher crystals | Sertoli cell tumour. These structures are not true crystals or crystalloids, but represent aggregates of cytofilaments |
| Charcot-Leyden crystals | Histiocytosis X and granulocytic leukaemias |
| Auer bodies | Acute myeloblastic and promyelocytic leukaemias. Fig. 28.4 |
| Lysosomal granules | Mononuclear phagocytic tumours. Figs. 20.9 and 27.22 Granulocytic leukaemias; Figs. 28.1–28.3 Granular cell tumours (multiple autophagosomal granules). See Figs. 18.12 and 18.13 Benign clear cell tumour (sugar tumour) of lung; (membrane-bound glycogen – see Fig. 2.16) |
| Immunoglobulin granules | Lymphoplasmacytic tumours. Fig. 27.15 |

**Table 2.6    Occurrence of intracellular crystalloids and crystals in tumours**

| Intracellular localization and tumour | Comments and figure numbers |
| --- | --- |
| *WITHIN NUCLEI* | |
| As for intranuclear fibrillary inclusions | See Table 1.1 and Fig. 1.10. Intranuclear crystalline inclusions are thought to be related to fibrillary inclusions, the crystalline pattern resulting from crossing of filaments in the plane of section |
| *IN CISTERNAE OF ROUGH ENDOPLASMIC RETICULUM\** | |
| Lymphoproliferative disorders, including: | |
| B-lymphocytic lymphoma-leukaemia | Figs 27.14 and 28.7 |
| Plasma cell myeloma | Fig. 27.29 |
| *MEMBRANE-BOUND CRYSTALLOIDS†* | |
| Warthin's tumour | — |
| Pancreatic B-cell tumours (insulinomas) | Figs. 14.1 and 14.3 |
| Juxtaglomerular cell tumour | Figs. 15.1 and 15.2 |
| Alveolar soft part sarcoma | Figs. 24.1 and 24.2 |
| Chondromatous pulmonary hamartoma | Clara cell-type granules in epithelial component. Fig. 5.13 |
| Clara cell adenocarcinoma | Fig. 5.31 |
| Other adenocarcinomas | Fig. 5.12 |
| Schwannoma | — |
| Oligodendroglioma | — |
| Ependymoma | Fig. 17.10 |
| Glioblastoma multiforme | Fig. 17.7 |
| Acute myeloblastic leukaemia | Auer bodies |
| Acute promyelocytic leukaemia | Auer bodies. Fig. 28.4 |
| *IN MITOCHONDRIA* | |
| Rhabdomyomas | Fig. 2.5 |
| Benign hepatomas | In women taking oral contraceptives |
| Hepatocellular carcinoma | — |
| Prostatic adenocarcinoma | See Fig. 5.19 |
| *NON-MEMBRANE-BOUND CYTOPLASMIC CRYSTALS* | |
| Leydig-hilus cell tumours or components of tumours | Reinke crystals.§ Figs. 30.1 and 30.2 |
| Pancreatic B-cell tumour | Reinke-like crystals |

\*Dissolution of membranes may release crystalline material into cytoplasmic matrix. †Presumably derived from Golgi apparatus. §Rarely intranuclear

(Modified from Marcus et al[2087] and published by permission)

References: 749, 2087, 3095

**Table 2.7 Cytoplasmic filaments in tumours**

| Filament types | Diameter of filaments | Representative tumours | Comments |
| --- | --- | --- | --- |
| 1. *MICROFILAMENTS* (thin myofilaments; actin-like filaments) | 5—7 nm | Smooth muscle neoplasms Myofibroblastic tumours Striated muscle tumours Epithelial and leukopoietic tumours Others | See Tables 3.5, 3.6 and 21.1. See also Introduction, and Chapters 2, 4, 8, 20, 21, 22 and 23 |
| 2. *THICK MYOFILAMENTS* (myosin filaments) | 15 nm | Striated muscle tumours Smooth muscle tumours rarely | See Chapter 22 |
| 3. *INTERMEDIATE FILAMENTS* | | | |
| 3.1 Tonofilaments | 7.5–9 nm | Squamous cell tumours Thymoma Other epithelial tumours | Also known as 'cytokeratin', 'keratin' and 'prekeratin' filaments (see text, Chapter 4). See Table 2.8 |
| | | | Bundles of tonofilaments convering onto desmosomes to produce desmosome-tonofilament complexes are a major feature of squamous cell tumours (see Chapter 4) |
| 3.2 Vimentin filaments | 10 nm | Many mesenchymal tumours Others | See Table 2.8, and Fig. 20.10 |
| 3.3 Desmin | 10 nm | Myoid tumours | See Table 2.8 |
| 3.4 Glial filaments — glial fibrillary acidic protein | 10 nm | Astrocytic tumours Ependymal neoplasms Ganglioglioma | See Chapter 17 and Table 2.8 |
| 3.5 Neurofilaments | 10 nm | Neuritic tumours | See Chapters 13 and 17, and Tables 2.8 and 29.1 |

**Table 2.8 Principal types of intermediate filaments***

| Filament | Diameter | Representative cell types | Remarks |
|---|---|---|---|
| Tonofilaments (cytokeratin filaments) | 7.5–9 nm | Most epithelial cell lines, notably squamous and thymic epithelium, and mesothelial cells | Cytokeratins represent an extremely complex group of intermediate filament proteins and include multiple polypeptides with molecular weights in the range 40 000–70 000 Daltons. Nineteen distinct components are recognized, different types being characteristic of various epithelia. Components 8, 18 and 19 characterize small and large intestinal mucosa and are also found in adenocarcinomas from a variety of anatomical sites. Hepatocellular carcinomas contain cytokeratins 8 and 18, as in normal hepatocytes. High molecular weight fractions 1 and 2 appear to typify keratinizing squamous epithelia, and are also found in ectocervical and anal epithelium. Squamous carcinomas tend to be characterized by cytokeratins 5 and 6, together with some acidic components (14 and 17). Monoclonal antibodies against these components can be generated; in the future they may prove invaluable, not only in typing poorly differentiated carcinomas, but also in determining the source of metastases |
| Vimentin | 10 nm; reported range 7–11 nm | Many. Mesenchymal cells especially, including endothelium, fibroblasts, macrophages and chondrocytes. Vimentin also occurs in lymphocytes as well as in ganglionic, glial, meningothelial and myogenic cells. Although usually undetectable in epithelia, vimentin has been recorded in melanocytes and renal adenocarcinoma cells; in melanocytes the vimentin occurred in the absence of cytokeratins, whereas the two coexisted in renal adenocarcinoma, sometimes within the same cell | M. Wt. 57 000–58 000 Daltons. Filaments tend to be perinuclear in distribution and are associated with lateral 'whisker' filaments |
| Desmin | 10 nm | Muscle – smooth, cardiac and voluntary | M. Wt. 50 000–55 000 Daltons. Thought to have a cytoskeletal function, interconnecting myofilaments at the level of Z-discs and attaching them to the sarcolemma; also appears to anchor actin filaments to Z-lines. Probably identical to skeletin. Other intermediate filament-associated proteins have also been identified in muscle. Synemin is a distinct protein, being associated with desmin and vimentin; paramenin is a similar protein. See Table 21.1 for a discussion of actin filaments and their related proteins |
| Glial filaments – GFAP | 10 nm | Glial cells – astrocytes and ependymal cells, but not oligodendrocytes | Have been found in astrocytomas, ependymomas and medulloblastoma. Glioma cells contain both glial fibrillary acidic protein (GFAP) and vimentin (which has also been demonstrated in normal fetal glial cells). GFAP has a molecular weight of 49 000–51 000 Daltons. S-100 protein has also been detected in astrocytes, as well as in oligodendrocytes and Schwann cells |
| Neurofilaments | 10 nm | Neurones | Tubular in cross section. Component proteins have molecular weights of 200 000, 150 000 and 68 000 Daltons |

*As listed in this table, five types of intermediate filaments are generally recognized. Recent amino acid sequencing studies indicate that desmin, vimentin, GFAP and the 68 kiloDalton fraction of neurofilaments 'are distinct but related members of a multigene family expressed in a cell type-specific manner.'[272]

Investigation of intermediate filaments and their associated proteins is one of the most rapidly developing topics in cell biology, but is fraught with inconsistencies, unsolved problems and lack of a uniform nomenclature. Many of the recognized subclasses have been defined by immunocytochemical methods and only a few (such as tonofilaments) have characteristic ultrastructural appearances, the nature of the filaments in other instances being inferred from the type of cell which they inhabit

Clathrin forms a fuzzy perivesicular basket-like lattice to produce coated vesicles (acanthosomes), but does not occur as elongated filaments and is not usually included in the intermediate filament class

A variety of cytoskeletal-cytocontractile proteins have been identified in the microvillar cores of intestinal epithelial cells by biochemical and immunocytochemical techniques. Some appear to represent bridging or linker molecules, binding filaments to each other and/or the plasmalemma. They include proteins with such euphonious names as calmodulin, villin, vinculin, tropomyosin, actin, $\alpha$-actinin and 110K protein. It is likely that there are topographical differences in the distribution of these proteins. For example, microvilli from the upper respiratory tract display greater morphological diversity than intestinal microvilli and appear to lack microfilamentous cores. In the future, some of these regional differences may be used for diagnostic purposes.

References: 39, 45, 47, 180, 236, 238, 240–242, 245, 255, 260, 269, 272, 278, 296, 297, 2183, 2212

**Table 2.9   Some tumours containing intracytoplasmic filamentous bodies**

| Tumour | Diameter of filaments | Comments |
|---|---|---|
| Pituitary adenomas containing growth hormone cells or their precursors | 10–13 nm; associated with microtubules 20–40 nm in diameter | See Table 10.1 and Fig. 10.3. In general, whorling intermediate filaments associated with secretory granules appear to be characteristic of polypeptide-producing endocrine tumours. The filaments are located close to the microtubular system, and may be instrumental in the transport and release of granules |
| Medullary carcinoma of thyroid | 7.5–10 nm | Filaments do not react for calcitonin by immuno-electron microscopy |
| Follicular carcinoma of thyroid* | 10 nm | — |
| Insulin-secreting pancreatic islet tumours | Approximately 7–10 nm | See Fig. 14.1 |
| Glucagonoma | 10 nm | — |
| Gastroduodenal endocrine tumours, including duodenal carcinoid tumour | 10 nm | Extracellular filaments also found in some tumours |
| Bronchial, rectal, ovarian and cervical carcinoid tumours | 5–10 nm | See Fig. 16.6 |
| Juxtaglomerular cell tumour | — | See Fig. 15.3 |
| Paraganglioma | 10 nm | — |
| Neuroblastoma | — | Closely associated with whorled microtubules 20 nm in diameter |
| Merkel cell carcinoma of skin | 10 nm | Filamentous aggregates often concentrated in paranuclear region. See Figs. 6.3 and 6.4 |

The fibrous bodies in the tumours detailed above form whorled collections closely associated with granules and microtubules, but those listed below often form other patterns, including parallel sheaves of filaments

| Tumour | Diameter of filaments | Comments |
|---|---|---|
| Papillary carcinoma of thyroid | 6–9 nm | — |
| Giant cell carcinoma of lung | 6–8 nm | — |
| Hepatocellular carcinoma | Approximately 10 nm | Ultrastructurally identical to Mallory's alcoholic hyalin; diameters variously estimated at 8–20 nm in literature |
| Carcinoma of breast | 11 nm | In tissue culture |
| Endometrial adenocarcinoma | 8 nm | Concentrated in perinuclear area |
| Fibrillocaveolated cell carcinoma of midgut | 7.5–10 nm | Filaments mostly straight, forming sheaves, and occasionally arranged in spirals. High urinary 5-HIAA levels, suggesting a relationship to the enterochromaffin system,[818] a view supported by the finding of similar filaments in a gastric carcinoid tumour[804] |
| 'Hyaline' cells in: | 10–12.5 nm | |
|    Mixed salivary tumours | | — |
|    Islet cell tumours | | — |
|    Basal cell carcinoma | | — |
|    Epithelioid leiomyoma | | — |
|    Hepatic apudoma | | — |
| Malignant rhabdoid tumour of kidney | 4–10 nm | See text, Chapter 30 |
| Synovial sarcoma | 10 nm | Constituent intermediate filaments formed circumscribed aggregates. Not seen in original biopsy; followed intra-arterial chemotherapy[2558] |
| Fibrous histiocytomas | 10 nm | Filaments correspond to presence of vimentin. See Fig. 20.10 |
| Dermatofibrosarcoma protuberans | 5–10 nm | In tissue culture |
| Epithelioid sarcoma | 3–10 nm | See Fig. 24.5 |
| Clear cell sarcoma | — | Tumour of thoracic spinal nerve root; melanosomes in neoplastic cells[2217] |
| Angiosarcoma | 10 nm | — |
| Neural tumour in von Recklinghausen's neurofibromatosis | 6–9 nm and 11–15 nm | Spheroidal filamentous inclusions composed of radiating filaments |
| Follicular centre cell lymphoma | — | Subset of so-called signet-ring cell lymphoma. See Fig. 27.16 |
| Myeloblasts in acute leukaemia | 10 nm | Filaments often parallel, sometimes whorling |

*Henderson, Papadimitriou & Coleman, unpublished observation

References: 45, 64, 251, 294, 379, 439, 594, 804, 818, 819, 878, 888, 976, 988, 1152, 1155, 1176, 1354, 1513, 1521, 1665, 1679, 1681, 1703, 1713, 1716, 1727, 1754, 1880, 1890, 1896, 2053, 2193, 2212, 2216–2218, 2226, 2558

**Table 2.10  Some tumours characterized by glycogen accumulation**

| Tumour | Comments |
|---|---|
| Ewing's sarcoma | Neoplastic cells classically contain copious glycogen, forming 'lakes' and present in the form of rosettes (see Figs. 25.7 and 25.8, and Table 29.1). |
| | The presence of glycogen is one of several features used to distinguish Ewing's sarcoma from neuroblastoma, but up to 10 per cent of neuroblastomas contain considerable quantities of glycogen.[1876,1880] Conversely, in one series of Ewing's tumours, glycogen granules were infrequent in 33 per cent, and rare in 14 per cent.[2611] In a more recent study, Llombart-Bosch et al[2605] mention that 30 per cent of otherwise typical Ewing's sarcomas lack glycogen (see Fig. 25.9) |
| Erythroleukaemia | Presence of glycogen in proerythroblastic cells aids in distinguishing erythroleukaemia from other leukaemias (see Table 28.1) |
| Benign clear cell tumour of lung (sugar tumour) | Membrane-bound collections of monoparticulate and rosetted glycogen may be present.[570] See Fig. 2.16 (intralysosomal glycogen in a pinealoma) |
| Smooth muscle tumours | — |
| Striated muscle tumours | Glycogen usually present in monoparticulate form. Peripheral 'lakes' of glycogen in cardiac rhabdomyomas[2450] and adult-type rhabdomyomas[2431] account for the appearance of so-called 'spider web cells'. See Fig. 22.1 |
| Chondroid tumours | See Fig. 25.2 (chondrosarcoma of bone) |
| Chordoma | See Fig. 25.10 |
| Oncocytic tumours | Glycogen may be partly intramitochondrial in location |
| Hepatocellular carcinoma | See Fig. 5.33 |
| Hepatoblastoma | — |
| Clear cell adenomas and carcinomas of various sites, including: | |
|    Parathyroid tumours | See Table 12.1 and Fig. 12.2 |
|    Renal adenocarcinoma | Lipid droplets typically also present. See Figs. 5.15 and 5.16 |
|    Squamous cell tumours | Variable |
|    Clear cell carcinomas of vagina, uterus, ovary and breast | See Fig. 5.27 |
|    Clear cell carcinomas of lung | Includes glycogen-rich so-called Clara cell carcinoma |
|    Clear cell tumours of salivary glands | Monogranular glycogen and adenosquamous features illustrated by Chaudhry et al[701] |
| Endodermal sinus tumour (yolk sac carcinoma) | See Fig. 30.5 |
| Malignant mesothelioma | See Fig. 9.2 |
| Seminoma and dysgerminoma | See Fig. 30.3 |

References: 45, 64, 86, 443, 570, 575, 650, 701, 745, 890, 896, 907, 1030, 1140, 1141, 1152, 1153, 1155, 1156, 1159, 1170, 1250, 1251, 1288, 1316, 1317, 1370, 1791, 1803, 1876, 1880, 1922, 2194, 2207, 2431, 2450, 2570, 2605, 2611, 2631, 2741, 2865

**Table 2.11  Examples of tumours and tumour-like disorders consistently or occasionally containing abundant lipid**

*MESENCHYMAL LESIONS*

Lipomas, all types
Hibernoma
Liposarcomas, all types (Fig. 19.1)

Elastofibroma
Fibrous histiocytomas, benign and malignant (Fig. 20.13)
Mesenchymoma
Myelolipomas
Lipoleiomyoma of uterus
Angiomyolipoma of kidney
Haemangioblastoma (Fig 23.10)
Rhabdomyosarcoma

*MIXED EPITHELIO-ADIPOSE LESIONS*

Liponeuronaevus of skin
Thyrolipoma
Parathyroid lipoadenoma
Adenolipoma mammae

*EPITHELIAL TUMOURS*

Carcinomas of skin with sebaceous differentiation
Sebaceous adenoma of parotid gland
Parathyroid tumours
Adrenal cortical adenomas and carcinomas (Figs. 2.19, 13.1 and 13.2)
Lipid-rich mammary carcinoma
Hepatocellular carcinoma
Renal adenocarcinoma (Figs. 5.16 and 5.17)
Prostatic adenocarcinoma (Fig. 5.19)

*NEURAL TUMOURS*

Ependymoma
Cellular Schwannoma*

*GONADAL TUMOURS*

Ovarian thecoma (Fig. 2.20)
Folliculome lipidique of ovary
Sertoli-Leydig cell tumour of ovary
Leydig/hilar cell tumour of testis/ovary
Trophoblastic tumours such as hydatidiform mole

*LYMPHOHAEMOPOIETIC LESIONS*

Thymolipoma
Burkitt's lymphoma (Fig. 27.18)

*Henderson, Papadimitriou & Coleman, unpublished observation

**Table 2.13  Intercellular junctions in tumours**

| Type of junction | Representative tumours |
|---|---|
| Junctional complex (JC) | Absorptive/secretory glandular epithelial tumours (adenomas and adenocarcinomas)<br>Endocrine adenomas and adenocarcinomas<br>So-called APUD tumours<br>Transitional cell (urothelial) tumours<br>Mesotheliomas (epithelioid component)<br>Adenomatoid tumour of genital tract<br>Biphasic synovial sarcoma<br>Craniopharyngioma<br>Ependymoma<br>Choroid plexus tumours<br>Neuroblastoma with olfactory rosettes<br>Retinoblastoma |
| Tight junction | As for JC<br>Endothelial tumours, including:<br>  Kaposi's sarcoma<br>  So-called intravascular bronchiolo-alveolar tumour<br>  Lymphangiosarcoma<br>  Haemangiopericytoma |
| Intermediate junction* | Numerous epithelial, epithelioid, neural and mesenchymal tumours, but not lymphomas and leukaemias |
| Desmosome | As for JC<br>Squamous cell tumours<br>Thymoma and thymic carcinoma<br>Follicular centre cell lymphomas†<br>Meningiomas<br>So-called sclerosing haemangioma of lung[514]<br>Trophoblastic tumours |
| Gap junction* | Epithelioid and glandular epithelial neoplasms, as for JC<br>Smooth muscle tumours<br>Hibernoma<br>Cardiac rhabdomyoma<br>Meningiomas<br>Other (many) |

*By themselves, intermediate and gap junctions have little diagnostic value; junctional complexes and desmosomes are the most important junctions in tumour diagnosis

†In follicular centre cell lymphomas, desmosomal junctions *may* be seen between dendritic cells, but are typically *not present between lymphocytoid cells*

References: 39, 44–47, 63, 64, 84–87, 97, 109, 119, 126, 514, 1719, 2226

**Table 2.12  Types of intercellular junctions**

Tight junction (*zonula occludens*) ┐
Intermediate junction (*zonula adhaerens*) ┤ Junctional complex (terminal bar; *Schlussleisten; bandes de fermeture*)
Desmosome (*macula adhaerens*) ┘

Gap junction (*nexus*)
Septate junction*
*Zonula continua**
Hemidesmosome†

*Not normally present in tissues of vertebrates. However, intracellular septate junctions are recorded in the myofibroblasts of a simple ameloblastoma.[686] In addition, intracytoplasmic junctions similar to septate junctions and referred to as 'zipper-like structures' are found very rarely between lysosomes;[273] these structures are described in the hepatocytes of patients with intrahepatic tumours, including metastases and hepatocellular carcinoma. Similar interlysosomal junctions have also been found in clear cell adenocarcinoma of the genital tract, pleural mesothelioma, pulmonary squamous carcinoma and a pituitary adenoma.[256,299] 'Zipper-like structures' of this type appear to be curiosities without diagnostic value

†Not actually an intercellular junction; promotes adherence of cells to external lamina

All desmosomes contain the protein desmoplakin; the filaments inserting into desmosomes between epithelial cells represent cytokeratins, whereas those in meningothelial cells contain vimentin, and those in the intercalated discs of cardiac muscle possess desmin

References: 39, 45, 180, 189, 249, 256, 273, 299, 686

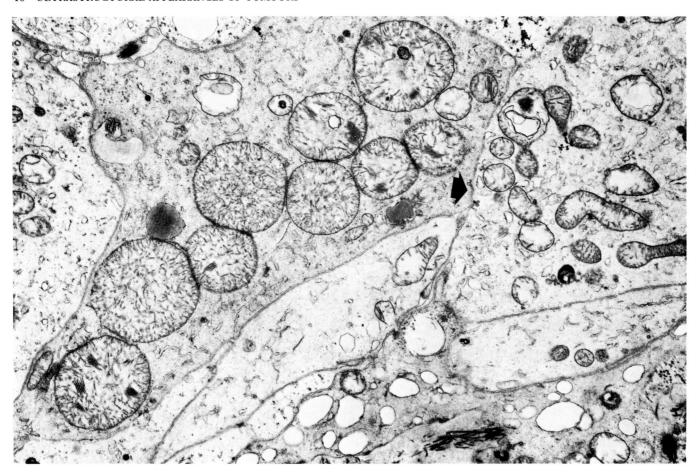

**Fig. 2.1  Mitochondrial pleomorphism: Smooth muscle tumour**

A variety of mitochondrial alterations has been described in neoplastic cells, including hydropic changes, pleomorphism, gigantism, and inclusions. Perhaps the most striking is the remarkable mitochondrial hyperplasia and hypertrophy characteristic of oncocytic tumours (see Figs. 11.1, 12.3 and 12.4, and Table 2.1). None of these alterations is specific for malignancy, or even for neoplasia, and they may be encountered in diverse pathological states and in apparently normal tissues.

Most of the mitochondria depicted here are spheroidal, with irregular lamellar cristae, while those in an adjoining cell are smaller and more variable in shape (bold arrow). (×9600)

References: 44, 47, 58, 288, 291, 1758

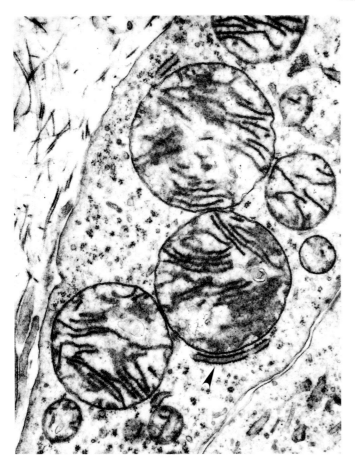

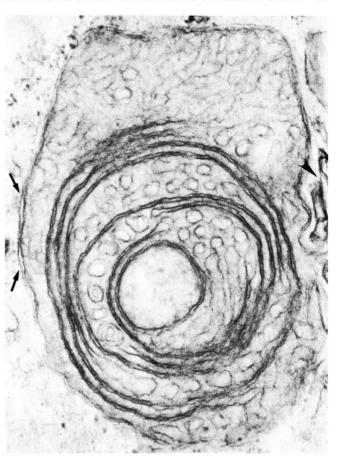

**Fig. 2.2   Mitochondrial pleomorphism: Leiomyosarcoma**

Metastasizing gastric leiomyosarcoma from a 62-year-old woman. These rounded mitochondria vary considerably in size, the diameters ranging from about 490–1950 nm. Most of the mitochondria in this case approximated the smaller profiles depicted here. The lamellar cristae are seen in various planes of section, and a strand of RER is closely apposed to one of the large mitochondria (arrowhead). Most cells in this sarcoma contained few myofilaments. (×21 900)

**Fig. 2.3   Mitochondrion: Renal adenocarcinoma**

Pleural metastasis from a 74-year-old man who presented with a pleural effusion. The patient had an occupational history of asbestos exposure, with pleural plaques on chest X-ray and asbestos bodies in the sputum. In the pleural biopsy the neoplasm had a focal clear cell pattern, but in other regions there was a spindle cell component mimicking sarcomatoid mesothelioma. Ultrastructural examination of a clear cell area disclosed glandular epithelial differentiation with copious cytoplasmic glycogen and lipid (see Figs. 5.15 and 5.16). He subsequently developed hypercalcaemia, and a primary renal carcinoma was confirmed at autopsy.

This atypical mitochondrion contains both tubular and concentric lamellar cristae. The outer membrane forms a poorly developed myelin figure (arrowhead), attributable to glutaraldehyde fixation. Even when greatly distorted and enlarged, mitochondria can usually be recognized as such by remnants of the cristae and/or the double boundary membrane (arrows); the nucleus is the only other cell component with a double membrane. Mitochondria with tubular cristae are particularly found in neoplasms of the female reproductive system, the steroid-secreting cells of the adrenal gland (see Fig. 13.3) and in some testicular tumours. (×69 200)

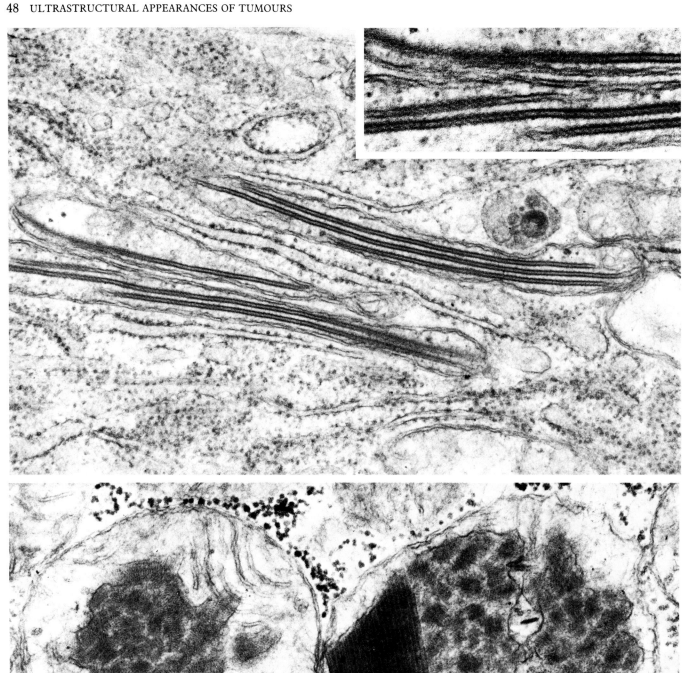

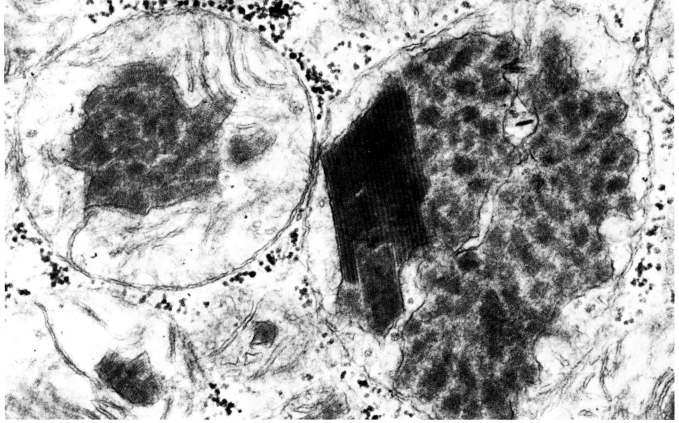

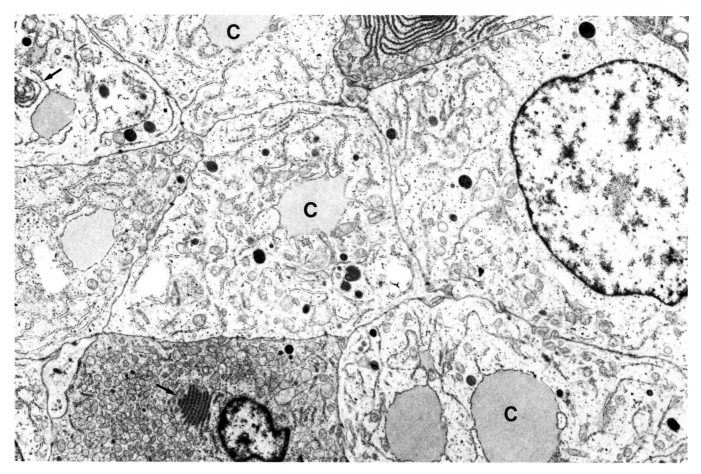

**Fig. 2.6  Dilatation of rough endoplasmic reticulum, and annulate lamellae: Adenocarcinoma of lung**

Moderate quantities of rough endoplasmic reticulum are present in the malignant cells, with focal dilatation of cisternae (C). Two sets of annulate lamellae (arrows) are also evident.(×6900)

See also Figs. 11.4, 20.11, 27.14, 27.27, 27.29 and 30.7.
References: 39, 44, 47, 291

**Fig. 2.4** *(Facing page — top)*  **Septate mitochondrial cristae: Adenocarcinoma of lung**

These rod-like structures average 22 nm in diameter, appear to be continuous with mitochondrial cristae, and show transverse and oblique periodicity of 15–20 nm (inset). In transverse section, inclusions of this type have been reported to be cylindrical, with thin walls, and diameters up to 50 nm; they contain moderately electron-dense material, and sometimes have axial cores. (×68 000. Inset: ×124 200)

**Discussion:** The significance of these atypical cristae is unknown. They have been found in up to 40 per cent of mammary carcinomas, about 10–15 per cent of benign breast lesions,[280] and in both normal astrocytes and glioblastoma cells.[289] Septate cristae have also been recorded in both olfactory and adrenal neuroblastoma,[239,1834] an oligodendroglioma[1944] and an oxyphilic parathyroid adenoma.[1799] Similar structures occur in HeLa cells treated with anti-HeLa serum and in the livers of women taking oral contraceptives.[280] Brown & Mackay[239] suggested that enlargement and elongation of mitochondria preceded the development of these altered cristae, which measured 30 nm in transverse diameter and were thought to have a helical substructure.

Identical mitochondria are also described in the pneumocytes of newts.[301] In this setting the cristae seem to lack a helical substructure; instead, Witaliński & Goniakowska-Witalińska[301] suggest that the appearances result from oblique septation, characterized by a periodicity of approximately 14 nm and inclined at 45° to the cristal long axis. The septa are 4–6 nm in thickness and the cristae measure about 22.5 nm in diameter.

Such septate cristae may be related to the mitochondria with longitudinally-orientated cristae recorded in a variety of non-neoplastic tissues and which are associated with an altered enzyme profile. Mitochondria of this type have been found in renal adenocarcinoma and ovarian carcinoma.[47]

References: 31, 44, 47, 239, 280, 289, 301, 1799, 1834, 1944

**Fig. 2.5** *(Facing page — bottom)*  **Crystalline mitochondrial inclusions: Adult rhabdomyoma**

The inclusions consist of curved interweaving parallel aggregates of filaments/tubules which average 6 nm in diameter. They are surrounded by irregular membranes, suggesting an origin within, and expansion of, the cristae. A regular linear parallel crystalline inclusion is also present. (×72 100)

Intramitochondrial crystalline inclusions are frequent in seemingly normal hepatocytes and a variety of disorders including alcoholic liver disease. They are also recorded in focal nodular hyperplasia, the so-called 'hepatomas' of women taking oral contraceptives[39] and hepatocellular carcinoma, as well as in rhabdomyomas, the so-called mitochondrial myopathies and prostatic adenocarcinoma (see Fig. 5.19). Although probably proteinaceous, their exact nature and significance are obscure.

References: 31, 39, 44, 47, 246, 362, 907, 1085

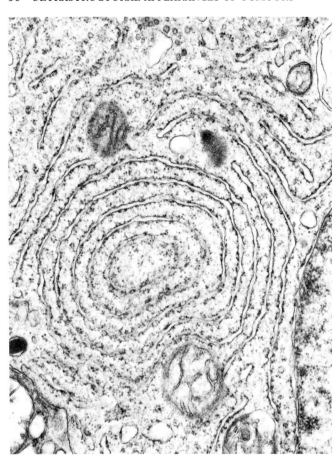

### Fig. 2.7 Concentric array of rough endoplasmic reticulum: Prolactin cell adenoma of adenohypophysis

Targetoid membranous arrays formed by the RER and SER occur in a variety of tumours. As illustrated here, those derived from the RER are often referred to as *Nebenkern* or concentric lamellar bodies. Compare with the ribosome-lamella complex shown in Fig. 28.17. Membranous whorls of SER are frequently seen in Leydig cell tumours and pituitary adenomas; spironolactone bodies also possess concentric closely packed peripheral lamellae of SER (see Fig. 13.1). (×23 900)

References: 39, 47, 109

### Fig. 2.8 Annulate lamellae: Duodenal smooth muscle tumour

In this electron micrograph a set of six annulate lamellae is seen in profile, adjacent to a group of lipid droplets (L). (×65 900)

**Discussion:** First described in the oocytes of marine invertebrates, annulate lamellae are considered to represent distinctive organelles characterized by intracytoplasmic parallel cisternal arrays showing regularly spaced annuli resembling nuclear pores. Continuity with both the endoplasmic reticulum and the nuclear envelope has been demonstrated in different cases. The significance of annulate lamellae is poorly understood, but they have been found in a variety of animal and human tissues. Annulate lamellae appear to be frequent in animal tumours, and they have been reported in a variety of benign and malignant human neoplasms (Table 2.2).

See also Fig. 30.3.

References: 312–322, 1551, 1802, 1922, 1930, 2296, 2914

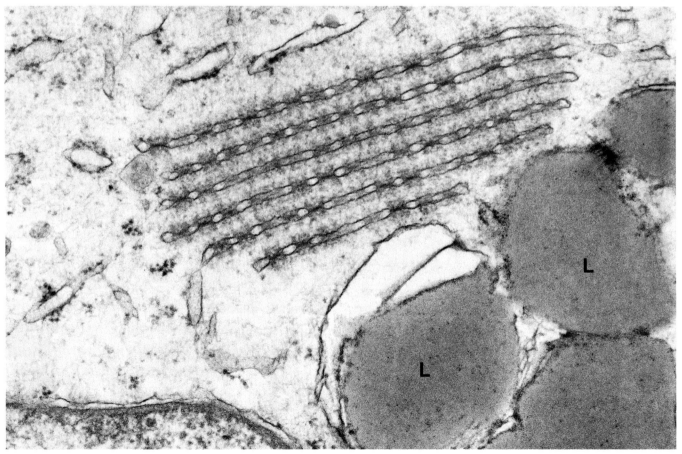

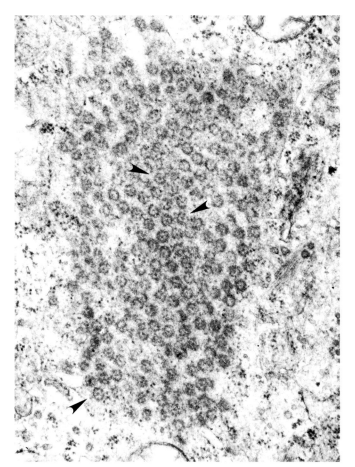

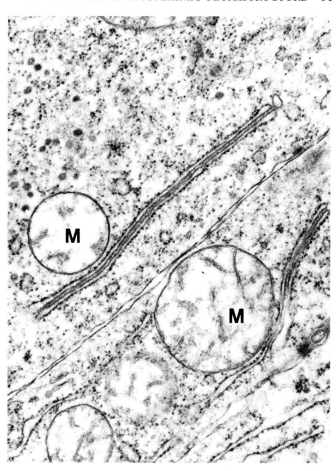

**Fig. 2.9    Annulate lamellae: Pulmonary adenocarcinoma**

When seen *en face*, as in this view, tangentially sectioned annulate lamellae may be mistaken for viral particles, but are distinguished by their resemblance to nuclear pore annuli, including a central electron-dense granule (arrowheads). They are not found budding into the endoplasmic reticulum. Annulate lamellae were remarkably frequent in this case, being found in approximately 20 per cent of the cell population examined. (×36 300)

**Fig. 2.10    Confronting cisternae of endoplasmic reticulum: Small cell anaplastic carcinoma of lung**

Two sets of confronting cisternae are apparent in adjoining cells, close to swollen mitochondria (M). Ribosomes stud the outer membranes but are conspicuously absent from the apposed lamellae. (×31 900)

**Discussion:** Although detected in normal cells, confronting cisternae have most often been found in neoplastic cells, including those of fibromyxosarcoma, rhabdomyosarcoma, giant cell tumour of bone, osteogenic sarcoma, malignant lymphoma, rectal adenocarcinoma and Wilms' tumour.

Confronting cisternae are rarely seen in continuity with the nuclear envelope, annulate lamellae, or tubuloreticular arrays. Occasionally more than two cisternae are involved in the confrontation, producing 'triple cisternae' or 'pentalaminar membranous structures'.[47] An association with mitosis has been noted but they also occur in interphase cells (as in this case). Their mode of formation and functional significance are unclear.

References: 39, 44, 47, 1026

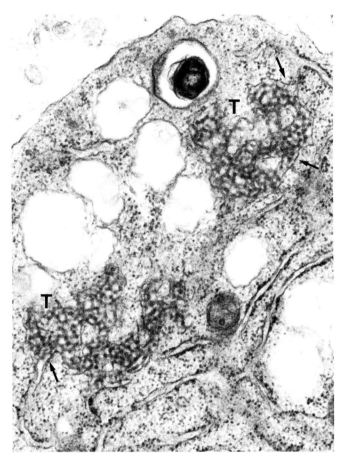

### Fig. 2.11 Tubuloreticular arrays: Glioblastoma multiforme

Within the neoplastic cell there are two apparently separate tubuloreticular arrays (T), consisting of coiled, branching tubular structures averaging 23 nm in diameter, which are located within expanded cisternae of the rough endoplasmic reticulum (arrows). (×41 800)

**Discussion:** Although characteristically present in glomerular endothelial cells in systemic lupus erythematosus, tubuloreticular arrays (TRA) have been described in a variety of pathological processes, most often in cells of mesodermal derivation, particularly endothelium. They have also been found in the neoplastic cells, stromal vascular endothelium, or other stromal elements in many different tumours (Table 2.3), although their identification may require a prolonged search.

Because TRA resemble Paramyxovirus nucleocapsids, it has been suggested that they represent viral particles, perhaps in incomplete form. However, their morphology, and their occurrence in many seemingly unrelated conditions, together with electron-histochemical studies and the absence of significant antibody titres against viral antigens in the patients investigated, indicate that they are non-viral (Table 2.4). They probably reflect a non-specific reaction of endoplasmic reticulum to a variety of stimuli.

References: 44, 47, 303–311, 438

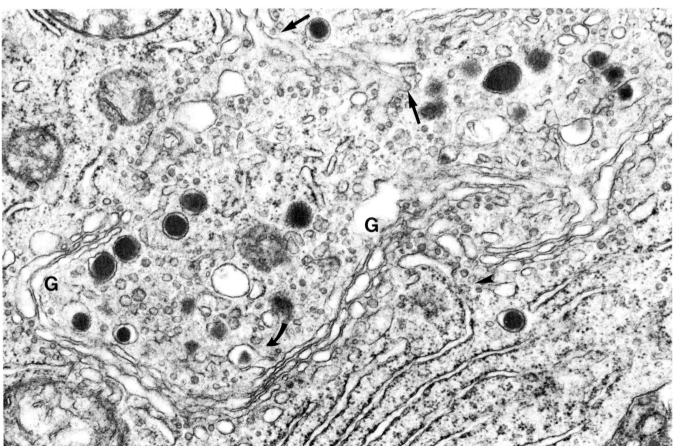

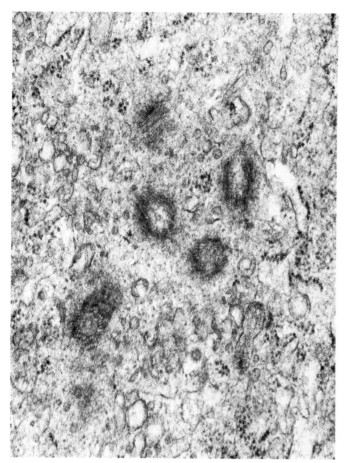

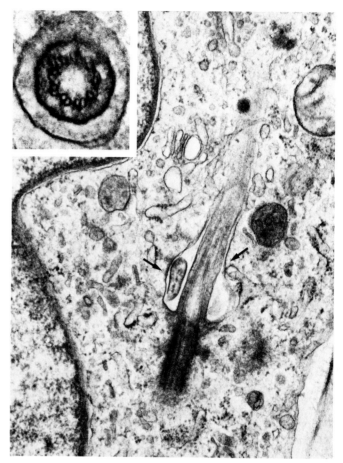

**Fig. 2.13  Multiple centrioles: Osteogenic sarcoma**

Five centriolar profiles are present in the paranuclear cytoplasm of an apparently mononuclear sarcomatous cell, suggesting centriolar division before an abnormal mitosis, or a consequence of cell fusion. (×50 300)

Multiple abnormal centrioles concentrated in large centrospheres may be present in tumour giant cells, but this appears to be a variable phenomenon and Friedländer[1941] could not find more than four centrioles within centrospheres in the giant cells of human gliomas.

References: 44, 47, 1941

**Fig. 2.14  Oligociliogenesis: Duodenal smooth muscle tumour, and small cell anaplastic carcinoma of lung**

Apart from the multiple surface cilia of ciliated epithelia, the development of 'oligocilia'[44] has been recorded in many different neoplastic and non-neoplastic mesenchymal and epithelial cells. They may be deeply situated, as shown in this field, and they are typically seen in close association with invaginating vacuolar membranes (arrows). These cilia develop from structures resembling centrioles in the paranuclear region. They occur singly or, less often, in small groups; in contrast to the 9+2 tubular pattern of classical cilia, they generally have a 9+0 configuration in transverse section, as shown in the inset, from a small cell anaplastic carcinoma of lung. In addition, dynein arms may be absent, indicating that such cilia are dysfunctional (see Fig. 5.28, inset). (×33 400. Inset: × 100 000)

See also Figs. 5.15, 7.8, 8.7, 17.9 and 24.3.

References: 39, 44, 180, 1745, 1779, 1918, 2034, 2505, 2547

**Fig. 2.12** *(Facing page — bottom)*  **Secretory apparatus: Prolactin cell adenoma of adenohypophysis**

The RER-Golgi apparatus-secretory granule complex is common to a variety of secretory epithelial and non-epithelial cells. As depicted in this pituitary adenoma, the lamellae of the RER are closely related to the outer convex *(cis)* aspect of the Golgi complex (G), also known as the 'maturing' face. The RER in one area appears to be continuous with the Golgi saccules (arrowhead). After concentration and packaging in the Golgi apparatus, the RER-derived secretory product emanates from the inner concave aspect (also referred to as the 'forming' or *trans* face) in the form of secretory granules of variable size. Portion of the Golgi-ER-lysosome (GERL) complex is also present (straight arrows); this is thought to represent a distinctive Golgi-related organelle implicated in the packaging of lysosomal material. Note the differences in the cores of the granules; presumably immature granules possess small, relatively lucent cores (curved arrow), while the mature forms have larger denser contents. Minute vesicles are also present in relation to the Golgi saccules. (×32 900)

Hypertrophy, depletion, dilatation and distortion of the Golgi apparatus in neoplasms represent non-specific alterations, being found in a variety of secretory and apparently non-secretory cells.

References: 39, 47, 180, 250

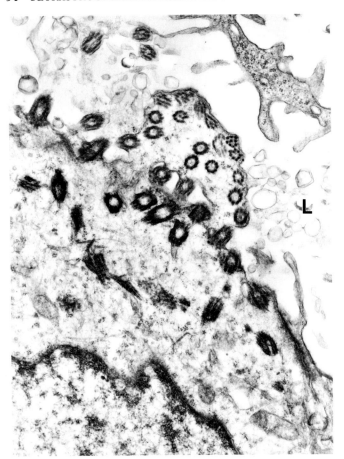

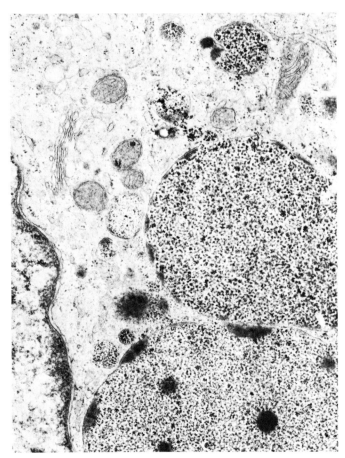

**Fig. 2.15  Abnormal ciliogenesis: Adenocarcinoma of cervix**

The luminal portion of this malignant cell exhibits basal bodies and a few of these have formed cilia. The majority, however, aggregate beneath the plasmalemma without forming well constructed cilia. Cell debris is present in the lumen (L). (×20 000)

**Discussion:** Ciliated cells are common in highly differentiated epithelial neoplasms of the thyroid gland and female genital tract; these include papillary and follicular thyroid carcinomas, serous cystadenoma and low-grade serous cystadenocarcinoma of ovary, and endometrial and cervical adenocarcinomas. However, cilial frequency is greatly reduced in poorly differentiated carcinomas.[1342] Ciliogenesis is also recorded in Brenner tumour of the ovary, ependymoma, choroid plexus papilloma and carcinoma, pineoblastoma and retinoblastoma. It is notable that the carcinomas which develop in relation to respiratory epithelium are usually devoid of cilia.

See also Fig. 5.28.

References: 1342, 1975

**Fig. 2.16: Pinealoma: Intralysosomal glycogen**

The lysosomes in this tumour were enlarged, some measuring more than 4 $\mu$m in diameter. As shown here, they are loaded with glycogen, although there is little in the ground substance of the cell. (×28 900)

**Discussion:** The accumulation of glycogen in lysosomes, presumably due to autophagocytosis, is not necessarily pathological and is described in several experimental models.[247] Although recorded in Hurler's disease, intralysosomal glycogen is a characteristic and prominent feature of type II glycogenosis (Pompe's disease) where its presence is the result of a lysosomal enzyme deficiency (acid $\alpha$-glucosidase).

In tumours, intralysosomal glycogen characterizes benign clear cell tumour of lung (so-called sugar tumour), but the lysosomal bodies are more uniform in size than those shown here.

Glycogen in cells may be seen in two forms: monogranular ($\beta$-particles 15–30 nm in diameter) and rosetted ($\alpha$-particles 80–100 nm in diameter). The particles may be intralysosomal in location or – far more commonly – free in the cytoplasm. Glycogen granules are distinguishable from ribosomes by their slightly larger size and greater electron-density, the assessment being facilitated by comparison of the particles with the ribosomes studding the lamellae of the RER. In addition, glycogen tends to form circumscribed closely packed aggregates; it is extracted from cells by overstaining with uranyl acetate, and its optimal preservation requires special fixation and staining techniques (for further details see caption to Fig. 25.8).

See also Figs. 5.15, 5.16, 5.27, 5.33, 12.2, 22.1, 25.2, 25.8 and 30.3, and Table 2.10.

References: 39, 44, 45, 47, 247, 443, 570

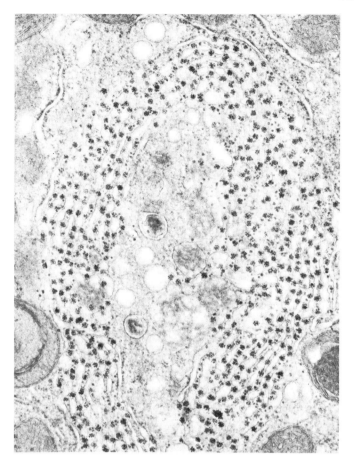

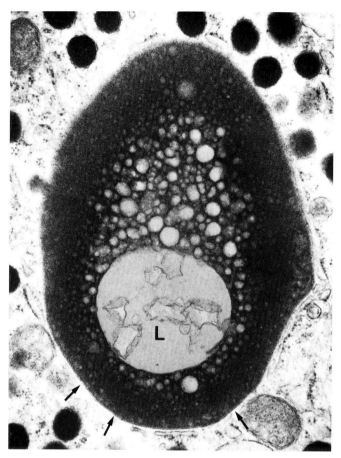

**Fig. 2.17 Glycogen-membrane complex (glycogen body): Hepato-cellular carcinoma**

Prominent glycogen rosettes are interspersed between concentric lamellae of endoplasmic reticulum forming a *Nebenkern* pattern. Such glycogen bodies should not be misinterpreted as ribosome-lamella complexes (compare with Fig. 28.17). (×18 000)

**Fig. 2.18 Lipofuscin body: Adenoma-hyperplasia of adeno-hypophysis**

Pituitary lesion from a 26-year-old woman with the galactorrhoea-amenorrhoea syndrome. The resected adenohypophyseal tissue consisted predominantly of densely granulated prolactin cells, with sporadic cells showing immunoreactivity for growth and luteinizing hormones (see Chapter 10).

Segments of membrane (arrows) are evident at the periphery of this lipofuscin body, which consists of finely granular electron-dense matter associated with more lucent lipid (L) droplets of varying size. Membrane-bound secretory granules inhabit the surrounding cytoplasm. (×29 000)

**Discussion:** Lipofuscin bodies, probably resulting from autophagocytosis, are frequent in a variety of neoplasms; accumulation of these bodies in adrenal cortical adenomas may occasionally be so extreme that pigmentation is evident to the naked eye (so-called black adenomas). The orange pigment sometimes found overlying malignant melanomas of the uveal tract has also been reported to represent lipofuscin. In the pituitary, similar large spheroidal lysosomal bodies with an electron-lucent lipidic centre and a dense rim are sometimes referred to as 'enigmatic bodies';[1623] they are usually located close to the nucleus and Golgi complex.

See also Figs. 10.1, 12.2, 13.2 and 18.2.

References: 44, 47, 1569, 1623, 1827, 1831, 1838, 2146

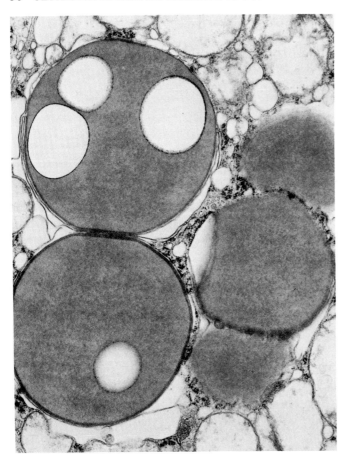

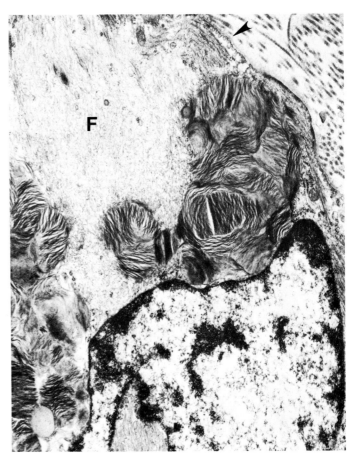

**Fig. 2.19 Lipid: Adrenal cortical adenoma**

Several moderately dense, membrane-bound lipid droplets are illustrated, two of which contain lucent vacuoles. (×20 400)

Lipid droplets show considerable variability in electron-density, reflecting the concentration of unsaturated fatty acids which are blackened as a result of reduction by osmium. In contrast, highly saturated lipids appear relatively lucent. They are easily distinguished from other granular elements of the cytoplasm by their size and amorphous 'glassy' contents.

See also Table 2.11 and Figs. 5.16, 5.17, 12.1, 13.1, 13.2, 19.1, 20.13, 23.10 and 25.9.

References: 180, 1030, 1031, 1508, 1509, 2328–2348

**Fig. 2.20 Ovarian thecoma: Intralysosomal lamellated lipid**

Leaflets of phospholipid membranes are enclosed within autophagosomes, closely resembling the appearances seen in Fabry's disease; similar 'zebra bodies' also occur in the neurones in Hurler's disease and in Sandhoff's disease (a form of $GM_2$-gangliosidosis). The ultrastructure of the lipid in this case is exceptional; the lipid droplets typical of ovarian thecoma resemble those depicted in Fig. 2.19. Note also the filaments (F) and micropinocytotic vesicles (arrowhead). (×20 300)

References: 47, 247

# 3 Stromal ultrastructure

The stroma of most tumours consists of a mass of mesenchymal, inflammatory, and vascular elements in varying proportions. In general, however, the stroma lacks diagnostic significance apart from the notable exceptions of the granulofibrillary matrix typical of chondroid tumours, the deposition of hydroxyapatite crystals on stromal collagen in osteoblastic tumours, and the occurrence of amyloid fibrils in some tumours, such as polypeptide-producing endocrine neoplasms (Tables 3.2 and 3.3).

## VASCULATURE

The degree of vascularization of neoplasms varies, and in general the vessels consist of endothelium-lined sinusoids of variable size. Often there are no unusual endothelial appearances, but the cells may be plump, with correspondingly reduced vascular luminal calibre, in areas of neovascularization. Fenestrated endothelium may be seen, particularly in endocrine tumours (Fig. 3.4); however, normally fenestrated endothelium may be lost in neoplasia — as in a disseminated choroid plexus 'papilloma'[2021] — or the fenestrations may be reduced in frequency.[377] Multiple external laminae often surround the endothelial cells, apparently as a result of repetitive vascular injury.[332,337,377,404] Abluminal projections from the endothelial cells occasionally penetrate the external lamina; these are probably associated with neovascularization.

Pericytes and smooth muscle cells are uncommonly found in the vicinity of stromal blood vessels. Nerve endings are usually absent, not only in the vicinity of the sinusoidal vessels, but also throughout the neoplastic mass. Lymphatics similarly are rare, apart from the periphery of the neoplasm.

## INFLAMMATORY CELLS

Various inflammatory cells may be seen in the stroma; these include polymorphonuclear leukocytes, mononuclear phagocytes, lymphocytes, and plasma cells. Mast cells are also frequent in some neoplasms.[30,356,1023,2188,2510]

## FIBROBLASTS AND MYOFIBROBLASTS

Fibroblasts and myofibroblasts are important cellular components of the stroma, their numbers and proportions being subject to great variation. The concentration of myofibroblasts in carcinomas appears to be proportional to the degree of desmoplasia; their occurrence in invasive carcinomas is thought to represent an adaptive stromal response, ultimately leading to tissue retraction in some cases. Following invasion a succession of changes is thought to occur, including a granulation tissue-like reaction and myofibroblast induction with type III collagen synthesis, followed by a transition to type I collagen.[371] Smooth muscle, fibroblasts and primitive mesenchymal cells have each been proposed as myofibroblast precursors. Myofibroblasts often display intermediate junctions (Fig. 3.16) and are associated with fragmented external laminal material; they should not be misinterpreted as poorly differentiated epithelial cells in so-called spindle cell carcinomas.

## EXTRACELLULAR MATRIX: COLLAGEN, ELASTIN AND EXTERNAL LAMINA

The stroma also contains variable quantities of extracellular matrix composed of differing proportions of collagens, elastin, proteoglycans, glycoproteins and external (basal) lamina.

The collagen fibres usually display the classical 64 nm periodicity and are 20–120 nm in diameter. In some instances fibrous long-spacing collagen (FLSC)[47] can be recognized; this form is possibly related to type IV collagen, and has a transverse periodicity of 90–120 nm instead of the classical banding of 64 nm. It has been particularly reported in neural neoplasms, notably Schwannoma and meningioma, but it may be seen in a variety of tumours (Table 3.4). FLSC is also present in normal lymph nodes, where it is concentrated in relation to vascular components, including perivascular connective tissue such as medullary perivenous tissue and the vicinity of the marginal sinus.[360] In pathological lymph nodes, FLSC has been found in reactive lymphadenopathies,[360] immunoblastic lymphadenopathy, Hodgkin's disease and non-Hodgkin's lymphomas (Table 3.4). We have also identified FLSC in pulmonary sarcoidosis, and pigmented villonodular synovitis. Nevertheless, the occurrence of large quantities of FLSC forming circumscribed Luse bodies is highly characteristic of *benign* nerve sheath cell tumours, especially Schwannomas (see Fig. 18.2).

Giant collagen fibres (amianthoid fibres) — 6 to 10 times thicker than native collagen fibres and with a periodicity of 56–62 nm,[47] — have been reported in chondrosarcoma,[47] synovial sarcoma,[362] malignant Schwannoma[362] and a peculiar soft tissue tumour designated by Connolly[331] as an 'amian-thioma'; we have also identified this form of collagen in an unusual intermediate filament-rich cerebral tumour of uncertain type, resembling the malignant rhabdoid tumour of kidney. Other unusual patterns include 'spiralled' and 'spiny' collagen;[47] the spiralled form has been recorded in elasto-fibroma[47] and spiny collagen has been identified in an infantile mesenchymal tumour of the kidney, medullary carcinoma of the thyroid and Hodgkin's disease.[45] Numerous elastin fibres may also be present, particularly in infiltrating mammary carcinomas (Fig. 3.18).

*External laminae* surround stromal vessels and are often present adjacent to the neoplastic cells, particularly epithelial cells. However, external lamina (EL) also occurs in association with mesenchymal cells such as lipoblasts and lipocytes, myofibroblasts, smooth and striated muscle, endothelium and pericytes, as well as nerve sheath cells. The extent of development of these laminae is quite variable in tumours; they are often inconspicuous in highly anaplastic neoplasms and may be absent from invasive malignant cells, notably in mammary carcinomas. Some tumour cells characteristically lack EL (Table 3.1), while nodular multilayered accumulations of EL typify adenoid cystic carcinoma (Fig. 3.17),[737] basal cell adenoma of the parotid gland,[700] adenoid cystic-like areas of mixed parotid tumours, eccrine cylindroma of skin, gynandroblastoma and ovarian sex cord tumour with annular tubules.[1356] Breaks in the basal lamina at the epithelio-stromal interface may also be seen in a variety of epithelial tumours, both benign[404] and malignant.

External laminae constitute ubiquitous extracellular matrices which normally function by acting as barriers and filters, and by facilitating cell-substratum adherence, thereby promoting the development and organization of tissues (see Introduction). Such laminae consist of a complex of macromolecules,[329] including glycosaminoglycans, glyco-proteins and type IV collagen (which retains its telopeptide moiety and does not aggregate to form classical collagen fibres with their 64 nm periodicity). The non-collagenous components include fibronectin, laminin (GP-2) and entactin (a sulphated glycoprotein), as well as heparan sulphate. Laminin may be instrumental in the attachment of epithelial cells to type IV collagen, and in determining cell polarity, but its exact role is uncertain.[329] Fibronectin (M.Wt. 440 000) appears to represent a 'molecular glue',[355] the facilitation of cell-substratum adherence being one of its many properties.[329,334,336] Cartilage lacks dimeric fibronectin; instead, chondrocytes elaborate the closely related protein chondronectin (M.Wt. 180 000), which attaches them to collagen.[352]

Apart from the Latin expression *lamina externa*, a variety of other terms have been used for EL, including 'basement membrane' and 'basal lamina'. Two objections have been levelled at these expressions:[45,180]

1. External lamina bears no resemblance to trilaminar plasma membranes.
2. Although the laminae are 'basal' in normal epithelia, this topographical relationship is disturbed in many neoplasms and is essentially meaningless in mesenchymal and neural tissues.

'External lamina' is therefore the most accurate terminology,[45,180] but 'basal lamina' is also entrenched in the literature and these terms can be used interchangeably; throughout this work we have used both, but have tended to reserve the description 'basal' for those instances where this polarized relationship to the cell surface can be recognized with ease.

Finally, fibrin tactoids with a transverse periodicity of 20 nm may also be present in tumour matrices, especially in areas of necrosis and haemorrhage.

## STROMAL AMYLOID

Stromal amyloid deposits are well documented in lymphoplasmacytic and polypeptide-producing endocrine tumours (see Figs. 11.7 and 16.2) and are occasionally seen in other neoplasms (Table 3.3). Representing a conglomerate of β-pleated fibrillary proteins, amyloid is characterized in its ultrastructure by haphazard fibrils which are classically 10 nm in diameter;[47] it is impossible to predict the clinicopathological type of amyloid or its chemical characteristics by the morphology of the fibrils. In the case of polypeptide-producing endocrine neoplasms such as medullary carcinoma of thyroid,

**Table 3.1 Tumours devoid of external lamina***

Astrocytomas†
Seminoma-dysgerminoma
Leydig and ovarian hilar cell tumours
Endometrial stromal sarcomas
Fibroblastoid tumours lacking myofibroblasts
Epithelioid sarcoma
Alveolar soft part sarcoma
Chordoma
Cartilaginous tumours
Osteoblastic tumours lacking myofibroblasts
Ewing's sarcoma
Histiocytosis X
Malignant histiocytosis
Hodgkin's disease
Non-Hodgkin's lymphomas
Plasmacytic tumours
Leukaemias, all types

*This list excludes stromal elements such as blood vessels and refers only to the neoplastic cells

†Except those differentiating as the subpial astrocytic layer (Fig. 17.5)

**Table 3.2 Distinctive stromal components in tumours**

| Stromal component | Tumours |
|---|---|
| Amyloid fibrils | Plasmacytic tumours<br>Lymphomas<br>So-called apudomas, including medullary carcinoma of thyroid (Figs. 11.7 and 16.2)<br>Others (see Table 3.3) |
| Hydroxyapatite deposits on collagen fibres | Osteoblastic tumours, notably osteogenic sarcoma (Fig. 25.6) |
| Granulofibrillary matrix ± amianthoid fibres | Chondrocytic and chondroblastic neoplasms (Figs. 25.1–25.3) |

the fibrils seem to represent polymerized secretory products, while in plasmacytic tumours they are related to immunoglobulin light chains. Amyloid-like intrafollicular filaments 7.5–10 nm in diameter are recorded in parathyroid adenoma, but Altenähr[1799] regarded the identity of this material as an 'open question'; systemic amyloid is not seen with such adenomas and it is probable that the filaments comprise polymerized parathormone.

The nature of the extracellular hyaline material accumulating in the calcifying epithelial odontogenic tumour of Pindborg (and adenomatoid odontogenic tumour) and its possible relationship to amyloid are discussed in Chapter 4.

## CALCIFIC DEPOSITS

Areas of calcium deposition may be present.[821,1361,2034] Calcium salts can occur within cytoplasmic organelles (such as lysosomes, secretory granules, autophagosomes and mitochondria), or lie free within the cytoplasm or acini; deposits of poorly soluble calcium salts may otherwise be found in the stroma.

**Table 3.3   Tumours consistently, occasionally or rarely containing stromal amyloid**

*LYMPHOPROLIFERATIVE DISORDERS*

Multiple myeloma-plasmacytoma
Waldenström's macroglobulinaemia
Hodgkin's disease
Non-Hodgkin's lymphomas
Immunoblastic lymphadenopathy

*ENDOCRINE TUMOURS*

Pituitary adenomas:
Growth hormone cell adenoma
Prolactin cell adenoma
Melanocorticotrophinoma
Medullary carcinoma of thyroid and related tumours, including:
Bronchial carcinoid tumour (medullary carcinoma-like tumour)
Strumal carcinoid tumour of ovary
Cervical carcinoid tumour
Mixed papillary and follicular carcinoma of thyroid
Parathyroid adenoma
Pancreatic islet tumours, including:
Insulinoma
Gastrinoma
Paraganglioma-phaeochromocytoma

*ODONTOGENIC TUMOURS*

Calcifying epithelial odontogenic tumour of Pindborg*
Adenomatoid odontogenic tumour*

*MISCELLANEOUS EPITHELIAL TUMOURS*

Small cell carcinoma of lung
Thymoma
Renal adenocarcinoma
Urothelial carcinoma
Prostatic carcinoma
Adenocarcinoma of uterine cervix
Mucoepidermoid carcinoma of parotid gland
Papillary adenocarcinoma of parotid gland†
Tubular carcinoma of palate
Oesophageal squamous cell carcinoma
Gastric adenocarcinoma
Basal cell carcinoma of skin
Adnexal tumours of skin

*See text, Chapter 4

†Randomly orientated 10 nm amyloid fibrils found in stroma and intraluminal corpora amylacea; postulated that this β-fibrillosis resulted from apoptosis and dissolution of tumour cells, with release and conglomeration of intermediate filaments[713]

References: 64, 333, 487, 672, 685, 689, 713, 918, 1173, 1475, 1640, 1644, 1646, 1694, 1731, 1752, 1754, 1774, 1793

**Table 3.4   Fibrous long-spacing collagen in tumours and tumour-like conditions**

*NEURAL TUMOURS*

Schwannoma (Fig. 18.2)
Neurofibroma
Granular cell tumour
Peripheral neural tumour in von Recklinghausen's neurofibromatosis
Meningioma
Meningeal melanocytoma
Malignant astrocytoma
Cerebellar haemangioblastoma (Fig. 23.10)*
Pinealoma

*EPITHELIAL/EPITHELIOID TUMOURS*

Pituitary chromophobe adenoma
Transitional oxyphilic parathyroid adenoma*
Parathyroid carcinoma†
Thymoma
Blue naevus
Malignant melanoma
Basal cell carcinoma of skin
Merkel cell carcinoma*
Wilms' tumour*
Adenocarcinoma of prostate (lymph node metastasis)*
Yolk sac carcinoma

*QUASI-NEOPLASTIC FIBROPROLIFERATIONS*

Proliferative fasciitis
Fibromatosis hyalinica multiplex juvenilis

*MESENCHYMAL TUMOURS AND TUMOUR-LIKE CONDITIONS*

Xanthelasma
Ovarian thecoma*
Pigmented villonodular synovitis
Malignant fibrous histiocytoma (Fig. 20.6)
Haemangiopericytoma (Fig. 3.18)
Angiosarcoma
Vascular leiomyosarcoma
Alveolar rhabdomyosarcoma
Extraskeletal myxoid chondrosarcoma
Alveolar soft part sarcoma

*LYMPHOHAEMOPOIETIC DISORDERS*

Immunoblastic lymphadenopathy
Malignant lymphomas with sclerosis
Hodgkin's disease (nodular sclerosis; mixed cellularity; lymphocyte depletion)
Lymphoma of mononuclear phagocytes
Mycosis fungoides
Hairy cell leukaemia§
Chronic granulocytic leukaemia§
Myelofibrosis

*Henderson, Papadimitriou & Coleman, unpublished observations

†Oxyphilic parathyroid carcinoma; the collagen formed sharply demarcated collections with a periodicity of 73.5 nm, resembling that illustrated in Fig. 20.6 (malignant fibrous histiocytoma)[1823]

§Tissue infiltrates

References: 45, 64, 324, 344, 357, 360, 576, 708, 1146, 1682, 1823, 2037, 2065, 2110, 2115, 2132, 2252, 2312, 2321, 2385, 2758, 2769, 2778, 2833

**Table 3.5** **Myofibroblasts (MFB) in tumours and tumour-like conditions I: Benign/non-metastasizing mesenchymal proliferations**

| Condition | Remarks |
|---|---|
| *REACTIVE FIBROPROLIFERATIONS* | |
| Nodular fasciitis | — |
| Proliferative fasciitis | The large ballooned cells represent MFB |
| Myositis ossificans/ossifying fasciitis | — |
| Elastofibroma | — |
| *FIBROMATOSES* | |
| Fibrous hamartoma of infancy | — |
| Congenital generalized and localized fibromatosis (infantile myofibromatosis) | Spontaneous regression of one case, designated as multiple congenital mesenchymal hamartomas, attributed to contractile properties of MFB,[2247] but Bhawan et al[2248] considered the evidence to be unconvincing. We have also observed numerous MFB in a congenital localized fibromatosis of bone |
| Fibromatosis hyalinica multiplex juvenilis | |
| Infantile digital fibroma | The intracytoplasmic inclusions are often continuous with cytoplasmic microfilaments 5–7 nm in diameter, presumably contractile and with associated dense bodies.[2279,2298] Growth of inclusions takes place by accretion of filaments.[2248] The component cells are widely considered to represent MFB, but this has been disputed.[2264] See Fig. 20.3 |
| Juvenile aponeurotic fibroma | — |
| Nasopharyngeal angiofibroma | See Fig. 20.1 |
| Dupuytren's contracture | — |
| Desmoid fibromatosis | — |
| Desmoplastic fibroma of bone | — |
| *BENIGN MESENCHYMAL TUMOURS/TUMOUR-LIKE CONDITIONS* | |
| Ossifying and non-ossifying fibroma of bone | — |
| Fibroma of tendon sheath | Most of the cells are MFB |
| Dermatofibroma | — |
| Giant cell fibroma of oral mucosa | — |
| Benign spindle cell tumour of breast | Resembled spindle cell lipoma. EM revealed a population of fibroblasts, MFB, smooth muscle cells and undifferentiated mesenchymal cells[1446] |
| Smooth muscle tumours | — |
| Plexiform tumourlet of myometrium | Ultrastructurally the plexiform tumourlet is predominantly a smooth muscle lesion |
| Disseminated peritoneal leiomyomatosis | — |
| Lymphangiomyoma and lymphangiomyomatosis | — |
| Cardiac myxoma | See text, Chapter 24 |

References: 64, 323, 347, 349, 351, 359, 364, 365, 370–372, 380, 413, 417, 422, 647, 1177, 1221, 1244, 1400, 1446, 2179, 2196, 2221, 2226, 2227, 2247, 2248, 2252–2254, 2257, 2260, 2264, 2265, 2268, 2269, 2271, 2278, 2279, 2285, 2294, 2298, 2299, 2303, 2306, 2309, 2315, 2318, 2325, 2388, 2506, 2600, 2622, 2626, 2647, 2657, 2847

**Table 3.6  Myofibroblasts (MFB) in tumours and tumour-like conditions II: Atypical/malignant tumours**

| Tumour | Remarks |
|---|---|
| *ATYPICAL/MALIGNANT MESENCHYMAL TUMOURS* | |
| Congenital mesoblastic nephroma | — |
| Aggressive angiomyxoma of female pelvis and perineum | — |
| Atypical fibroxanthoma of skin | — |
| Malignant fibrous histiocytoma | Found in all 30 tumours examined in one series,[347] while Tsuneyoshi et al[2315] identified MFB in 12 of 17 cases. See Chapter 20 |
| Fibrosarcoma | — |
| Myxofibrosarcoma | — |
| Sclerosing liposarcoma | MFB most numerous in desmoplastic areas[347] |
| Pleomorphic liposarcoma | — |
| Leiomyosarcoma | See text, Chapter 21 |
| Alveolar and so-called pleomorphic rhabdomyosarcoma | — |
| Malignant haemangiopericytoma | — |
| Stromal sarcoma of breast | — |
| Metastasizing pleural sarcoma | MFB predominated[2179] |
| Synovial sarcoma | — |
| Osteogenic sarcoma ('conventional' type) | MFB constitute a small proportion of the neoplastic cells, in contrast to parosteal osteosarcoma (see below) |
| Parosteal osteosarcoma | MFB concentrated at periphery of tumour;[2657] in one case they represented 90 per cent of the neoplastic cells[349] |
| *BIMORPHIC EPITHELIO-MESENCHYMAL TUMOURS* | |
| Fibroadenoma of breast | In stromal component |
| Cystosarcoma phyllodes | In stromal component; smooth muscle cells also present |
| Carcinosarcoma of uterine cervix | — |
| 'Nasal blastoma'[413] | Diagnosis questioned; may represent a mixed salivary-type tumour[417,422] |
| Malignant mesothelioma | MFB in mesotheliomas are usually either not mentioned or are said to be absent,[2179] but they are clearly illustrated in the article by Suzuki et al,[647] published before the heyday of the myofibroblast. See Table 9.1 |
| EPITHELIAL/EPITHELIOID NEOPLASMS | |
| Desmoplastic spindle cell melanoma | See Figs. 8.7 and 8.8 |
| Adamantinoma of long bones | — |
| Neuroblastoma | — |
| Testicular choriocarcinoma | Figs. 3.14 and 3.15 |
| Stroma of invasive carcinomas, including primary carcinomas of breast, stomach, colon, lung, thyroid, renal pelvis and the ampulla of Vater, as well as a variety of metastatic carcinomas in different organs | Fig. 3.16 (infiltrating duct carcinoma of breast) |
| *LYMPHOPROLIFERATIVE DISORDERS* | |
| Nodular sclerosing Hodgkin's disease | MFB found in lymph nodes in all 10 cases examined in one series (lymph nodes normally lack MFB)[371] |

References: See Table 3.5

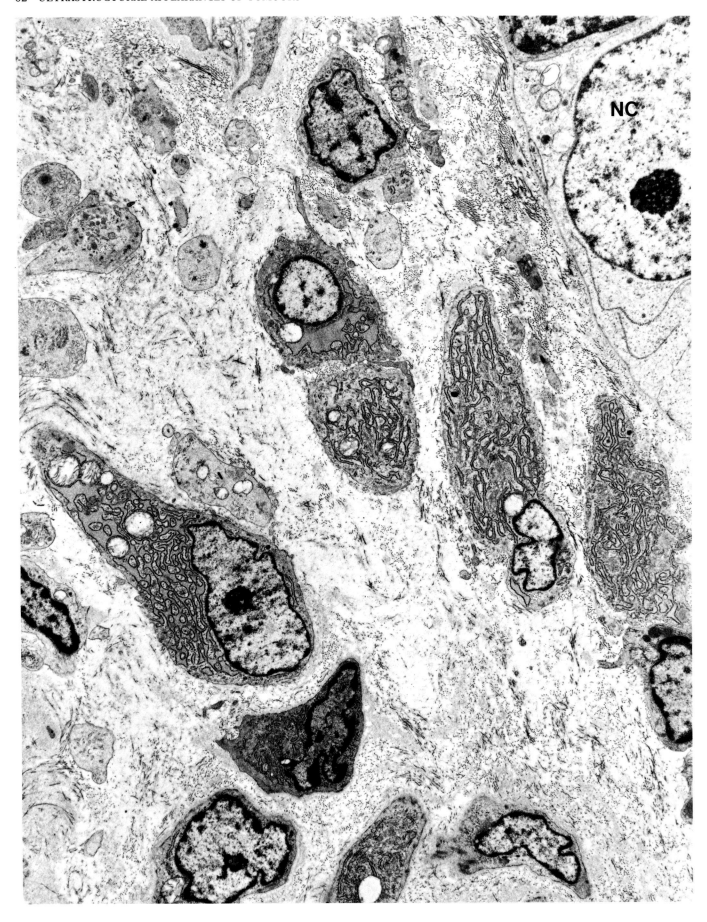

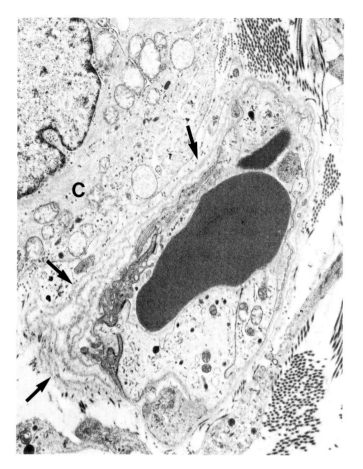

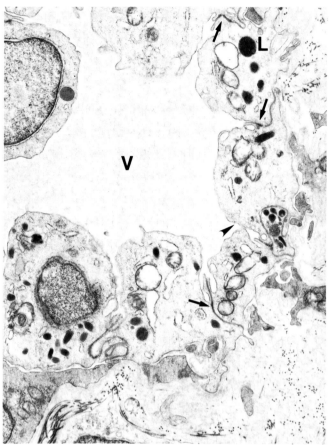

**Fig. 3.2    Stromal capillary: Infiltrating duct carcinoma of breast**

A carcinomatous cell (C) is in close proximity to the stromal capillary, which contains red blood cells. The endothelium displays focal swelling, with lucency of the cytoplasm. The vascular external lamina close to the neoplastic cell is reduplicated, forming multiple laminae (arrows), consistent with repetitive vascular injury associated with malignant invasion. In comparison, the external lamina furthest from the infiltrating cell is affected to a lesser degree. (×8900)

References: 332, 337, 340, 350, 361, 378, 1363, 1745, 1976, 2017, 2076, 2522

**Fig. 3.3    Blood vessel: Immunoblastic lymphadenopathy**

The vascular lumen (V) is surrounded by plump endothelial cells resembling those of postcapillary venules. Junctions link adjoining cells (arrows) and there are a few collections of micropinocytotic vesicles (arrowhead). The endothelial cytoplasm also contains dense Weibel-Palade bodies, which are either rounded or elongated, depending on the plane of section. A lysosome (L) is also evident. Adjacent collagen fibres, external laminal material and portions of smooth muscle cells are included in the field. Frequent endothelial tubuloreticular arrays were also found in this case (see Table 2.3 and Fig. 2.11). (×9800)

**Fig. 3.1** *(Facing page)*    **Survey of stroma: Adenocarcinoma**

Portion of a group of neoplastic cells (NC) can be seen, but most of the field is occupied by fibroblasts with copious and often dilated RER. Collagen fibres are evident within the abundant intercellular matrix. (×7000)

Reference: 356

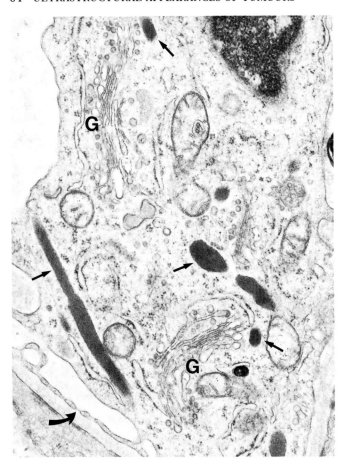

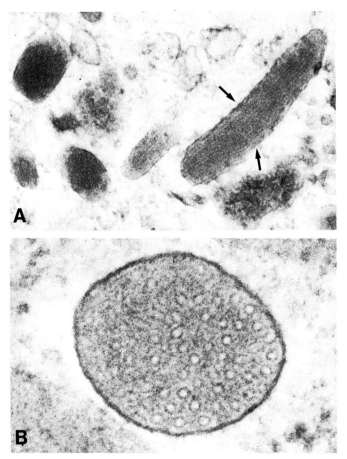

**Fig. 3.4 Endothelial Weibel-Palade bodies I: Parathyroid adenoma**

Several Weibel-Palade bodies (straight arrows) inhabit the endothelial cytoplasm, some situated in proximity to the Golgi complexes (G) from which they are probably derived. Sectioned longitudinally, the largest body has an elongated rod-shaped profile. Fenestrations (curved arrow) are evident in the attenuated cytoplasm. (×24 400)

Weibel-Palade bodies represent a reliable ultrastructural marker for endothelium and they have not been convincingly identified in other cell types. Their numbers may reflect endothelial maturity and they are usually sparse or absent in both benign and malignant vasoformative tumours. Their function is uncertain, but it has been suggested that they may contain a procoagulant substance such as platelet factor 3,[2481] while immunocytochemical analysis indicates the presence of von Willebrand factor. Others[179] have speculated that they may participate in defences against spontaneous thrombosis.

See also text, Chapter 23, and Figs. 23.3 and 23.5.

References: 39, 44, 45, 179, 345, 2478, 2481, 2516

**Fig. 3.5 Weibel-Palade bodies II: Immunoblastic lymphadenopathy**

At high magnification Weibel-Palade bodies are seen to represent membrane-bound rod-shaped organelles with a tubular substructure.

**A:** In longitudinal section the component tubules produce a linear periodicity parallel to the long axis of the bodies (arrows). (×67 400)

**B:** In the near-transverse section shown here the tubules have ring-shaped profiles, with an average diameter of 18 nm and a range of 15–20 nm. (×172 800)

**Fig. 3.6** *(Facing page)* **Inflammatory cell infiltrate: Bronchogenic squamous cell carcinoma**

Several plasma cells with copious rough endoplasmic reticulum and the characteristic 'clock-face' pattern of marginated heterochromatin are evident in this field, together with a lymphocyte (L). Mononuclear phagocytes (MP) with interdigitating cytoplasmic flaps are also present. (×7400)

See also Fig. 30.3.

References: 45, 356

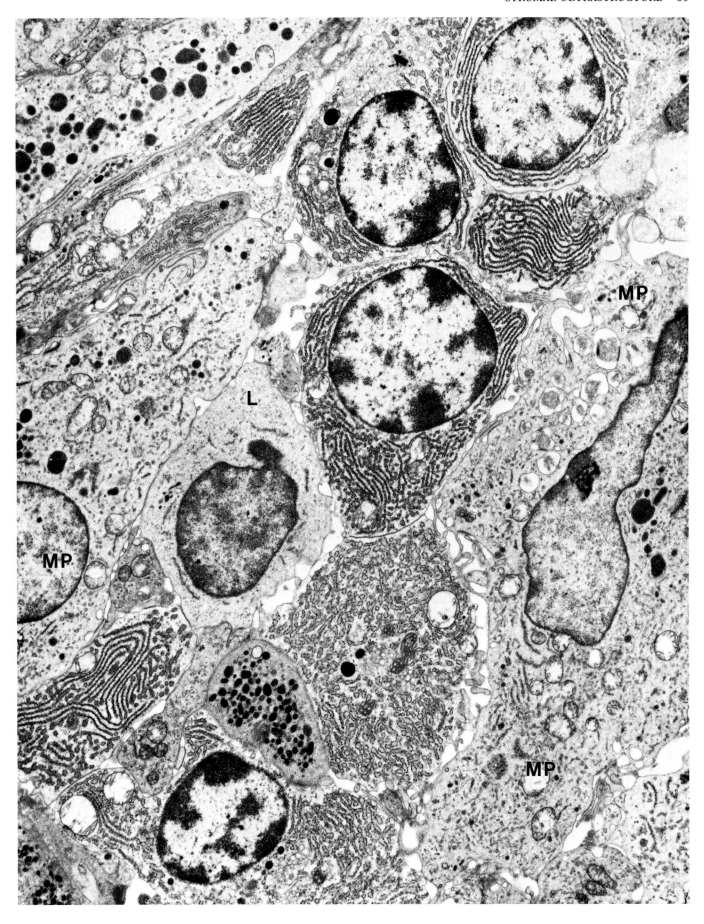

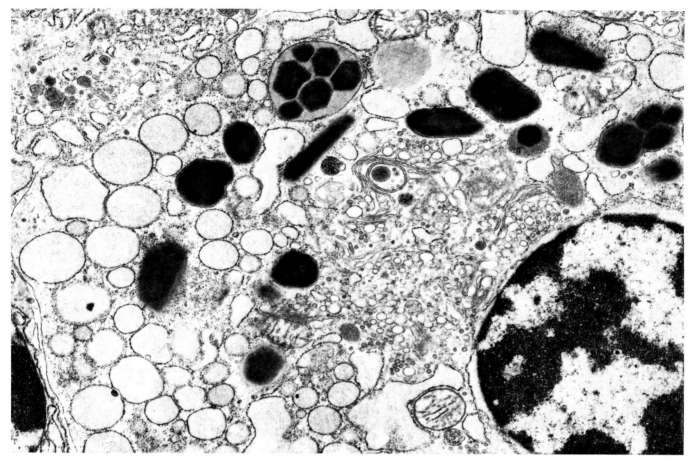

**Fig. 3.7   Stromal plasma cell I: Small cell anaplastic carcinoma of lung**

The cisternae of the RER are dilated and some contain electron-dense material consistent with proteinaceous secretion, presumably containing immunoglobulin. The intracisternal secretory product sometimes forms angulated polygonal patterns. The paranuclear Golgi complex is prominent. These appearances correspond to an early phase of Russell body formation. (×17 800)

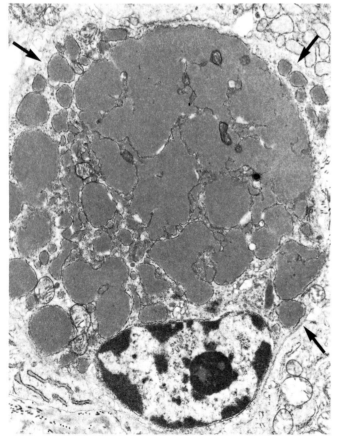

**Fig. 3.8   Stromal plasma cell II: Russell body: Adenocarcinoma of lung**

A later stage of Russell body development is depicted here. Accumulated moderately dense proteinaceous material occupies most of the cytoplasm, with displacement of the nucleus to the cell periphery. Dilated cisternae are discernible (arrows), but elsewhere apparent dissolution of cisternal membranes has resulted in coalescence of the secretory product. (×9400)

Such intracisternal material in Russell bodies is widely thought to represent an accumulation of immunoglobulin (IG). However, Hsu et al[341] could not identify IG determinants in Russell body cores by light- or electron-immunohistochemistry, suggesting that they either consisted of non-IG components or that any IG present existed in an altered unreactive state, but these findings have been questioned by others.[327] The presence of glycoprotein is recorded.[47]

References: 47, 327, 341

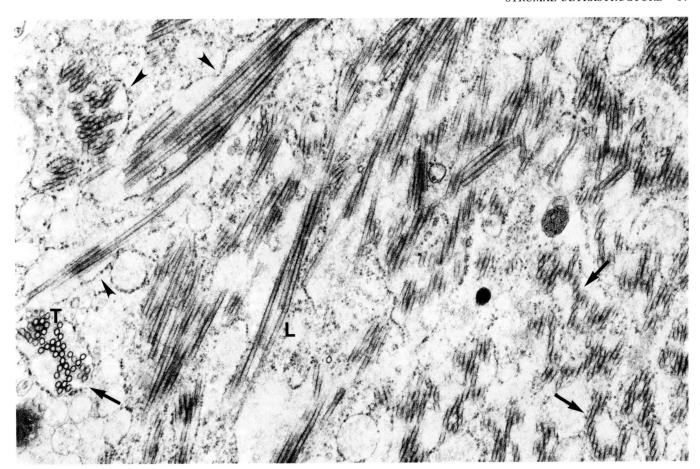

**Fig. 3.9   Crystalline arrays in stromal plasma cell: Squamous cell carcinoma**

Within the cytoplasm of the cell shown in this field there are numerous crystalline inclusions, which appear to be confined to the cisternae of the RER (arrowheads). As shown in both longitudinal (L) and transverse (T) section, they represent elongated cylinders averaging 50 nm in maximum diameter, sometimes arranged in an undulating/geometric pattern (arrows). Inclusions of this type probably represent crystallized immunoglobulin products. (×38 100)

   See also Figs. 27.14, 27.15 and 27.29.

   Reference: 285

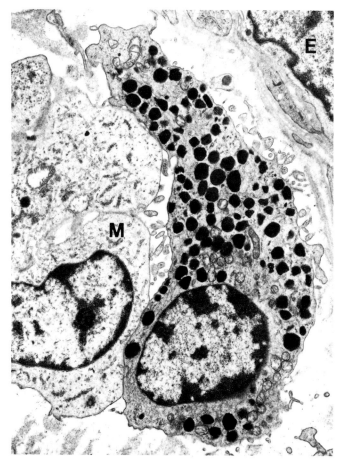

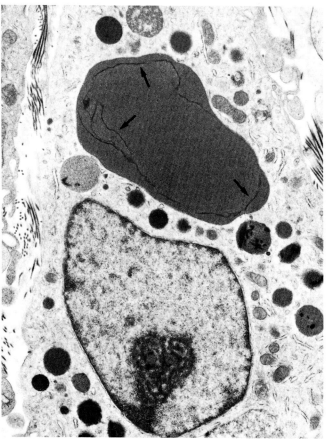

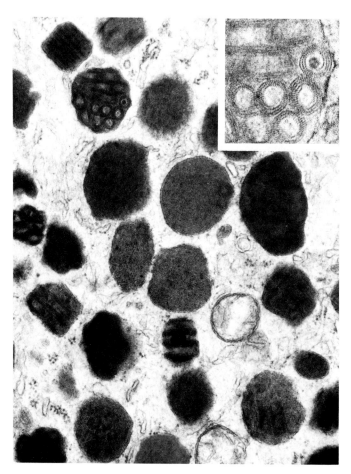

**Fig. 3.10** *(Top — left)* **Perivascular stromal mast cell: Carcinoid tumour**

The mast cell lies next to a mononuclear cell (M), shows prominent cell processes, and contains numerous pleomorphic osmiophilic granules. Portion of an endothelial cell (E) with its investing external lamina is also apparent. (×7300)

In an ultrastructural study of rectal signet-ring cell carcinomas, Shousha[863] found a close topographic relationship between argentaffin cells in the tumour and stromal mast cells. Pasyk et al[2510] described both elongated and rounded stromal mast cells in haemangiomas; the mast cells in growing haemangiomas contained variably developed simple granules, whereas those in involuting lesions tended to possess mature compound granules.

See also Fig. 24.3.

References: 328, 863, 2510

**Fig. 3.11** *(Top — right)* **Mast cell granules: Carcinoid tumour**

The granules show considerable variation in both density and morphology. Some have a membranous substructure, with the formation of tubular and scroll patterns. **Inset:** Scroll pattern in a mast cell granule. Same case as Fig. 3.10. (×34 000. Inset: ×92 000)

Although characteristic of human mast cells, scroll granules are not found in all species and they do not occur in the rat. Similarly, they are not present in circulating human basophil leukocytes and cells containing them are therefore designated as mast cells.

**Fig. 3.12** *(Bottom — left)* **Stromal histiocyte with erythrophagocytosis: Infiltrating carcinoma of breast**

This histiocyte contains numerous lysosomes of variable size and density. Degradative changes affect the ingested erythrocyte, with rupture and partial collapse of its membrane (arrows). (×9100)

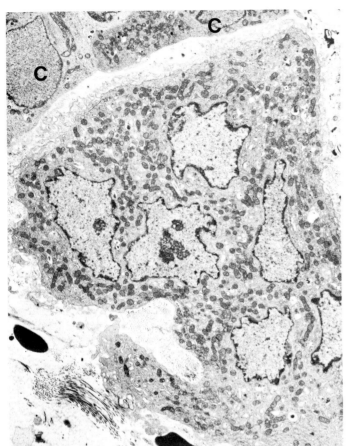

### Fig. 3.13 Multinucleated stromal histiocytic giant cell: Infiltrating duct carcinoma of breast

Locally recurrent carcinoma from a 50-year-old woman; by LM the stromal giant cells were a striking feature, often overshadowing the ductal component. The giant cell portrayed here has a histiocytic appearance (compare with the histiocytic giant cell in Fig. 20.13). Six nuclear profiles are evident and there are numerous mitochondria. Many plasmalemmal ruffles emanate from the periphery of the cell; these appear to be most elaborate adjacent to the group of carcinomatous cells (C) occupying the upper left corner of the micrograph. (×3800)

See also Chapter 7.
References: 330, 335, 1358, 1381, 1386, 1439

### Fig. 3.14 Stromal myofibroblasts I: Testicular choriocarcinoma

The myofibroblasts illustrated have appearances intermediate between fibroblasts and smooth muscle; they contain numerous fine actin-like filaments with dense bodies (arrowheads) and peripheral attachment zones, together with RER. The largest cell displays nuclear crenellation, perhaps attributable to contraction, and there are two nuclear bodies. Micropinocytotic vesicles are situated beneath the plasma membrane in some regions (arrows), and both collagen fibres and external laminal material (E) are closely related to the cells. (×12 800)

Myofibroblasts have been described in three main pathological settings, namely inflammatory and repair phenomena, quasineoplastic fibroproliferative disorders and neoplasia (Tables 3.5 and 3.6).

See also Figs. 4.5 and 5.6.
References: 323, 351, 364, 365, 370–372, 380, 1421, 1499, 2247, 2252, 2265, 2268, 2271, 2294, 2388, 2657

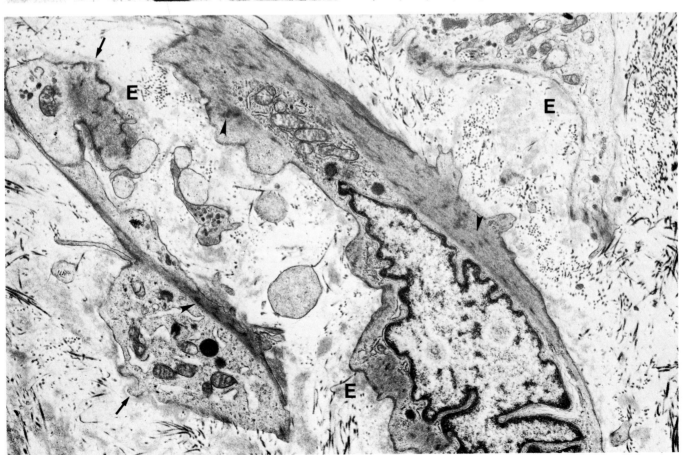

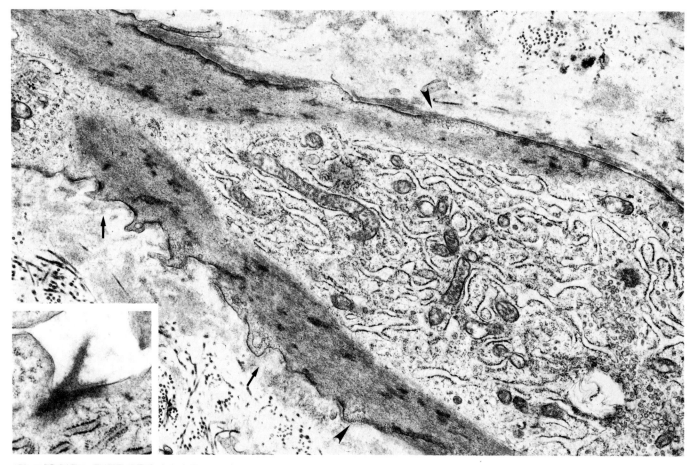

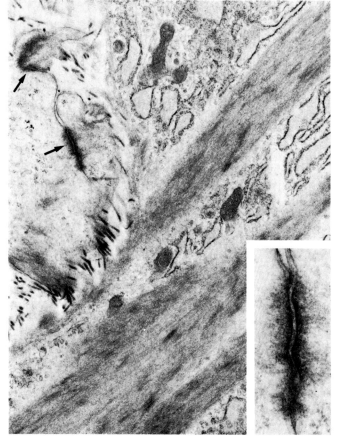

**Fig. 3.15 Stromal myofibroblasts II: Testicular choriocarcinoma, and adenocarcinoma of lung**

Cytoplasmic detail of a myofibroblast is illustrated. Fine filaments with dense bodies and subplasmalemmal linear densities are shown, and micropinocytotic vesicles are also apparent (arrowheads). External lamina lies adjacent to the cell in some areas (arrows), and the cytoplasm contains moderate quantities of RER. **Inset:** Microtendon attached to the region of a subplasmalemmal linear density of a stromal myofibroblast in a pulmonary adenocarcinoma. (×16 700. Inset: ×25 900)

**Fig. 3.16 Stromal myofibroblasts III: Infiltrating duct carcinoma of breast**

Bundles of thin myofilaments with dense bodies are disposed in the long axis of the myofibroblast; a small amount of RER is also included in this field.

Intermediate junctions (arrows) link adjoining plasma membranes; when well developed, junctions of this type can be mistaken for desmosomes, but at high magnification (inset) they lack the characteristic morphology and intercellular linear densities of desmosomes as illustrated in Fig. 4.3. They should not be misconstrued as evidence of epithelial differentiation. (×15 900. Inset: ×54 600)

See also Figs. 4.5 and 20.7.

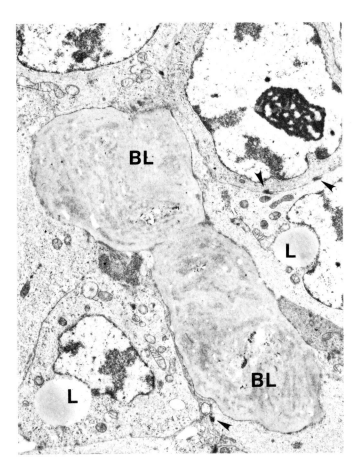

### Fig. 3.17 Adenoid cystic carcinoma (solid variant): Nodular accumulation of basal lamina

The intercellular space is expanded by a nodular mass of inhomogeneous but non-fibrillated basal lamina (BL) in which a few collagen fibres are embedded. In adenoid cystic carcinoma the laminal replication classically has a distinctly fibrillated and multilayered appearance. By LM the PAS-positivity of such nodules may be misinterpreted as mucin within acini. A few lipid droplets (L) and desmosomes (arrowheads) are also present. (×11 600)

References: 700, 705, 724, 725, 727–729, 737, 741, 744, 748, 750, 762, 786, 1049, 1184, 1405, 1428

### Fig. 3.18 Stromal collagen and elastin: Infiltrating duct carcinoma of breast, and haemangiopericytoma

Both collagen (C) and elastin (E) fibres are evident adjacent to a stromal blood vessel in an infiltrating mammary carcinoma. (×17 300)

**Inset:** Fibrous long-spacing collagen showing the characteristic 100 nm periodicity, in a presacral haemangiopericytoma. (×31 000)

**Discussion:** Although usually absent in benign breast disorders, stromal elastosis has been ultrastructurally documented in infiltrating ductal and lobular carcinomas; local elastosis has also been found in intraductal carcinomas, but appears to be more 'orderly' than that encountered in infiltrating tumours.[354] Medullary carcinoma elicits only a minimal stromal elastotic response. The possibility that the elastic fibres are produced by the carcinomatous cells has been raised; however, both fibroblasts and myofibroblasts constitute more important sources, being both abundant and closely associated with the elastin fibres.[354]

See also Figs. 18.2 and 20.6.

References: 324, 354, 356, 360, 375, 1361, 1376, 1435, 2270, 2758, 2769, 2778

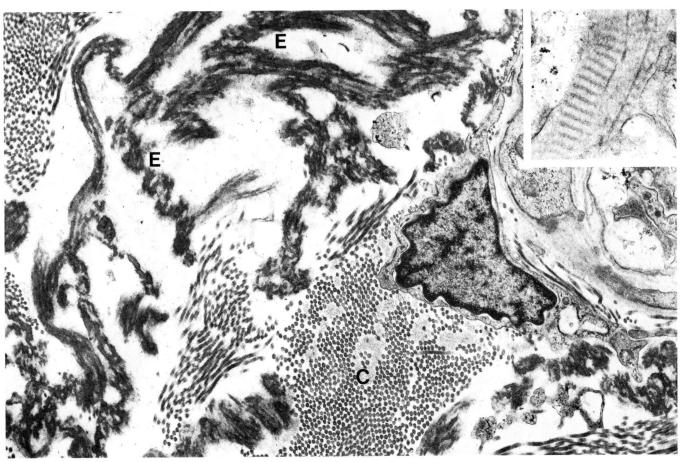

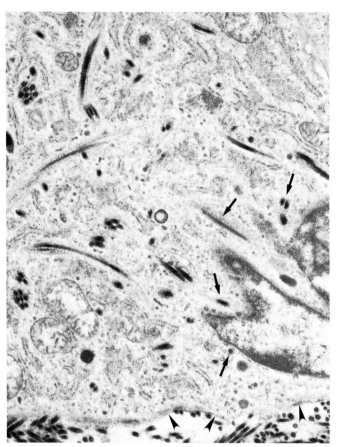

### Fig. 3.19 Fibroblast with intracytoplasmic collagen: Colonic adenocarcinoma

The cytoplasm of this stromal fibroblast contains numerous membrane-bound collections of collagen fibres, possibly intracisternal in location and raising the possibility of intracellular collagen synthesis. The profusion of the fibres and their proximity to the nucleus (arrows) indicate that they are truly intracellular, instead of representing tangential sections of extracellular fibres enfolded by cytoplasmic flaps; this interpretation is reinforced by the relatively smooth outline of the plasma membrane (arrowheads), but in other instances the distinction requires serial sectioning. (×14 700)

**Discussion:** Intracytoplasmic collagen is also recorded in the fibroblastoid cells of fibrohistiocytic tumours such as fibrous histiocytomas and the fibromatoses, occasionally including the fibrous long-spacing variety.[2299] In non-neoplastic disorders characterized by rapid dissolution of connective tissue, collagen has been identified in both macrophages and fibroblasts, within lysosome-like vacuoles containing acid phosphatase. The participation of macrophages in the removal of collagen fibres by way of phagocytosis and subsequent intralysosomal digestion has therefore been invoked.[47] It is conceivable that similar degradative activity occurs in tumours, accounting for some instances of intracellular collagen.

See also Figs. 9.6 and 20.5.
References: 47, 2204, 2243, 2270, 2299

### Fig. 3.20 Stromal calcification: Infiltrating duct carcinoma of breast

Calcification appears to have occurred in successive layers, and a peripheral electron-dense layer of hydroxyapatite crystals is present. In epithelial tumours calcification may also occur within the neoplastic cells (for example in matrical dense bodies of mitochondria and in areas of cytoplasmic electron-lucency),[808] or in their secretory products. In sarcomas the deposition of hydroxyapatite crystals on collagen fibres is characteristic of osteogenic sarcoma (see Chapter 25). (×17 000)

See also Figs. 14.7, 17.21 and 25.6.
References: 671, 685, 808, 826, 1227, 1283, 1361, 1719, 1746, 2034, 2042, 2047, 2051, 2602, 2659

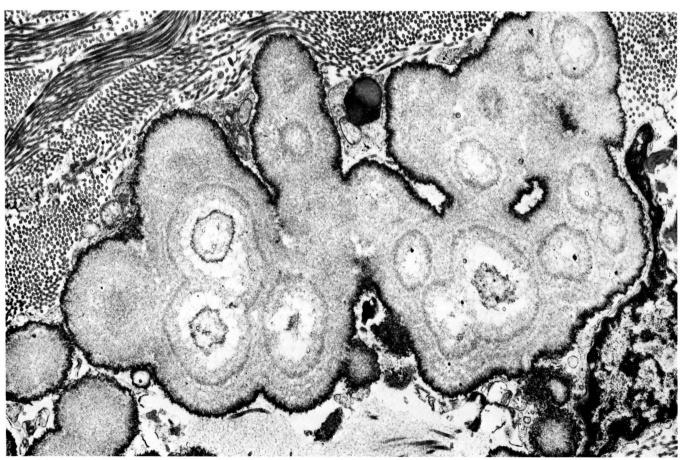

# PART TWO

## The Special Fine Structure of Neoplasia

# 4  Squamous and transitional cell tumours

## SQUAMOUS CELL CARCINOMAS

Squamous cell carcinomas generally show close morphological similarities to each other, irrespective of their site of origin,[86] but different features vary in prevalence and prominence according to the degree of differentiation. Electron microscopy is extremely valuable in establishing the diagnosis in poorly differentiated tumours such as nasopharyngeal carcinoma. Ultrastructural studies have also established that so-called large cell undifferentiated carcinoma of lung represents a heterogeneous collection of extremely poorly differentiated carcinomas, with squamous or composite adenosquamous features being found in about half the cases examined[468,507] (see Chapter 7). Similar results have been obtained for apparently undifferentiated carcinomas of the uterine cervix, where the squamous tumours predominate[1152] (see Table 30.1).

Although not as frequent as in normal squamous epithelia, desmosomes are a major feature of squamous cell carcinomas.[86,298,468] The desmosomes are often incompletely developed, especially in poorly differentiated carcinomas, but enough with the typical appearances can usually be found to establish the diagnosis. Intracytoplasmic desmosomes are not infrequent, but their mode of formation is uncertain.[44,45]

Bundles of tonofilaments are also characteristic of squamous carcinomas. Such tonofibrillar bundles may be small and disarrayed, and it is imperative that they be distinguished from other filamentous components of the cytoplasm by their convergence towards desmosomes. Thinner, less osmiophilic actin-like filaments with associated dense zones are also described in squamous cell carcinomas,[254] and are distinguished from tonofibrils by their morphology, peripheral distribution and parallelism with the cell surface (Fig. 4.6). Similar differences in the distribution of tonofilaments and actin filaments have been detected in the cells of pleomorphic salivary adenomas by immuno-electron microscopy.[698]

Tonofilaments are sometimes referred to as 'keratin',[86] 'cytokeratin' or 'prekeratin' filaments, but these appellations are imprecise, as emphasized by Ghadially.[47] For example, keratin is rich in sulphur whereas tonofilaments are not, and normal keratinization involves an intermediary step, namely the development of keratohyaline granules, which form a substrate for the accumulation of keratins.* The expression 'prekeratin filament' is perhaps less objectionable and the filaments appear to be spatially associated with immunoreactivity for so-called prekeratin antibody. The

situation is further complicated by the recognition that the 'cytokeratins' characteristic of all epithelia have multiple components which vary with the type of epithelium;[272] thus high molecular weight components appear to be specific for keratinizing squamous epithelia, and ectocervical and anal epithelia, whereas other components typify non-squamous epithelia (see Table 2.8). Confusion has also arisen through use of the term 'keratin' in two separate ways:

1.  For the keratinous end-product of epidermis and certain squamous neoplasms; we use 'keratin' and 'keratinization' exclusively in this sense.
2.  For a cytoskeletal constituent characteristic of a variety of epithelial cells, whether keratinizing or not.[276]

As well as differences in their subfractions, there is evidence that immunoreactive cytokeratins differ in both quantity and distribution in the above two situations. In view of the foregoing, we prefer to use the traditional non-committal term 'tonofilament' as a purely ultrastructural description for this class of intermediate filament (Fig. 4.2), reserving 'prekeratin' and 'cytokeratins' as immunocytochemical terms.

Keratohyaline granules, distinguished by their electron-density and oblong shapes (Fig. 4.2), are occasionally seen in squamous carcinomas, but are usually undetectable in poorly differentiated tumours, and keratinosomes (membrane-coating granules; lamellar granules) are unlikely to be found. In addition, some cells may show keratinization, characterized by low- to high-density filaments replacing the cytoplasmic contents (Fig. 4.7).

Cytoplasmic glycogen is sometimes prominent, perhaps due to phosphorylase deficiency.[1461] The development of other cytoplasmic organelles and components is dependent on the degree of differentiation, but these are of limited value in diagnostic evaluation.

Basal laminae are usually present around aggregates of squamous cells and may show attachment to cells by hemidesmosomes; the laminae vary in thickness and are often incomplete — especially in poorly differentiated squamous

---

*The synthesis of keratohyalin and keratins by keratinocytes is a complex process which has yet to be fully elucidated; nevertheless, there have been major recent advances in our understanding of the process, as reviewed by Baden.[3144] Keratohyalin consists of histidine-rich proteins produced in the upper stratum spinosum and the stratum granulosum of the epidermis. The development of keratohyaline granules appears to involve the participation of basic proteins known as filaggrins,[3144] which form a matrix for the fibrous protein, organizing it into aggregates.[3144] The formation of the cornified envelopes in the stratum corneum is apparently related to cross-linkage of the proteins keratolynin and involucrin by the enzyme transglutaminase.[3144]

carcinomas — while prominent reduplication of basal lamina is described in verrucous carcinoma.[669] The spaces between adjacent neoplastic squamous cells may be wide (perhaps attributable in part to artefactual shrinkage, and/or disintegration of necrotic tumour cells), and contain many cell processes; the appearances may then simulate acini with microvilli (Fig. 4.8), but absence of the junctional complexes characteristic of acinus formation and other indicators of glandular epithelial differentiation (see Chapter 5) help to make the distinction from adenocarcinoma. Rarely, the processes are so numerous and elongated that they simulate mesothelial differentiation (so-called 'anemone' cells),[421,423,424] but once again junctional complexes are not present.

*Minimal criteria for the ultrastructural identification of squamous differentiation:* Desmosome-tonofilament complexes and cytoplasmic tonofibrils, as illustrated in Figs. 4.1–4.11, are essential features. These characteristics must be present in pure form for a diagnosis of squamous cell carcinoma; the additional finding of other forms of differentiation indicates a composite carcinoma (for example, adenosquamous carcinoma; see Chapter 7). Desmosomes and tonofilaments are also encountered in other neoplasms such as adenocarcinoma without necessarily implying squamous differentiation, but in these circumstances they are neither as numerous nor well constructed as in squamous carcinomas of equivalent differentiation.

## SPINDLE CELL SQUAMOUS CARCINOMA

Squamous cell carcinomas with an extensive spindle cell component are well documented in the skin, pharynx, larynx, oesophagus and breast.[1387,1474] The nature of the spindle cells has long been the subject of speculation and controversy. A number of ultrastructural studies have reported evidence of squamous differentiation in the spindle cells.[1474,1494] Some, published before the heyday of the myofibroblast, can be discounted; they embody misinterpretation of intermediate junctions, longitudinal cytoplasmic actin-like filaments and even fragmentary external lamina possessed by myofibroblasts, as evidence of squamous properties. Nevertheless, unequivocal squamous features have been documented by EM,[1157,1474] an observation supported by the immunocytochemical detection of cytokeratins.[1157,1512] In other cases the spindle cells have been found to have mesenchymal characteristics,[1474] with varying proportions of undifferentiated cells, fibroblasts, myofibroblasts and histiocytes. Finally, an admixture of squamous and mesenchymal cells may be found occasionally, sometimes with the simultaneous expression of both myofibroblastic and squamous epithelial properties by single cells, as indicated by the dual presence of abundant myofilaments and desmosome-tonofilament complexes. We have observed both squamous and fibrohistiocytic differentiation in our cases and agree with both Battifora[1457] and Harris[1474] that the findings are explicable on the basis of mesenchymal metaplasia developing in, and to varying degrees effacing, an original clone of squamous cells.

Actin is a constituent of many non-myoid cell lines, presumably being related to contractile and locomotor functions. Small numbers of actin-like microfilaments are also common in epithelial neoplasms including squamous cell carcinoma and malignant melanoma (Figs. 4.6 and 8.6), and there are indications that some epithelial cells can also synthesize collagen.[52] Whether or not such properties should be regarded as evidence of 'mesenchymal metaplasia' is open to speculation, and on a philosophical plane they pose fundamental questions as to what constitutes a 'differentiation' characteristic. However, these observations do serve to blur the traditionally sharp distinction between mesenchymal and epithelial tissues, and suggest that a spindle cell component in epithelial tumours sometimes reflects derepression of mesenchymal potentialities, which usually are only minimally expressed, if at all.

## BASAL CELL CARCINOMA OF SKIN

The diagnosis of cutaneous basal cell carcinoma is ordinarily straightforward, but occasionally there are difficulties in deciding whether a tumour represents a basal or squamous cell carcinoma. EM is unlikely to resolve this issue, since the tumour cells in basal cell carcinoma have squamoid appearances in the form of cell processes traversing a relatively wide intercellular space, cytoplasmic tonofibrils, and desmosome-tonofilament complexes. The nuclei are large in proportion to the cytoplasm and contain abundant euchromatin; they vary from rounded to fusiform, with only slight irregularity. An admixture of other 'intruder' cell types may be found; thus Macadam[1497] detected Langerhans' cells in 20 of 32 basal cell carcinomas, while eight contained melanocytes, and Merkel cells were seen in one case. The nests of tumour cells are invested by basal lamina; myofibroblasts or amyloid may be seen in the stroma.[1475,1499]

## CRANIOPHARYNGIOMA

The craniopharyngioma is composed predominantly of squamous cells, with varying proportions of glial, vascular and connective tissue elements.[1623] Microcysts (acinar spaces) lined by cells with numerous microvilli and subluminal junctional complexes are also described.[1719] The squamous epithelium in one case we studied by EM closely simulated the maturation of fetal epidermis, while keratinization is said to be a characteristic finding.[1623] The diagnosis of craniopharyngioma is achieved by light microscopy.

## ODONTOGENIC TUMOURS

The diagnosis of odontogenic tumours is established by LM; EM has little, if any, place in this exercise, but may be of value in elucidating the nature of some of the cellular or stromal components.

The *ameloblastoma* exhibits squamous epithelial features, sometimes with a layer of columnar cells at the periphery of the cell nests, corresponding to the zonal appearances on LM. Scattered 'dark' cells are also present, especially in areas of cystic change.[681] In an analysis of 21 cases, Nasu & Ishikawa[683] subdivided ameloblastoma into plexiform and follicular types, the former consisting only of squamous cells. The follicular type was additionally characterized by columnar cells at the periphery of the follicles and resembled the enamel organ; intracytoplasmic lumina were also described, but there were no subluminal secretory granules. Langerhans' histiocytes have also been recorded in a 'simple' ameloblastoma.[681] The hyalinized zone surrounding the epithelial nests is seen by EM to consist of varying quantities of amorphous to finely granular material[681] admixed with collagen fibres, as well as anchoring fibrils and fine 100–150 nm fibrils (possibly oxytalan);[675] the fibrils tend to fuse with the fragmentary external lamina at the epithelio-stromal interface.[675] Stromal myofibroblasts may also be seen, and in one reported case of simple ameloblastoma they possessed intracellular septate junctions.[686]

The *calcifying epithelial odontogenic tumour of Pindborg* is also composed of squamous cells; these are characteristically associated with fibrillary, focally calcifying extracellular material, which has been designated as 'amyloid' largely on the basis of staining characteristics. Page et al[685] could not demonstrate well-formed fibrils by EM; instead, the hyaline masses had a poorly defined granulofibrillary appearance with a laminar conformation. It was suggested that this 'amyloid' may be a protein product of the enamel organ, different to conventional fibrillary amyloid, and that its accumulation was the dual result of active secretion and cell death. The 'amyloid' found in *adenomatoid odontogenic tumour* may also be derived from enamel protein (which can have a β-protein

configuration), and well-formed fibrils 10 nm in diameter are described.[689]

The nature of the adamantinoma of long bones is discussed in Chapter 25.

## TRANSITIONAL CELL TUMOURS

Transitional cell carcinomas recapitulate to varying degrees the normal features of urothelium.[1057,1080,1081] The surface epithelium is characterized by ridges and microvilli, but in contrast with normal transitional cells, deep vesicles are quite uncommon. The intercellular junctions include desmosomes, while junctional complexes occur at the free surface. Plasma membrane interleaving is usually present and the intermediary cells are separated by a comparatively wide intercellular space. A fragmentary basal lamina separates the cells from the subjacent stroma. Intercellular and subcellular crypts may be found,[1044] many probably representing irregular extensions of the surface membrane. In such circumstances, the distinction from adenocarcinoma is based on the relative paucity of the Golgi complexes and secretory granules.

Adenocarcinomas of the urinary bladder are often associated with foci of urothelial differentiation, but have no ultrastructural features peculiar to this site (see Chapter 5). The plasma membranes form microvilli with a prominent glycocalyx.[1047] Junctional complexes are present between adjoining cells; in freeze-fracture preparations the tight junctions are proliferated, but poorly formed, while gap junctions are small and sparse.[1047]

We have also identified bimorphic glandular and urothelial differentiation in an ultrastructural study of an inverted urinary papilloma, as reported earlier by Alroy and associates[1043] (Figs. 4.16–4.18).

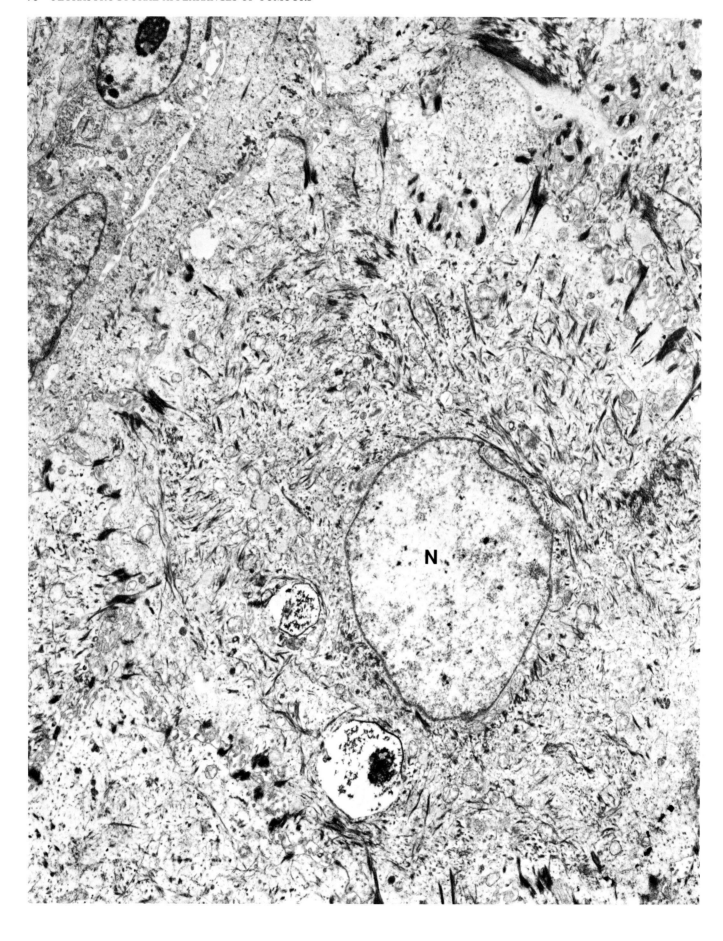

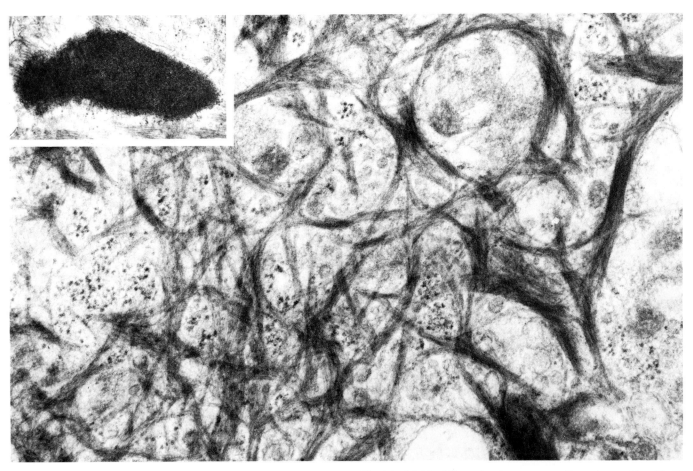

**Fig. 4.2   Highly differentiated squamous cell carcinoma: Tonofibrils and keratohyaline granule**

The tonofibrillar bundles consist of sheaves of tonofilaments averaging 7.5 nm in diameter. In comparison to the appearances seen in normal keratinocytes, the bundles show considerable disarray; in some tumours they form a distinct perinuclear wreath. ($\times 64\ 900$)

**Inset:** Osmiophilic keratohyaline granule from a squamous cell carcinoma. The granule shows no evidence of a filamentous substructure. ($\times 32\ 600$)

**Fig. 4.1** *(Facing page)*   **Highly differentiated squamous cell carcinoma: Survey**

Bronchogenic carcinoma in a 64-year-old man. Even at this low magnification, numerous electron-dense tonofibrils are apparent, many converging perpendicularly onto desmosomes at the apices of cell processes. The nucleus (N) is only slightly irregular, but contains abundant euchromatin. ($\times 8600$)

References: 45, 109, 257, 468, 534, 538, 539, 548, 669, 783, 784, 1066, 1174, 1175, 1386, 1457, 1474, 2152

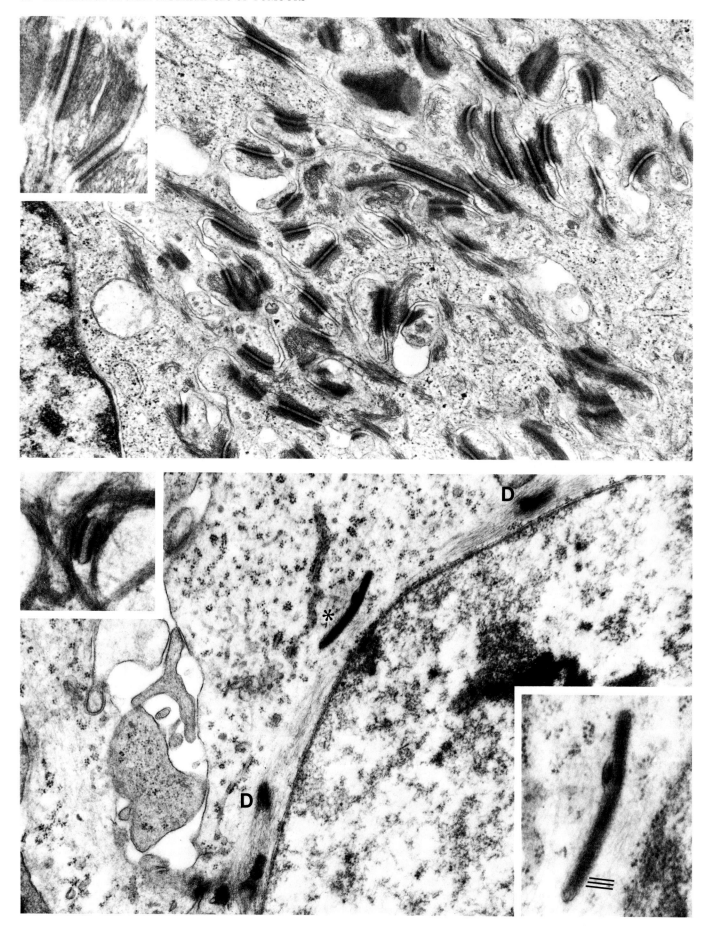

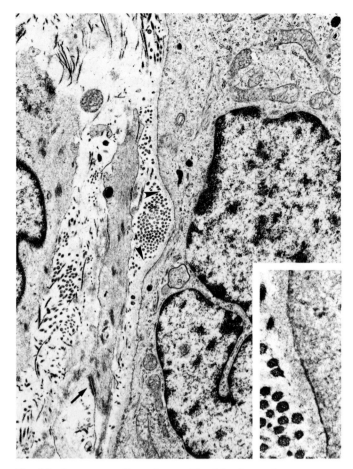

**Fig. 4.5 Squamous cell carcinoma: Basal lamina and stroma**

A layer of grey basal lamina (arrowheads) invests one of a group of squamous cells. Myofibroblasts are present in the adjacent stroma, where two of their plasma membranes are attached by an intermediate junction (arrow), and collagen fibres are also evident. **Inset:** the basal lamina at higher magnification, showing a suggestion of a fibrillary substructure. (×13 000. Inset: ×52 800)

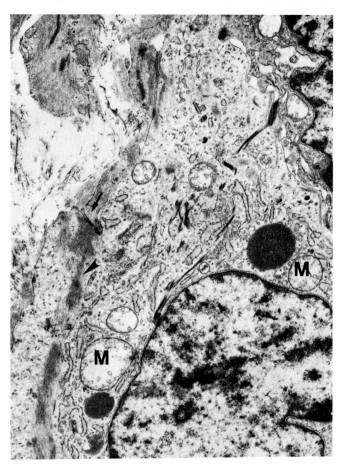

**Fig. 4.6 Moderately differentiated bronchogenic squamous cell carcinoma: Actin-like microfilaments**

Two adjoining neoplastic cells are attached by desmosomes; osmiophilic tonofibrils converge on the desmosomes, and are also seen in the paranuclear region. The peripheral cytoplasm contains aggregates of microfilaments; these tend to be longitudinally orientated, have a 'softer' appearance than the tonofibrils and form less discrete bundles. Individual filaments cannot be resolved at this magnification, but associated dense zones are evident (arrowhead), and the nearby plasma membranes sometimes form intermediate junctions (arrow). Swollen mitochondria (M) can also be seen. (×11 300)
    Reference: 254

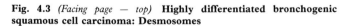

**Fig. 4.4** *(Facing page — bottom)* **Squamous cell carcinoma: Intracytoplasmic desmosomes**

Poorly differentiated bronchogenic tumour in a 71-year-old male. Intracytoplasmic desmosomes (D) with associated tonofilaments lie adjacent to the outer nuclear envelope. One of these has been sectioned tangentially (*) and is shown in detail in the inset (lower right) where it displays transverse periodicity (bars). Another intracytoplasmic desmosome (inset, upper left) shows typical desmosome morphology and is surrounded by sheaves of tonofilaments. (× 27 500. Inset, lower right: × 57 700. Inset upper left: × 80 900)

Intracytoplasmic desmosomes in syncytiotrophoblast are attributable to fusion of cytotrophoblastic cells, but their manner of development in seemingly mononuclear neoplastic cells is unclear. They have also been found in an apudoma and a phaeochromocytoma, and we have found large aggregates of intracytoplasmic desmosomes in a poorly differentiated adenocarcinoma of lung with atypical giant cell formation.
    References: 44, 45, 47

**Fig. 4.3** *(Facing page — top)* **Highly differentiated bronchogenic squamous cell carcinoma: Desmosomes**

There are numerous interweaving cell processes with long desmosomes, some of which have been sectioned tangentially. (×41 100)

**Inset:** Desmosomes at higher magnification, showing the characteristic appearances. The paradesmosomal cytoplasm displays plate-like thickening, with converging tonofilaments. The intercellular spaces are approximately 25 nm wide, and contain moderately electron-dense material in which there are linear densities. (×78 000)
    References: 39, 45, 259, 266, 298

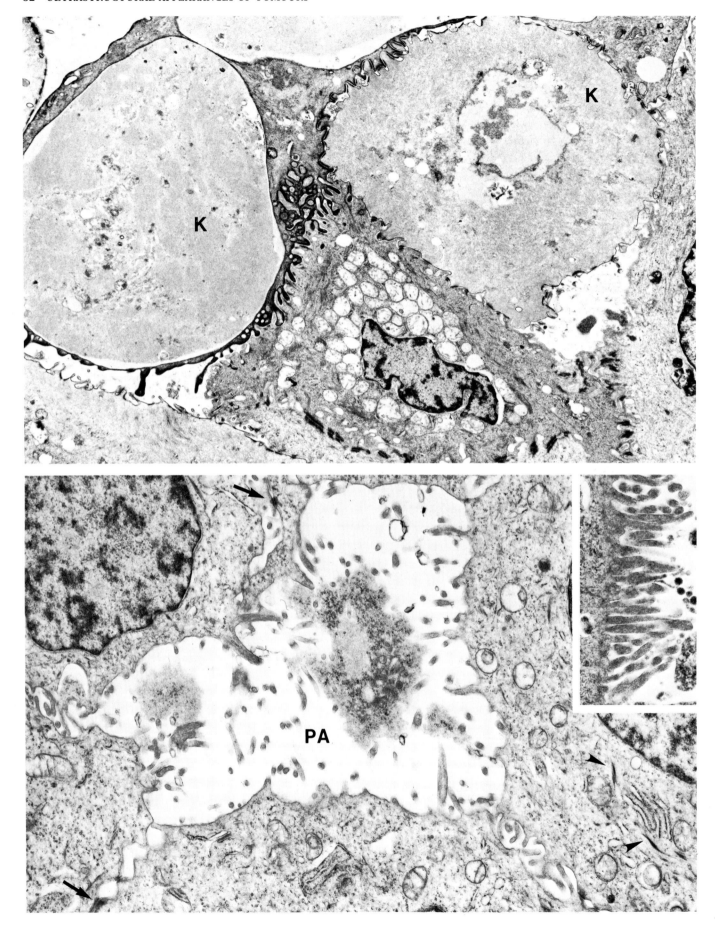

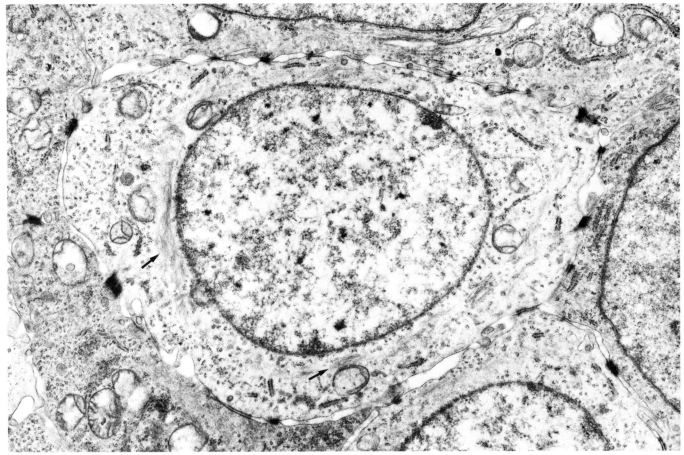

**Fig. 4.9 Poorly differentiated squamous cell carcinoma: Cell relationships and morphology**

Tumour of left lower lobar bronchus in a 51-year-old man. In contrast to the highly and moderately differentiated carcinomas illustrated in the preceding figures, the cells are more closely apposed, with a corresponding diminution in the intercellular spaces, while cell processes are both fewer and shorter. Apical desmosomes are apparent, but there are only a few small bundles of paranuclear tonofilaments (arrows). ($\times$14 400)

**Fig. 4.8** *(Facing page — bottom)* **Squamous cell carcinoma: Pseudoacinar space and microvillous processes**

Metastatic carcinoma in an axillary lymph node of a man aged 83 years. Pseudoacinar expansions (PA) of the intercellular space are not infrequent in squamous cell carcinomas, some apparently resulting from necrosis and 'drop-out' of tumour cells. Although desmosomes (arrows) are present, the absence of subluminal junctional complexes distinguishes such spaces from true acini (see Chapter 5). Tonofilaments (arrowheads) are also evident. ($\times$12 600)

**Inset:** Orderly microvillous processes may also occur in squamous cell carcinomas. Once again, the distinction from adenocarcinoma is based primarily on the lack of junctional complexes. In addition, membrane-bound secretory granules, a terminal filamentous web, penetrating microvillous core rootlets and surface glycocalyx are all absent. Bronchogenic squamous cell carcinoma. ($\times$14 500)

References: 468, 470

**Fig. 4.7** *(Facing page — top)* **Highly differentiated squamous cell carcinoma: Keratinization**

There is an accumulation of low-density filaments replacing most of the cytoplasmic contents (K), indicating early keratinization. The plasma membrane regions of the intervening cells are often extremely osmiophilic. The appearances closely resemble those of the final stages of maturation of epidermal keratinocytes. ($\times$8200)

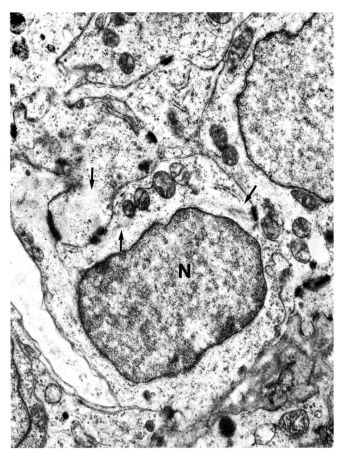

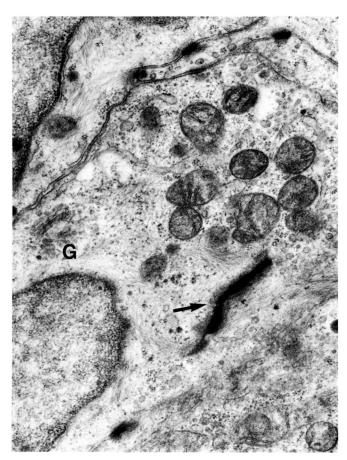

**Fig. 4.10  Nasopharyngeal carcinoma I: Cell morphology, including desmosomes**

Ultrastructural investigations have demonstrated the squamous nature of this neoplasm, although the degree of differentiation varies. In this field only a narrow rim of cytoplasm surrounds the slightly irregular nucleus (N). Desmosomes are prominent, but the bundles of tonofilaments (arrows) are poorly developed. Keratinosomes have been reported, while intracisternal tubular inclusions are not uncommon in the cytoplasm of the malignant cells. Elaborate elongated cell processes simulating mesothelial differentiation have also been described. Tumour from a middle-aged Chinese man. (×12 100)

References: 392, 397, 406, 421

**Fig. 4.11  Nasopharyngeal carcinoma II: Cell detail**

Same case as Fig. 4.10. There is an intracytoplasmic desmosome (arrow) in this neoplastic cell; a small Golgi apparatus (G) is also present. (×19 400)

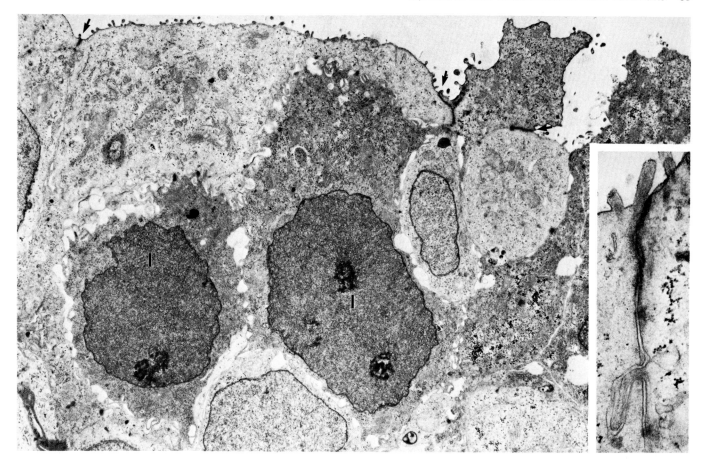

## Fig. 4.12 Moderately differentiated transitional cell (urothelial) carcinoma: Architecture and junctional complex

Papillary tumour of urinary bladder (W.H.O. Grade II). The surface epithelium forms cytoplasmic ridges and microvilli, and there are superficial junctional complexes (arrows), one of which is detailed in the inset. Note that asymmetrical unit membranes and precursor discoid vesicles are not present. Two intermediary cells (I) are evident, and some cells contain glycogen. (×5500. Inset: ×32 100)

Scanning EM of the surface of such tumours reveals pleomorphic microvilli — which appear to be a constant feature, irrespective of tumour grade[1065] — and a network of microridges. Other findings include superficial dark cells, as well as abnormalities of the junctional complexes and subjacent basal lamina.[1077] The tumour cells have been·divided into a number of subtypes depending on microvillar morphology and frequency, but this exercise lacks practical value.

References: 1044, 1046, 1057, 1068, 1079–1082

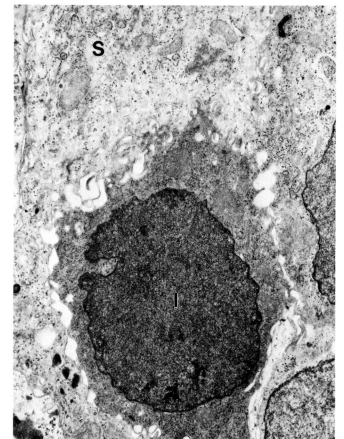

## Fig. 4.13 Moderately differentiated transitional cell carcinoma: Intermediary cell

This intermediary cell (I) shows greater electron-density than the superficial epithelial cell (S), beneath which it is situated. The intercellular space is relatively wide, and is bridged by short cytoplasmic processes. (×7600)

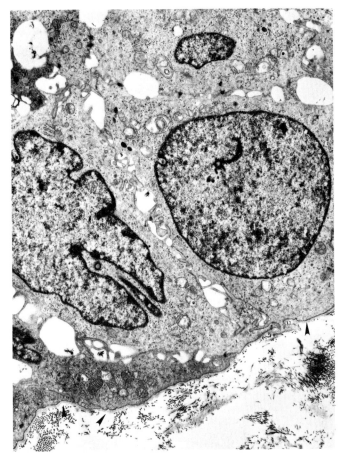

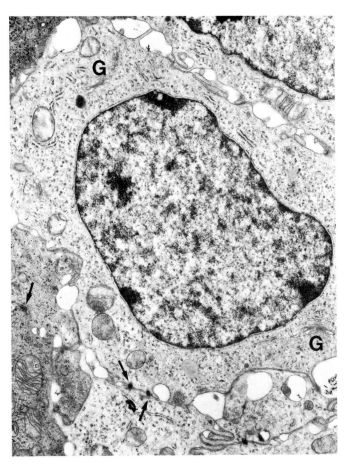

**Fig. 4.14 Invasive poorly differentiated transitional cell carcinoma: Architecture**

Retroperitoneal recurrence of a previously resected infiltrating carcinoma of the ureter. This cell nest is invested by basal lamina (arrowheads); the intercellular spaces are quite wide and are interrupted by short desmosomes and interdigitating cytoplasmic processes. Tonofilaments are not evident. Compare with squamous cell carcinoma (Fig. 4.9). (×5900)

**Fig. 4.15 Poorly differentiated transitional cell carcinoma: Cell morphology**

The Golgi apparatus (G) is apparent and there are numerous polyribosomes. Short strands of RER can also be seen, but there are no tonofilaments, secretory granules or microvilli. However, the cells form frequent processes interdigitating across the extracellular space. Intermittent desmosomes (arrows) join the plasma membranes. Compare with Fig. 4.13. (×9700)

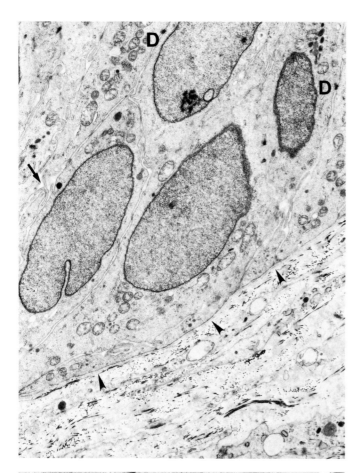

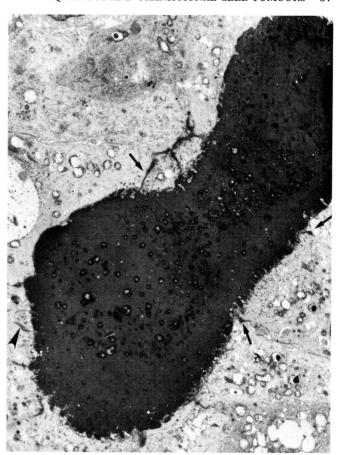

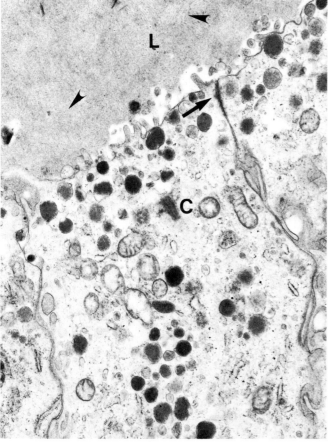

**Fig. 4.16** *(Top — left)* **Inverted urinary papilloma: Urothelial cells and epithelio-stromal interface**

Prolapsed pedunculated tumour from the bladder neck of a man aged 46 years. Although numerous elsewhere, only a few desmosomes (D) are included in this field. Cytoplasmic processes protrude into the intercellular space (arrow). The nuclei contain plentiful euchromatin, while the cytoplasm is devoid of tonofibrils. Basal lamina (arrowheads) separates the urothelial cells from the collagen-containing stroma, but there is no laminal reduplication as described by Alroy et al.[1043] (×6900)

Figs. 4.16–4.18 are all from the same case.

References: 1043, 1064, 1069

**Fig. 4.17** *(Top — right)* **Inverted urinary papilloma: Acinus I**

The acinus depicted here at low magnification corresponds to the presence of microglandular structures containing eosinophilic colloid-like secretion on LM. The lumen is filled with electron-dense matter into which microvilli project. A few microvillar core rootlets (arrowhead) are evident, as are subluminal junctional complexes (arrows). The appearances indicate glandular differentiation. (×4700)

**Fig. 4.18** *(Bottom — left)* **Inverted urinary papilloma: Acinus II**

Portion of another crypt lumen (L) is shown at higher magnification, together with detail of the apical cytoplasm of the lining epithelial cells. Numerous membrane-bound secretory granules of varying size and electron-density inhabit the cytoplasm, and a centriole (C) is also present. A tight junction of a junctional complex is indicated by the arrow. The cells possess irregular surface microvilli, while the intraluminal secretion sometimes forms paracrystalline arrays (arrowheads); the filaments comprising these arrays average about 25 nm in diameter, while in a report of two cases documenting almost identical appearances, Iwata et al[1064] give an average diameter of 30 nm. (×13 700)

Reference: 1064

# 5  Glandular epithelial tumours

## GENERAL REMARKS ON GLANDULAR EPITHELIAL TUMOURS

Adenocarcinomas are characterized by acinus formation, but in poorly differentiated tumours the acini may be small and only distinguishable by ultrastructural techniques.[86,468] Variable numbers of short, blunt microvilli project into the lumina and may be covered by glycocalyx. The combination of membrane-associated glycocalyceal bodies and microvillar filamentous cores penetrating underlying cytoplasm is valuable in identifying tumours differentiating as intestinal-type epithelium (Fig. 5.7). A terminal web containing actin, actomyosin complexes and intermediate filaments may also be seen in the cytoplasm immediately adjacent to the luminal microvilli.[39] Junctional complexes are found in the subluminal region between the cells forming the acini (Fig. 5.3), while intermediate junctions and desmosomes occur elsewhere on the cell periphery.

Intracellular crypts (neolumina) may sometimes be found, and are also lined by short blunt microvilli coated with glycocalyceal material (Fig. 5.5). The mode of development of these intracytoplasmic neolumina is uncertain. Step sections have sometimes demonstrated continuity between the crypt and the extracellular space, indicating a process of plasma membrane inversion (Fig. 5.21).[1044] In other cases, the neolumina may represent sequestrated intracytoplasmic microacini,[1044] perhaps resulting from progressive distension of Golgi complexes; the possibility of an origin from agglomerated mucin granules has also been raised.[47]

Secretory products may accumulate in the intracellular crypts as well as in the intercellular acinar spaces. Accumulation of mucin within neolumina and/or aggregates of cytoplasmic mucin granules correspond to the presence of intracytoplasmic mucin droplets by LM, which can therefore be interpreted as evidence of glandular differentiation in an otherwise undifferentiated carcinoma. Signet-ring cells are ultrastructurally typified by abundant intracytoplasmic mucin granules of varying size, displacing the nucleus to the periphery of the cell; the plasma membranes are often smooth and devoid of an associated external lamina, but laminal material is seen occasionally (Fig. 5.10) and is sometimes reduplicated.[1047]

Secretory granules vary in dimensions and morphology, but tend to concentrate in the vicinity of the acinar lumen or intracellular canaliculus. Mucin is a common secretory product, but the amounts produced can be small. The morphological characteristics of mucin-containing granules vary greatly (Figs. 5.8–5.11). They may be punctate or flocculent, while dense cores, skein-like substructures, and even electron-lucent material may be present;[47,55] neighbouring granules are often closely apposed and even partly fused. Distinctive elongated membrane-bound fibrillary bodies thought to represent mucin granules are sometimes seen in endocervical adenocarcinomas (Fig. 5.11).[39,1154] Small electron-dense immature mucin granules about 100–300 nm in diameter occur in gastrointestinal adenocarcinomas; they may closely resemble neurosecretory granules,[39] but are recognizable in part by their concentration in the subluminal cytoplasm, where they are often closely related to the penetrating filamentous cores of microvilli. The morphology of other secretory granules is sometimes distinctive, as with the large osmiophilic granules typical of acinic cell tumours (Fig. 5.14), lamellar granules in alveolar type II cell carcinomas, and the paracrystalline granules of so-called Clara cell carcinomas (Table 5.3). Often, it is impossible to determine the nature of the secretory products solely on the basis of granule morphology.

Intracellular polarity is also reflected by the localization of the Golgi complexes relative to the secretory granules and the abortive lumina. In secretory cells the Golgi apparatus is generally well developed and is roughly proportional to the mass of secretory granules.

Cellular apposition in adenocarcinomas is close, often with focal plasma membrane interdigitation. In addition, fragmentary basal laminal material may be found at the periphery of cell clusters, but is often absent from the pericellular region of infiltrating cells in invasive carcinomas, notably in mammary carcinomas (but see Fig. 5.22).

Mixed patterns of differentiation are occasionally seen, notably Paneth cell and enterochromaffin cell differentiation in gastrointestinal adenocarcinoma (see Chapter 7). Composite squamous and acinar differentiation characterizes adenosquamous and mucoepidermoid tumours, and mixed patterns of epithelial differentiation have also been reported in ovarian cystadenomas (see Table 30.2).[1153]

*Minimal criteria required for the ultrastructural recognition of glandular epithelial differentiation:* Definite acini and/or intracytoplasmic neolumina in an appropriate cellular environment, taking into account the tumours listed in Table

5.1. Unequivocal mucin granules in an epithelial neoplasm also establish glandular differentiation.

## MAMMARY CARCINOMAS

The fine structure of breast tumours has been the subject of several reviews.[1361,1385,1419,1423] EM is of diagnostic importance in only a small proportion of cases (for example, the distinction between medullary carcinoma and malignant lymphoma), and is usually of most value in casting new light on problems in cell biology.[1419]

Both *ductal and lobular carcinomas* predictably exhibit glandular-tubular differentiation. In general, infiltrating duct carcinomas have more intracytoplasmic lumina, less complex plasmalemmal interdigitation and more cytoplasmic filaments than their intraductal counterparts.[1419] Myoepithelial cells are usually absent from areas of infiltration, where there is disruption of the epithelial-stromal interface. In intraductal carcinomas, cytoplasmic protrusions through gaps in the investing basal lamina may indicate early invasion.[1419] Absence of basal lamina in tubular carcinoma is said to be a useful feature distinguishing this lesion from benign processes such as sclerosing adenosis.[1419] Apocrine differentiation in mammary ductal carcinomas is ultrastructurally characterized by extensive RER, abundant mitochondria and numerous electron-dense granules 400–600 nm in diameter.[1413] Lobular carcinomas usually contain more frequent intracytoplasmic crypts than ductal carcinomas, but they are distinguished from each other by LM.

*Medullary carcinoma* is composed of light and dark epithelial cells with ovoid to irregular nuclei containing abundant

---

**Table 5.1  Tumours consistently or occasionally containing acini and intracytoplasmic neolumina (crypts)**

*ACINAR SPACES*

Glandular epithelial neoplasms (adenomas and adenocarcinomas)
Endocrine adenomas and carcinomas
Transitional cell (urothelial) tumours, including inverted urinary papilloma (Figs. 4.17 and 4.18)
Brenner tumour of ovary
Mesotheliomas
Adenomatoid tumour of genital tract
So-called sclerosing haemangioma of lung
Craniopharyngioma
Ependymoma
Glandular Schwannoma
Neuroblastoma with olfactory rosettes
Retinoblastoma
Biphasic synovial sarcoma

*INTRACYTOPLASMIC NEOLUMINA*

Adenocarcinoma-large cell undifferentiated carcinomas of lung and other sites
Carcinoma of breast (various types, especially lobular)
Clear cell carcinoma of female genital tract
Choriocarcinoma
Brenner tumour of ovary
Renal adenoma and adenocarcinoma
Adenocarcinoma of prostate
Adenocarcinoma of salivary gland
Apparently undifferentiated carcinoma of stomach
Hepatocellular carcinoma
Oxyphilic thyroid carcinoma
Phaeochromocytoma
B-cell pancreatic islet tumour
Mesotheliomas
Adenomatoid tumour of genital tract
So-called sclerosing haemangioma of lung
Ameloblastoma (follicular type)
Pseudopsammomatous meningioma
Metastatic malignant melanoma (one case)[3150]

Eccrine spiradenoma
Eccrine poroma
Poroepithelioma
Syringoma
Syringocystadenoma papilliferum
Sweat gland carcinoma with syringomatous features
Metastasizing porocarcinoma

(Angiosarcoma)*
(So-called intravascular bronchiolo-alveolar tumour)*
(Follicular lymphoma with signet-ring cell features)†

---

*The crypts in these endothelial tumours do not constitute true intracellular microacini; they lack luminal microvilli and appear to represent intracytoplasmic vascular lumina.  †The vacuoles in these lymphomas also lack luminal microvilli and may represent giant multivesicular bodies; see Fig. 27.13

**Table 5.2** **Tumours in which glycocalyceal bodies and microvillous core rootlets have been demonstrated**

---

*GLYCOCALYCEAL BODIES*

1. *Tumours of the gut and its embryological derivatives*

   Oesophageal adenocarcinoma
   Intestinal-type gastric adenocarcinoma
   Adenosquamous carcinoma of stomach
   Small intestinal adenocarcinomas
   Large intestinal polyps and adenocarcinomas
   Anal gland carcinoma*
   Large pancreatic ductal adenocarcinomas
   Intestinal-type gallbladder carcinoma
   Pulmonary adenocarcinomas
   Bronchial carcinoid tumour
   Pulmonary blastoma
   Urachal-type bladder carcinoma

2. *Female genital tract tumours*

   Mucus-producing Müllerian epithelial tumours or components of tumours
   Strumal ovarian carcinoid tumours

*MICROVILLOUS CORE ROOTLETS*

1. *Tumours containing glycocalyceal bodies (see above)*

2. *Tumours in which unequivocal glycocalyceal bodies have not been demonstrated*

   Enteric nasal adenocarcinoma
   Gastrointestinal carcinoid tumours
   Pancreatic islet tumour (Fig. 14.7)
   Hepatoma
   Bile duct carcinoma
   Endodermal sinus tumour

---

*Marcus, personal communication, 1983
(Modified from the review by Marcus[660] and published by permission)
References: 660, 661, 806

euchromatin and prominent nucleoli. Cytoplasmic organelles vary in frequency and may be sparse, with ribosomes, polyribosomes and Golgi complexes often predominating; intracytoplasmic neolumina and filaments are generally not conspicuous, but varying numbers of desmosomes are recorded.[1419] Lymphocytes, plasma cells and macrophages dominate the stroma, and the lymphocytes are often intimately apposed to the neoplastic cells. In an ultrastructural study of three cases of typical medullary carcinoma, Ahmed[1363] suggests that the following combination of features is specific for this tumour: light and dark neoplastic cells with abundant organelles but absent secretory activity, macrophage-lymphocyte aggregates, and stromal venules lined by the high endothelium thought to facilitate transfer of lymphocytes.

The fine structure of *secretory carcinoma* is characterized by abundant secretory vacuoles and granules in addition to secretory material within both acinar spaces and large intracytoplasmic neolumina.[1365]

The pathological status of *'carcinoid' tumours of the breast* is controversial, and some investigators[1368,1429,1443] believe that they represent lobular and ductal carcinomas, or tumours with composite differentiation, as supported by the detection of oestrogen receptor protein in one case.[1443] The presence of argyrophilic granules in mammary tumours does not in itself necessarily constitute evidence of neuroendocrine properties. Immunoreactive lactalbumin has been demonstrated in the secretory granules of an argyrophilic breast carcinoma by LM and EM; in contrast, reactions for gastrin, insulin, calcitonin,

somatostatin, glucagon, ACTH, prolactin, and pancreatic polypeptide were all negative.[1374] However, in a report of 14 argyrophilic non-argentaffin breast tumours with carcinoid-like appearances, Azzopardi and associates[1368] argue that the presence of oestrogen receptor protein does not preclude neuroendocrine differentiation, as oestrogen receptors have been detected in gastrointestinal carcinoid tumours. They suggest that these argyrophilic carcinomas share endocrine properties with features of in situ and invasive lobular and ductal carcinomas. Four of their tumours examined by EM possessed rounded cytoplasmic dense-core granules of varying sizes, and five contained mucin. By their estimation, argyrophilic carcinomas represent approximately 5 per cent of breast carcinomas, while Min[1411] detected argyrophilia in 32 of 50 consecutive cases. In a recent study, Raju & Fine[1429] compared seven carcinoid-like tumours with nine unselected carcinomas of breast; they demonstrated argyrophilia, dense-core granules and a similar immunocytochemical profile in both groups, and concluded that carcinoid-like tumours represent variants of conventional mammary carcinomas.

'Lobular endocrine neoplasia' (LEN) in fibroadenoma of the breast has also been described. The ultrastructural appearances include evidence of glandular epithelial differentiation with intracytoplasmic lumina, and dense-core granules 200–330 nm in diameter, with a mean of 208 nm. On the basis of these observations Govoni et al[1395] suggested that LEN is a form of in situ lobular carcinoma with endocrine differentiation (see above).

**Table 5.3  Putative fine-structural classification of bronchiolo-alveolar tumours**

| Tumour | Comments |
|---|---|
| 1. Mucinous bronchiolar adenocarcinoma | See Fig. 5.9 |
| 2. Non-ciliated non-mucinous bronchiolar carcinoma (so-called Clara cell adenocarcinoma) | Characterized by microvillous cell population containing secretory granules with myelinoid and 'finger print'-like paracrystalline substructure. See Figs. 5.13 and 5.31. |
| | Although widely accepted, the status of Clara cell carcinoma does not appear to have been established unequivocally by the published data. In addition to the morphology of the secretory granules, proof of Clara cell differentiation would require further histochemical evaluation of the normal Clara cell, as well as these carcinomas |
| 3. Alveolar cell carcinoma (type II pneumocytic carcinoma) | Characterized by cells with electron-dense lamelliform inclusions conforming to those of type II pneumocytes (Figs. 0.4 and 5.30), but must be distinguished from reactive type II cell proliferation at the periphery of other pulmonary mass lesions (Fig. 0.4). The very existence of alveolar cell carcinoma has been disputed, but the data on recently reported cases are convincing, and include persistence of type II cell morphology in long-term tissue culture,[457] and the presence of lamellar bodies in regional lymph node metastases.[550] Alveolar cell carcinoma has been reported to fill alveoli occasionally with confluent sheets of cells, and must then be distinguished from other large cell carcinomas which are undifferentiated by LM[482] |
| | A surfactant-specific apoprotein has been identified in alveolar cell carcinoma and may prove useful in immunocytochemical diagnosis.[476,577] In addition, phospholipids, including dipalmitoyl phosphatidylcholine, have been detected biochemically in a bronchiolo-alveolar carcinoma with a mixed population of lamelliform and mucous granules[556] |
| 4. Bronchiolo-alveolar carcinoma with mixed granule population | See Fig. 5.30. A mixture of lamellar and electron-dense granules is also recorded in a papillary adenoma of lung, interpreted by the authors as evidence of combined Clara cell and type II pneumocytic differentiation[479] |
| 5. Type I (membranous) pneumocytic carcinoma | Listed here only as a theoretical possibility. An acceptable case of a type I pneumocytic tumour does not seem to be recorded. Normal type I pneumocytes are thought to be incapable of mitosis, and any neoplasm expressing this pattern of differentiation could therefore be expected also to show evidence of type I precursor cells such as type II pneumocytes and/or fetal pulmonary epithelium. In such circumstances it is likely that the tumour could be recognized as a type I cell carcinoma only with great difficulty, if at all in view of the non-diagnostic organelle-poor morphology of type I cell cytoplasm |
| (Intravascular bronchiolo-alveolar tumour–IVBAT) | Listed parenthetically here only because of its nomenclature. Recent studies prove that IVBAT is unrelated to bronchiolo-alveolar epithelial differentiation and that it represents a low-grade interstitial epithelioid angiosarcoma, as discussed in Chapter 23 |

References: 45, 445, 449, 457, 472, 476, 479, 482, 492, 509, 521, 523, 525, 526, 549, 550, 556, 557, 575, 577, 602

**THE ELECTRON MICROGRAPHS IN THIS CHAPTER ARE ARRANGED IN THREE BROAD GROUPS:**

1. **FIGS. 5.1–5.7 ILLUSTRATE THE ARCHITECTURAL AND CELL SURFACE-ASSOCIATED FEATURES OF ADENOCARCINOMAS IN A SEQUENCE OF DIMINISHING DIFFERENTIATION.**

2. **FIGS. 5.8–5.14 DEPICT DIFFERENT TYPES OF SECRETORY GRANULES FOUND IN ADENOCARCINOMAS.**

3. **FINALLY A VARIETY OF DISTINCTIVE ADENOCARCINOMAS IS ILLUSTRATED IN FIGS. 5.15–5.34.**

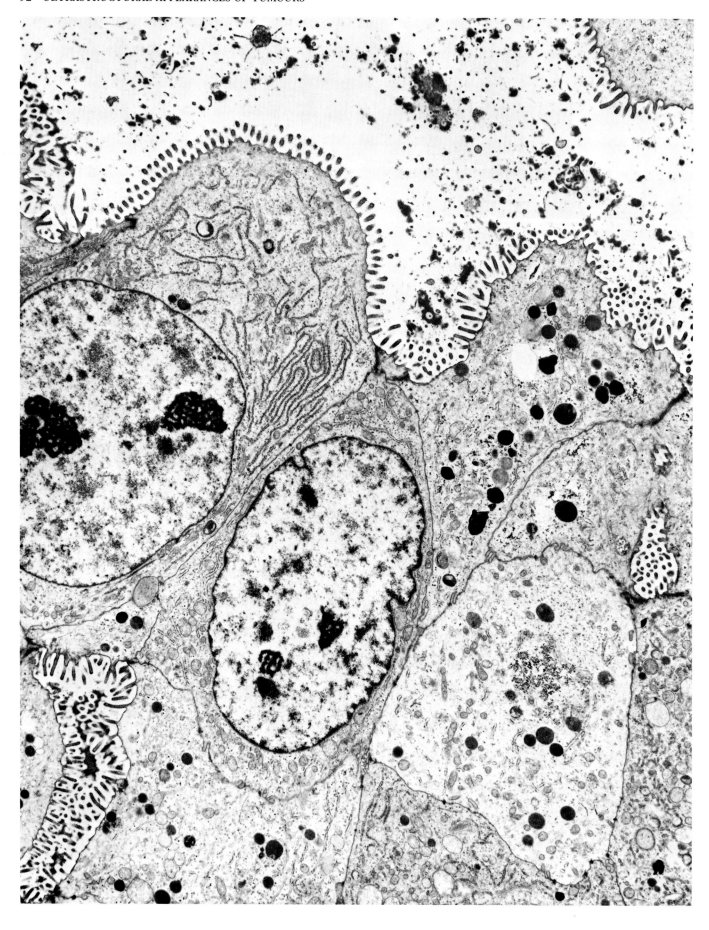

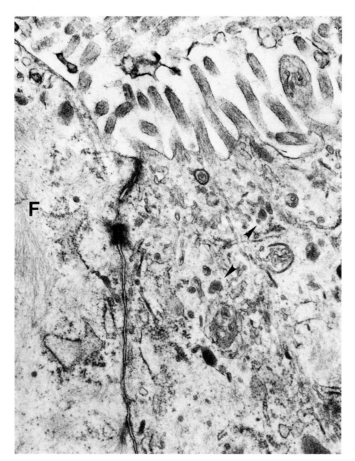

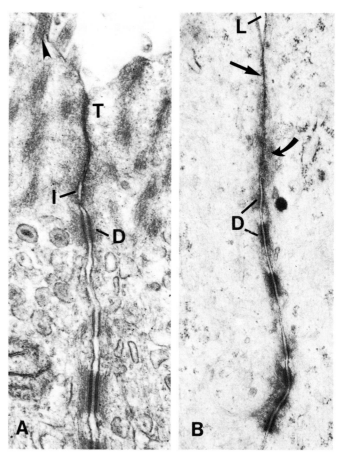

**Fig. 5.2  Adenocarcinoma of lung: Acinus and junctional complex**

The cells bordering the acinar lumen are attached by a junctional complex (consisting of a tight junction, intermediate junction and desmosome in sequence). The cells contain fine filaments (F) and microvilli line the lumen; the microvilli in brush borders are normally stabilized by a core of about 20 actin filaments,[180] which may also be present in adenocarcinomas, particularly intestinal tumours. Minute secretory granules (arrowheads) are present near the free surface. (×27 500)

References: 39, 180

**Fig. 5.3  Colonic adenocarcinoma and infiltrating duct carcinoma of breast: Junctional complexes**

**A:** The tight (T), intermediate (I) and desmosomal (D) junctions forming a junctional complex can all be discerned in this colonic adenocarcinoma. Note also the filamentous cores of the microvilli (arrowhead). Microvillar core filaments may be seen converging onto the intermediate junctions in tumours differentiating as intestinal epithelium. (×43 500)

**B:** Classical junctional complexes are seen uncommonly in adenocarcinomas, for two reasons:
1. The assembly of such junctions is often defective, especially in poorly differentiated carcinomas.
2. Variable obliquity of sectioning; a complete longitudinal section through all three components of the complex is infrequent, unless a goniometer stage is used to tilt the section.[39]

In the region of the tight junction (straight arrow) beneath the acinar lumen (L), the plasma membranes are closely apposed and the intercellular space is narrowed to approximately 6–8 nm. A pentalaminar configuration resulting from fusion of membranes is not apparent, suggesting that the junction may be leaky; a focus of possible membrane fusion in the uppermost portion is probably due to obliquity of sectioning. The intermediate junction is not demonstrated, and the plasma membranes in its expected location are indistinct (curved arrow), reflecting an oblique plane of section. In contrast, desmosomes (D), the last of the three components, are easily recognized. (×23 300)

References: 39, 45, 64, 249

**Fig. 5.1** *(Facing page)* **Highly differentiated adenocarcinoma: Cell relationships**

Peripheral adenocarcinoma of lung in a 77-year-old man. Intercellular acinar spaces are readily apparent. The cell membranes are closely apposed, with scattered membrane interdigitations and short desmosomes, while junctional complexes are present near the acini. The cells have numerous short luminal microvilli, and small quantities of secretion can be seen within the acini. (×6800)

References: 39, 45, 63, 64, 85, 86, 91, 119, 534, 563, 564

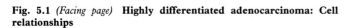

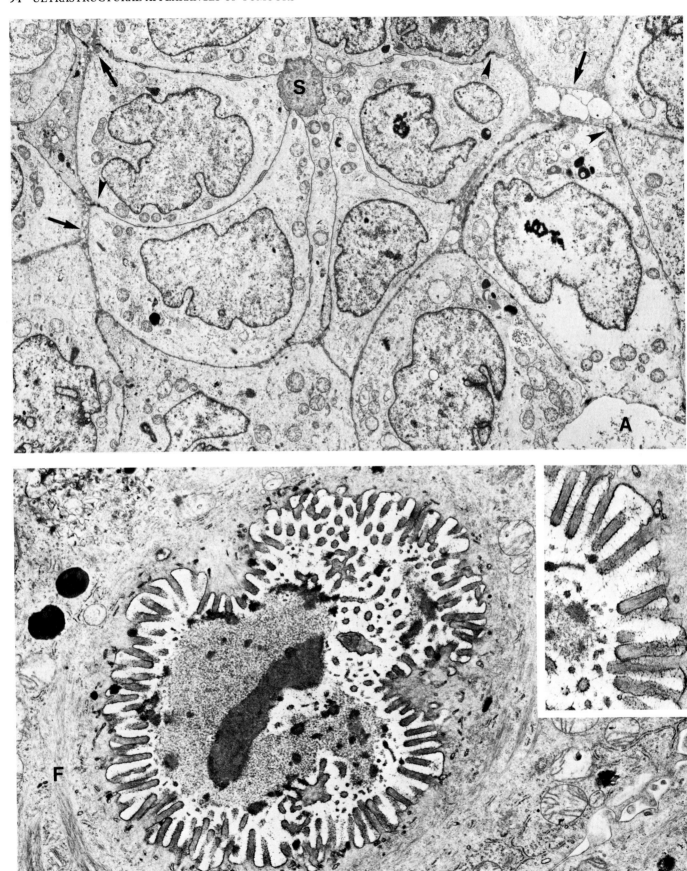

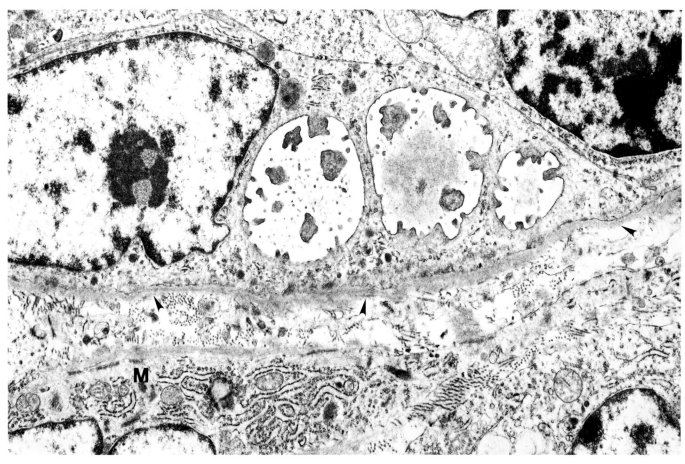

## Fig. 5.6 Poorly differentiated adenocarcinoma of lung: Intracytoplasmic crypt formation

Tumour of right upper lobe of lung discovered on routine chest X-ray. Light-microscopic examination of the resected lobe revealed a large cell undifferentiated carcinoma, but EM demonstrated a few intracellular crypts, consistent with the suggestion that a proportion of large cell undifferentiated carcinomas of lung represent very poorly differentiated adenocarcinomas (see Chapter 7). The crypt profiles are lined by poorly developed microvilli. Adjacent external lamina is apparent (arrowheads), and there is a myofibroblast (M) in the stroma. (Formalin fixation, × 15 800)

**Discussion:** In seemingly undifferentiated carcinomas such crypts containing microvilli are considered to indicate glandular epithelial differentiation, but similar neolumina may be found in a variety of tumours (Table 5.1). Nevertheless, their presence excludes alternative diagnoses such as squamous cell carcinoma and malignant lymphoma,[283] and they are vanishingly rare in melanocytic neoplasia, being described in the pulmonary metastasis of a single case of malignant melanoma.[3150]

References: 283, 468, 488, 507, 3150

## Fig. 5.4 (Facing page — top) Poorly differentiated adenocarcinoma of lung: Survey

The rounded structure (S) simulating an acinar space probably represents a stromal pocket, as indicated by absence of junctional complexes from this region. In contrast, most of the true acinar spaces are reduced to slit-like lumina (arrows) containing a few distorted microvilli; subluminal junctional complexes (arrowheads) — although not fully resolved at this low magnification — betray their nature, while portion of a more easily recognizable acinus (A) occupies the lower right corner. Compare with the highly differentiated adenocarcinoma illustrated in Fig. 5.1. (× 5500)

## Fig. 5.5 (Facing page — bottom) Poorly differentiated adenocarcinoma of pancreas: Intracytoplasmic crypt

The crypt (neolumen) contains electron-dense secretion, and is lined by microvilli with a prominent glycocalyx; the microvillous lining is shown at higher magnification in the inset, where the glycocalyx can be seen to have a granular configuration. The cytoplasm also contains bundles of filaments (F) which tend to be arranged circumferentially around the crypt. (× 14 400. Inset: × 25 700)

Reference: 939

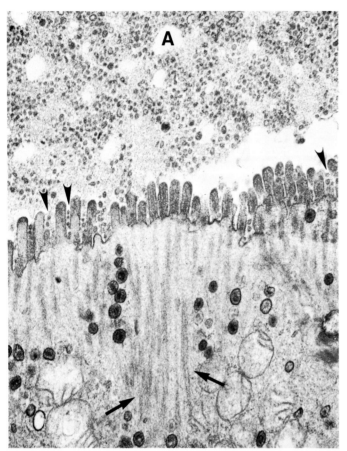

**Fig. 5.7** *(Left)* **Colonic adenocarcinoma: Glycocalyceal bodies and penetrating microvillous core rootlets**

Moderately differentiated carcinoma of the sigmoid colon. The acinar space (A) contains innumerable small rounded glycocalyceal bodies averaging 55 nm in diameter, with a range of 35–90 nm. A few such bodies also occupy the intervillous spaces (arrowheads). The filamentous core rootlets of the microvilli penetrate deeply into the cytoplasm (arrows). These appearances strongly indicate differentiation as intestinal epithelium or its derivatives. Small dense immature mucin granules are also present in the apical cytoplasm, averaging 145 nm in diameter, with a range of 100–180 nm; compare with the more 'mature' granules shown in Fig. 5.8. (×26 900)

**Discussion:** Synonyms for glycocalyceal bodies (GCB) include coccoid or 'C' bodies, intermicrovillous particles and membrane bodies. They consist of spherical or elliptical vesicles with a trilaminar boundary membrane and a fine coating of glycocalyx. Their diameters range from 20–130 nm, with an average of about 50 nm. They are usually arranged in rows and clusters, often being closely associated with the apical plasma membrane and forming intervillous arrays; aggregates may also be seen lying free within luminal spaces. GCB need to be distinguished from viral particles and collections of inspissated glycocalyx (clavate fimbriae); in carcinomas, degenerative changes afflicting microvilli can also produce vesicles, but these are larger and more pleomorphic than GCB, the diameters often exceeding those of microvilli.

Although GCB represent a useful marker for intestinal epithelium, their genesis and function are obscure. Development by budding from apical plasma membranes or by discharge from cytoplasmic vesicles has been postulated. At present the evidence is more in favour of an origin from a type of multivesicular body known as an R body. Different from lysosomal multivesicular bodies, R bodies contain small elongated vesicles 100–250 nm in length and 50 nm in width. However, R bodies are seldom numerous — even when GCB are present in profusion — and miniaturized R bodies may represent more important sources of GCB. The manner in which R bodies are formed is uncertain.

The extensive review on this subject by Marcus[660] is recommended to the interested reader.

References: 660, 661

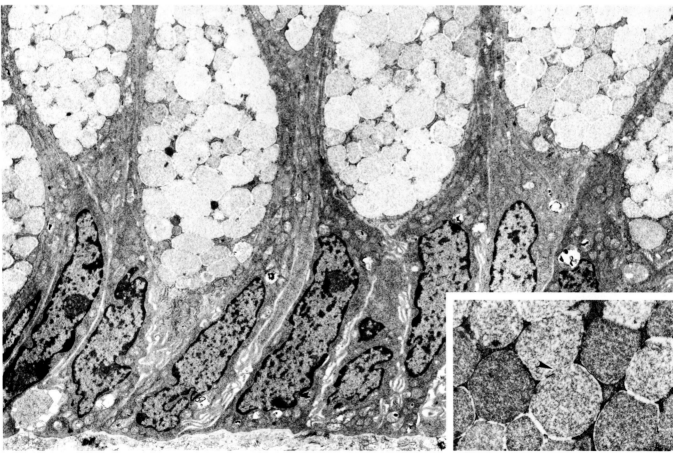

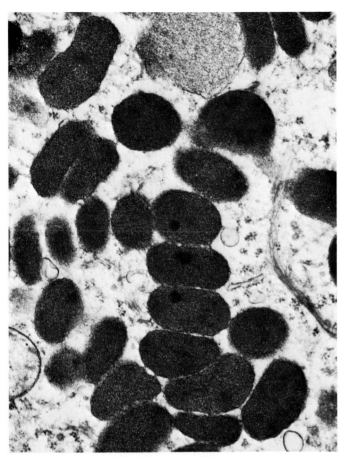

**Fig. 5.9 Mucinous bronchiolar carcinoma: Mucin granules II**

The granules are denser than those of the hindgut tumour illustrated in Fig. 5.8. Some have an eccentric osmiophilic core; when well developed dense cores are present, a so-called 'bull's eye' configuration is produced. (×32 600)

References: 45–47, 563

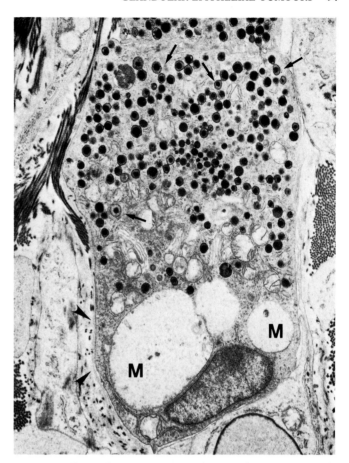

**Fig. 5.10 Signet-ring cell adenocarcinoma of stomach: Mucin granules III**

Tumour from the gastric cardia of a 76-year-old woman. This infiltrating cell was selected because of its content of immature small dense mucin granules. Other cells contained numerous large pale granules similar to those shown in Fig. 5.8 — or a mixture of the two forms — presumably corresponding to the signet-ring cell morphology on LM; in addition, intracytoplasmic neolumina were also seen.

These granules average 290 nm in diameter, with a range of 185–415 nm. The dense cores are often eccentric in location, and are surrounded by a relatively wide zone of medium electron-density (arrows), aiding the distinction from neurosecretory granules. The diminutive nucleus is situated at the periphery of the cell. The lucent paranuclear vacuoles represent ballooned mitochondria (M). The Golgi apparatus is prominent, and the cell possesses an external lamina (arrowheads). Note the apparent polarization of the subcellular components. (×8800)

See also Fig. 5.7.

References: 812, 816, 863, 1047, 1060

**Fig. 5.8** *(Facing page — bottom)* **Highly differentiated colonic adenocarcinoma: Mucin granules I**

The neoplastic epithelium is aligned in a 'picket-fence' pattern and contains apical collections of mucin granules. **Inset:** the mucin granules are moderately dense, have a delicate flocculent or reticulated appearance, and coalesce (arrowhead). Such apparent fusion may in part represent a fixation artefact related to the hydrophilic properties of mucin granules;[39] nevertheless, it represents a diagnostically valuable finding. (×5700. Inset: ×11 700)

References: 39, 45, 55

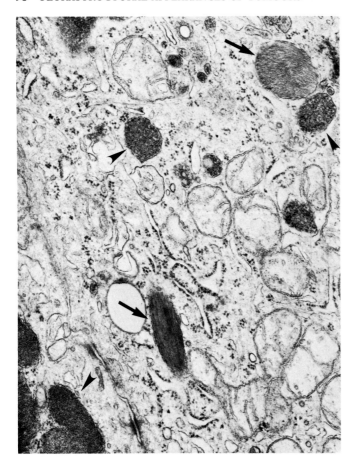

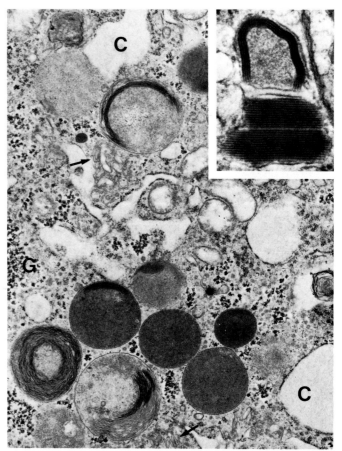

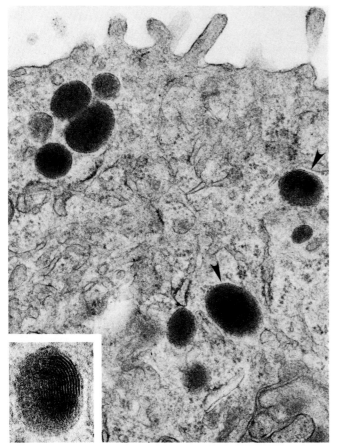

**Fig. 5.11** *(Top — left)* **Adenocarcinoma of uterine cervix: Fibrillary granules**

Thought to be specific for normal and neoplastic endocervical epithelium in the human, these membrane-bound granules have a fibrillary substructure (arrows). 'Conventional' mucin granules (arrowheads) are also present. Sporadic desmosomes link adjoining plasma membranes. (×18 000)
 (Case contributed by Dr. C.M. Fenoglio).
 See Table 30.1.
 References: 39, 1154

**Fig. 5.12** *(Top — right)* **Adenocarcinoma: Secretory granules**

Secretory granules in a non-mucinous adenocarcinoma of lung. Some of the granules have a membranous internal substructure, producing myelinoid figures. Glycogen (G) is also evident, as are dilated cisternae (C) of the RER and small Golgi complexes (arrows). (×16 100)
 **Inset:** Paracrystalline granules in a peripheral pulmonary adenocarcinoma with Clara cell features, from a 70-year-old man. These membrane-bound granules display linear periodicity with a spacing of approximately 10 nm. (×64 200)
 Reference: 563

**Fig. 5.13** *(Bottom — left)* **Lipochondroadenoma of lung (so-called chondromatous hamartoma): Clara cell granules**

This micrograph is included to depict the typical features of Clara cell granules within the terminal airway epithelial component of the lesion. Note the internal periodicity in two of the granules (arrowheads). The diameters are in the range 170–465 nm. The cell has a microvillous non-ciliated surface. (×38 700)
 **Inset:** Detail of a Clara cell granule. (×73 500)
 References: 508, 580, 583, 602

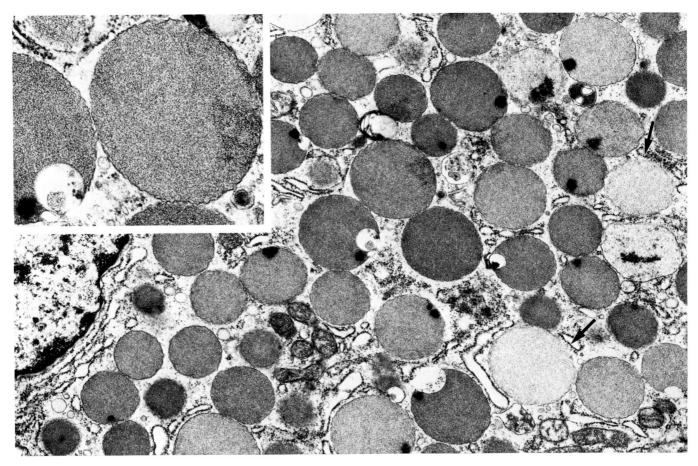

**Fig. 5.14 Acinic cell adenocarcinoma of parotid gland: Granule morphology**

The serous cells of salivary acinic cell tumours typically contain numerous round secretory (zymogen) granules measuring 300–1000 nm in diameter. The granules depicted here have cores of medium density with frequent eccentric denser foci. As detailed in the inset, the contents are finely granular (compare with mucin granules in Figs. 5.8 and 5.9). Scattered more lucent granules are usually present (arrows), while in some cases the granules are extremely dense. They are probably best preserved by glutaraldehyde fixation, and the use of other primary fixatives such as osmium tetroxide may result in considerable extraction of their contents, with loss of up to 70 per cent of enzymic protein. Tumour from a 66-year-old woman. (×17 300. Inset: ×38 500)

(Case contributed by Prof. R.L. Kempson).

**Discussion:** Although these low-grade neoplasms occur predominantly in the parotid gland, similar acinic cell tumours have also been recorded in extrasalivary tissues such as the respiratory tract and pancreas. The granules in pancreatic acinic cell carcinoma have been recorded to vary from 200 to 6000 nm in diameter. Zymogen granules have also been described in a basal cell adenoma of the parotid gland,[758] pancreatoblastoma[945] and a composite acinar-endocrine pancreatic tumour.[984] Paneth cells contain similar electron-dense granules rich in lysozyme; although pure Paneth cell carcinomas do not seem to have been recorded, apparently neoplastic Paneth cells are occasionally found in gastrointestinal adenomas and adenocarcinomas, and rarely are quite numerous (see Table 7.2).

References: 30, 86, 414, 425, 481, 512, 717, 719, 731, 758, 764, 923, 944, 945, 962, 984

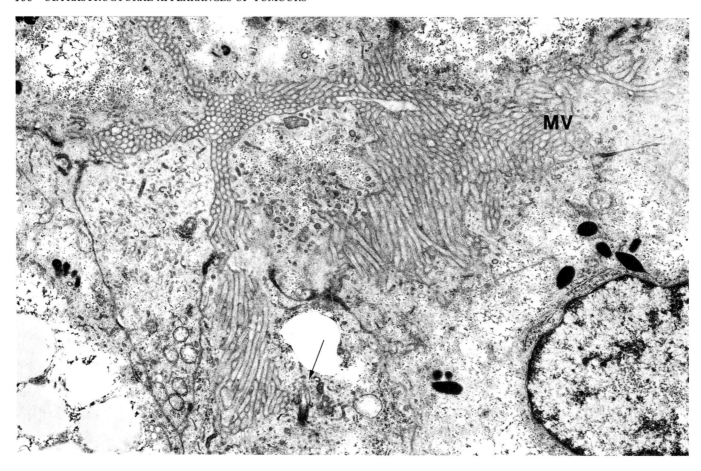

## Fig. 5.15   Renal adenocarcinoma: Tubular differentiation with microvilli

The irregular intercellular space is almost totally filled by numerous microvilli (MV), which are seen in both longitudinal and transverse section. Scanning EM of such tumours reveals numerous well separated blunt microvilli with considerable variation in pattern.[1032] There are junctional complexes between adjoining cells and portions of budding cilia are also present (arrow). (×13 000)

References: 994, 1002, 1010, 1024, 1030–1033, 1041

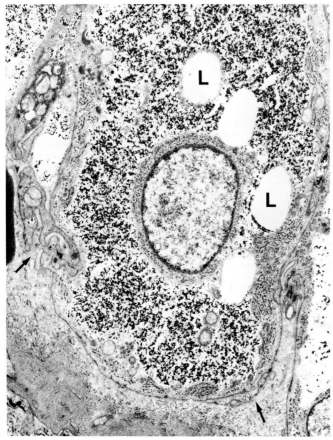

## Fig. 5.16   Renal adenocarcinoma: Glycogen and infolding of basal plasma membrane

Clear cell carcinoma in a 70-year-old man who presented with peritoneal metastases. The basal plasmalemma is focally infolded (arrows) in a pattern reminiscent of normal tubular epithelium. The cytoplasm contains abundant glycogen and a few lucent lipid droplets (L). (×7400)

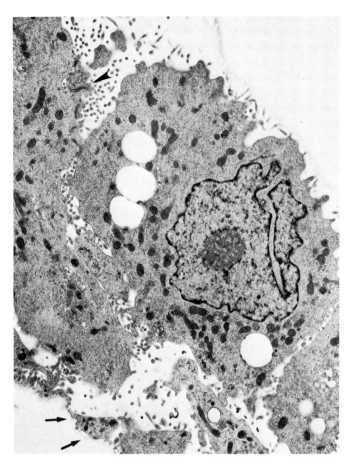

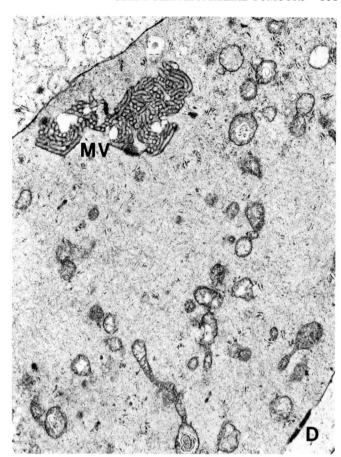

**Fig. 5.17 Renal adenocarcinoma: Tubular differentiation and depletion of glycogen**

Fine needle aspiration biopsy specimen. These neoplastic cells resemble renal tubular epithelium. One contains an irregular nucleus with a prominent nucleolus, as well as lucent lipid droplets within the cytoplasm. Moderate numbers of mitochondria are also present, but glycogen is inconspicuous. Microvillous processes protrude from the cell periphery, and portion of an apical junctional complex (arrowhead) can be seen. Basal lamina (arrows) is situated at the inferior aspect of the cell aggregate. (×7600)

**Fig. 5.18 Renal adenocarcinoma: Granular cell with intracytoplasmic microvilli**

A collection of interweaving microvilli (MV) has invaginated into the cell; the cytoplasm contains mitochondria, but these do not nearly reach oncocytic proportions in this instance; however oxyphilic cells ultrastructurally indistinguishable from those of renal oncocytoma may occur in renal adenocarcinoma (see Table 2.1). In contrast to Figs. 5.15 and 5.16, glycogen and lipid are not apparent. A desmosome (D) is also illustrated. (×8800)

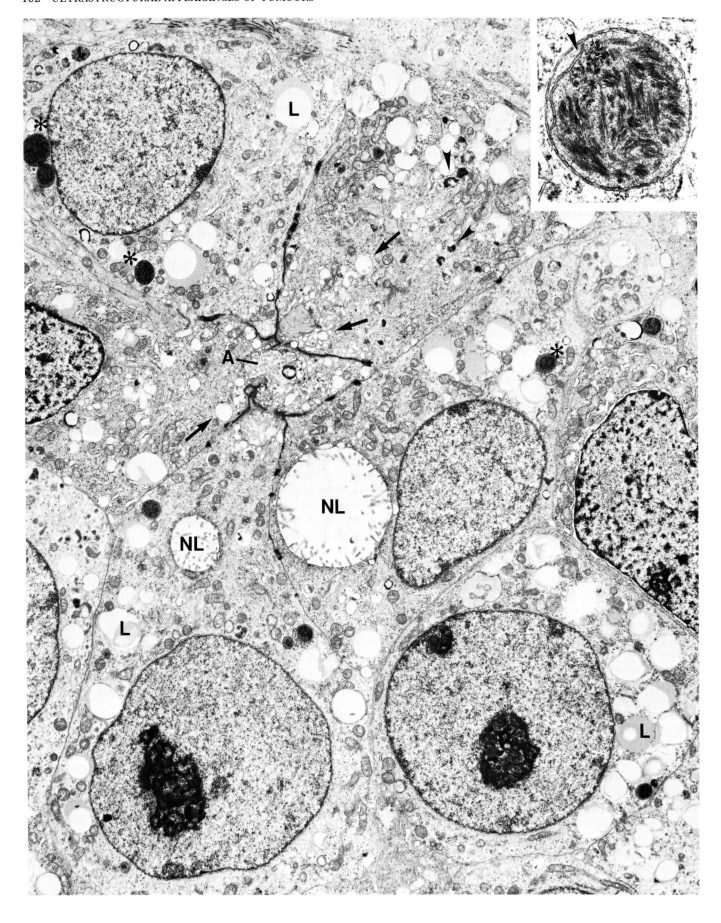

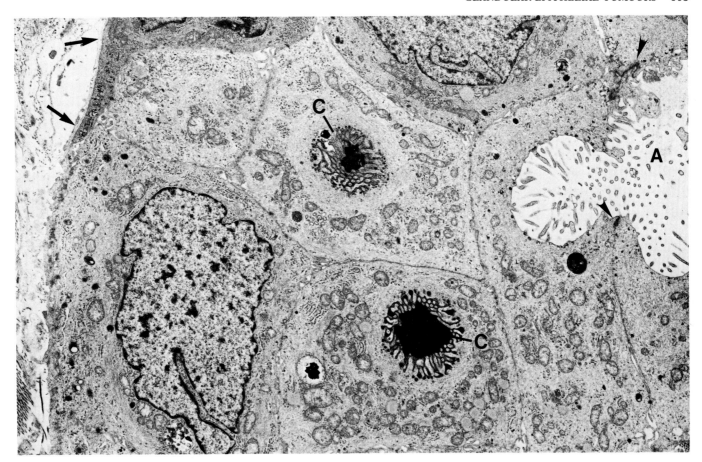

**Fig. 5.20  Infiltrating duct carcinoma of breast: Cell morphology**

A polycellular acinus (A) and two intracytoplasmic crypts (C) are evident in this collection of closely apposed neoplastic cells. Junctional complexes (arrowheads) border the acinar space, while the crypts contain electron-dense secretion and are also lined by microvilli. Small secretory granules are located beneath the crypt microvilli, and the surrounding cytoplasm contains circumferentially arranged filaments, with displacement of organelles. A fragmentary basal lamina (arrows) lies next to the cell nest in one area, but is absent elsewhere. (×6600)

References: 1359, 1361, 1362, 1368, 1369, 1374, 1385, 1391, 1393, 1413, 1417, 1419, 1423, 1424, 1443

**Fig. 5.19** *(Facing page)*  **Prostatic adenocarcinoma: Architecture and mitochondrion**

Cervical lymph node biopsy from a patient who presented with a neck mass. On the basis of the ultrastructural findings, prostate was predicted to be the source of the metastasis and a subsequent needle biopsy of prostate revealed adenocarcinoma. Immunocytochemistry demonstrated prostatic acid phosphatase and prostate-specific antigen in both specimens.

The rounded nuclei possess abundant euchromatin and prominent nucleoli. Intracytoplasmic neolumina (NL) are evident, while prominent junctional complexes border the intercellular acinus (A). Lucent membrane-bound secretory vesicles (arrows) can be seen in the cytoplasm and are clustered near the acinus. Small dense lysosomal bodies (arrowheads) are also present. Lipid droplets (L) are increased in comparison to normal prostatic epithelium. (×6900)

**Inset:** In this case the cells also contain large rounded bodies (*); as detailed here, their double boundary membranes and occasional remnants of cristae (arrowhead) prove that they represent mitochondria with a paracrystalline substructure — thought by Brandes & Kirchheim[1085] to result from closely packed filamentous cristae. (×39 300)

(Case contributed by Dr. E.J. Wills).

**Discussion:** Other alterations reported in prostatic carcinoma include loss of organellar polarity — particularly affecting Golgi complexes and secretory vacuoles — hypertrophy and dilatation of the Golgi apparatus, and depleted basal lamina. Increased numbers of mitochondria, intranuclear mitochondria, tubuloreticular arrays and intracisternal 'virus-like' particles are also described; so too are intracisternal tubules, as well as striated and lattice-like structures.

Acid phosphatase activity is thought to be localized to the secretory vacuoles and lysosomes. Evidence indicates that on a weight-for-weight basis acid phosphatase is *reduced* in carcinoma of prostate, compared to normal prostatic glands — implying that elevated acid phosphatase levels in the blood are explicable by an increased cell mass and/or enhanced enzyme release.

References: 280, 1085, 1087, 1088, 1091–1096, 1100, 1101, 1104–1106

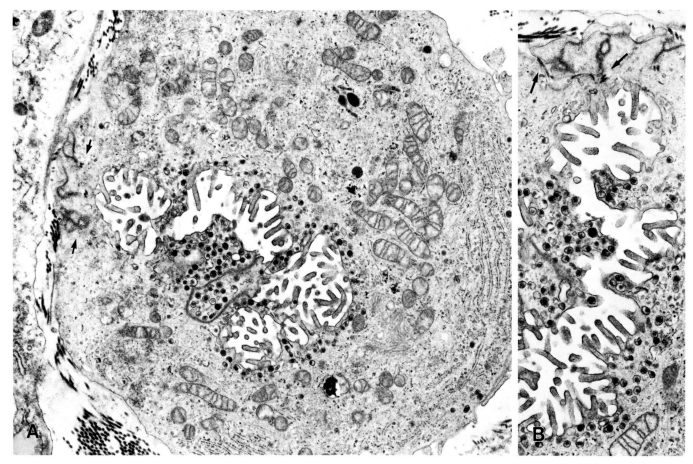

**Fig. 5.21   Infiltrating mammary carcinoma: Intracytoplasmic crypt and secretory granules**

**A:** There is evidence of continuity between the external plasma membrane and the neolumen (arrows), suggesting that the crypt has developed by a process of membrane infolding. The neolumen is lined by microvilli, and there are small subluminal secretory granules. (×12 300)

**B:** Portion of the crypt, showing the infolded cell membrane with associated collagen fibres (arrows), together with microvilli and secretory granules. (×14 900)

There is evidence of a significant correlation between the frequency of intracytoplasmic vacuoles and positive oestrogen receptor status in breast carcinomas.[1451]

Reference: 1451

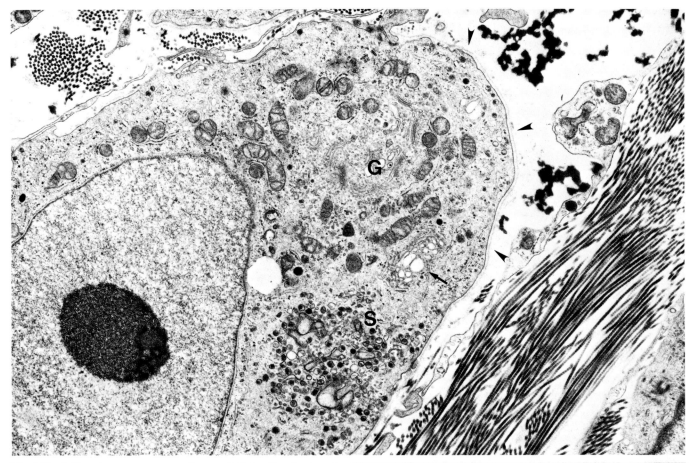

**Fig. 5.22   Infiltrating mammary carcinoma: Cell detail and external lamina**

Portion of an extraductal infiltrating cell is illustrated. The Golgi complex (G) is prominent, and is dilated in one area (arrow); beneath this there is a collection of secretory granules (S). Although usually absent in infiltrating mammary carcinomas, external lamina (arrowheads) surrounds most of the cell. In non-infiltrating carcinomas the extent of development of the basal lamina appears to be proportional to the myoepithelial cell component.[1393] Numerous nucleolar ribosomes are present, while the stroma contains elastin and collagen fibres. (×15 700)

Reference: 1393

**Fig. 5.23   In situ and infiltrating duct carcinoma of breast: Myoepithelial cell**

Same case as Fig. 5.20. An elongated myoepithelial cell — containing fine actin-like filaments with dense bodies — traverses the field obliquely. A desmosomal junction (arrow) with an adjoining neoplastic epithelial cell (E) is apparent. Although fine filaments are present in the epithelial cell cytoplasm, they are far less numerous than in the myoepithelial cell. A prominent basal lamina (arrowheads) can also be seen. (×28 300)

**Discussion:** Myoepithelial cells are usually absent from areas of invasion in ductal carcinomas; however, infiltrating mammary carcinoma cells are known to contain augmented quantities of contractile proteins, which may be organized into a peripheral myofilamentous apparatus (see Fig. 7.3), especially in lobular carcinoma cells.[1424] Myoepithelial properties are sometimes attributed to such cells. Nevertheless, Ozzello[1424] cautions that the simple presence of contractile proteins is insufficient for the identification of myoepithelium, and he suggests that all mammary carcinomas may derive from a single epithelial or indeterminate cell type which can express various patterns of differentiation, including myoepithelium-like properties. Such filament-rich malignant cells need to be distinguished from non-neoplastic myoepithelium at the periphery of ducts and ductules containing in situ carcinomas.[1424] The elongated cell depicted here is thought to represent a residual duct myoepithelial cell, in view of its apparent compression by the neoplastic epithelium and the well developed basal lamina.

References: 1361, 1371, 1372, 1379, 1388, 1393, 1394, 1403, 1419, 1421, 1424

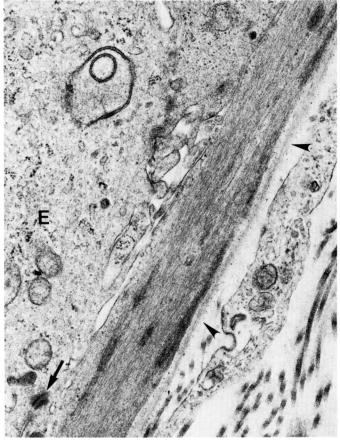

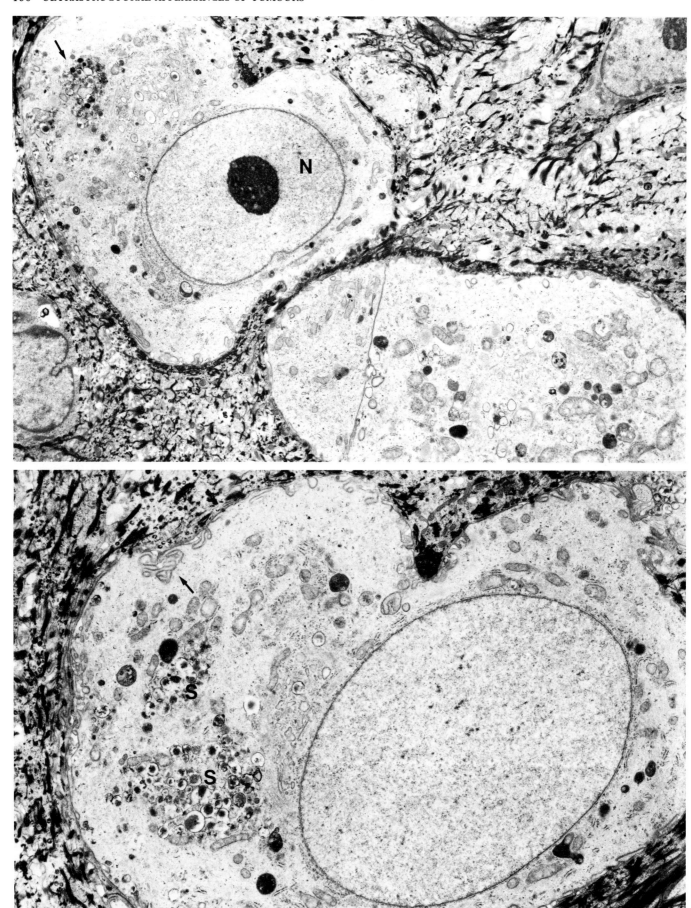

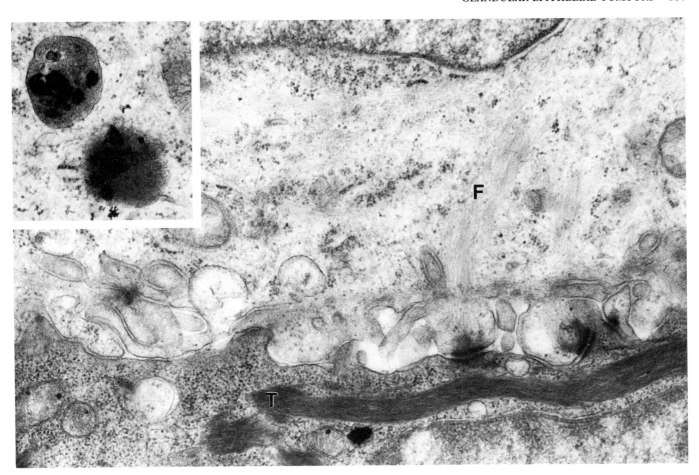

**Fig. 5.26 Extramammary Paget's disease: Intercellular junctions and melanin granules**

Peripheral microvillous processes of a Paget cell form an interleaving pattern with the processes of an adjacent epidermal cell in which a tonofibrillar bundle (T) can be seen. Desmosomes are evident between the cells. Tonofilaments (F) within the Paget cell converge onto the desmosomes. **Inset:** Melanin granules in the form of compound melanosomes within a Paget cell; stage II melanosomes were not present. Same case as Figs. 5.24 and 5.25. (×34 000. Inset: ×40 200)

**Fig. 5.24** *(Facing page — top)* **Cutaneous Paget's disease: Survey of Pagetoid cells**

Extramammary Paget's disease of scrotum, in a 62-year-old. The pale Paget cells are surrounded by epidermal keratinocytes, which in contrast contain numerous bundles of tonofilaments. The ovoid nucleus (N) of one of the Paget cells contains a prominent nucleolus, but there is little heterochromatin. Secretory granules can be seen (arrow). (×5700)

Ultrastructural studies have shown the close similarity of the component cells in both mammary and extramammary Paget's disease. The neoplastic cells show glandular epithelial differentiation: a significant proportion contain secretory granules and intracytoplasmic neolumina are occasionally present. In addition, CEA is consistently demonstrable in the Paget cells of both the mammary and extramammary types, but not in the adjacent keratinocytes and melanocytes.[1507] However, the dispute over the site of origin of Paget's disease unassociated with underlying ductal neoplasia still awaits resolution.

References: 1361, 1423, 1458, 1464, 1466, 1470, 1491, 1492, 1502, 1505, 1507, 1517

**Fig. 5.25** *(Facing page — bottom)* **Extramammary Paget's disease: Paget cell**

The ovoid nucleus is almost devoid of heterochromatin. Groups of secretory granules (S) are present within the cytoplasm, and the cell membrane forms peripheral microvilli and focal infoldings (arrow). (×9000)

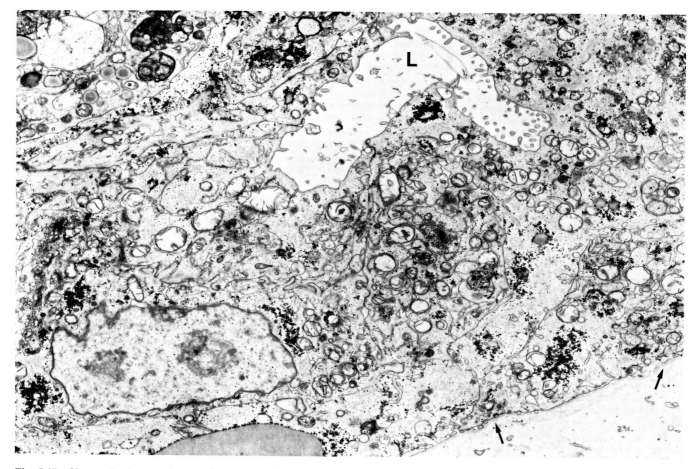

**Fig. 5.27  Clear cell adenocarcinoma of cervix: Architecture and glycogen**

Portion of a neoplastic gland is shown, with a distinct lumen (L) and an external lamina (arrows). Pleomorphic microvilli protrude into the lumen, while aggregates of cytoplasmic glycogen are plentiful. Profuse elongated microvilli are described in a clear cell adenocarcinoma of the female urethra.[1078] Lipid globules are also present, and are often surrounded by glycogen granules. (×7000)

References: 1078, 1152, 1153, 1156, 1159, 1175, 1191, 1250, 1251

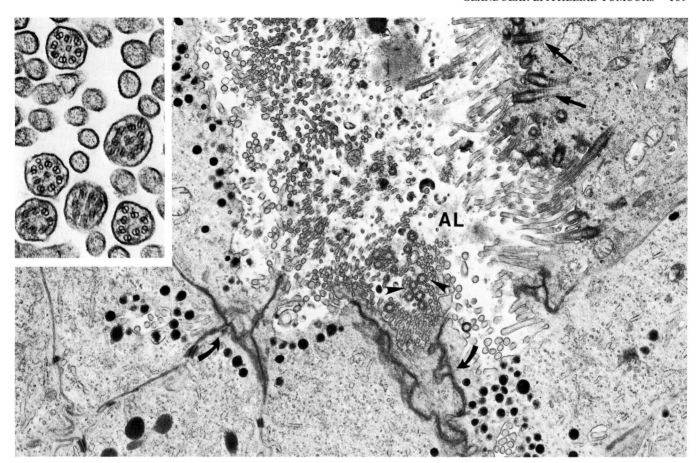

**Fig. 5.28  Endometrial adenocarcinoma: Ciliated and microvillous cells forming acinus**

Highly differentiated invasive adenocarcinoma of endometrium, from a patient aged 48 years. The acinar lumen (AL) contains innumerable microvilli in various planes of section. The cells in two areas also possess cilia; the longitudinally sectioned cilia display basal bodies and rootlets (straight arrows), and a few are seen in near-transverse section (arrowheads). The neoplastic cells in other regions contained intracytoplasmic aggregates of disarrayed basal bodies and rootlets, without constructing cilia. Most numerous in well differentiated carcinomas, both cilia and microvilli are depleted in poorly differentiated tumours, and cilia may be absent in such cases. Paranuclear collections of intermediate filaments are another feature of low-grade endometrial carcinomas. Electron-dense secretory granules inhabit the apical cytoplasm of the non-ciliated cells in this field, and junctional complexes (curved arrows) are also present. (×12 800)

**Inset:** Transverse sections of the cilia in this case reveal anomalous axonemal substructure. Malposition of outer tubular doublets and deletion of both outer and central tubules can be seen. Instead of the normal 9+2 configuration, the majority of cilia in this case had a variable 5–8+0–2 pattern. Note also displacement and absence of the dynein arms, indicating cilial immotility. (×64 500)

References: 1152–1155, 1218, 1219, 1223, 1227, 1229, 1234, 1255

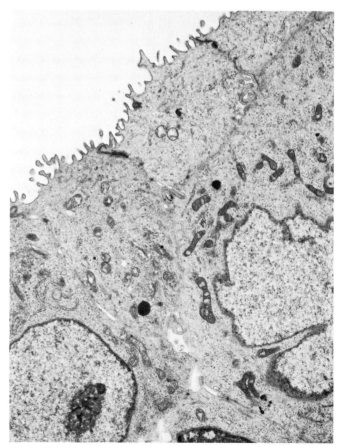

**Fig. 5.29  Endometrial adenocarcinoma: Acinus**

The luminal microvilli in this moderately differentiated carcinoma are distorted and poorly developed, in contrast to the profuse microvilli in the highly differentiated tumour illustrated in Fig. 5.28. Although detected elsewhere, cilia are not present in this area, and there are no apical secretory granules. (×6800)

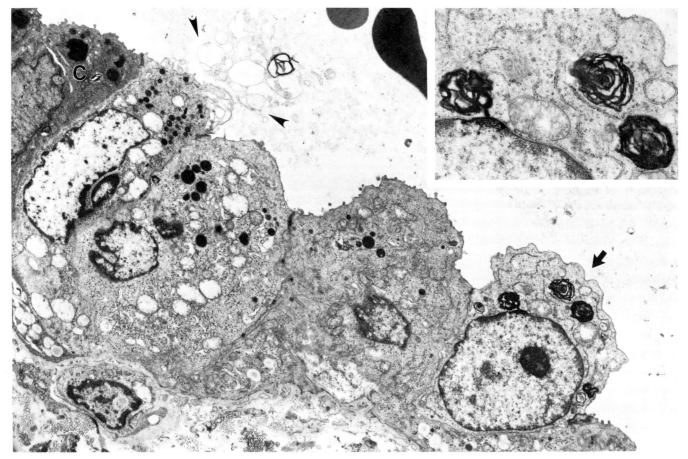

## Fig. 5.30 Bronchiolo-alveolar cell carcinoma: Survey and mixed granules

The neoplastic cells are arrayed along an alveolar wall, and one contains lamelliform electron-dense inclusions (arrow and inset). The other cells contain non-lamellar secretory granules and one has cytoplasmic clefts (C). Another cell shows evidence of probable apocrine secretion (arrowheads). Only a few short, irregular microvillous processes are formed at the apices of the cells, and there are no cilia. (×5600. Inset: ×11 800)

In alveolar cell carcinomas containing osmiophilic lamellar granules (type II pneumocyte carcinomas) the diagnosis can be further supported by the immunocytochemical demonstration of surfactant-specific apoprotein.[476,577]

See also Table 5.3.

References: 204, 233, 442, 445, 457, 472, 476, 482, 492, 496, 509, 521, 523, 525, 548–550, 556, 557, 563, 575, 577, 580

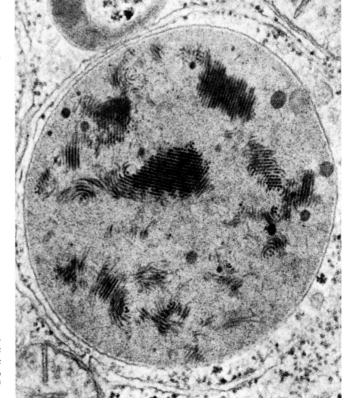

## Fig. 5.31 Bronchiolo-alveolar cell carcinoma: Secretory granule

The secretory granule shown here has a striking paracrystalline substructure, with a point-to-point spacing of approximately 14 nm. The appearances are similar to those described in some so-called Clara cell adenocarcinomas (see also Fig. 5.13 and Table 5.3). The pulmonary interstitial cells in this case also contained unusual complex fibrillary granules with a targetoid substructure.[64]
(×69 900)

Reference: 64

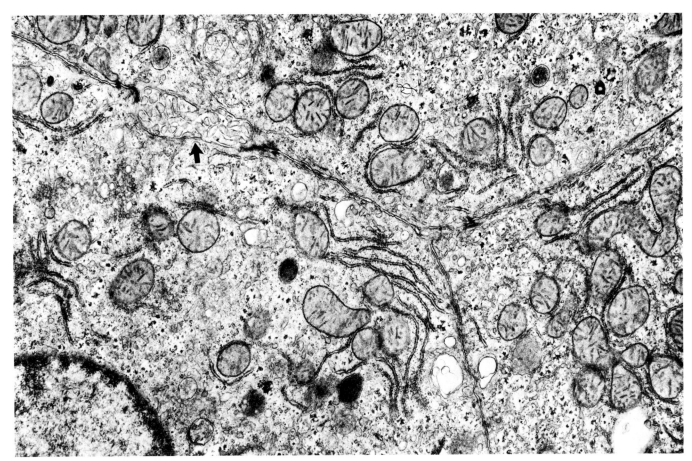

**Fig. 5.32 Hepatocellular carcinoma: Cell morphology and bile canaliculus**

In this field the neoplastic cells resemble normal hepatocytes, and a bile canaliculus has formed (arrow). Lysosomes and microbodies are few. (×21 200)

**Discussion:** Bile canaliculi are generally not numerous in hepatomas, and can be delineated by 5–6 cells. Sinusoids and a space of Disse may occur in highly differentiated cases, as well as bile pigment. Generally, the elements of the endoplasmic reticulum and glycogen aggregates are less prominent in more anaplastic tumours. Lobulated nuclei, nuclear pseudoinclusions, whorled collections of both RER and SER, autophagic vacuoles and virus-like particles have also been described. Large mitochondria wth paracrystalline inclusions have been observed, as have filamentous aggregates identical to so-called Mallory bodies, and membrane-bound pigment bodies similar to those of the Dubin-Johnson syndrome.[901] Nakanuma et al[893] also record rounded membrane-bound cytoplasmic structures with finely granular matrices, corresponding to the presence of pale eosinophilic inclusions on LM. An et al[867] describe the development of such hyaline globular inclusions, suggesting that they result from accumulation of granular material within intracytoplasmic lumina lined by microvilli; histochemical analysis of these inclusions demonstrates the presence of $\alpha$–fetoprotein, $\alpha_1$–antitrypsin ($\alpha_1$–antiprotease) and $\alpha_2$–macroglobulin.

Carcinoid components, including cytoplasmic neurosecretory granules approximately 210 nm in diameter, have additionally been reported in hepatocellular carcinoma.[871] Oncocytic cells with non-crystalline mitochondrial inclusions also occur in fibrolamellar hepatoma, as well as a characteristic interposition of fibroblasts between the oncocytes and the collagenous stroma.

In hepatomas arising in the aged there are more mitochondria and the endoplasmic reticulum is more irregular than in those seen in infancy and childhood. Hepatoblastomas contain both fetal and embryonic cells; the fetal cells often contain glycogen and bile, while abundance of both glycogen and lipid may produce a so-called hypernephroid appearance. The embryonic cells are less differentiated and possess relatively few mitochondria and other organelles.[896]

References: 867, 871, 872, 875, 878, 879, 882, 884–886, 888, 893, 896, 897, 901, 902, 904, 907, 908, 913, 914

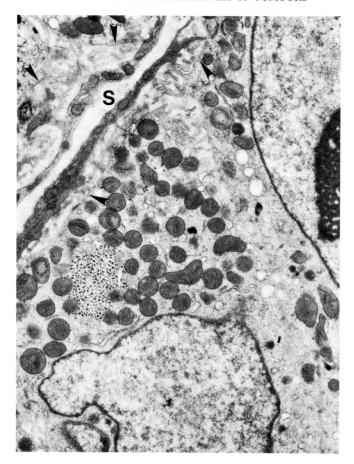

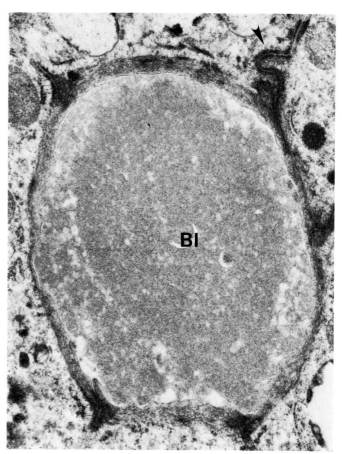

**Fig. 5.33  Hepatocellular carcinoma: Space of Disse**

A sinusoidal circulation often persists in this neoplasm and here a distinct space of Disse (arrowheads) can be identified around the cells lining the narrow sinusoidal lumen (S). The cytoplasmic characteristics are generally similar to those of normal hepatocytes although nuclear irregularity, increased amounts of euchromatin and large nucleoli are typically present. (×8100)

**Fig. 5.34  Hepatocellular carcinoma: Intracanalicular bile**

Multifocal hepatoma from a 63-year-old man. This collection of bile (BI) consists of granular material of medium electron-density, distending the bile canaliculus. Although luminal microvilli are not present, subluminal junctional complexes (arrowhead) border the space. Note the concentration of microfilaments in the periluminal cytoplasm. Lipid droplets and intranuclear cytoplasmic pseudoinclusions were prominent features of this case. (×18 900)

Bile pigment is usually restricted to highly differentiated hepatomas, occurring within canaliculi, the cytoplasm, or both; its electron-density is variable but is often intense.

By use of freeze-fracture techniques, the pericanalicular junctions in hepatocellular carcinoma are seen to be disorganized; the tight junctions show loss of orientation, with focal discontinuities and proliferations, while gap junctions are small and infrequent.[906]

Reference: 906

# 6 Small cell carcinomas

## SMALL CELL CARCINOMAS OF LUNG AND OTHER SITES

Electron microscopy is often of decisive value in assessing differentiation in small cell carcinomas. Squamous cell carcinomas can be excluded, while neoplasms of neuroendrocrine (APUD; paraneurone) cells can be positively identified by the detection of typical neurosecretory granules (NSG) (Tables 6.1, 6.2, 26.1 and 29.2).

Although most small cell carcinomas arise in the respiratory tract, similar primary tumours have now been recorded in many anatomical sites (Table 6.3). Small cell carcinomas are ultrastructurally distinguished from carcinoid tumours by a relative paucity of NSG and their fine structure is compared with other small cell tumours in Tables 29.1 and 29.2. Not all small cell carcinomas represent neuroendocrine tumours, and some may show evidence of squamous or glandular epithelial differentiation by EM.[470] Conversely, some apparently non-neuroendocrine tumours (such as squamous carcinomas) may occasionally contain membrane-bound bodies indistinguishable from NSG,[470] a situation perhaps analogous to the mixed patterns of differentiation found occasionally in gastrointestinal carcinomas (see Chapter 7). NSG and mucin granules, as well as tonofilaments and cilia, have been identified in single cells in some pulmonary and extra-pulmonary neuroendocrine tumours, suggesting multi-directional differentiation.[541,542,567,781]

There is therefore increasing evidence that 'small cell carcinoma' is a heterogeneous category of tumours analogous in this respect to large cell undifferentiated carcinoma of lung.

### Table 6.1 Ultrastructural classification of bronchopulmonary small cell carcinomas

1. Small cell neuroendocrine carcinoma (true oat cell carcinoma)
2. Small cell carcinoma without neurosecretory granules (NSG)*
3. Small cell squamous carcinoma
4. Small cell adenocarcinoma
5. Bipartite carcinomas:
    5.1 Neuroendocrine-squamous carcinoma
    5.2 Neuroendocrine-adeno-carcinoma
6. Tripartite neuroendocrine-adeno-squamous carcinomas

*The frequency of NSG in neuroendocrine carcinomas is variable, presumably reflecting a spectrum of cytodifferentiation (see Table 6.2). Failure to identify NSG in small cell carcinomas otherwise resembling neuroendocrine carcinoma *may* be explained by their extreme rarity in very poorly differentiated tumours
References: 447, 453, 455, 464, 470, 473, 483, 493, 497, 498, 506, 529, 530, 536, 541–543, 552, 567

### Table 6.2 Sequence of diminishing differentiation in bronchopulmonary neuroendocrine tumours

| Tumour | Frequency of NSG |
|---|---|
| Typical carcinoid tumour | |
| Atypical carcinoid tumour* | |
| Neuroendocrine carcinoma, intermediate cell type | |
| Neuroendocrine carcinoma, small cell type | |
| Small cell carcinoma without NSG (?) | |

*Gould et al[489] tentatively designate most of these tumours as well differentiated neuroendocrine carcinomas (see Table 16.3). Some neuroendocrine carcinomas have an undifferentiated large cell pattern by LM; in this scheme such tumours would be included in the intermediate cell category

References: 437, 447, 448, 453, 455, 456, 460, 467, 473, 483, 486, 489, 491, 495, 519, 536, 543, 547, 552, 566

### Table 6.3 Sites of origin of undifferentiated small cell carcinomas

Trachea, bronchus and lung

Paranasal sinus
Larynx
Thyroid gland*
Thymus
Salivary gland
Oesophagus
Stomach
Small bowel
Colon
Pancreas
Urinary bladder
Prostate
Uterine cervix
Endometrium†
Skin§
Breast (?)[1452]

*Most small cell tumours of thyroid represent lymphomas; see text, Chapter 11. †Neuroendocrine differentiation proven by the presence of cytoplasmic neurosecretory granules 100–160 nm in diameter.[1246] §Merkel cell carcinoma

Of the 29 cases of small cell anaplastic lung carcinomas reported by Li et al[530] only 19 (66 per cent) contained NSG on ultrastructural examination; the remaining 10 tumours were designated variously as squamous, adenosquamous, adeno- and bronchiolo-alveolar carcinoma, 'reserve cell' and undifferentiated carcinoma, and malignant lymphoma. Recognition of non-neuroendocrine small cell carcinomas may have prognostic significance. Twelve patients in this series underwent pulmonary resection; five of the six with non-neuroendocrine carcinomas survived more than 2 years, compared to only two out of six with 'oat cell' carcinomas containing NSG.

Bolen & Thorning[453] more recently have reported similar conclusions concerning classification, based on an analysis of 46 small cell carcinomas and 5 carcinoid tumours of lung. Twenty-two of the small cell tumours were neuroendocrine in type, containing NSG 100-180 nm in diameter, often concentrated in short cell processes; a considerable range of differentiation was encountered in this group, partly expressed by the frequency of NSG. Six of the carcinomas were squamous and two represented 'mucus secretory' adenocarcinomas, while 16 were too poorly differentiated to be assigned to the first three categories and were designated as null cell carcinomas.

To the best of our knowledge there is no published evidence to suggest that predominantly non-neuroendocrine (squamous and/or glandular) carcinomas containing sporadic clusters of NSG should be reclassified as small cell neuroendocrine carcinomas, with the prognostic and therapeutic implications of that diagnosis. It is our belief that such an approach may have disastrous consequences for patient management, and that therapy should be based on the predominant pattern(s) of differentiation as determined by both LM and EM. Finally, it is cautioned that the size and morphology of structures resembling NSG require careful assessment to ensure that other granular cytoplasmic constituents, such as lysosomes or Clara cell-like granules, are not misinterpreted as NSG (see also Chapter 2).

## NEUROENDOCRINE (MERKEL CELL) CARCINOMA OF SKIN

The histomorphological spectrum of the recently delineated cutaneous neuroendocrine carcinomas ranges from tumours composed of intermediate-sized cells with a carcinoid-like arrangement, to small cell neoplasms reminiscent of oat cell carcinoma of lung.[1472] The designation Merkel cell carcinoma (MCC) is most often applied to the small cell subgroup, but is also used for the whole class of cutaneous neuroendocrine carcinomas. In the past these tumours have also been reported as trabecular carcinoma,[1528] small cell neuroepithelial tumour of skin, and peripheral adult neuroblastoma.[1535,1852]

A definitive diagnosis of MCC is facilitated by electron microscopy (Figs. 6.3 and 6.4).[1521,1538] The cells are classically polyhedral and loosely cohesive, with sporadic intermediate-type junctions. Moderate numbers of rounded neurosecretory

granules (NSG) 80–200 nm in diameter constitute the outstanding cytoplasmic feature (see Table 29.2); these are concentrated at the cell periphery, often forming linear subplasmalemmal arrays,[1521] but they also occur in cytoplasmic processes.[1523] Paranuclear aggregates of intermediate filaments also typify MCC, being found in 23 of 24 cases in two combined series;[1469,1538] immunocytochemical analysis of one case indicates that the filaments represent neurofilaments in the absence of detectable cytokeratins or vimentin.[1503] Sporadic microvillous processes may also be found, but true acini have never been reported.[1538] The NSG distinguish MCC from other neoplasms such as squamous and sweat gland carcinomas, malignant lymphomas and Ewing's sarcoma. The ultrastructural distinction from metastatic oat cell carcinoma of lung (and other sites) and neuroblastoma potentially poses greater difficulties, and is discussed in detail in Tables 29.1 and 29.2.

The cell now bearing his name was described by Merkel in 1895, in a study of epidermal terminal neurites in the snout skin of the mole; together with neuronal processes these cells form complexes designated as *Tastzellen*.[1521] In human skin the complexes are usually related to either hair follicles[1518] or epidermis; they are thought to represent slowly reacting mechanoreceptors and it is possible that Merkel cells exert a modulating influence on nerve fibre function.[1469] Ultrastructural examination of Merkel cells reveals cytoplasmic NSG, as well as cell processes and collections of intermediate filaments; MCC has similar neuroendocrine appearances, but there is no proof that these neoplasms originate from Merkel cells,[1472] and the less committal expression 'neuroendocrine carcinoma' seems preferable. Merkel cells normally contain met-enkephalin,[1521] and the demonstration of this substance in MCC would be valuable confirmatory evidence of *bona fide* Merkel cell differentiation. Melanosomes have also been recorded in cutaneous neuroendocrine carcinomas,[1629] as have neurone-specific enolase[1490,1538] and polypeptides such as calcitonin, somatostatin and ACTH.[1486,1629] MCC is therefore appropriately included in the broadening spectrum of neuroendocrine carcinomas of skin, lung, endocrine organs, gastrointestinal tract and other sites. Up to one-third of cases of MCC are associated with synchronous or metachronous squamous cell carcinomas;[1469,1471] the synchronous tumours occasionally develop in the same anatomical site, with admixture of the squamous and neuroendocrine cells. In two such cases, Gomez et al[1471] found that each component remained distinct, without convincing cellular transitions. However, this association suggests bidirectional differentiation, and casts some doubt on the postulated neural crest derivation of Merkel cells.[1469]

*Minimal criteria for the ultrastructural diagnosis of neuroendocrine (Merkel cell) carcinoma of skin:* Unequivocal neurosecretory granules in the appropriate cellular environment of a primary cutaneous carcinoma.

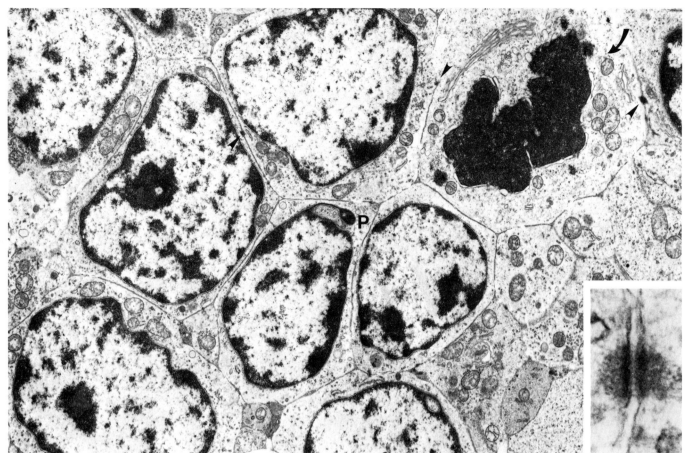

## Fig. 6.1 Small cell neuroendocrine carcinoma of lung: Topography and desmosome

The neoplastic cells are tightly packed and attached by scattered desomosomes (arrowheads and inset). The nuclei contain moderate quantities of heterochromatin, and occasional nucleoli; a nuclear projection (P) is also apparent. The nuclear heterochromatin in these carcinomas is often clumped, producing a leopard skin-like pattern. One of the cells (curved arrow) is in mitosis, with scattered separate chromatin collections. Cytoplasm is generally small in amount, and contains few organelles. Cell processes in cross-section are evident, but at this power neurosecretory granules cannot be readily identified.

**Inset:** Desmosome in the same tumour at high magnification, showing the plate-like thickening of the paradesmosomal cytoplasm. Tight junctions in the absence of gap junctions are also described.[552] (×8600. Inset: ×119 800)

See Tables 6.1—6.3, 16.1, 26.1 and 29.1–29.3.

References: 258, 385, 398, 408, 409, 435, 447, 453, 461, 464, 483, 488, 489, 493, 498, 506, 536, 552, 735, 736, 771, 776, 780–782, 787, 792, 794, 828, 848, 1053, 1055, 1182, 1204, 1246, 1277, 1452, 1453, 2684, 2692

## Fig. 6.2 Small cell neuroendocrine carcinoma of lung: Neurosecretory granules

Oat cell carcinoma from a 53-year-old woman, who had a six-year history of a myasthenic syndrome, which had been unsuccessfully treated by thymectomy; when a carcinoma of the lung was finally discovered, her electromyogram was typical of the so-called Eaton-Lambert syndrome.

Most neoplastic cells had few granules or none at all, but some contained small numbers of dense-core membrane-bound neurosecretory granules (NSG), averaging 155 nm in diameter, as shown here (arrows). Note the thin lucent haloes between the cores of the granules and the surrounding membranes, especially in the inset. Although fewer than in carcinoid tumours, the number of NSG in such neuroendocrine small cell carcinomas varies considerably and their detection may require a prolonged search. (×45 200. Inset: ×73 100)

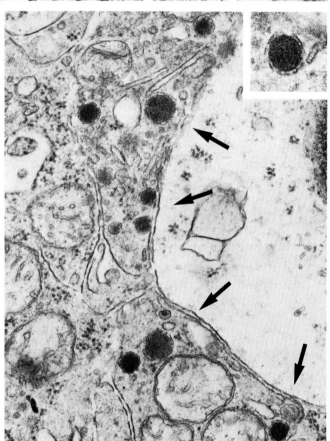

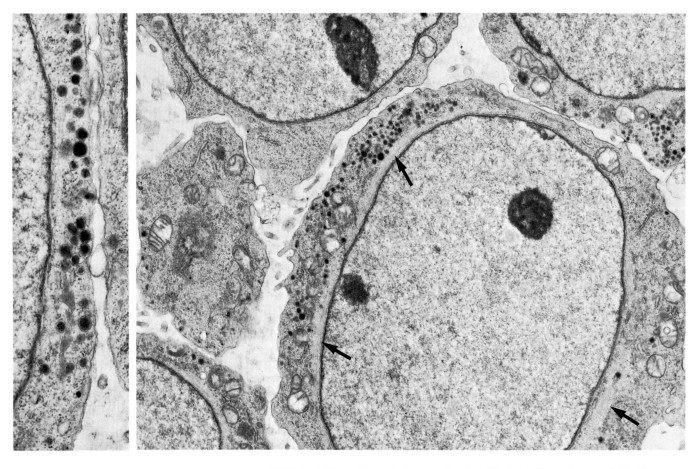

**Fig. 6.3 Neuroendocrine (Merkel cell) carcinoma of skin: Survey**

This neoplasm typically consists of rounded cells with spherical nuclei which possess small nucleoli. Perinuclear bundles of intermediate filaments are present (arrows), while numerous small electron-dense granules are polarized in segments of the cytoplasm. Intercellular junctions are usually small and infrequent; none is present in this field. (×10 400)

**Inset:** Subplasmalemmal array of granules, some displaying a distinct electron-dense core. (×23 100)

References: 1469, 1471, 1472, 1486, 1487, 1490, 1503, 1513, 1521–1523, 1527–1529, 1535, 1538, 1541

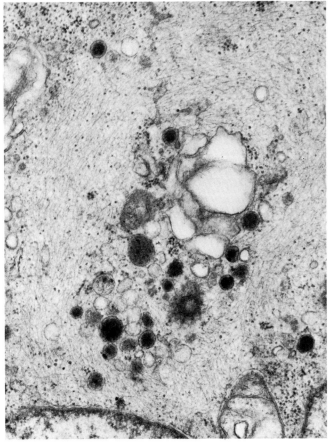

**Fig. 6.4 Cutaneous neuroendocrine (Merkel cell) carcinoma: Cytoplasmic detail**

A whorl of cytoplasmic filaments surrounds elements of the Golgi zone together with neurosecretory granules and a few other cytoplasmic organelles. (×32 000)

# 7 Miscellaneous epithelial tumours – large cell undifferentiated, giant cell, and composite carcinomas; sweat gland tumours and mixed epithelio-mesenchymal neoplasms

## LARGE CELL UNDIFFERENTIATED CARCINOMA OF LUNG

Although so-called large cell undifferentiated carcinomas of lung consist mainly of primitive cells without identifying features, focal squamous or glandular differentiation, or both, can be recognized ultrastructurally in the majority of cases.[468,507,582] Such observations may have prognostic relevance; accordingly, Horie & Ohta[507] have identified four subtypes of large cell carcinoma of lung with corresponding prognostic differences, based on a study of 26 cases:

1. Squamous carcinomas: Most favourable prognosis (5 cases).
2. Adenosquamous carcinoma: Poor prognosis (10 cases). These tumours need to be distinguished by LM from mucoepidermoid carcinoma which has a far more favourable prognosis.
3. Adenocarcinoma: Poor prognosis (9 cases).
4. Giant cell carcinoma (considered to represent a special type of squamous or undifferentiated carcinoma; see below): Fulminant course (2 cases).

Finally, EM uncommonly demonstrates neurosecretory granules within large cell carcinomas, indicating that these cases represent one form of neuroendocrine carcinoma (see Chapter 6).

## GIANT CELL CARCINOMAS

Excluding the skeleton and soft tissues, tumours characterized by multinucleated giant cells have been described in several visceral sites including breast, thyroid, pancreas, lung, ovary

**Table 7.1 Ultrastructural differential diagnosis of undifferentiated large cell carcinomas**

Carcinomas: Adenocarcinoma
Adenosquamous carcinoma
Squamous cell carcinoma
Neuroendocrine carcinoma
Urothelial carcinoma
Unclassifiable undifferentiated carcinoma
Malignant melanoma
Non-Hodgkin's lymphomas
Plasma cell myeloma
Granulocytic sarcomas
Seminoma-dysgerminoma
Ewing's sarcoma, large cell type
Sympathicoblastoma
Undifferentiated unclassifiable malignancy

and kidney. They comprise a heterogeneous group in which three main categories can be discerned:

### 1. Carcinomas with malignant epithelial giant cells

This group is exemplified by the distinctive pleomorphic giant cell carcinoma of lung which may be regarded as a special variant of large cell undifferentiated carcinoma,[507] in which squamous and glandular patterns of differentiation have been demonstrated. However, Wang et al[594] have described an apparently 'pure' form of pulmonary giant cell carcinoma with 'unique' ultrastructural features including concentric whorls of tonofilament-like cytoplasmic fibrils, abundant mitochondria and aggregates of multiple pairs of centrioles in cells lacking surface specializations. It is likely that such tumours simply reflect extreme anaplasia within the spectrum of squamous and glandular differentiation.

Epithelial differentiation with giant cell formation is also described in similar neoplasms in other sites such as parotid gland,[723] thyroid,[1746,1753] pancreas,[917,985] and ovary.[1275] Furthermore, syncytiotrophoblastic giant cells may occur in gonadal and extragenital germ cell tumours, and also in gastrointestinal carcinomas with focal trophoblastic differentiation.[810]

### 2. Carcinomas containing banal stromal osteoclast-like or histiocytic giant cells

Neoplasms in this group usually consist of a readily identifiable carcinomatous component associated with benign multinucleated histiocytoid giant cells resembling osteoclasts and located within the stroma. The polykaryons in these cases are most probably reactive to either the tumour cells and their products, to stromal constituents, or to associated haemorrhage and necrosis. Such tumours have been described in the breast[1358,1439] and pancreas.[917,983] The giant cell component may be diffuse, or form a discrete focus which merges with or lies adjacent to the carcinomatous region, as recorded in the pancreas,[966] lung[560] and ovary.[1334] In these cases the osteoclastoid zones resemble giant cell tumours ('osteoclastomas') of bone. Sometimes this component predominates and may overshadow the epithelial foci; such lesions merge with the next category of giant cell neoplasms.

### 3. Primary visceral giant cell tumours indistinguishable from giant cell tumour of bone

These enigmatic neoplasms, in which there is no LM evidence of epithelial differentiation, occur in the pancreas,[917,970,971] liver,[892] thyroid,[1728] breast,[1408] and kidney.[1013] In these reports, the ultrastructural characteristics of both the mononuclear and giant cell components have been variously interpreted as histiocytic, osteoclastic and epithelial; however, the accompanying descriptions and illustrations have often been ambiguous and in some cases histiocytic cells have been misinterpreted as epithelial, because of the identification of occasional non-desmosomal junctions. Nonetheless, epithelial features have been demonstrated in both the mononuclear and giant cell components in some studies, notably that of Rosai.[971] Such observations, coupled with the identification of transitional cases in category 2 above, suggest that visceral osteoclastoma-like giant cell tumours are probably carcinomas dramatically modified by histiocytic metaplasia affecting the neoplastic cells.

Composite giant cell carcinomas including both tumour giant cells and reactive stromal histiocytic giant cells have rarely been documented.[1386] Giant cell carcinomas need to be distinguished from other neoplasms containing giant cells, notably fibrohistiocytic tumours and other soft tissue sarcomas. Interlobular stromal giant cell aggregates have been described in association with breast carcinomas in areas remote from tumour, and also in non-tumour-bearing breasts.[1433]

## TUMOURS WITH MULTIDIRECTIONAL EPITHELIAL DIFFERENTIATION I: GENERAL REMARKS

The recognition of divergent epithelial differentiation in single human neoplasms is now commonplace. For example, squamous, glandular and neuroendocrine differentiation may be seen in various combinations in a broad range of epithelial tumours from diverse primary sites. In such instances most cells contain only one type of secretory product, but single cells exhibiting a composite phenotype may be demonstrated; examples include the coexistence of mucous and neurosecretory granules within individual cells in mucinous carcinoid tumours of the appendix and colon, and both zymogenic and neurosecretory granules in a pancreatic tumour showing acinic and neuroendocrine differentiation. Indeed, the once strict separation of adenocarcinomas and neuroendocrine tumours of the gastrointestinal tract has needed to be modified as increasing numbers of tumours with composite characteristics have been reported; these form a spectrum of differentiation from classical carcinoid tumours at one end, to classical adenocarcinomas at the other. Even more complex admixtures of endocrine, mucin-secreting, absorptive and Paneth cells are sometimes demonstrable in gastrointestinal neoplasms, as well as in other sites (see Table 7.2 and Fig. 7.1).[420,984] It is worthwhile distinguishing between 'composite' tumours where the different components are restricted to distinct areas, and truly 'mixed' tumours with a diffuse and intimate admixture of different cell types.

The controversial problem of argyrophilia in breast carcinomas is considered in Chapter 5.

## TUMOURS WITH MULTIDIRECTIONAL EPITHELIAL DIFFERENTIATION II: MELANOTIC NEUROENDOCRINE CARCINOMAS

Melanin-containing neuroendocrine tumours have been found in the skin,[1629] thyroid (medullary carcinoma),[1629,1770] bronchus[462,490] and gastrointestinal tract.[1629]

Gould and associates[1629] have lucidly reported four such tumours which contained two or more polypeptides; somatostatin was demonstrated in all four cases, while ACTH and calcitonin were present in three. Neurosecretory granules 200–300 nm in diameter and melanosomes were generally found in different cells, but occasionally coexisted within the same cell. The authors considered a variety of explanations to account for this association, including transfer of melanin from nearby melanocytes into the carcinomatous cells, incorporation of non-neoplastic bystander melanocytes into the carcinomas, so-called collision tumours, and transformation of melanocytes into malignant cells due to 'horizontal induction' by the carcinomas. They favoured the hypothesis that these neoplasms are complex neuroendocrine carcinomas with composite differentiation, as indicated by polypeptide and melanin production.

## SWEAT GLAND TUMOURS

The diagnosis of most sweat gland tumours is established by LM. However, EM may occasionally be of diagnostic value in poorly differentiated sweat gland carcinomas by detecting ductal-acinar structures or adenosquamous appearances, thereby facilitating the distinction from other skin tumours such as Merkel cell carcinoma. Composite ductal-squamous features have been described in a variety of sweat gland tumours; these include eccrine spiradenoma,[1480] cylindroma,[1480] eccrine acrospiroma (clear cell hidradenoma),[1477] eccrine poroma,[1480] chondroid syringoma,[1533] malignant chondroid syringoma,[1515] syringoma,[1480] sweat gland carcinoma with syringomatous features[1495] and mucin-producing adenosquamous carcinoma of the vulva.[1532] Well developed squamous characteristics are also recorded in a malignant acrospiroma.[1484] In addition to desmosome-tonofilament complexes and cytoplasmic tonofibrils, the squamous cells may contain keratohyaline granules and show evidence of keratinization, as described in syringoma.[1476,1480] The occurrence of periluminal tonofilaments, lysosomes, keratohyaline granules and keratinization in cells bordering duct lumina is said to be characteristic of immature eccrine intra-epidermal cells;[1476] intracytoplasmic neolumina also appear to indicate eccrine duct differentiation. In a study of a metastasizing porocarcinoma, Turner et al[1531] mention that 'intracytoplasmic lumina in cells with squamous features appear to be highly characteristic of eccrine duct tumours with poral differentiation'. Such adenosquamous cells are also reported in eccrine poroma, syringoma, sweat gland carcinoma with syringomatous features, and poroepithelioma.[1531] Intra-

**Table 7.2  Examples of tumours exhibiting multidirectional epithelial differentiation**

| Patterns of differentiation | Typical anatomical sites | Remarks |
|---|---|---|
| Mucoepidermoid or adenosquamous carcinoma (or adenoacanthoma) | Respiratory tract | — |
| | Salivary glands | Oncocytic change is recorded in a parotid mucoepidermoid carcinoma[755] |
| | Pancreas | — |
| | Small intestine | — |
| | Endometrium | — |
| | Skin (vulva) | — |
| *Neuroendocrine cells in mucosubstance-producing adenomas and adenocarcinomas | Respiratory tract | — |
| | Gastrointestinal tract | Multiple neuroendocrine products may be demonstrable within single composite neoplasms. For example, cells containing serotonin, somatostatin, gastrin, motilin, secretin and neurotensin are described in a colonic adenocarcinoma containing argentaffin cells[865] |
| | Pancreas | — |
| | Uterine cervix | — |
| | Ovary | See below |
| | Prostate | Argentaffin cells found in 8 per cent of prostatic carcinomas in one study[1084] |
| *Neuroendocrine carcinomas with focal glandular or squamous differentiation | Larynx | — |
| | Lung | — |
| | Oesophagus | — |
| | Stomach | — |
| | Colon | — |
| | Skin | — |
| | Cervix | — |
| | Prostate | — |
| | Thyroid | — |
| Mucinous carcinoid tumours (goblet cell carcinoids) | Appendix and colon | Single cells with composite phenotypes (mucoendocrine cells) are described in both sites |
| Melanotic neuroendocrine carcinomas | Skin | See text, this chapter |
| | Thyroid | — |
| | Bronchus | See also Table 16.3 |
| | Gastrointestinal tract | — |
| Basal and squamous cell carcinomas with admixed neuroendocrine (Merkel) cells | Skin | — |
| Complex intestinal-type epithelial differentiation, including various combinations of goblet, resorptive, neuroendocrine and Paneth cells | Ovary | As part of mucinous cystadenomas and cystadenocarcinomas in particular. The neuroendocrine elements may be admixed with the cyst lining epithelium, or may form discrete foci of carcinoid tumour.[1352] The coexistence of Brenner tumours with mucinous ovarian neoplasms,[1351] and with a neuroendocrine cell component[1310] is also recorded. Strumal carcinoids are considered in Table 30.2 |
| | Gastrointestinal tract | Proliferations of Paneth cells have been documented in the following: carcinoma of stomach, adenomas and carcinomas of small and large intestine, the lesions of familial and juvenile polyposis coli, an adenocarcinoma of Meckel's diverticulum, and a papilloma of gall bladder.[797,854,862] In a Paneth cell-rich papillary adenocarcinoma, single cells containing both mucous and Paneth-type granules have been identified[862] |
| | Nasal cavity and paranasal sinuses | Some primary adenocarcinomas in these sites mimic colonic adenocarcinoma. Schmid et al[420] reported a highly differentiated villoglandular enteric-type carcinoma of the nasal mucosa containing Paneth-like cells and cells containing gastrin and glucagon – with 7 different neuroendocrine cell subtypes on EM, including cells with composite endo- and exo-crine morphology |
| Trophoblastic differentiation in: | | |
| 1. Seminomas-germinomas | Gonadal and extragonadal | — |
| 2. Extragenital carcinomas | Gastrointestinal tract, notably stomach | Confirmed by detection of intracellular human chorionic gonadotrophin ($\beta$-subunit)[810] |

*The distinction between these two categories is based on the proportions of the various cell types in a particular tumour

References: 52, 398, 418, 420, 462, 490, 522, 740, 755, 781, 797, 803, 810, 817, 830, 831, 834, 850, 854, 862, 865, 951, 973, 984, 1084, 1185, 1208, 1264, 1280, 1281, 1306, 1310, 1351, 1352, 1497, 1629, 1740, 1770

cytoplasmic lumina are additionally documented in chondroid syringoma[1533] and in a single cell of an eccrine spiradenoma.[1461]

Myoepithelial cells may also be seen in sweat gland neoplasms. In *chondroid syringoma* they form the outer layer of the ductal elements,[1533] and myoepithelium-like cells also occur in the chondroid areas[1533] (as in pleomorphic salivary adenomas).

Hashimoto & Lever[1480] subdivided the cells comprising *eccrine spiradenoma* into multiple types, including basal and intermediate cells, and luminal cells with ductal or secretory features; histiocytes and a few immature myoepithelial cells were also identified. Some of the luminal cells were devoid of ductal differentiation, lacking both microvilli and secretory granules, while others possessed microvillous apices; periluminal tonofilaments were also seen.

Hashimoto & Lever[1480] also divided the cells of *cylindroma* into a number of subtypes, including dark basal cells, and lighter indeterminate cells, as well as ductal and secretory cells. The lumina were slit-like and bordered by microvillous cells; some of the lining cells possessed dark secretory granules reminiscent of apocrine epithelium. The basal laminae were reduplicated and associated with anchoring fibrils.

*Apocrine tumours* are characterized by numerous, often bizarre mitochondria and large secretory granules which are probably lysosomal; annulate lamellae may also be present.[1473] In addition, large secretory granules and annulate lamellae may be found in eccrine acrospiroma.[1477] The cytoplasmic clarity of some sweat gland tumours is attributable to the accumulation of glycogen.[1477,1480] Admixed Langerhans' histiocytes are also recorded in several categories of sweat gland tumour (see Table 28.3).

The 'histogenetic' implications of these ultrastructural observations are discussed in detail in the original articles.[1476,1477,1479,1480]

## MIXED EPITHELIO-MESENCHYMAL TUMOURS

Neoplasms with composite epithelial and mesenchymal differentiation occur in several organs and tissues, notably the reproductive tract (see Chapter 30). Most of these diverse tumours are illustrated and described in other sections of this atlas; only two examples are shown here, namely so-called cystosarcoma phyllodes (Figs. 7.4 and 7.5) and mixed salivary tumours (Figs. 7.6–7.8).

## MIXED SALIVARY TUMOURS AND SALIVARY GLAND CARCINOMAS

The 'histogenesis' of pleomorphic salivary adenomas has excited much interest and controversy, but has not been clearly defined; a derivation from either duct epithelial or myoepithelial cells has been invoked.[709] The ultrastructural appearances are variable, with a morphological continuum from epithelial to mesenchymal cells.[743] Some adenomas consist mainly of myoepithelial cells, but these may not always be identifiable; myoepithelial and myoepithelium-like cells are principally encountered in myxoid or chondroid areas, where undifferentiated cells are also evident. Chondrocytic cells are also described in cartilaginous areas, although only a minority have pericellular lacunae.[743] 'Hyaline' cells rich in intermediate filaments may also occur in salivary adenomas.[294]

In an ultrastructural investigation of both epithelial and mesenchymal (stromal) regions of 24 pleomorphic salivary adenomas, Dardick et al[707,708] propose a central role for modified myoepithelial cells in the continuum between epithelial and stromal tissue. They describe both luminal epithelial and myoepithelial cells in cellular epithelial areas, organized in mimicry of normal ductal-acinar units, with the myoepithelial cells frequently undergoing squamous metaplasia. Representing a transitional zone between the epithelial and stromal elements, the periphery of these cellular areas is characterized by myoepithelial dedifferentiation with depletion of squamous features, and an accumulation of extracellular matrix between the modified myoepithelial cells, forming 'microcystic' stromal aggregates bordered by basal lamina. Further accumulation of the matrix produces the characteristic myxoid and chondromyxoid areas, but even here the authors describe myoepithelium-like features, including a fragmentary basal lamina and tonofilaments. A major problem with this hypothesis concerns the criteria used to define a modified myoepithelial cell (Fig. 7.8). As the authors point out, these cells usually lack the microfilamentous apparatus of classical myoepithelial cells, being characterized instead by intermediate and tono-filaments, polarized basal lamina, desmosomes and hemidesmosomes, and cytoplasmic processes; therefore, others may designate them as duct epithelial in type. Nevertheless, this study represents an important attempt to interrelate the cell types in pleomorphic adenomas and is recommended to the interested reader.

*Adenoid cystic carcinomas* have uniform ultrastructural appearances, whether they arise in salivary gland or extrasalivary sites such as breast, lung and uterine cervix.[737] They are characterized by the combination of pseudocysts, marked basal laminal replication, and intercellular spaces including acini. The pseudocysts mimic acini on LM and contain PAS-positive material, but in fact represent nodular replications of truly 'basal' lamina within the extracellular matrix, bordered by the basal region of epithelial cells (see Fig. 3.17).[737] Fine actin-like filaments, possibly indicating myoepithelial differentiation, are also recorded.[737]

In an ultrastructural analysis of 'undifferentiated' parotid gland carcinomas, Donath et al[715] recognized five cell types: undifferentiated epithelial cells, undifferentiated duct cells, secretory epithelial cells, and squamous and myoepithelial cells. Based on the proportions of these, the tumours could be divided into two major types:

1. Squamous cell carcinomas.
2. Salivary duct carcinomas (containing myoepithelial and squamous cells, together with undifferentiated duct/epithelial cells).

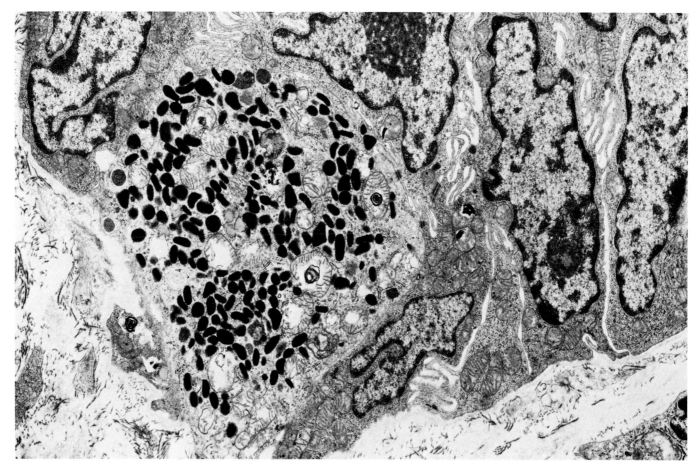

**Fig. 7.1 Colonic adenocarcinoma with mixed cell population: Enterochromaffin cell**

An enterochromaffin cell with pleomorphic osmiophilic membrane-bound granules resembling mid-gut granules (see Table 16.1) is evident in this colonic adenocarcinoma. Although this finding might be interpreted as a residual enterochromaffin cell included within the carcinoma, the granule morphology is dissimilar to that of hind-gut granules. (×13 300)

References: 803, 862, 865

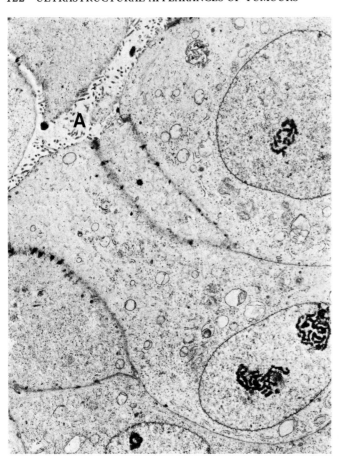

**Fig. 7.2 Infiltrating duct carcinoma of breast: Adenosquamous differentiation I**

These malignant cells display glandular epithelial differentiation with acinus (A) formation. Note also the abundance of nuclear euchromatin and the filamentous nucleoli. (× 4500)

**Fig. 7.3 Infiltrating duct carcinoma of breast: Adenosquamous differentiation II, and microfilaments**

In contrast to the glandular-ductular differentiation shown in Fig. 7.2, a different area of the same carcinoma is characterized by squamous features, as indicated by desmosome-tonofilament complexes (arrows) and numerous cytoplasmic tonofibrils (T). 'Softer' actin-like microfilaments (arrowheads) can also be seen, producing a myoepithelium-like morphology. Nuclear bodies (N) are also present. (×9500)

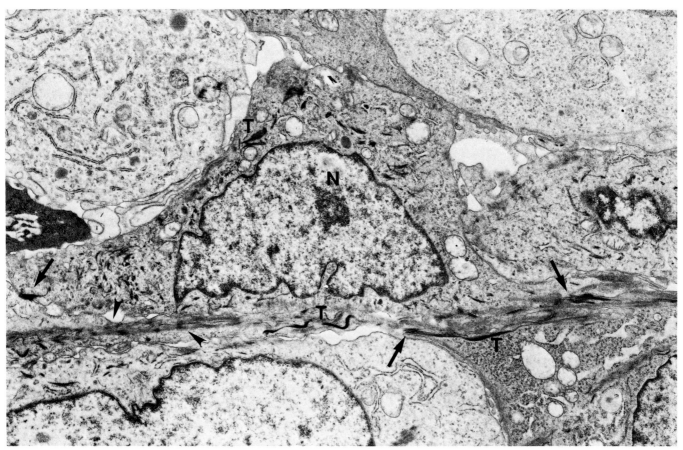

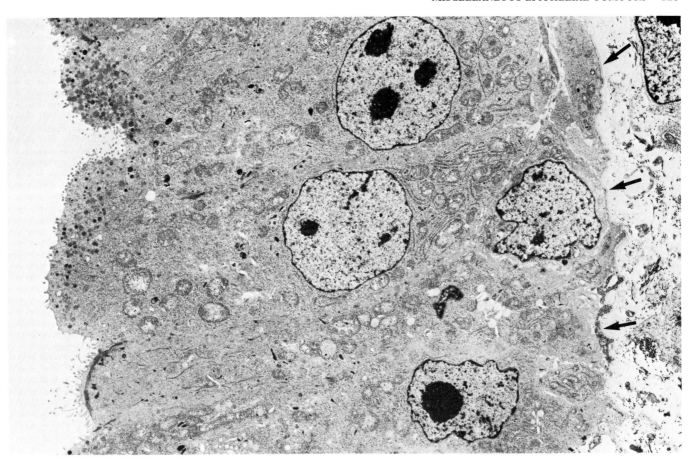

### Fig. 7.4 Giant cellular fibroadenoma of breast (so-called cystosarcoma phyllodes) I: Ductal component

Tumour from the axillary tail of breast of a 53-year-old woman. A continuous basal lamina (arrows) is situated at the epithelio-stromal interface. The epithelial cells have rounded to slightly irregular nuclei with large nucleoli. Secretory granules are concentrated in the apical cytoplasm, and there are numerous luminal microvilli. ($\times 4100$)

In general the ultrastructural appearances of cystosarcoma phyllodes do not deviate significantly from those of ordinary fibroadenomas.[1424] The issue of malignancy is determined by LM.

References: 1361, 1383, 1400, 1424, 1427

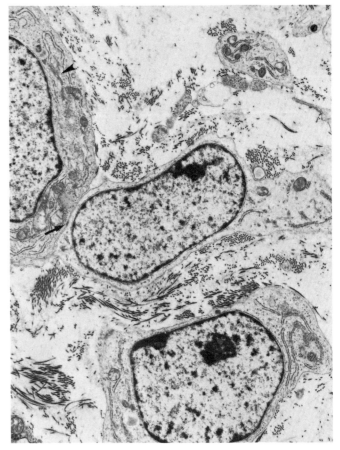

### Fig. 7.5 Giant cellular fibroadenoma of breast II: Mesenchymal component

Same case as Fig. 7.4. These stromal cells have the characteristics of active fibroblasts, and possess prominent strands of RER. The Golgi apparatus in such cells is often well formed,[1424] but only a small complex (arrowhead) is present in this field. A single junction (arrow) has developed between closely apposed plasma membranes. The extracellular matrix contains both collagen fibres and flocculent proteoglycans. Many of the collagen fibres are closely related to the cell borders. ($\times 6700$)

Myofibroblasts and smooth muscle may be found in the mesenchymal component of these tumours.[1400] Cartilage and bone are present on rare occasions;[1361,1424] lipoblastic and rhabdomyoblastic elements are also recorded.[1427]

References: 1361, 1400, 1424, 1427

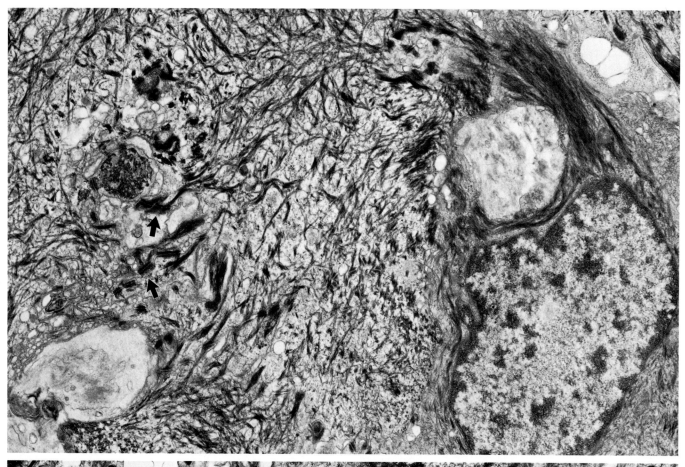

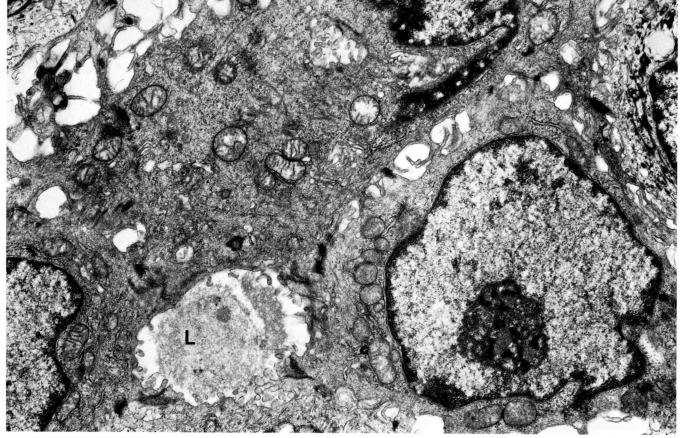

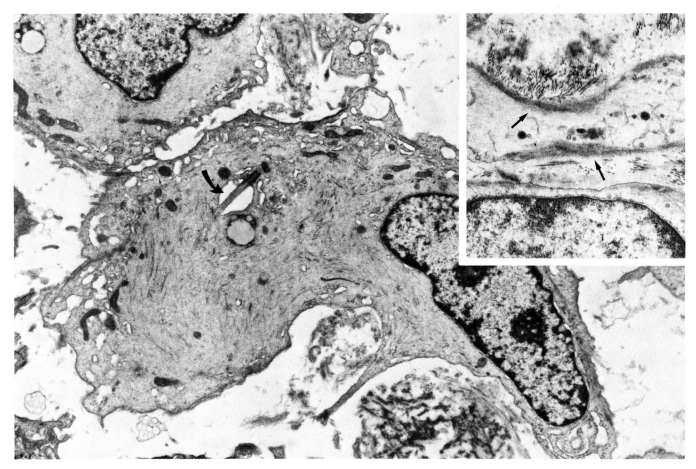

**Fig. 7.8   Mixed salivary tumour: Myoepithelium-like cells**

Myoepithelium-like cells characterized by many fine cytoplasmic filaments are also frequently found, especially in areas where the connective tissue appears on light microscopy to be hyalinized. They contain lipofuscin bodies, and cilia are occasionally present (curved arrow). Observe the loose texture of the connective tissue fibres and filaments. Some of these may show distinct periodicity, presumably representing poorly formed collagen in a matrix of proteoglycans. The latter is probably represented by the amorphous material in the interstices of the formed elements. (×8000)

   **Inset:**  Peripherally   concentrated   fine   filaments   (arrows)   in   a myoepithelium-like cell. (×14 100)
   References: 707–709, 716

**Fig. 7.6** *(Facing page — top)*  **Mixed salivary tumour: Squamous differentiation**

The cells in some parts of these neoplasms have squamous characteristics, including well formed desmosomes (arrows) between adjacent cells, and many cytoplasmic tonofilaments. (×14 800)
   Glandular   epithelial   cells,   as   well   as   'hyaline',   myoepithelial, myoepithelium-like, undifferentiated and even chondrocytic cells may be found in varying proportions.
   References: 288, 294, 697, 702, 704, 707–709, 714, 716, 718, 721, 733, 743

**Fig. 7.7** *(Facing page — bottom)*  **Mixed salivary tumour: Ductular differentiation**

Ductular structures with a distinct lumen (L) and periluminal junctional complexes are also found. Secretory granules can occur, but cytoplasmic filaments are few. (×14 800)

# 8 Melanocytic tumours

## MALIGNANT MELANOMA

In most cases the diagnosis of melanocytic neoplasia is readily achieved by light microscopy, but the amount of melanin produced by some malignant melanomas may be so minute that its detection by routine LM techniques is impossible. In these cases the melanocytic nature of the neoplastic cells may be confirmed by the detection of melanosomes — organelles characteristic of melanocytic differentiation, despite their infrequent description in other neoplasms (Table 8.1). These organelles consist of membrane-limited vesicles with a distinctive internal structure (Figs. 8.2–8.4). Depending on the stage of development, there may be parallel lamellae, or helical or zigzag structures with a periodicity of 8–10 nm.[39,45,47] Some studies suggest that the melanosomes in lentigo maligna melanoma are usually ellipsoidal and resemble those of normal melanocytes, while those in superficial spreading and nodular melanomas are usually spheroidal and abnormal in appearance.[1581] Other investigators have found variable and often aberrant melanosome morphology,[1591] and have indicated that structural differences are unreliable in distinguishing between malignant melanoma and benign melanocytic lesions.[1594]

Melanosomes cannot be found in some cases of undoubted malignant melanoma, while in other instances their identification requires a prolonged search. The morphology of melanosome-like bodies in tumours should also be assessed critically, to ensure that other structures such as lysosomes are not erroneously identified as melanosomes. It is also emphasized that compound melanosomes have no diagnostic significance whatsoever; they can be found in a variety of non-melanocytic cells (see Fig. 5.26), especially macrophages,[45] as a result of phagocytosis or passive transfer. Melanin transfer has also been invoked to explain the presence of stage II melanosomes in extraordinary circumstances such as a melanotic adenocarcinoma of the ano-rectum (Table 8.1); *therefore, in order to have unquestionable discriminant value, melanosomes should be evaluated in the light of their microenvironment to determine that this is 'appropriate', even if non-melanocytic* (see Table 8.1, and Chapter 7).

The Golgi complex of melanoma cells is moderately well developed and microfilaments occur in the cytoplasm occasionally. Intermediate filaments are also described; according to one report,[1560] they consist of vimentin only. Intercellular junctions are infrequent, the intermediate type

predominating, while external laminae may be poorly developed or undetectable.

Straight intracisternal tubules with a fuzzy coating are occasionally present in the RER,[1590] sometimes forming geometric aggregates (Fig. 8.5). These coated parallel tubules (CPT) have most often been found in malignant melanoma, and Mackay[85] has suggested that they may have diagnostic value in the absence of demonstrable melanosomes. However, they have also been reported in adrenal cortical adenoma, Müllerian adenosarcoma of the uterus, osteogenic sarcoma,[2613] extraskeletal myxoid chondrosarcoma,[2181] chondroid chordoma[2655] and a thyroid carcinoma. Nevertheless, these tumours are easily distinguished from malignant melanoma by LM; in malignancies resembling melanomas, CPT may therefore be suggestive of that diagnosis, if not of decisive confirmatory value.

*Minimal criteria required for the ultrastructural recognition of melanocytic differentiation:* Stage II melanosomes in an appropriate cellular environment, taking into account the exceptions listed in Table 8.1. Coated parallel tubules in melanocyte-like cells lacking melanosomes are highly suggestive of melanocytic differentiation, but are not pathognomonic.

## DESMOPLASTIC SPINDLE CELL MELANOMA

The precise nature of so-called desmoplastic spindle cell melanoma is unclear, and there have been relatively few published ultrastructural studies of this tumour.[1564,1588,1617] The spindle cells have generally been devoid of melanosomes and instead have resembled fibroblasts, myofibroblasts or even smooth muscle cells. Bundles of closely apposed elongated cells with Schwannian characteristics in the absence of identifiable melanosomes were also reported by DiMaio et al[1564] in an analysis of six cases, and were interpreted as neurosarcomatous transformation.

A local fibroxanthoma-like desmoplastic response to cutaneous melanoma has been invoked to account for these observations.[1588] However, persistence of mesenchymal morphology in the absence of identifiable melanocytes in the metastases of one of our cases (Fig. 8.7) militates against this interpretation. The metastatic tumour in another of our cases represented a composite of melanosome-containing epithelioid malignancy resembling conventional melanoma, and

126

unmelanized spindle cell areas (Fig. 8.8). Other cases in our experience have contained cells with perineurial features, and in one instance we have found stage II melanosomes within the spindle cells after a prolonged search of many tissue blocks. Sobel et al[2226] also detected melanosomes in one of four cases.

We consider these findings to be explicable on the basis of mesenchymal and/or nerve sheath cell differentiation, developing in and replacing to varying degrees an original clone of melanocytic cells — a proposal analogous to the mesenchymal metaplasia hypothesis advanced in the case of spindle cell squamous carcinoma (see Chapter 4). Apart from the possible 'histogenetic' implications, documentation of the vimentin filaments characteristic of glial and mesenchymal cells in conventional malignant melanoma[1560] might also be interpreted as a subliminal indicator of such neuro-mesenchymal potentialities.

**Table 8.1  Tumours reported to contain melanosomes***

| Tumour | Comments |
| --- | --- |
| Naevocellular and blue naevi, and fibrotic papule of nose | Balloon cell changes in naevi and malignant melanomas are attributable to vacuolation of melanosomes,[1613] and perhaps to lipid accumulation in some instances.[2146] Schwannian features are described in the melanosome-containing cells of blue naevi of the uterine cervix[1587] |
| Malignant melanoma | Including melanomas arising in the uveal tract.[2146] However, in the published accounts of desmoplastic spindle cell melanoma, the spindle cells generally appear to be mesenchymal or neural in type by EM and devoid of melanosomes (see text, this chapter, and Figs. 8.7 and 8.8) |
| Ovarian teratoma | In melanocytic cells in epidermal component[1311] |
| Clear cell sarcoma of tendons and aponeuroses | See text, Chapter 24, and Figs. 24.6 and 24.7 |
| Dermatofibrosarcoma protuberans (DFSP) | Within melanocytic cells deep in tumour;[2197] in this study the tumour cells were thought to have perineurial and endoneurial cell features. Others have described fibrohistiocytic characteristics and Yoshida et al[2326] also demonstrated acid phosphatase and non-specific esterase activity, as well as Fc and C3 receptors and phagocytic properties in tumour cells maintained in tissue culture. Mature melanosomes have also been detected in a pigmented DFSP (Bednář tumour), in which the cells had the features of fibroblasts and Schwann cells[2261] |
| Melanotic Schwannoma | Melanosomes in varying stages of maturation have been identified in cells whose other ultrastructural appearances conformed to those of Schwann cells (Figs. 18.4 and 18.5);[1998,2089] Webb[2106] also found them in cells with perineurial features |
| Melanizing retinoblastoma | Melanosomes observed in cells maintained in tissue culture for 2 years; melanin pigment evident in original enucleation specimen by LM[2161] |
| Melanotic medulloblastoma | — |
| Meningeal melanocytoma | By LM the tumour resembled a cellular blue naevus and spindle cell A melanoma of uveal tract[2037] |
| Malignant melanocytic tumour of sympathetic ganglia | LM appearances resembled cellular and malignant blue naevus[1592] |
| Melanotic neuroectodermal tumour of infancy | Cell population includes melanocytic and neuroblast-like cells |
| Malignant melanotic neuroectodermal tumour of infancy | Melanosomes seen in varying stages of maturation. In its final stages the tumour resembled a conventional neuroblastoma[1563] |
| Melanotic carcinoid tumour of bronchus/lung | Grazer et al[490] found both neurosecretory granules 80–400 nm in diameter and granular but non-laminated melanosomes within single cells. See Table 16.3 |
| Neuroendocrine carcinomas of thyroid (medullary carcinoma), bronchus and skin | See text, Chapter 6 (so-called Merkel cell carcinoma) and Chapter 7 |
| Melanotic adenocarcinoma of the anorectum | One case.[841] Ultrastructural study revealed 3 types of cells:<br>1. Glandular epithelial cells with mucin granules and compound melanosomes<br>2. Melanocytes admixed with the tumour cells<br>3. Rare epithelial cells containing both mucin granules and stage II melanosomes<br>The appearances were explained by transfer or ingestion of melanosomes, rather than melanin synthesis by the glandular cells |
| Pigmented squamous cell carcinoma | Stage II-IV melanosomes detected in neoplastic squamous cells; presumably acquired by transfer of melanosomes from neighbouring non-neoplastic melanocytes[1616] |

*Unless stated otherwise, this table lists only tumours in which ultrastructural examination has demonstrated stage II-III melanosomes with the characteristic internal periodicity (Figs. 8.2, 8.3, 8.4, 8,8. 18.5, 24.6 and 24.7): it excludes tumours in which only compound melanosomes may be encountered (Fig. 5.26), as these are devoid of diagnostic significance. Curtis & Rubinstein[390] identified a melanin-like substance in a pigmented olfactory neuroblastoma without detectable melanosomes and suggested that the pigment represented a catecholamine degradation product

References: 39, 45, 64, 109, 390, 462, 490, 790, 841, 1311, 1541, 1551, 1563, 1571–1573, 1587, 1588, 1592, 1595, 1597, 1599, 1601, 1605, 1610, 1613, 1616, 1617, 1629, 1770, 1931, 1998, 2026, 2037, 2089, 2106, 2146, 2161, 2170, 2173, 2197, 2198, 2232, 2261, 2326, 2542

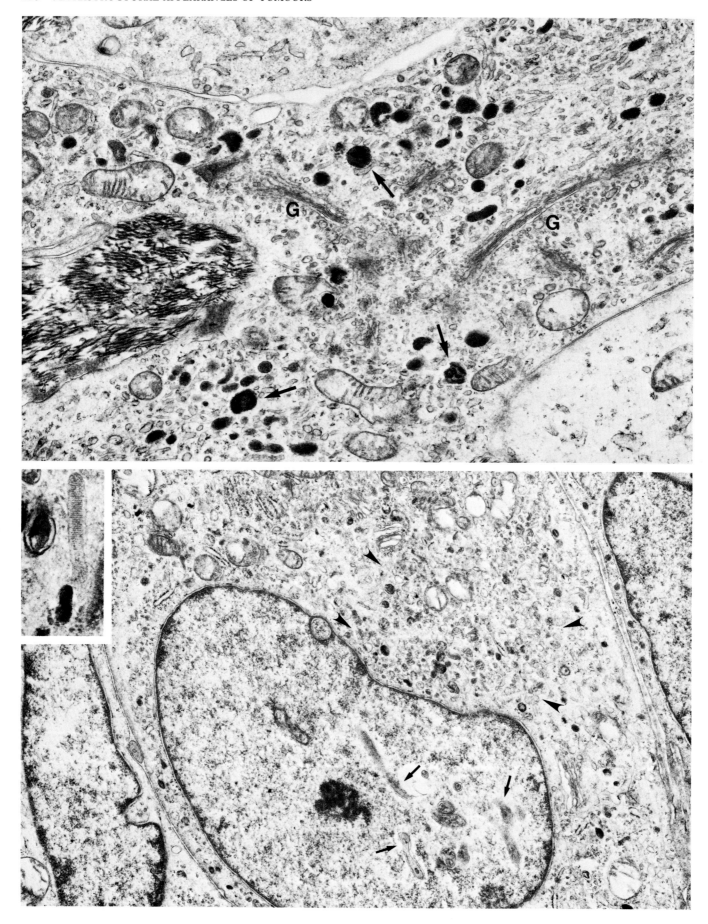

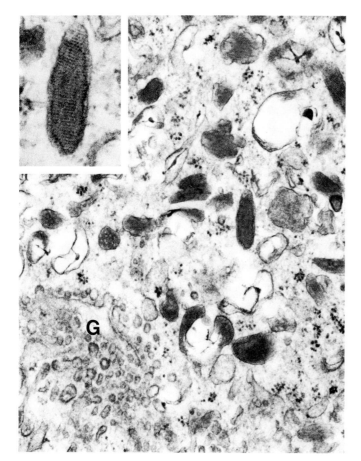

**Fig. 8.3    Malignant melanoma: Melanosomes I**

Cervical lymph node metastasis from an amelanotic epithelioid tumour of the scalp. Portion of the Golgi complex (G) with associated vesicles is apparent, and there are several stage II melanosomes showing the characteristic internal helical-transverse periodicity of 8–10 nm. One of these is shown at higher magnification in the inset. (× 41 000. Inset: × 89 600)

See also Table 8.1

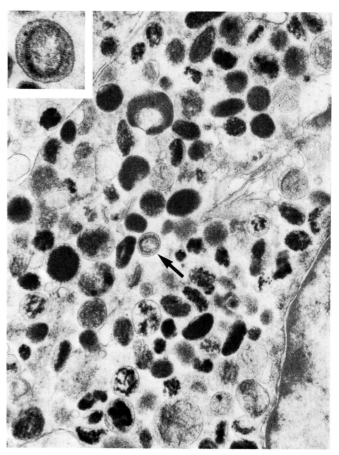

**Fig. 8.4    Malignant melanoma: Melanosomes II**

Lymph node metastasis from a cutaneous melanoma, in a man aged 62 years. Melanosomes in malignant melanomas often show considerable deviations from the classical morphology, with both pleomorphism and aberrant internal substructure. A prolonged search may be necessary to identify unequivocal stage II melanosomes among such atypical and variant forms, even when frequent melanized granules suggest the diagnosis, as in this case. Of the many melanized melanosomes illustrated, only one (arrow and inset) exhibits the internal periodicity characteristic of stage II melanosomes. (× 26 900; Inset: × 54 800)

Giant melanosomes have also been recorded in naevi and malignant melanoma, including both benign and dysplastic naevi in the B-K mole syndrome.[1558,1577] Such rounded giant melanosomes lack the typical helical-filamentous substructure and contain vesicles 30 nm in diameter.

Further variations on melanosome morphology are shown in Figs. 8.8, 18.5, 24.6 and 24.7.

References: 1558, 1577, 1591

**Fig. 8.1** *(Facing page — top)*    **Malignant melanoma: Organelles**

Metastatic tumour in the pubic ramus of a woman aged 54 years. The Golgi apparatus (G) is prominent, with many adjacent small vesicles. There are also numerous denser melanosomes (arrows), with patterned matrices and varying degrees of melanization, but transverse periodicity is not evident. Stromal collagen fibres can also be seen. There are no tonofibrillar bundles. (×17 700)

In malignant melanomas the neoplastic cells often form clusters, and dendritic processes can be found in most cases; Mazur & Katzenstein[1591] also reported microvilli. External lamina and cell junctions are often present, but may be poorly developed.

References: 39, 45, 47, 775, 1161, 1162, 1550–1552, 1554, 1559, 1562, 1568, 1571, 1574, 1578–1582, 1589, 1591, 1593, 1595, 1602, 1605, 1606, 1610, 1613, 1614, 2037, 3150

**Fig. 8.2** *(Facing page — bottom)* **Malignant melanoma: Poorly melanized cell**

Amelanotic cerebral metastasis of undetermined origin, from a 64-year-old man. There are only a few small electron-dense melanosomes in the cytoplasm, but numerous more lucent immature granules and vesicles are concentrated near one of the Golgi complexes and in the paranuclear region (arrowheads). In our experience, stage II melanosomes in poorly melanized tumours are most likely to be found in the peri-Golgian region or at the periphery of the cell. An intranuclear (pseudo)inclusion is also evident (arrows). (× 14 500)

**Inset:** Stage II-III melanosomes in the same case. (× 67 000)

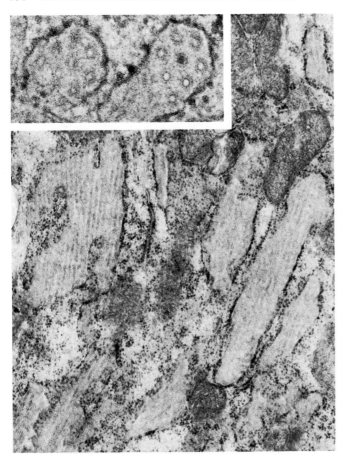

**Fig. 8.5 Malignant melanoma: Coated parallel tubules**

In this melanocytic cell the cisternae of the RER are distended with sheaves of fuzzy tubules, shown here in longitudinal section. (× 33 700)

**Inset:** In transverse section each tubule has a fuzzy outer coating and a lucent core, the internal diameter approximating 15 nm. The tubules are spaced at regular intervals. (× 120 400)

References: 85, 1590

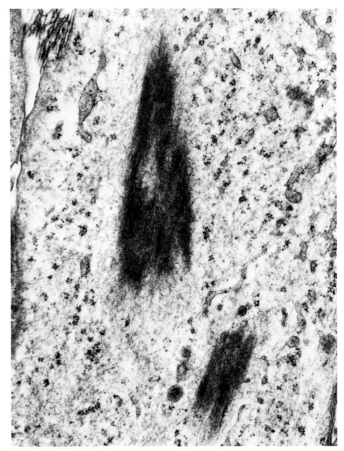

**Fig. 8.6 Malignant melanoma: Cytofilaments**

Intermediate cytoskeletal (vimentin) filaments are occasionally encountered in melanocytic cells and may be numerous; there is little or no tendency to aggregate into tonofibril-like bundles, and according to Caselitz et al[1560] cytokeratins are undetectable. Fine filaments which label with anti-actin antibody have also been recorded in malignant melanoma; the thin filaments illustrated here average 6–7 nm in diameter. (× 25 700)

References: 254, 1560

**Fig. 8.7** *(Facing page)* **Desmoplastic spindle cell melanoma: Myofibroblastic and myoid cells in regional lymph node metastases**

A melanotic freckle of Hutchinson was excised from the malar region of a 67-year-old man. A small area of ulceration with surrounding amelanotic sclerosing spindle cell proliferation was apparent within the macule. The spindle cell proliferation recurred locally and was re-excised, but one year later the patient developed cervical lymph node metastases and a block dissection was carried out. The metastases consisted of an amelanotic spindle cell malignancy, histologically identical to the locally recurrent tumour. The ultrastructural appearances of the metastatic neoplasm are shown in Figs. A to C.

**A:** In spite of a prolonged search, melanosomes were not found in the metastases. The malignant cells appear mesenchymal in character, with

elongated profiles. The cytoplasm often contains fine filaments — which have not been resolved at this magnification — together with peripheral condensations (arrow). A budding cilium (C) and several lysosomes are also present. (× 16 100)

**B:** In this field the cytoplasm appears myoid, with numerous filaments, peripheral condensations and intermediate junctions (arrows). There is little rough endoplasmic reticulum. (× 19 400)

**C:** The spindle cells in this area contain moderate amounts of RER and lysosomes; peripheral filaments (arrows) with subplasmalemmal linear densities and foci of external lamina (arrowhead) are also present, in keeping with myofibroblastic differentiation (see Table 3.6). (× 6700)

References: 1557, 1561, 1564, 1588, 1617, 1621, 2226

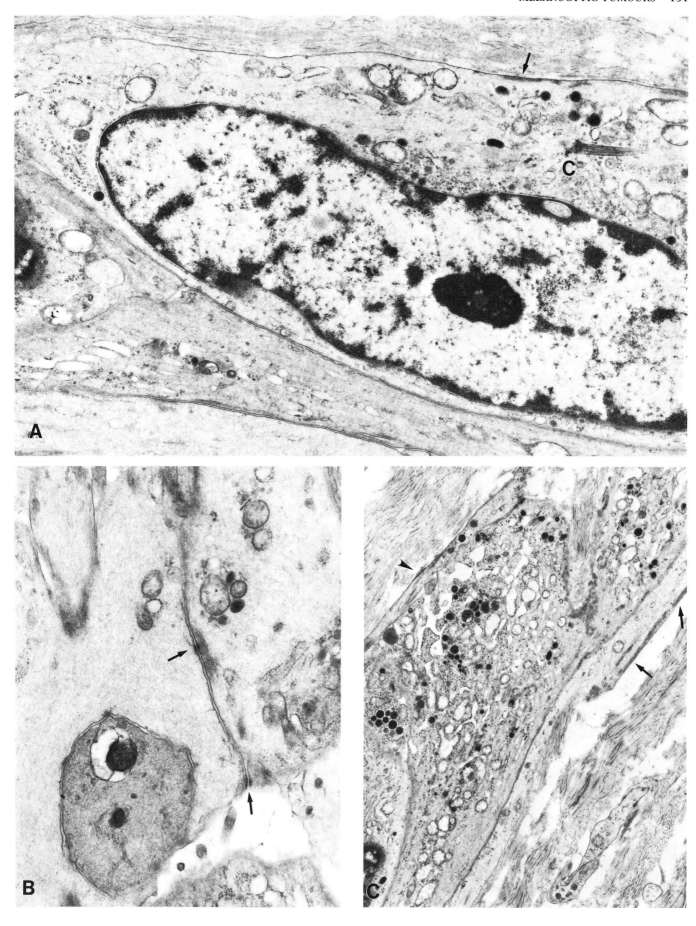

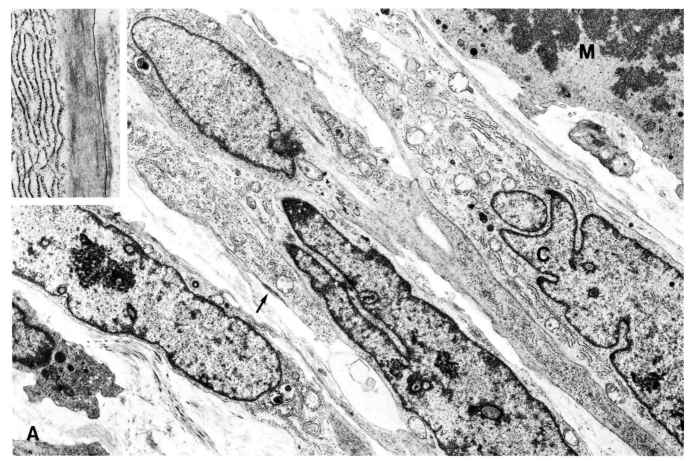

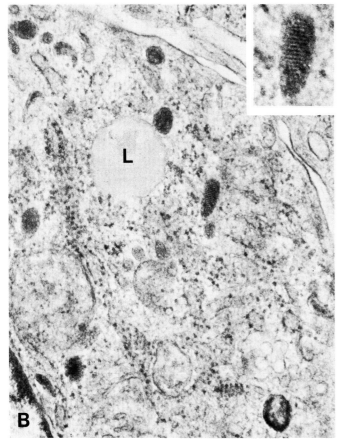

## Fig. 8.8 Desmoplastic spindle cell melanoma: Myofibroblasts and melanocytic cells

Sclerosing spindle cell malignancy from the dorsum of the left 4th toe, histologically resembling a smooth muscle tumour, with bimorphic spindle cell and epithelioid metastases to inguinal lymph nodes, in a 77-year-old woman.

**A:** Portion of the primary tumour from the toe is illustrated here. Despite an exhaustive search, no ultrastructural evidence of melanocytic differentiation could be found. The component cells appear mesenchymal, with elongated profiles. The nuclei are focally crenellated (C). The cytoplasm contains small to moderate quantities of rough endoplasmic reticulum, and there are groups of peripheral fine actin-like filaments (which cannot be individually resolved at this magnification). Peripheral attachment zones and foci of external lamina (arrow) can be seen. Portion of a mitosis (M) is also evident. **Inset:** Detail of one of the participating myofibroblasts, showing the RER, microfilaments with dense areas, and external lamina. (× 6100. Inset: × 20 400)

**B:** The epithelioid component of the inguinal lymph node metastases is depicted. At low power the neoplastic cells had polygonal outlines, with adjacent external lamina. Plasma membranes were closely apposed, but there were no specialized junctions. The cells were characterized by a paucity of RER and absence of myoid filaments.

As shown in this micrograph, one of the metastatic cells contains melanosomes, including striated (stage II) forms. A lipid droplet (L) is also apparent. **Inset:** One of the melanosomes at high magnification, demonstrating the characteristic transverse periodicity of 8–10 nm. (× 56 200. Inset: × 119 200)

Compare with Fig. 8.6

# 9 Mesothelial tumours

## MESOTHELIOMAS: GENERAL REMARKS

Mesothelial neoplasms are typified by attenuated mesothelial cells with epithelial features, either enclosing luminal spaces or situated on the surface of cellular aggregates. Innumerable long slender microvilli generally protrude from the cell surface (Fig. 9.2)[652] and can be demonstrated by both transmission and scanning EM;[616] however, they are sometimes neither well developed nor numerous,[642] and a distinction from adenocarcinoma may be impossible.

In effusions, fine-structural differences between benign, atypical and degenerate mesothelial cells are described.[98] The benign cells usually have smooth round or oval nuclei with eccentric nucleoli; the cytoplasm is plentiful and contains bundles of perinuclear intermediate filaments. By way of contrast, atypical mesothelial cells have nuclear invaginations and an elevated nuclear:cytoplasmic ratio. The degenerate cells exhibit lipidic and hydropic vacuolation, with subplasmalemmal ballooning. Nevertheless, the ultrastructural distinction between malignant mesothelioma and a reactive mesothelial hyperplasia (accompanying, for example, metastatic carcinoma) in effusion fluids remains problematical, as Mukherjee[98] has emphasized.

There are also claimed to be differences in the organization of intercellular junctions in mesothelioma and adenocarcinoma, as revealed by freeze-fracture. Thus Mukherjee[98] states that incorporation of gap junctions into the tight junctional network is a constant feature of mesothelioma, but is seen only occasionally in adenocarcinoma, and that gap junctions occur on the lateral plasma membranes in mesothelioma but not in adenocarcinoma; however, this claim needs to be more widely substantiated before it can be accepted unreservedly.

The epithelioid cells of malignant mesothelioma may rest directly on a basal lamina, but one or two layers of less differentiated cells are often interposed between the surface layer and the subjacent lamina. Tight junctions between adjoining cells are found near the luminal space; intermediate junctions and desmosomes are generally also present, with the formation of junctional complexes. Small bundles of filaments, predominantly intermediate (10 nm) in type,[631] occur in the cytoplasm and correlate with the presence of cytokeratins. Aggregates of glycogen — including both $\alpha$ and $\beta$ particles — may be prominent, while multivesicular bodies and lysosomes are often present. Osculati et al[640] also described membrane-bound dense granules, possibly secretory, in seven of eight cases examined; these ranged from 80–600 nm in diameter and had a paracrystalline or geometrical substructure. Apart from this study, secretory granules have been reported only rarely in mesothelioma[609] and their absence is one of several features used in the distinction from adenocarcinoma (Table 9.1). Osculati and associates[640] have also suggested that prominent RER and hypertrophied Golgi complexes together with amorphous extracellular material bathing the microvilli may correlate with glycosaminoglycan production.

In addition to the mesothelial cells, submesothelial and fibroblastoid cells are seen in varying proportions (Figs. 9.1 and 9.6). The fibroblastoid cells sometimes predominate; only sporadic mesothelial features may be retained in such cases, a diligent search being required to find them.

*Minimal criteria for the ultrastructural recognition of mesothelial differentiation:* Elongated slender microvilli in the absence of an underlying terminal filamentous web or typical mucin granules, in an appropriate cellular environment, as illustrated in Figs. 9.1–9.8 and discussed in Table 9.1.

## ADENOMATOID TUMOUR AND SO-CALLED MESOTHELIOMA OF ATRIOVENTRICULAR NODE

Ultrastructural investigations have also established that the adenomatoid tumour of genital and extragenital sites is a mesothelial neoplasm (Figs. 9.7 and 9.8).[638] This view is supported by immunocytochemical studies revealing the presence of cytokeratins, with negative reactions for vimentin and factor VIII-related antigen, and negative binding by *Ulex europaeus I*-lectin (UEA I), the last two being markers for endothelium.[632] Nevertheless, endothelial differentiation has recently been reported in some tumours thought to be 'adenomatoid' neoplasms.[606,615] However, it is worth emphasizing that by light microscopy adenomatoid tumours are easily confused with angiomas, especially lymphangiomas;[1228] the value of EM thus lies in facilitating this distinction, rather than creating a specious sub-class of adenomatoid tumour.

Similar appearances, including surface microvilli and complex intercellular junctions, were reported in so-called mesothelioma of the atrioventricular node by Fenoglio et al[620] and were thought suggestive of mesothelial differentiation. On the other hand, squamoid appearances are recognized in these lesions, and Paulson & Kristensen[641] demonstrated both epithelial mucin and carcinoembryonic antigen in the

**Table 9.1  Comparative histochemistry, immunocytochemistry and ultrastructure of mesothelioma and mucin-secreting adenocarcinoma**

|  | Mesothelioma* | Mucinous adenocarcinoma |
|---|---|---|
| *HISTOCHEMISTRY* | | |
| Secretory products | Hyaluronic acid often present. See footnote | Neutral mucosubstances |
| PAS-diastase | Negative | Positive |
| Alcian blue | Often positive | Positive |
| Alcian blue after hyaluronidase digestion | Negative | Positive |
| *IMMUNOCYTOCHEMISTRY* | | |
| Carcinoembryonic antigen | Generally negative, occasionally weakly positive | Frequently positive |
| Cytokeratins | Often strongly positive | Frequently positive, but immunoreactivity is usually sporadic and weak |
| Epithelial membrane antigen | Negative, or focal weak to strong positivity | Strongly positive |
| *ULTRASTRUCTURE* | | |
| External lamina | Present | Present |
| Desmosomes | Present | Present |
| Junctional complexes | Present | Present |
| Acinar spaces | Present | Present |
| Intracytoplasmic neolumina | Present | Present |
| Microvilli | Usually numerous, delicate and elongated (see Figs. 9.2, 9.3, 9.7 and 9.8). In a comparative study of 10 mesotheliomas and 10 adenocarcinomas, Warhol et al[652] reported a mean microvillous length:diameter ratio (MLDR) of $11.9 \pm 5.87$ (range 4.8–21.3) in the mesothelioma group, as opposed to an MLDR of $5.28 \pm 2.3$ (range 2.3–10.0) for the adenocarcinomas | Fewer and shorter than those classically seen in mesotheliomas (see Figs. 5.1 and 5.7) |
| Terminal filamentous web | Absent | May be present, especially in gastrointestinal adenocarcinomas (see Figs. 5.3A and 5.7) |
| Intermediate filaments | Present, usually more abundant than in adenocarcinomas | Present, number variable |
| Mucin-like granules | Typically absent. Lucent vacuoles presumably corresponding to mucolipid production are recorded,[609] as are dense granules[640] | Present |
| Other granules and vesicles | Lysosomes, osmiophilic lamellar granules and vacuoles often present | Variable, depending on pattern of cell differentiation |
| Glycogen | Often prominent | Variable |
| Other characteristics of infiltrating cells and stroma | May show microvilli interweaving with adjacent collagen fibres<br><br>Spectrum of appearances from epithelium-like cells to fibroblastoid cells, and sporadic epithelial features have been described even in predominantly fibrous mesothelioma<br><br>Myofibroblasts are also recorded, but are usually not numerous<br><br>The principal ultrastructural findings favouring a diagnosis of mesothelioma are the number, length and complexity of microvilli, absence of microvillous core rootlets and plentiful intermediate filaments. Such features are found not only in 'conventional' mesotheliomas, but also in benign cystic and papillary peritoneal mesotheliomas, and adenomatoid tumour of the genital tract | Fibroblasts and myofibroblasts in stroma |

*In mesotheliomas only glycosaminoglycans associated with epithelioid cell cytoplasm and/or acini have diagnostic significance, whereas their presence in sarcomatoid mesotheliomas (and in the stroma of carcinomas) lacks discriminant value. The ultrastructural appearances listed here also refer to epithelioid cells unless stated otherwise; these features are most obvious in highly differentiated tumours and are depleted to varying degrees in poorly differentiated mesotheliomas

(Modified from the review by Henderson[623] and published by permission)

References: 64, 528, 568, 608, 609, 622, 623, 626, 633, 635, 637, 638, 640, 643–645, 647, 650, 652, 2226 component cells. At the fine-structural level, the cells had luminal microvilli, junctional complexes and a basal lamina. There were also numerous cytoplasmic tonofibrils, presumably reflecting the squamoid morphology on LM. The findings were considered to indicate an epithelial lesion developing during cardiac organogenesis from sequestered foregut endoderm.

Finally, Katzenstein et al[514] have adduced evidence that the so-called sclerosing haemangioma of lung may represent a mesothelial tumour (see text of Chapter 23).

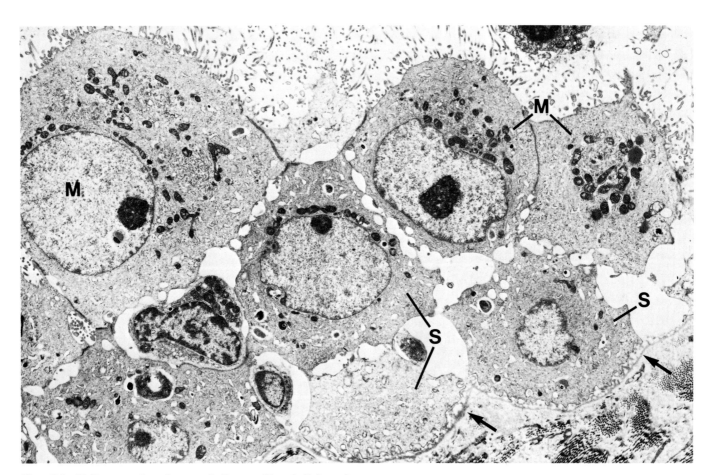

**Fig. 9.1 Malignant pleural mesothelioma: Mesothelial and submesothelial cells**

Submesothelial cells (S) with few microvillous processes are situated between the superficial mesothelial cells (M) and the underlying basal lamina (arrows). (×5400)

**Discussion:** Three main cell types can be recognized in mesotheliomas: mesothelial, submesothelial and fibroblastoid cells. The mesothelial cells are characterized by long microvilli, are closely apposed and are attached to each other by junctional complexes and desmosomes. Submesothelial cells (atypical mesothelial cells) have fewer microvilli, but these may be focally prominent; cytoplasmic filaments are more abundant than in mesothelial cells and intracytoplasmic neolumina are sometimes present. A spectrum of cytodifferentiation can be traced in many mesotheliomas, ranging from typical mesothelial cells to fibroblastoid cells, with transitional forms. Myofibroblasts may be present[608,647] and predominated in one metastasizing pleural sarcoma[2179] but are usually inconspicuous.

References: 605, 608, 613, 616, 618–620, 624, 628–631, 634, 635, 639, 640, 642, 646–648, 650–652, 2179, 2226

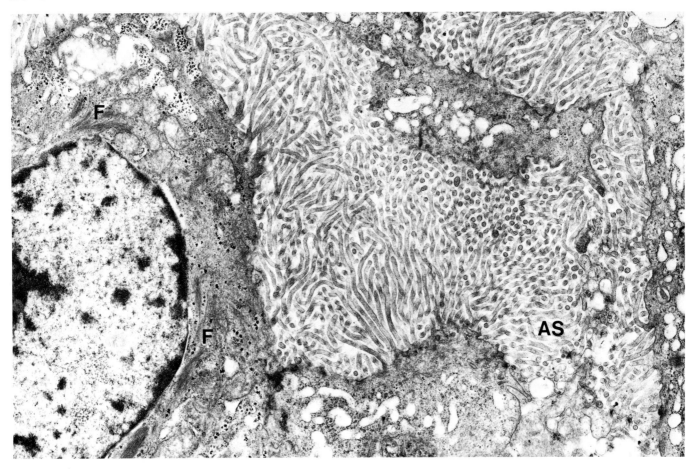

## Fig. 9.2 Malignant pleural mesothelioma: Microvilli

The acinar space (AS) contains countless delicate elongated microvilli, some of which have central filamentous cores. Compare with the stubbier microvilli typically found in adenocarcinomas (Figs. 5.1 and 5.2). Glycogen rosettes and bundles of intermediate filaments (F) are also present. (×14 600)

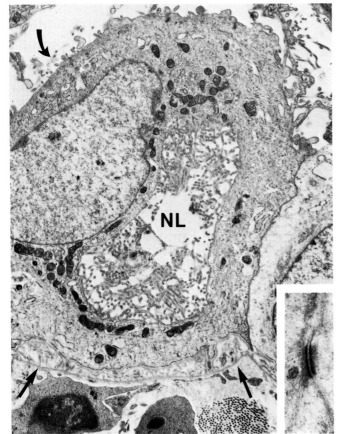

## Fig. 9.3 Malignant pleural mesothelioma: Atypical mesothelial cell with intracytoplasmic neolumen, and desmosome

Mesothelioma from a 39-year-old woman who had been exposed environmentally to asbestos as an adolescent.

Although few microvilli protrude from the surface of this mesothelial cell (curved arrow), there are many within the neolumen (NL). Filaments are inconspicuous and there are no secretory granules. The cell rests on a reduplicated basal lamina (straight arrows). One of the well constructed desmosomes in this tumour is shown in the inset. Subluminal junctional complexes were also found easily. (×6200. Inset: ×25 000)

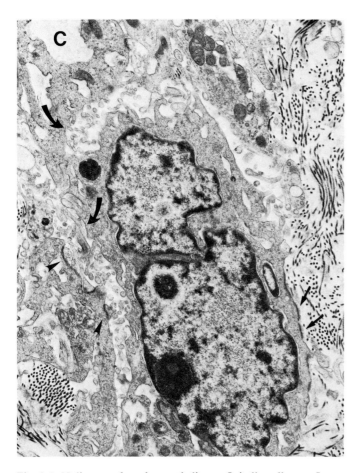

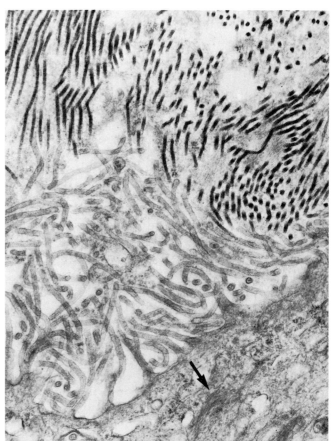

**Fig. 9.4  Malignant pleural mesothelioma: Spindle cell  area I**

Spindle cell focus in a predominantly epithelioid mesothelioma. Fibroblastoid cells are often numerous in the spindle cell areas of mesotheliomas and predominate in fibrous mesotheliomas. Nevertheless, cells with mesothelial features may still be detected in such tumours. Intermediate cells combining fibroblastoid properties with sporadic microvillous membrane specializations may also suggest the diagnosis.

These elongated infiltrating cells are surrounded by stromal collagen fibres, but nevertheless they possess microvillous processes (curved arrows). Intercellular junctions (arrowheads) and hemidesmosome-like subplasmalemmal densities with an associated fragmentary external lamina (straight arrows) are also evident. Dilated cisternae of RER (C) inhabit the cytoplasm. Note the prominent nucleolus and nuclear bodies. (×10 200)

References: 608, 623

**Fig. 9.5** *(Top — right)*  **Malignant pleural mesothelioma: Spindle cell area II**

Periphery of an infiltrative cell similar to that shown in Fig. 9.4. Numerous elongated microvilli project into the stroma, intermingling with the collagen fibres. Bundles of filaments (arrow) are present in the cytoplasm. (×22 900)

**Fig. 9.6** *(Bottom — right)*  **Malignant pleural mesothelioma: Spindle cell area III**

Collagen fibres are closely related to the periphery of this infiltrative cell. Membrane-bound collagen fibres (straight arrows) are present within the cell borders and in at least one area (curved arrow) these may represent intracytoplasmic collagen, rather than extracellular collagen enfolded by plasmalemmal flaps (see Fig. 3.19). Desmosomes (arrowheads) link the cell with a neighbour, and are shown at higher magnification in the inset. These appearances may reflect bimorphic epithelioid-fibroblastoid differentiation. RER, mitochondria, a Golgi complex and prominent filaments also occupy the cytoplasm. (×16 700. Inset: ×23 500)

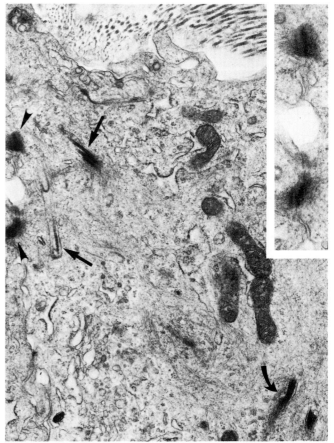

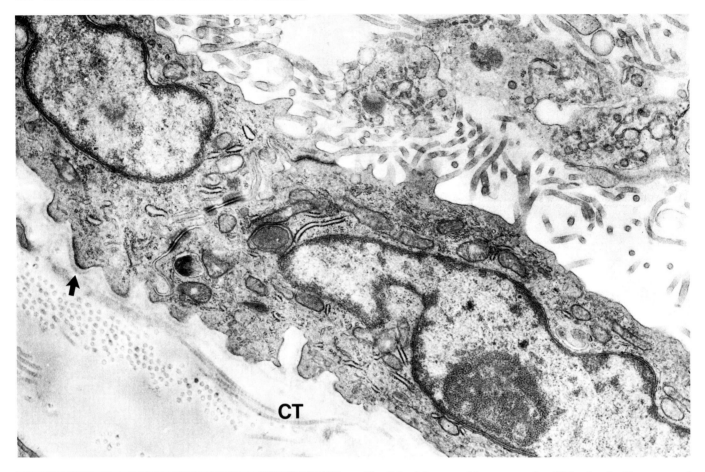

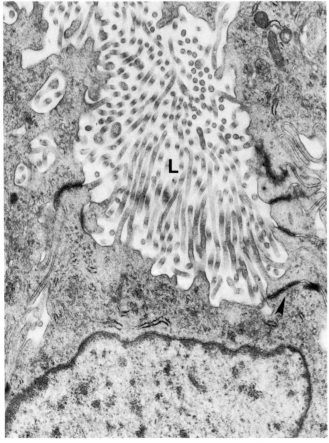

**Fig. 9.7 Adenomatoid tumour of epididymis: Architecture and mesothelial cells**

A single layer of plump mesothelial cells with a distinct basal lamina (arrow) rests on fibrous connective tissue (CT). The nuclei are slightly irregular and possess prominent euchromatin and nucleoli. Long slender microvilli protrude into the luminal space, and portion of a junctional complex can be seen between the adjoining cells; desmosomes also link the plasma membranes. ($\times 16\ 300$)

References: 604, 612, 621, 632–634, 638, 643–645, 649

**Fig. 9.8 Adenomatoid tumour of epididymis: Mesothelial cells**

Plump mesothelial cells surround the small luminal space (L) into which long slender microvilli project. The Golgi apparatus of these cells was moderately well developed. Short strands of RER and ribosomal rosettes are present in the cytoplasm. Note also the subluminal junctional complexes (arrowhead) in various planes of section. ($\times 21\ 100$)

## SECTION TWO
## EPITHELIAL NEOPLASMS II: ENDOCRINE TUMOURS

# 10 General features of endocrine neoplasms, and pituitary tumours

## GENERAL FEATURES OF ENDOCRINE NEOPLASMS

Electron microscopy may be useful in characterizing endocrine tumours developing in endocrine organs, especially in those normally containing multiple cell types, notably the pancreatic islets (see Chapter 14). Similarly, in a variety of non-endocrine organs, neoplasms differentiating as neuroendocrine (APUD) cells are recognizable by their characteristic subcellular morphology. Conversely, non-endocrine tumours arising in endocrine glands will also be detected.

In their ultrastructure the cells of many endocrine tumours closely resemble their normal counterparts, although organellar polarity may be disturbed to varying degrees. Diagnostic emphasis is often placed on the characteristics of the secretory granules, which are usually situated in the portion of the cell nearest a blood vessel, one exception being thyroid follicular epithelial tumours, where the granules tend to surround luminal spaces. The concentration of cytoplasmic granules varies greatly and many highly active endocrine tumours are poorly granulated, presumably because of rapid granule production and secretion. In some instances the granule morphology assumes specific configurations, allowing precise classification on the basis of the secretory products, but the granules in other cases are unfortunately abnormal and non-diagnostic. The situation is further complicated by tumours in which the component cells contain a mixture of both typical and atypical granules (see Table 14.3). *Identification of secretory products by immunocytochemistry is vital in the assessment of such tumours,[167,173] and is essential for the detection of multiple hormone-specific cell types in single neoplasms, for example in pancreatic islet tumours (see Chapter 14).*

The formation of acini may be seen in a variety of endocrine tumours, and intracytoplasmic neolumina and cytoplasmic filamentous bodies may be present. Whorled concentric aggregates of intermediate filaments, often containing enmeshed granules, are a frequent finding in polypeptide-producing endocrine tumours (see Table 2.9); in pituitary adenomas they indicate the presence of growth hormone cells (Fig. 10.3).[1681] The filaments are probably associated with the microtubular system and may be involved in the intracellular transport of granules.[986]

Ultrastructural examination easily identifies oncocytomas of endocrine organs such as oxyphilic adenomas of the thyroid gland, as these neoplasms consist of cells replete with mitochondria (see Fig. 11.1 and Table 2.1).

The neoplastic cells in endocrine tumours are joined by intermediate junctions and desmosomes, while subluminal junctional complexes are seen in areas of follicular-acinar differentiation. Basal laminae surround the cellular aggregates, and the stromal vasculature generally has fenestrated endothelium. Secretory granules are sometimes seen within vascular lumina and stromal connective tissues. Stromal amyloid fibrils may also be found (see Table 3.3).

In summary, the role of EM in the diagnosis of endocrine tumours lies in a two-stage assessment, namely:

1. *Determining that the neoplasm is indeed endocrine.[64,933]*
2. *Ascertaining whether the cytoplasmic granules have the characteristic morphology which may in some (but not all) cases allow the prediction of a particular secretory product.[64,933]* This is particularly the case with the halo granules typical of noradrenaline, the crystalline cores of classical insulin granules, and the rhomboidal granules indicative of renin production (see Figs. 13.4, 14.3, 15.1 and 15.2).

See also Tables 2.1 (oncocytic tumours), 2.9 (intracytoplasmic filamentous bodies), 10.1–10.3 (pituitary adenomas), 12.1 (parathyroid adenomas), 13.1 (spironolactone bodies) and 14.1–14.3 (pancreatic islet tumours).

## PITUITARY TUMOURS

In combination with immunocytochemistry, EM has contributed significantly to the specific typing of pituitary adenomas, as shown in Tables 10.1–10.3. These techniques have emphasized the limitations of LM alone, and it is notable that *cytoplasmic acidophilia or chromophobia primarily reflects the secretory granule mass — which is largely a product of granule frequency and size — and is unrelated to the specific hormonal contents of the granules; occasionally, acidophilia is related in whole or part to an abundance of mitochondria.*

The classification of pituitary tumours detailed in Tables 10.1–10.3 might be criticized on the grounds that the neoplasms are categorized according to their secretory products rather than cell morphology. Nevertheless, the ultrastructural appearances and immunohistology often correlate closely and adenomas producing multiple hormones do not seem to constitute a nosological problem of quite the same magnitude as gastroenteropancreatic endocrine tumours, because the range of hormones produced is more restricted. A mixture of cell types has been found in up to 20 per cent of pituitary adenomas, usually including 2 to 3 cell lines. Martinez & Barthe[1695] report that mammosomatotrophic adenomas are the most common mixed adenoma, but somatocorticotrophic and somatomammocorticotrophic adenomas also occur (mixed growth hormone-prolactin cell adenomas need to be distinguished from the recently described monomorphic mammosomatotrophic adenomas; see Table 10.2). Such heterogeneous tumours can be divided into two groups:

1. *Group A:* Adenomas with a predominant immunoreactive cell type (growth hormone, prolactin, corticotrophic, thyrotrophic or gonadotrophic cells) with a lesser component of one or more other cell lines.
2. *Group B:* Adenomas with a preponderance of non-immunoreactive cells (undifferentiated and/or oncocytic) with one or more less frequent immunoreactive specialized cell lines.

In addition, the documentation of multiple seemingly distinct specialized cell lines in single pituitary 'adenomas' serves to emphasize the difficulty of distinguishing between hyperplasia[1706] and neoplasia of endocrine tissues in general. This is illustrated by one of our recent cases of the galactorrhoea-amenorrhoea syndrome, in which a predominantly densely granulated prolactin cell proliferation without discrete tumour formation was accompanied by immunoreactive growth hormone and gonadotrophic cells.

The splitting of growth hormone and prolactin cell adenomas into densely (DG) and sparsely granulated (SG) types (Tables 10.1–10.3) is admittedly complex. However, these subcategories correlate with differences in both acidophilia-chromophobia and the intensity of immunoreactivity on LM. There are also significant ultrastructural differences, particularly in relation to granule frequency and dimensions. DG and SG adenomas are therefore listed separately in Tables 10.1–10.3 as opposite ends of a morphological spectrum. It is cautioned that ultrastructural evaluation of the granule characteristics alone is of quite limited value in predicting the type of hormone produced by SG adenomas, because granule frequency and size deviate from those of the corresponding normal pituicytes; in such circumstances, the diagnosis by EM must be based on other features such as fibrous (filamentous) bodies and misplaced exocytosis (Table 10.1). The secretory activity of pituitary adenomas as indicated by high blood hormone levels does not correlate directly with the numbers of cytoplasmic granules. Instead, prominence of both RER and Golgi complexes together with an abundance of nuclear euchromatin in sparsely granulated adenomas suggests a high order of endocrine activity (Fig. 10.6).

In some pituitary neoplasms, filaments compatible with amyloid deposits have been seen in the interstitium (Table 3.3),[1712] while in others, electron-dense deposits with the same antigenic characteristics as the secreted pituitary hormone have also been detected.

**Table 10.1    Comparison of anterior pituitary adenomas I: Growth hormone and prolactin cell adenomas**

| | Densely granulated growth hormone cell adenoma (DGGHA) | Sparsely granulated growth hormone cell adenoma (SGGHA) | Densely granulated prolactin cell adenoma (DGPCA) | Sparsely granulated prolactin cell adenoma (SGPCA) |
|---|---|---|---|---|
| Type of adenoma on routine light microscopy | Acidophilic | Chromophobic | Acidophilic | Chromophobic |
| Immunocytochemistry | Positive for growth hormone (GH) | Positive, but patchy, reaction for GH | Positive for prolactin | Positive reaction for prolactin; may be slight and patchy |
| Cell shape | Uniform, rounded or ovoid | Irregular and pleomorphic | Ovoid | Polyhedral; may have polarized, presumably apical, intertwining cell processes |
| Cytoplasmic granules | Numerous dense rounded membrane-bound granules. Diameters in range 300–600 nm, most measuring 350–450 nm. Giant granules up to 2000 nm in diameter and needle-shaped forms are rarely present. | Fewer and smaller than in DGGHA. Diameters in range 100–250 nm. Scattered cells may contain larger granules in range 450–500 nm | Numerous rounded or ovoid granules up to 1200 nm in diameter, and averaging up to 600 nm in diameter | Granules less numerous, and are smaller and more pleomorphic, than in DGPCA. Diameters in range 130–500 nm, averaging about 250 nm |
| Exocytosis | — | — | — | Misplaced exocytosis |
| Filaments and fibrous bodies | — | Frequent fibrous bodies, often associated with secretory granules and mitochondria. Component filaments approximately 11.5 nm in diameter. Present in more than half the cells of most adenomas | — | — |
| Organelles | Well developed RER. Prominent Golgi complexes | Prominent centrioles, sometimes multiple pairs; often situated near fibrous bodies. Mitochondria more pleomorphic than in DGGHA. Abundant RER, sometimes forming concentric lamellar bodies. SER also evident | Well developed RER. Prominent Golgi apparatus | Extensive RER, concentric lamellar bodies and prominent Golgi complexes |
| Nuclear morphology | Rounded or ovoid, centrally located. Dispersed chromatin | Pleomorphic, situated eccentrically, and with indentations and multiple profiles | Generally ovoid, may be pleomorphic | Ovoid or pleomorphic, with abundant euchromatin and small to prominent nucleoli |
| Remarks | Granule frequency and size are principal diagnostic features. Granules resemble normal GH cell granules  In rare instances the characteristic ultrastructural appearances are not present; an adenoma composed of a uniform cell population resembling TSH cells without GH cell-like features, but containing immunoreactive GH and $\beta$-TSH, is recorded[1682] See Fig. 10.1 | Fibrous bodies are the most prominent diagnostic feature; their occurrence indicates differentiation as GH cells or their precursors  Granules smaller than in DGGHA See Figs. 10.2-10.4 | Granule size is the principal diagnostic feature. Granules resemble normal prolactin granules See Figs. 2.18 and 10.5 | Misplaced exocytosis is the most characteristic feature  Granules smaller than in DGPCA See Figs. 2.7, 2.12 and 10.6 |

—=absent or inconspicuous

References: 1623, 1643, 1644, 1647–1658, 1660–1671, 1673, 1674, 1676, 1677, 1679–1692, 1694, 1695, 1697–1718, 3130

**Table 10.2  Comparison of anterior pituitary adenomas II: Mixed, stem cell and corticotrophic adenomas**

| | Mixed growth hormone and prolactin cell adenoma (MGH-PCA) | Monomorphic mammosomatotrophic adenoma (MMSA) | Acidophilic stem cell adenoma (ASCA) | Corticotroph cell adenoma (CCA) |
|---|---|---|---|---|
| Type of adenoma on routine light microscopy | Usually acidophilic, may be chromophobic | Acidophilic | Predominantly chromophobic, with infrequent acidophilic cells | Basophilic or chromophobic; some may be amphophilic |
| Immunocytochemistry | Positive for GH and prolactin in different cells | GH and prolactin present in the same (bihormonal) cells | Positive for GH and prolactin in varying numbers of cells | Positive reaction for ACTH; α- and β-endorphin and β-lipotropin/melanotropin usually also present |
| Cell shape | See remarks | Polyhedral | Elongated/irregular | Rounded or angular |
| Cytoplasmic granules | See remarks | Numerous, resembling appearances in DGGHA, but including large granules; measure 150–2000 nm in diameter. Large (>450 nm) or small (150–450 nm) granules often predominate in different cases. Pleomorphic and crystalloidal secretory bodies may also be seen | Granules not numerous, but present in every cell. Generally rounded, occasionally pleomorphic. Diameters in range 50–300 nm, and some may be up to 600 nm | Variable density. Diameters in range 120–700 nm, most being 120–350 nm in diameter. Commonly localized along cell membranes, but larger granules may be more evenly dispersed |
| Exocytosis | — | Present. Contents of subplasmalemmal granules often extruded into extracellular space through narrow funnels 25–100 nm wide | Misplaced exocytosis | — |
| Filaments and fibrous bodies | Present. See remarks for SGGHA | Not recorded | Present. See remarks for SGGHA | Bundles of fine perinuclear filaments averaging 7 nm in diameter may be present, and correspond to Crooke's hyalin |

| | | | | |
|---|---|---|---|---|
| **Organelles** | See remarks | RER well developed; moderate numbers of rounded mitochondria | RER poorly to moderately developed. Aggregates of SER present and may be a dominant feature. Golgi apparatus seldom prominent. Multiple centrioles<br><br>Mitochondria numerous, and may assume oncocytic proportions, but are generally small and rod-shaped, with focal swellings. Bizarre giant mitochondria may be found | Abundant RER. Prominent mitochondria; may show oncocytic characteristics |
| **Nuclear morphology** | See remarks | Rounded, similar to appearances in DGGHA; moderately prominent nucleoli | Large ovoid, or irregular; small nucleoli | Rounded or elongated |
| **Remarks** | Shows varying combinations of cells such as are seen in DGGHA, SGGHA, DGPCA and SGPCA<br><br>Other mixed-cell adenomas are also documented, but are not considered here (see text) | These adenomas resemble DGGHA, with the following exceptions:[1668]<br>1. Large secretory granules up to 2000 nm in diameter<br>2. Extrusion of granule contents through narrow channels<br>3. Presence of extracellular secretory material<br>4. Paracrystalline secretory structures in one case<br>They are distinguished from MGH-PCA by their monomorphic pattern and the occurrence of GH and prolactin in the same cells<br>Patients have acromegaly/gigantism, with elevated blood prolactin levels | Characteristics of GH cells and prolactin cells combined within the same cell<br><br>The combination of misplaced exocytosis, fibrous bodies, SER and megamitochondria is said to be characteristic[1671]<br><br>Tumours tend to be large and invasive, with a brief clinical history and low hormonal activity. Patients often have 'fugitive' acromegaly and hyperprolactinaemia | Some examples are sparsely granulated. Sporadic cells containing immunoreactive prolactin may also be present<br><br>The ACTH-secreting tumour in an 18-month-old infant reported by Saeger et al,[1707] was classified as a sparsely granulated mucoid cell adenoma by LM. On EM most cells lacked specific features; differentiated cells were confined to small foci, and contained bundles of filaments and secretory granules 140–260 nm in diameter<br><br>'Silent' corticotrophic adenomas are also recorded |

References:: See Table 10.1

**Table 10.3** Comparison of anterior pituitary adenomas III: Thyrotrophic, gonadotrophic and non-functional adenomas

| | Thyrotroph cell adenoma (TCA) | Gonadotroph cell adenoma (GCA) | Undifferentiated (null cell) adenoma (UA) | Oncocytoma (OC) |
|---|---|---|---|---|
| Type of adenoma on routine light microscopy | Generally chromophobic ± sporadic acidophilic cells. Mucoid characteristics also described | Chromophobic ± oncocytic cells | Chromophobic ± acidophilia due to oncocytic cells | Chromophobic to acidophilic |
| Immunocytochemistry | Variable. Negative in most cases, but sparse TSH reactivity may be seen. GH recorded in up to 10 per cent of cells[1705] | FSH, LH, or both. β-endorphin also recorded | Negative for all hormones (see remarks) | Negative for all hormones |
| Cell shape | Polyhedral to elongated, with cytoplasmic extensions | Elongated, with perivascular palisading | Polyhedral small cells | Light and dark large cells |
| Cytoplasmic granules | Not numerous, may be sparse. Concentrated along cell membranes. Diameters in range 100–200 nm, occasionally up to 400 nm | Generally not numerous. Diameters from < 100 nm, to 150–200 nm | Non-specific granules with diameters in range 100–250 nm; may be up to 500 nm in a few cells | Granules few or rare, and displaced to cell periphery. Diameters in range 100–350 nm |
| Exocytosis | Rare | Not illustrated | — | — |
| Filaments and fibrous bodies | Few filaments | Abundant microtubules, but neither filaments nor fibrous bodies, described by Trouillas et al[1718] | — | — |
| Organelles | Microtubules vary from sparse to prominent. Scattered profiles of RER. Mitochondria may occasionally reach oncocytic proportions | RER moderately to highly developed, sometimes forming parallel stacks and occasionally *Nebenkern* patterns. Golgi complexes usually not prominent. Perigolgian centrioles frequent, as are cilia. Lysosomes common. Mitochondria variable; generally sparse, but numerous in oncocytic cells. Tend to be rod-shaped, with lamellar cristae | Prominent Golgi complexes, but RER poorly developed. Numerous microtubules. Mitochondria may be prominent, and achieve oncocytic proportions. Annulate lamellae may be present | Mitochondria show pronounced hyperplasia, hypertrophy, and pleomorphism. Golgi apparatus may be well developed |
| Nuclear morphology | Varies from rounded to irregular, with small nucleoli | Ovoid, with plentiful euchromatin | Irregular, with indentations | Rounded, ovoid or irregular, with indentations. Pyknotic in condensed oncocytes |
| Remarks | Rare; less than 1 per cent of pituitary adenomas. Verification by elevated TSH levels in blood. Associated with thyroid deficiency[1681] or hyperthyroidism,[1705] and acromegalic features also reported (mixed adenoma)[1705]. In some cases the cells closely resemble normal TSH cells, but varying numbers of less differentiated cells with irregular nuclei, pleomorphic mitochondria and prominent Golgi complexes are usually present and may predominate | Tumours associated with hypogonadism. Few studies. Six of 495 surgically removed pituitary tumours reported by Horvath & Kovacs[1667] contained gonadotrophins, while Trouillas et al[1718] gave a frequency of 3.5 per cent. The tumours occurring in males consisted of undifferentiated cells by EM, whereas those in females were more differentiated (as indicated by the features listed above) | The functionless adenomas with small argyrophilic granules reported by Capella et al[1647] represent a variant of null cell adenoma; 33 such tumours were identified in a series of 200 pituitary adenomas (16.5 per cent). Immunoreactivity for glycoprotein α-chain was detected in 20 cases, and FSH β-chain was found in 11. Various mixtures of immature, oncocytic, and sparsely and densely granulated cells were found by EM; the granules varied from 120–180 nm. | Incidence variously reported as 5–18 per cent of pituitary adenomas. Although not an intrinsic pituitary tumour, myeloma may occasionally enter into the differential diagnosis of pituitary adenomas,[1699,3130] but is distinguished by the characteristically abundant RER, often showing varying degrees of cisternal dilatation; absence of appropriate secretory granules, and the characteristic nuclear heterochromatin pattern in some cases are additional distinguishing features (see Figs. 27.24–27.29) |

References: See Table 10.1

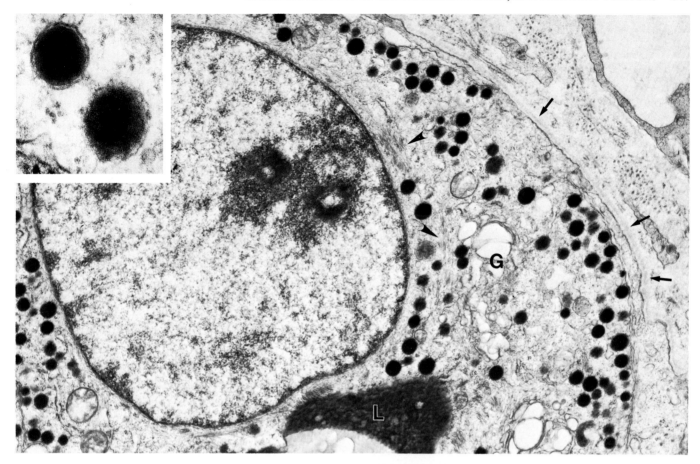

**Fig. 10.1 Acidophilic pituitary adenoma — Densely granulated growth hormone cell adenoma: Granule morphology**

In acidophilic adenomas the cytoplasmic granules usually resemble those of normal pituicytes and their morphology correlates with the hormone produced. There are many granules in this neoplastic cell, their diameters varying between 250–350 nm; however, these commonly range from 300–600 nm in diameter (Table 10.1). These dimensions are consistent with the granules seen in normal somatotrophs, in keeping with this patient's acromegaly. Bundles of cytoplasmic filaments (arrowheads) near the nucleus and Golgi apparatus (G), a lipofuscin body (L) and a distinct basal lamina (arrows) are also present. Reports indicate that diffuse electron-opacity of somatotrophs is seen only in neoplasms. **Inset:** The limiting membranes of these granules from the same cell closely surround the electron-dense contents. (× 17 000. Inset: × 66 500)

References: 306, 1623, 1656, 1666, 1681, 1686, 1689, 1694, 1697, 1713–1715, 1717

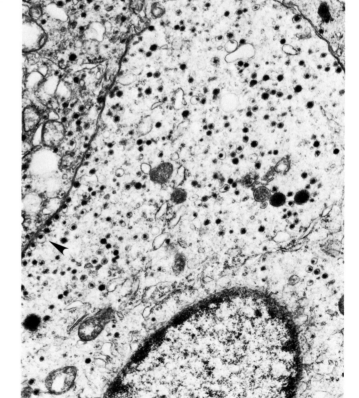

**Fig. 10.2 Pituitary chromophobe adenoma — Growth hormone cell adenoma: Granule morphology**

Acromegaly was the predominant clinical feature in this case. Small electron-dense granules measuring 150–200 nm are present, especially at the cell periphery (arrowhead). The correlation between functional disorders and the morphological appearances of granules is often misleading in chromophobe adenomas. Generally, the granules in such chromophobic cells are smaller than in normal pituicytes. (× 14 800)

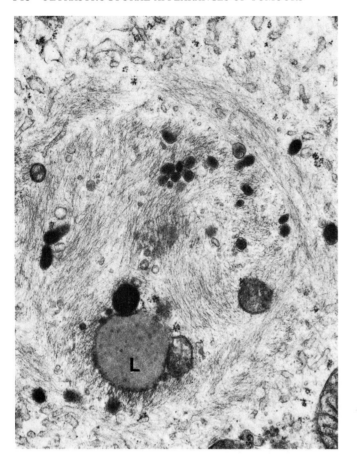

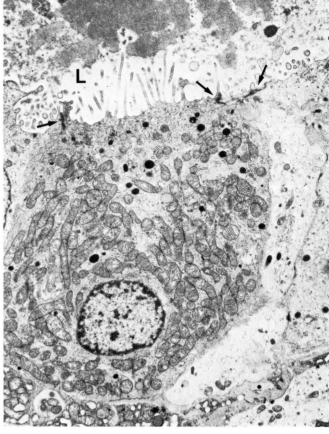

**Fig. 10.3** *(Top — left)* **Sparsely granulated growth hormone cell adenoma: Fibrous body**

Pituitary adenoma associated with acromegaly. This fibrous body consists of an aggregate of intermediate filaments approximately 10–12 nm in diameter, together with associated secretory granules and a lipid droplet (L). In pituitary adenomas, fibrous bodies of this type are characteristic of growth hormone production (see Tables 2.9 and 10.1). (× 21 700)

References: 1623, 1665, 1666, 1681, 1686, 1703, 1713

**Fig. 10.4** *(Top — right)* **Sparsely granulated growth hormone cell adenoma: Microfollicle and mitochondrial hyperplasia**

Tumour from a 56-year-old man with acromegaly; by LM the adenoma was predominantly chromophobic. On ultrastructural examination, both small and large secretory granules were found in the neoplastic cells; the former averaged 170 nm in diameter, with a range of 140–220 nm, while the larger granules averaged 380 nm (range 280–585 nm). Portion of a microfollicle in the adenoma is shown here. The lumen (L) contains granular grey material. The lining cells have luminal microvilli, and are linked by apical junctional complexes (arrows). There are scattered electron-dense secretory granules, and one cell shows considerable mitochondrial hyperplasia. (× 5200)

Follicles are also described in non-neoplastic adenohypophysis; the lining cells are usually agranular and their functional capacity is poorly understood. However, in one such instance we detected strong immunoreactivity for ACTH.

Reference: 1666

**Fig. 10.5** *(Bottom — left)* **Acidophilic pituitary adenoma — Densely granulated prolactin cell adenoma: Granule morphology**

Most granules in this adenoma varied between 400–800 nm in diameter. Tentative identification as a prolactin cell adenoma was made, and this correlated well with the endocrinological findings. (× 16 000)

References: 1623, 1655, 1666, 1676, 1681, 1686, 1694, 1700

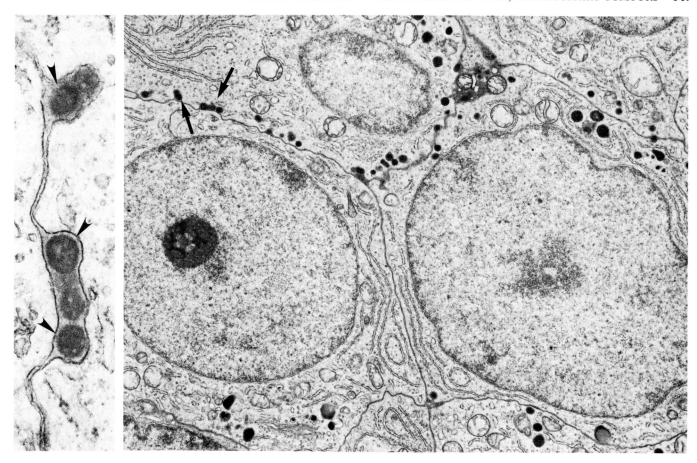

**Fig. 10.6 Sparsely granulated prolactin cell adenoma: Cell morphology and misplaced exocytosis**

Pituitary adenoma from a 55-year-old man who presented with *grand mal* epilepsy and was found to have hyperprolactinaemia. LM revealed a chromophobe adenoma.

The polygonal tumour cells generally had smooth plasma membranes, but polarized intertwining cytoplasmic processes were occasionally present. The ovoid nuclei contained abundant euchromatin and variably developed nucleoli, a moderately prominent nucleolus being depicted here.

Secretory granules were not numerous, and averaged 280 nm in diameter, with a range of 150–440 nm. Note their tendency to localize at the cell periphery. Misplaced exocytosis is a valuable marker for sparsely granulated prolactin cells and is indicated by the arrows; such inappropriately extruded granules are detailed in the inset (arrowheads), where they are seen to lie between adjoining plasmalemmae.

The cytoplasm also contains elongated and sometimes parallel strands of RER, and Golgi complexes, both of which were prominent in some cells (see Figs. 2.7 and 2.12). Mitochondria are also evident. (× 9300. Inset: × 50 400)

**Discussion:** The nucleocytoplasmic morphology shown here suggests a high level of metabolic-secretory activity. Dingemans and associates[1653] found that the endocrine activity of sparsely granulated prolactin cell adenoma correlated with a small number of secretory granules, the frequency of exocytosis and the amount of RER. There was no correlation with granule size, the extent of the Golgi apparatus, or the number of lysosomes. There was an inverse correlation with mitochondrial frequency. Lloyd et al[1694] found only slight endocrine activity in two densely granulated prolactin cell adenomas; the adenomas with marked secretory activity were sparsely granulated, with prominent Golgi complexes, abundant RER, large nuclei and prominent nucleoli.

References: 1623, 1653, 1666, 1680, 1681, 1694

# 11 Thyroid tumours

## FOLLICULAR AND PAPILLARY TUMOURS

Follicular thyroid tumours consist of cells resembling normal follicular epithelium, but disturbed cytoplasmic polarity is present, with distortion and maldistribution of organelles to varying degrees, depending on the level of differentiation. The recorded cytoplasmic derangements in follicular and papillary carcinomas[1750] include:

1. Proliferation of organelles such as mitochondria.
2. Varying proportions of RER, Golgi complexes and mitochondria.
3. Loss of cytoplasmic polarity.
4. Diminished frequency and even absence of some organelles.
5. Abnormal colloid structure.

Oxyphilic and toxic adenomas represent the only types of *follicular adenoma* with special ultrastructural features.[1757] Oxyphilic tumours are easily recognized by their profuse hypertrophied mitochondria and smooth surface membranes.[1739,1757] Toxic adenomas contain organelle-rich cells with abundant endoplasmic reticulum, irregular nuclei and apical microvilli.[1757]

The cells comprising follicular adenomas and carcinomas differ only slightly in appearance, and EM is generally of no value in distinguishing benign from malignant follicular tumours.[1758] Glycogen accumulation is seen in clear cell tumours, and an unusual clear cell-oxyphilic variant of papillary carcinoma is described, in which the component cells had clear apical zones, central nuclei and oxyphilic basal regions.[1736]

Either smooth or highly irregular nuclei with abundant euchromatin characterize *papillary carcinoma*, and intranuclear cytoplasmic inclusions are often present (Fig. 11.3). On scanning EM papillary carcinoma consists of convex and concave cells with apical microvilli (MV) and cilia. The MV are more profuse and pleomorphic than normal and are often club-shaped, whereas the cilia are reduced in frequency.[1787] Highly differentiated *follicular carcinomas* usually have more abundant cilia and fewer MV than papillary carcinoma, but their cilia are still less numerous and the MV more profuse than normal. Both cilia and MV are depleted in less differentiated tumours.[1756]

The MV in papillary carcinoma are more numerous and better developed in the cells bordering follicular areas than papillae.[1755] The number of MV is normally dependent on cyclic AMP levels, increased concentrations leading to a reduction in MV. This reciprocal relationship does not seem to apply in papillary carcinomas, where frequent MV are found in the face of high cyclic AMP levels. Spheroidal surface blebs and pseudopods are not numerous; these are normally formed by TSH stimulation and their scarcity may reflect low endocrine function in papillary carcinoma.[1755]

The ultrastructural appearances of well differentiated follicular and papillary tumours and their possible significance are discussed in depth by Johannessen & Sobrinho-Simoes[1758] in a critical review which is recommended to the interested reader.

## MEDULLARY CARCINOMA

Although stromal amyloid deposition has been reported in microfollicular carcinoma (see Table 3.3), the presence of amyloid fibrils together with cytoplasmic neurosecretory granules is highly characteristic of medullary carcinoma (Figs. 11.5–11.7). On the basis of size gradients, several groups of granules have been recognized,[1732] the diameters ranging from 60–550 nm, but calcitonin production cannot be equated with any single group. Calcitonin is constantly present in medullary carcinoma, but other polypeptides also occur. Memoli et al[1773] demonstrated leu-enkephalin in 50 per cent of cases, serotonin in 40 per cent, and bombesin in 30 per cent; ACTH, vasoactive intestinal polypeptide (VIP), substance P and somatostatin were detected less often.

Mixed medullary and follicular differentiation is now documented; Hales et al[1748] have reported a thyroid carcinoma with both medullary and follicular features on LM, containing immunoreactive calcitonin and thyroglobulin, and possessing neurosecretory granules on EM (see also strumal carcinoid tumour of ovary, Table 30.2). Mucin production and even squamous features are also described.[1740, 1772]

## ANAPLASTIC, SPINDLE AND GIANT CELL CARCINOMAS

Sporadic follicular foci in non-small cell anaplastic and spindle cell carcinomas ultrastructurally resemble follicular carcinomas. The cells otherwise have variable cytoplasmic morphology; Golgi complexes, filaments, microvilli and cilia have all been described, as have desmosomes and junctional complexes.[1746] These observations indicate epithelial differentiation (see Chapter 7), but should be evaluated with caution in at least a proportion of spindle and giant cell carcinomas. For example, we do not believe that the cells illustrated in some reports[1746] are convincingly epithelial; instead, myofibroblastic properties are depicted, emphasizing the problem of evaluating the fine structure of spindle cell carcinomas in general (see Chapter 4). The giant cells in anaplastic thyroid carcinomas are characterized by an abundance of mitochondria and RER; epithelial features are documented, but intercellular

junctions are not always found.[1746] So-called osteoclastoma-like tumours are discussed in Chaper 7.

Electron microscopy has also contributed to the recognition that most small cell tumours of the thyroid gland are in reality lymphomas rather than carcinomas.[1724,1726] Conversely, some small cell tumours resembling lymphomas by LM will be shown to be carcinomas.[1768] In such small cell carcinomas, rare intercellular acinar spaces lined by microvilli have been described,[1746] together with occasional foci of basal lamina, and some small cell carcinomas of thyroid have neuroendocrine features.

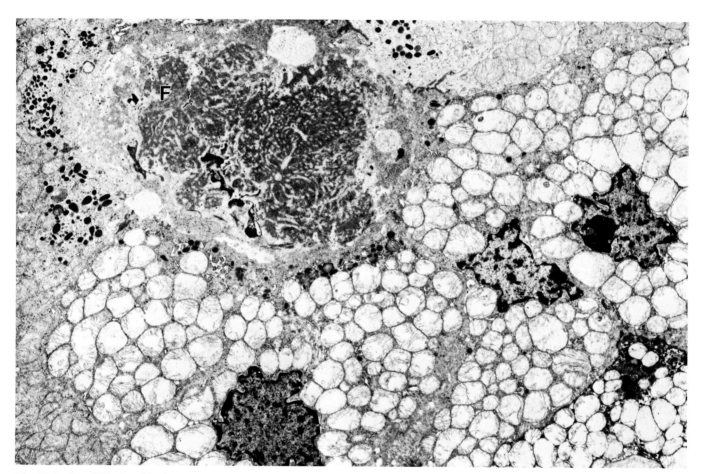

**Fig. 11.1 Oxyphilic thyroid adenoma (oncocytoma): Mitochondrial hyperplasia and microfollicle**

The oncocytes contain numerous hypertrophied mitochondria with generally clear matrices devoid of dense granules. The microfollicle (F) contains irregularly convoluted secretory material, and subluminal secretory granules are present in the lining follicular cells. (×5600)

Inclusions occasionally develop within the matrices of such mitochondria; they include electron-dense globules 100–300 nm in diameter and collections of filaments 6–8 nm in diameter. Paracrystalline patterns may also be seen.

See Table 2.1.

References: 1729, 1739, 1746, 1749, 1757, 1758, 1784

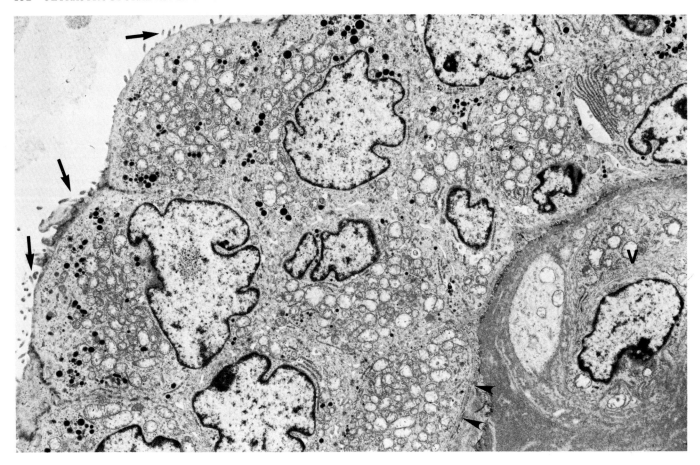

**Fig. 11.2   Papillary carcinoma of thyroid: Architecture**

These epithelial cells rest on a thin basal lamina (arrowheads), which is separated by a narrow layer of collagenous matrix from the reduplicated external lamina surrounding the stromal vessel (V). Poorly formed delicate microvilli project from the apical surface (arrows). Mitochondria vary greatly in number in papillary carcinomas; in this case they are abundant and crowded. Numerous rounded dense granules are also present, being concentrated in the apical cytoplasm; these dense bodies also vary in frequency and some are known to contain acid phosphatase. The irregular nuclei contain moderately abundant euchromatin. ($\times$ 5500)

**Discussion:** Prominent nuclear bodies and clustered large interchromatin graunles are often present in the nuclei, reflecting disturbed RNA metabolism, while nuclear pores may be less frequent than in normal follicular epithelium.[1746,1759]

The neoplastic cells characteristically rest on a basal lamina which is often thickened and reduplicated like the external lamina surrounding the stromal blood vessels. Interstitial microfibrils have also been identified[1746] and may represent a collagen precursor, or be related to the basal lamina.

References: 214, 215, 1720, 1722, 1727, 1736, 1745, 1746, 1755, 1758–1761, 1781, 1782, 1787, 1794

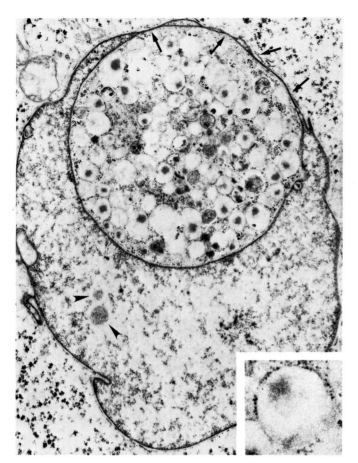

**Fig. 11.3 Papillary carcinoma of thyroid: Nucleus with cytoplasmic (pseudo)inclusion**

Note the slightly irregular periphery of this nucleus, as well as prominence of euchromatin and two nuclear bodies (arrowheads). The (pseudo)inclusion is enclosed by a thin layer of nuclear matrix and envelope (arrows); its contents include numerous vesicular structures known as M bodies, which often contain flocculent densities. (× 10 900)

**Inset:** M body at higher magnification. Ribosomes stud the surface of these bodies, suggesting that they develop by vesicular dilatation of RER. (× 36 000)

**Discussion:** The nuclei in papillary carcinomas have either smooth or irregular contours. The fine dispersal of chromatin is often assumed to correlate with the characteristic ground-glass ('Orphan Annie') morphology on LM. However, in an ultrastructural morphometric analysis of thyroid tumours Johannessen et al[1760] claimed that papillary carcinomas with numerous ground-glass nuclei *'did not seem to have particularly low densities of heterochromatin'*. Such optically clear nuclei need to be distinguished from intranuclear vacuoles,[1766] which occur in a far smaller proportion of cells. By EM these vacuoles are seen to represent membrane-bound spheroidal masses of cytoplasm intruding into nuclei. In some instances such (pseudo)inclusions represent cytoplasmic invaginations, and continuity with the main cytoplasmic mass can be demonstrated occasionally. Nevertheless, Carneiro et al[1727] have proposed that most of these inclusions represent 'true intranuclear inclusions'. In any event, it is likely that the sequestered contents differ physicochemically from the outer cytoplasm, as they are often more electron-dense; their rounded outlines may indicate either a higher internal pressure than the karyoplasm,[1746] or a surface tension phenomenon with minimal energy requirements. Their contents include RER, M bodies, lysosomes and intermediate filaments, sometimes forming concentric patterns; in addition, a sequence of degenerative changes can often be traced.

References: 196, 1727, 1746, 1758, 1760, 1766

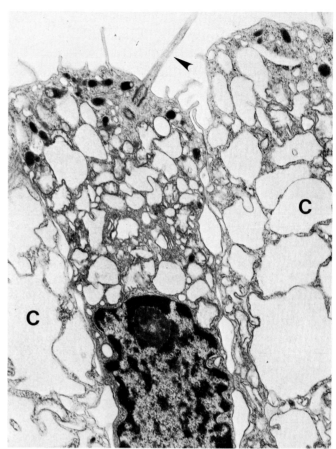

**Fig. 11.4 Follicular carcinoma of thyroid: Cell detail**

The columnar neoplastic cells in this field display basal, moderately irregular nuclei, dilated cisternae (C) of RER, and apical electron-dense secretory granules. A few microvilli and a solitary cilium (arrowhead) are present on the apical surface. (× 12 100)

The cells containing such dilated cisternae may appear oxyphilic by LM, but the distinction from the mitochondrial hyperplasia of true oncocytes is obvious by EM (compare with Fig. 11.1).

References: 1730, 1746, 1758, 1765, 1781, 1787

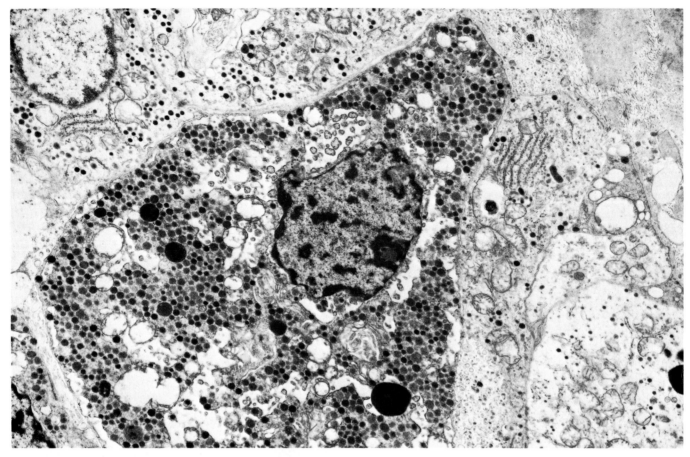

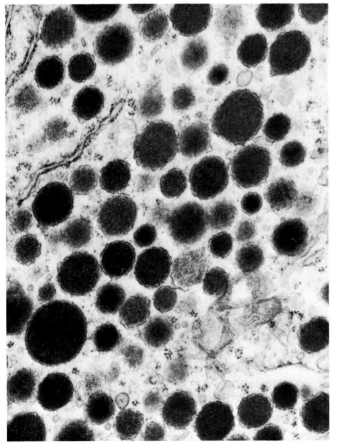

### Fig. 11.5 Medullary carcinoma of thyroid: Cell morphology

Thyroid mass from a 64-year-old woman. The cytoplasm of the central cell is packed with granules of varying density, averaging about 300 nm in diameter, with a range of 195–440 nm. In contrast, the granules in the surrounding cells are both fewer and smaller, averaging 150 nm, with a range of 120–185 nm. Despite heterogeneous size distributions of the granules in normal and hyperplastic C cells, the different granules have nevertheless been shown to label for calcitonin. (×8600)

**Discussion:** A variety of cytoplasmic inclusions mingling with the neurosecretory granules has been recorded in medullary carcinoma. Some represent small granules and vesicles, but rod-like and doughnut-shaped structures bordered by a trilaminar unit membrane have also been observed.[1762] The rod-like forms measured 200–800 nm in length and were 50–100 nm wide; they superficially resembled Langerhans' cell granules (see Fig. 28.22), but lacked a central lamella and were not attached to plasma membranes.

References: 1723, 1725, 1731–1734, 1740, 1744, 1746, 1748, 1751, 1752, 1762, 1764, 1770, 1772–1776, 1778, 1785, 1788, 1789, 1797

### Fig. 11.6 Medullary carcinoma of thyroid: Neurosecretory granules

At high power these granules show the characteristic appearances of neurosecretory granules, and consist of a delimiting membrane, a narrow internal lucent zone, and a central relatively uniform dense core. (×32 000)

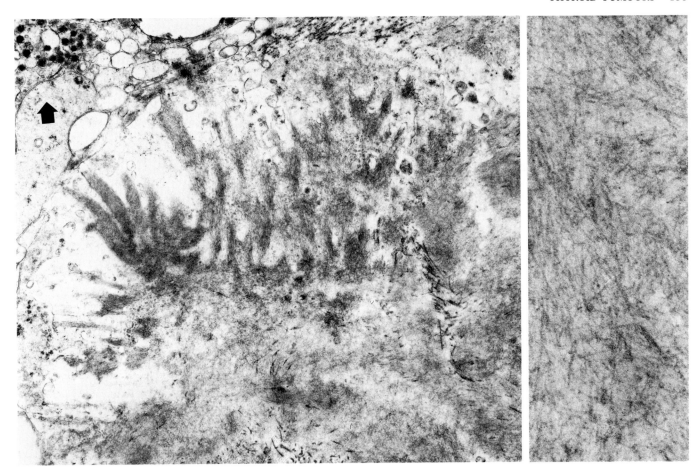

**Fig. 11.7  Medullary carcinoma of thyroid: Stromal amyloid**

The stroma contains masses of moderately dense amyloid, with admixed collagen fibres, while neurosecretory granules are evident in a nearby cell (bold arrow). At higher magnification (inset), the amyloid is seen to consist of randomly orientated non-branching fibrils averaging approximately 9—12 nm in this case. (×14 000. Inset: ×72 500)

See Table 3.3

# 12  Parathyroid tumours and hyperplasias

Current concepts indicate that the various cell types (such as oxyphilic and clear cells) identifiable in parathyroid tissue represent structural-functional modulations of chief cells, which are the only distinct parathyroid cell type.[1803] EM can facilitate distinction between the cell patterns, and has led to the recognition of transitional oxyphilic cells in hyperfunctional oxyphilic adenomas (Figs. 12.3–12.5).[1805,1816] The frequency of secretory granules and lipid globules, and the extent of development of the RER and Golgi apparatus also allow prediction of cellular metabolic-secretory activity.[1804]

The ultrastructural appearances of the cells in parathyroid adenomas and carcinomas resemble those of the corresponding normal cells, but varying degrees of organellar disarray can usually be appreciated; the fine structure of both adenomas and hyperplasias is discussed in detail in Table 12.1.

Few ultrastructural studies of *parathyroid carcinoma* have

**Table 12.1  Parathyroid cell types and related tumours and tumour-like disorders**

| Cell type | Functional phase | RER | Golgi complexes | Secretory granules | Mitochondria |
|---|---|---|---|---|---|
| Chief cell | Active | Prominent, forms parallel stacks | Prominent, multiple | Numerous; diameters in range 100–500 nm. Secretory granules are smaller and more uniform than lysosomes, which measure about 400–900 nm in diameter | Small |
| Chief cell | Resting | Poorly developed | Small | Infrequent | Small |
| Transitional oxyphilic cell | — | Present, may form parallel arrays | Moderately prominent | Present | Numerous, hypertrophied |
| Oxyphilic cell | — | Depleted | Depleted | Sparse | Numerous, hypertrophied |
| Water clear cell | — | Present | Present | Present | Present |

References: 1623, 1798–1824

156

been reported.[1811] The features observed include light and dark cells, microfollicle formation, tortuous plasma membranes, and desmosomes. Prominent and often pleomorphic mitochondria, RER and well developed Golgi complexes are typically present, as are lipid, lysosomes, glycogen granules and annulate lamellae. Secretory granules can be found in both the basal regions of the cells and in the apices bordering follicles. The nuclei may be either rounded or beset with deep invaginations, and contain variable chromatin patterns.[1799] As such, the appearances closely conform to those of parathyroid adenomas, and it is not possible to distinguish reliably between hyperplasia, adenoma and carcinoma by EM (with the exception of water clear cell hyperplasia; Table 12.1).

| Lipid/Lipofuscin | Glycogen | Pathological alterations | Comments |
|---|---|---|---|
| Depleted | Depleted. However, large aggregates in chronically stimulated chief cells may lead to formation of vacuolated chief cells | Hyperplasia, adenoma, carcinoma | Chief cells show gradations in the proportions of various organelles, comforming to resting, synthesizing, transferring, packaging, secretory and involuting phases. Packaging phase is characterized by tortuous cell membranes |
| | | | The combination of parallel arrays of RER, secretory granules, lipid droplets and glycogen is suggestive of parathyroid chief cell differentiation |
| | | | Cells of hyperplasia and adenoma are indistinguishable. Deranged relationships of organelles and morphological variability of chief cells are seen within a single tumour. Transitional oxyphilic cells and oxyphilic cells may also be present in varying numbers. Annulate lamellae can often be found and cilia with a 9 + 0 configuration are also described. Peculiar parallel granulo-membranous complexes related to the RER have been observed in a case of tertiary hyperparathyroidism; the possibility that the granules represented a proteinaceous deposit related to proparathormone was raised[1808] |
| | | | See Figs. 12.1 and 12.2 |
| Present. Prominent lipid droplets | Abundant | — | — |
| Present | Present | Hyperplasia, adenoma | Ultrastructural appearances are transitional between chief cells and oxyphilic cells |
| | | | See Figs. 12.3–12.5 |
| Inconspicuous | Present between mitochondria | Hyperplasia, adenoma, carcinoma | May be present in predominantly chief cell proliferations. Oxyphilic cells in functional adenomas and hyperplasias may have transitional oxyphilic appearances in the form of secretory granules, prominent Golgi complexes and conspicuous RER. Typical oncocytic cells can also be found and there is evidence that both classical and transitional oxyphilic cells are hormonally active |
| Rare | Present | Water clear cell hyperplasia | Ultrastructural appearances differ from those of any other hyperfunctional parathyroid disorder. Distinctive feature is the presence of numerous membrane-bound vacuoles, possibly derived from Golgi complexes and rarely containing amorphous or crystalline material |

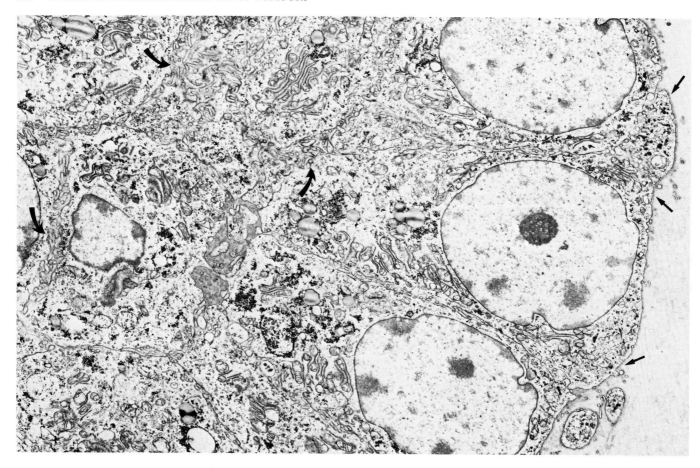

## Fig. 12.1  Parathyroid adenoma: Topography

This adenoma consists of aggregates of cuboidal to columnar cells enclosed by a basal lamina (straight arrows). Sometimes the neoplastic cells surround a small follicular lumen. Amyloid-like fibrils and corpora amylacea — as well as lipid vesicles and debris from disintegrated cells — may lie within the follicular lumina. The nuclei and granules are situated near the basal lamina, whereas stacks of RER, glycogen granules, and both lipid and lipofuscin globules are readily found in the apices. Microvilli (curved arrows) protrude from the surface of a few cells. Pleomorphic nuclei with indentations are also recorded. (× 9000)

Paired or fused smooth cisternae, annulate lamellae and invaginations of glycogen-rich ground substance within mitochondria have also been observed; so too have elongated rod-like mitochondrial cristae, and so-called chondriospheres consisting of spheroidal collections of one or more cup-shaped mitochondria enveloping a central mitochondrion.

See Table 12.1.

References: 47, 1799, 1803, 1804, 1806, 1807, 1809, 1810, 1812, 1813, 1815, 1817, 1820–1822

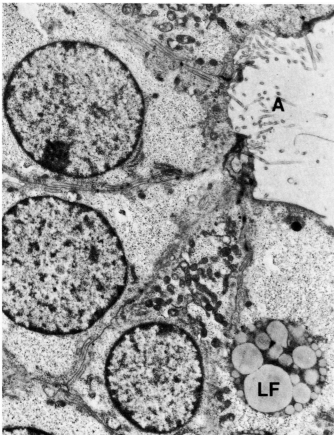

## Fig. 12.2 Parathyroid adenoma: Glycogen-rich cells

This aggregate of glycogen-rich cells is arranged in an acinar formation; microvilli project into the lumen of the acinus (A), while mitochondria and a lipofuscin body (LF) are also present. (× 10 000)

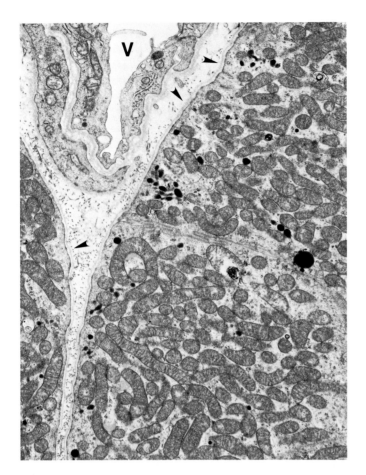

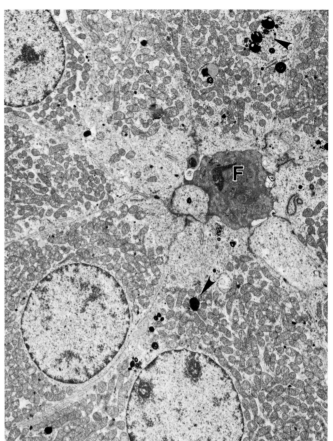

**Fig. 12.3** *(Top — left)* **Transitional oxyphilic parathyroid adenoma I: Mitochondria and secretory granules**

Oncocytic adenoma from a 58-year-old woman who presented with a depressive illness and was found to be hypercalcaemic.

EM reveals that the cells comprising hyperfunctional oxyphilic parathyroid adenomas often have features transitional between chief cells and classical oncocytes. They are distinguished from the latter by conspicuous RER, Golgi complexes and secretory granules (Table 12.1). The cells illustrated here contain numerous mitochondria, while the electron-dense secretory granules are polarized towards the base of the cells — and hence the stromal vasculature (V). A well defined basal lamina invests the cell nests (arrowheads). Although not seen here, Golgi complexes were easily found in other cells. (× 10 900)
References: 1798, 1800, 1805, 1816, 1819

**Fig. 12.4** *(Top — right)* **Transitional oxyphilic parathyroid adenoma II: Microfollicle**

The microfollicle (F) contains material of medium electron-density. Mitochondria are depleted from the apical cytoplasm of the surrounding cells. Several lysosomal bodies (arrowheads) are present. The ovoid nuclei contain plentiful euchromatin. (× 4600)

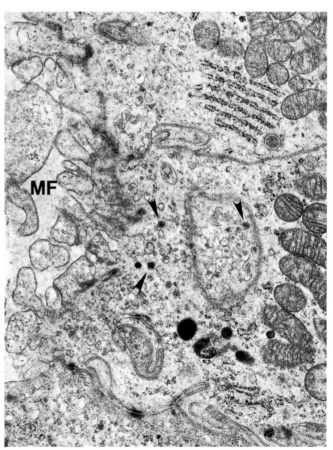

**Fig. 12.5** *(Bottom — right)* **Transitional oxyphilic parathyroid adenoma III: Secretory granules and RER**

Detail of cell bordering a microfollicle (MF). Small secretory granules — often electron-lucent, but with sporadic dense cores (arrowheads) — are concentrated in the apical cytoplasm. The lamellae of the RER are arranged in parallel. (× 16 900)

Figs. 12.3–12.5 are all from the same case; the nucleocytoplasmic features suggest a high level of metabolic activity.

# 13 Adrenal cortical and paraganglionic tumours

## ADRENAL CORTICAL NEOPLASMS

The cells of adrenal cortical tumours often contain appreciable quantities of SER, as in steroid hormone-producing cells in general. Concentric whorls of endoplasmic reticulum (spironolactone bodies) may be present in aldosterone-secreting adenomas from patients treated with spironolactone (Table 13.1 and Fig. 13.1).

**Table 13.1 Occurrence of spironolactone-type bodies in tissues**

| Tissue/occurrence | Comments |
|---|---|
| Adrenal cortex | Typically seen in zona glomerulosa, in patients treated with spironolactone. Occasionally found in deeper cortical layers. Similar bodies have been reported in adrenal cortical and luteal cells of rats treated with cycloheximide.[1848] A number of other chemical agents have been recorded to induce the formation of these structures and they have been identified in several organs of subjects treated with a coronary vasodilator |
| Adrenal cortical adenoma | Seen in patients with hyperaldosteronism (Conn's syndrome) treated with spironolactone. See Fig. 13.1 |
| Lipid cell tumour of ovary | Secondary amenorrhoea and hirsutism |
| Interstitial cell tumour of testis | In both masculinizing and feminizing Leydig cell tumours |

References: 1116, 1134, 1302, 1825, 1833, 1835, 1843, 1848, 1869

Mitochondria are usually numerous. In aldosterone-secreting adenomas, elongated 'sarcotubular' mitochondria with lamellar cristae resembling those of the normal zona glomerulosa may predominate. Similarly, adenomas associated with Cushing's syndrome may be characterized by mitochondria with tubular cristae similar to those of the zona fasciculata (Fig. 13.3). However, mixed and variant cristal patterns are frequent.[1854] Rarely, cortical adenomas contain abundant lipofuscin, which may be obvious on gross inspection (so-called black adenomas).[1827,1831,1838]

The fine structure of the malignant cells in *cortical carcinomas* may not differ significantly from those comprising adenomas. Silva et al[1870] have reported a range of ultrastructural appearances in a series of adrenal cortical carcinomas from 22 patients in whom there were only five cases with virilism and/or Cushing's syndrome. Distinctive markers of steroidogenic cells such as SER and mitochondria with tubular cristae were variable; tubular cristae, although identified in every case, were present in most cells of only 13

tumours. Similarly, SER was abundant in three carcinomas and lipid droplets in nine. The mitochondria sometimes contained dense matrical granules measuring up to 300 nm in diameter and a few 300–500 nm dense core granules, possibly lysosomal in character, were seen in three tumours. The characteristic appearances were depleted in recurrent tumours, which had a reduced organellar population; in two cases this changing morphology was accompanied by glycogen accumulation.

Adrenal cortical carcinomas producing Cushing's syndrome generally resemble each other, but the cytoplasmic characteristics can vary and mitochondria are sometimes more abundant than in adenomas. Complex folding of the plasmalemma and intranuclear cytoplasmic pseudoinclusions are described,[1873] and there may be disruption or absence of basal lamina.

## PHAEOCHROMOCYTOMA

Phaeochromocytomas are composed of cells containing cytoplasmic granules resembling those of normal chromaffin tissue. However, the granules in phaeochromocytomas tend to be abnormally large,[1871] perhaps reflecting failure of bio-synthetic regulation; thus Tannenbaum[1873] has recorded a mean granule diameter of 270 nm in adrenaline-secreting phaeochromocytomas — about 100 nm larger than in normal adrenal medulla. Varying proportions of membrane-bound noradrenaline and adrenaline granules are seen; the noradrenaline granules are characterized by dense, occasionally comma-shaped eccentric cores, bounded by wide haloes (Fig. 13.4). On the other hand, adrenaline granules usually have central, less dense cores with uniform thin submembranous haloes (Fig. 13.6).

## NEUROBLASTOMA AND GANGLIONEUROBLASTOMA

The ultrastructure of neuroblastoma is typified by cells with elaborate cytoplasmic processes in which microtubules, neurofilaments, and neurosecretory granules are concentrated (Figs. 13.7 and 13.8). Intercellular junctions may include synapses. Varying numbers of primitive embryonic cells devoid of distinctive features are also present and they may predominate. However, EM permits a diagnosis in the majority of cases, and has contributed to the recognition of neuroblastomas in adults[1852] (but see Chapter 29). The fine structure of neuroblastoma is discussed and compared with other small round cell tumours in Tables 29.1 and 29.2.

The cells comprising ganglioneuroblastoma may possess prominent mitochondria and a well developed paranuclear Golgi complex, together with pleomorphic granules 100–170 nm in diameter. Neuritic processes containing microtubules, filaments, vesicles and 100 nm granules are also present,[1873] and intracytoplasmic microtubular complexes are described.[1985] Schwann cells are also recorded in ganglioneuroblastoma and they may be seen in addition to perineurial cells in ganglioneuroma.[1867]

## EXTRA-ADRENAL PARAGANGLIOMAS

Irrespective of their anatomical location, paragangliomas are characterized by a *Zellballen* pattern in which chief cells containing neurosecretory granules are present.[1892] Sustentacular cells have also been reported, but may be absent.[1888,1894] A ribosome-lamella complex has been recorded in an abdominal paraganglioma (see Table 28.2).[1905]

Although a few large solitary pulmonary paragangliomas have been reported,[578] EM has established that so-called minute pulmonary chemodectomas are unrelated to paragangliomas.[469] Neurosecretory granules are not present; the cells comprising these lesions have elaborate processes with cytoplasmic filaments and desmosomal intercellular junctions — features reminiscent of meningiomas.[469,527] Although haemangiopericytic differentiation seems more plausible, the absence of thin myofilaments and pericellular external lamina, and the presence of desmosomes militate against this interpretation.[469] In addition, large primary pulmonary meningiomas are documented convincingly by both LM and EM; the tumour reported by Chumas & Lorelle[466] was closely related to the pleura, but the meningioma studied by Kemnitz et al[517] was situated more deeply.

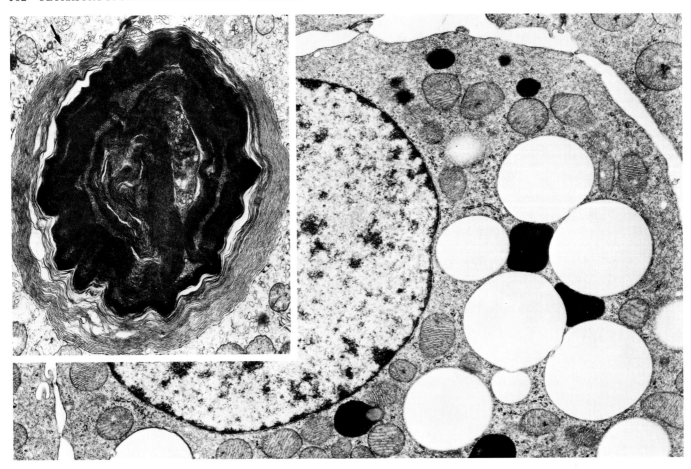

**Fig. 13.1   Adrenal adenoma associated with Conn's syndrome: Cell morphology and spironolactone body**

The cells of this adenoma had rounded, slightly eccentric nuclei with moderate amounts of euchromatin. The cytoplasmic lipid globules vary in size, and a few lipofuscin granules are also present; in some adenomas, however, the numbers of lipofuscin granules can be exceptionally high. The mitochondria possess lamellar cristae and scattered profiles of SER can also be discerned; the concentration of the latter may be high, while mitochondria with vesicular cristae resembling those of the normal zona fasciculata may also be encountered. The most frequent ultrastructural features, however, conform to those normally seen in cells of the adrenal zona glomerulosa. (×12 000)

**Inset:** This typical spironolactone body (S-body) consists of a whorling mass of membranes continuous with the SER (arrow) and has a central dense area. Although these structures are characteristically seen in the zona glomerulosa, and in adrenal cortical adenomas of patients treated with spironolactone (as in this case), they have been recorded in response to other chemical agents, and in other tissues and tumours (Table 13.1). (×11 600)

On the basis of enzyme histochemistry, enhanced but possibly abortive steroidogenic properties in S-body-containing cells have been postulated.[1825]

(Block of cortical adenoma with spironolactone bodies contributed by Dr. A. E. Seymour).

References: 1825, 1833, 1835, 1836, 1843, 1847, 1848, 1854, 1858, 1861, 1866, 1869, 1872, 1873, 1877

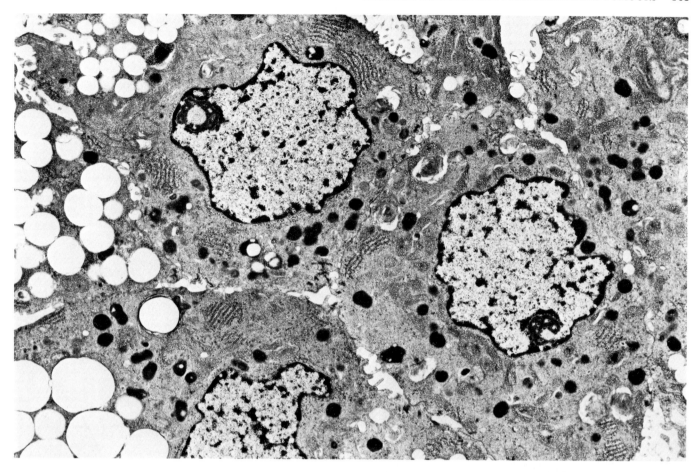

**Fig. 13.2  Adrenal adenoma associated with Cushing's syndrome: Organelles and lipid droplets**

The majority of the cells in this adenoma contained lipid globules of approximately similar dimensions. Abundant cytoplasmic lipid droplets sometimes produce irregularities of the nuclear contours. Lipofuscin granules, scattered mitochondria, and stacked lamellae of RER are also present. (× 7200)

References: 1844, 1855, 1858, 1862, 1866, 1872, 1873

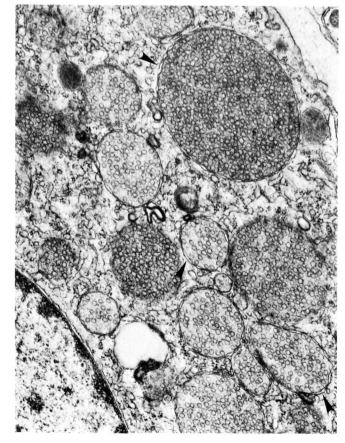

**Fig. 13.3  Adrenal adenoma associated with Cushing's syndrome: Mitochondria with tubular cristae**

The most prominent feature in this cell from an adrenal adenoma is the presence of mitochondria with tubular cristae; however, elongated mitochondria with lamellar cristae, similar to those of the normal zona glomerulosa, may also be present. Note the double outer mitochondrial membranes (arrowheads). Pleomorphic mitochondria with plentiful matrices and mitochondrial gigantism may also be encountered. The profiles of endoplasmic reticulum are both rough and smooth; SER is consistently present and may predominate. Crystalloids in the RER and filamentous structures in the cytoplasm have also been reported. The overall ultrastructural features are nevertheless those associated with cells of the zona fasciculata. (× 28 700)

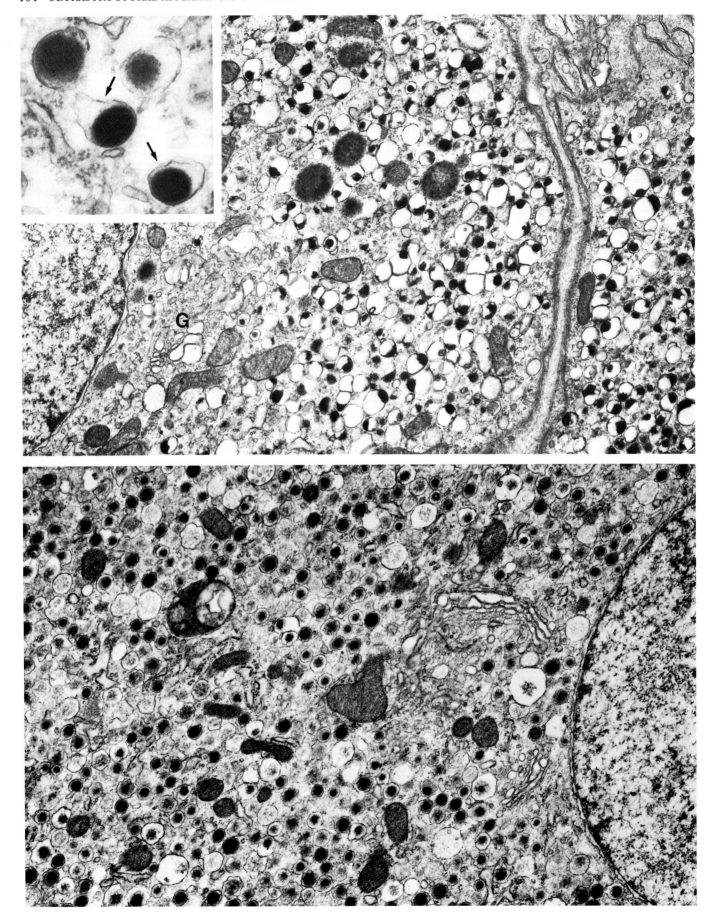

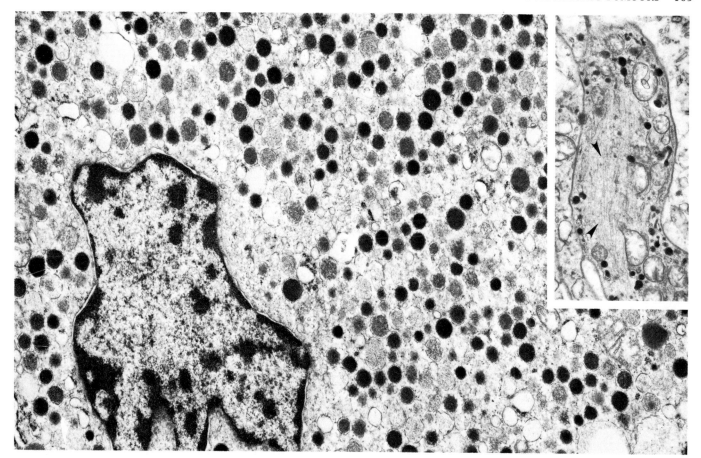

**Fig. 13.6 Phaeochromocytoma: Adrenaline granules and neuritic process**

These granules have a thin, uniform, lucent zone beneath the unit membrane, typical of adrenaline granules (compare with noradrenaline granules in Fig. 13.4). The mean diameter is 250 ± 60 nm; the profiles here are rounded, but ellipsoidal granules are also common. Adrenal tumour in a 39-year-old woman, whose differential plasma catecholamine assay showed an approximately ten-fold elevation of adrenaline above average. (× 22 000)

**Inset:** Adrenal tumour from a 10-year-old boy. Although recorded,[1832] neuritic (dendritic) processes with microtubules (arrowheads) and secretory granules are uncommon in phaeochromocytomas. It is conceivable that their presence in this case is related to the patient's age; nerve growth factor (NGF) is known to stimulate the formation of neuritic processes in cultured phaeochromocytes.[1915] However, such processes may be seen in a variety of neuroendocrine tumours – including medullary carcinoma of thyroid, carcinoid tumours and so-called Merkel cell carcinoma – as an in vivo phenomenon and in tissue cultures without the addition of NGF. (× 12 700)

References: 1832, 1915

**Fig. 13.4** *(Facing page — top)* **Adrenal phaeochromocytoma: Noradrenaline granules**

The cells of this tumour are characterized by many cytoplasmic granules ranging from 40–1000 nm in diameter; the majority, however, measure 200–300 nm. In this particular neoplasm, most secretory granules display an electron-dense, often eccentric, core. A few are comma-shaped with a protruding 'tail', as indicated by the arrows in the inset. Such granules indicate the production and storage of noradrenaline. In general, granule diameters in phaeochromocytomas exceed those of normal chromaffin tissue. Scattered lysosomal dense bodies, profiles of smooth endoplasmic reticulum, and mitochondria are also present, as well as a moderately well developed Golgi apparatus (G). (× 21 800. Inset: × 58 300)

Immunoreactive vasoactive intestinal polypeptide (VIP) and somatostatin have also been reported in one phaeochromocytoma; most cells contained noradrenaline granules 250–350 nm in diameter, while others possessed small granules 110–140 nm in diameter, possibly correlating with the VIP.[1865]

References: 295, 1829, 1830, 1832, 1840, 1850, 1856, 1864, 1865, 1868, 1871, 1873, 1878, 1879

**Fig. 13.5** *(Facing page — bottom)* **Adrenal phaeochromocytoma: Cell morphology**

Here the secretory granules are non-uniform. Some have an electron-dense core, indicating the production and storage of noradrenaline; others lack the peripheral halo, and the limiting membrane is closely related to the electron-dense contents, suggesting adrenaline-containing granules. Most neoplasms of this kind have both types of granules, albeit in varying proportions. Variations in cytoplasmic electron-density, intramitochondrial dense bodies, rodlets, and septate junctions between mitochondria have also been reported. In malignant phaeochromocytomas there is evidence to indicate much variation in the number, size, and electron-density of the granules, not only from cell to cell but also within single cells. (× 23 000)

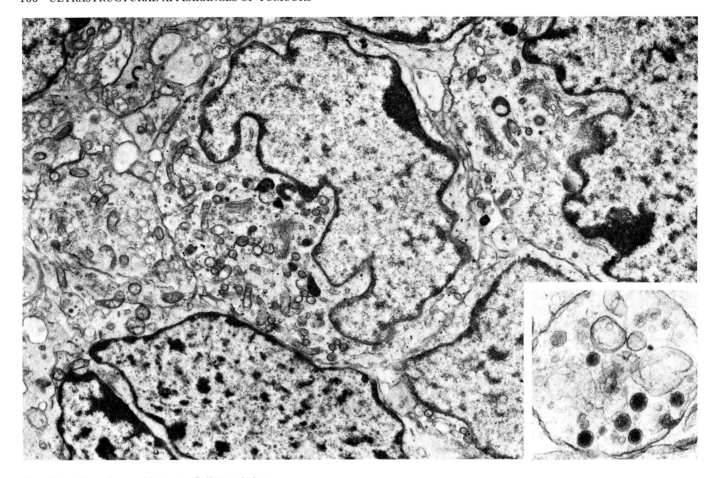

**Fig. 13.7 Adrenal neuroblastoma: Cell morphology**

The ultrastructural appearances of neuroblastoma vary with the degree of differentiation. There are usually tightly packed aggregates of cells with moderately irregular nuclei, and a small rim of surrounding cytoplasm. Typically, only minute amounts of glycogen can be detected. Few dense-core vesicles are seen in the body of the cell, despite the ease of their detection in the cytoplasmic extensions. (× 12 600)

**Inset:** Blunt processes are frequently found in some parts of this neoplasm, and these often contain the dense-core granules measuring 90–160 nm, which aid in the diagnosis. Such granules are smaller than those normally present in adrenal medulla; larger granules 250–550 nm in diameter may be found in the cell bodies. The concentration of granules generally correlates with the amounts of urinary catecholamine metabolites (× 42 000)

**Discussion:** Intermediate filaments (neurofilaments) also characterize the cytoplasm of neuroblastomas. These appear to be composed entirely of the 68 kiloDalton subunit and are additionally recorded in olfactory neuroblastoma, sometimes distending the cisternae of the RER. Labelling with monoclonal anti-neurofilament antibodies is described, along with negative reactions for vimentin and GFAP, supporting neuronal (neuritic) differentiation.[432] The immunohistochemical demonstration of neurone-specific enolase has been proposed as a further aid to the diagnosis of neuroblastoma as well as melanoma, Merkel cell carcinoma and apudomas.[168] Finally, Schwann cells have also been identified in neuroblastomas.[1874]

The ultrastructural appearances of *olfactory neuroblastoma (aesthesio-neuroblastoma)* are essentially identical to those of neuroblastomas developing in the adrenal gland and other sites, and therefore they are not depicted separately in this atlas.

See also Table 29.1.

References: 383, 388, 390, 399, 402, 407, 410, 425, 430, 432, 434 *(olfactory neuroblastoma)*; 239, 1249, 1834, 1837, 1845, 1846, 1849, 1852, 1853, 1856, 1857, 1863, 1867, 1871, 1873–1876, 1878, 1880 *(adrenal neuroblastoma)*; 1926, 1984, 1986, 1987, 1995, 2002, 2022–2024 *(cerebral neuroblastoma)*

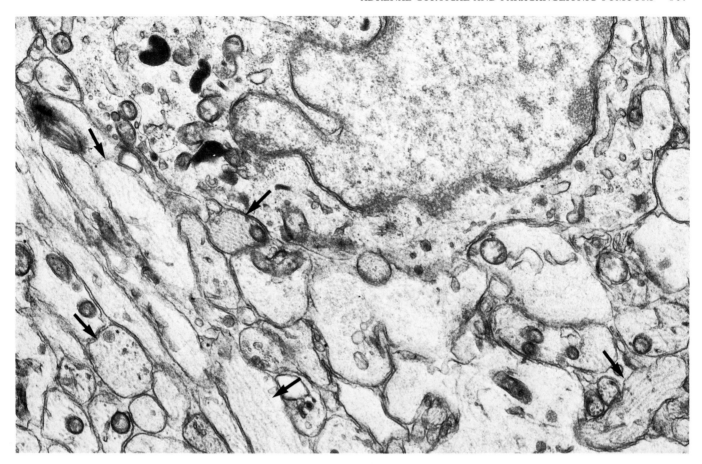

**Fig. 13.8   Adrenal neuroblastoma: Cell morphology**

Dendritic processes containing microtubules (arrows) are typical of these neoplasms. The processes interweave with each other and often are closely apposed, not only to other processes, but also to perikaryons. Generally, the number and length of dendritic processes relate to the differentiation of the neoplasm. Although desmosomes may be seen between adjacent cells, synapses are rare. Gap junctions, oblique septation of mitochondrial cristae (see Fig. 2.4) and so-called nematosomes (nucleolus-like bodies) in the cytoplasm have also been reported.[1834] (× 27 300)

The microtubules are most effectively demonstrated by glutaraldehyde fixation at room temperature instead of 4°C, and they are generally not evident in osmium tetroxide-fixed tissue.

Reference: 1834

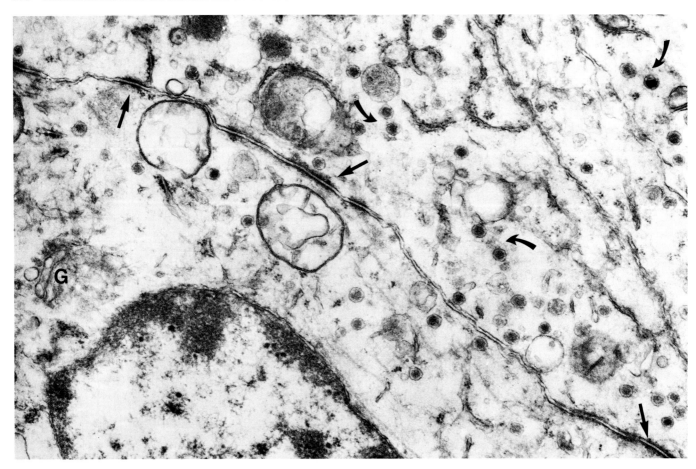

**Fig. 13.9   Paraganglioma (chemodectoma) of carotid body: Cell morphology**

These neoplasms consist of tightly packed cell bodies and their blunt processes. The nuclei contain moderate amounts of euchromatin. As well as dense-core granules 70–250 nm in diameter within both cell bodies and processes (curved arrows), there are microtubules, a moderately developed Golgi complex (G), lysosomal dense bodies and short strands of RER within the cytoplasm. Characteristically, there are desmosome-like junctions (straight arrows) between adjoining cells and their processes; synaptic contacts, however, have not been detected. Ribosome-lamella complexes have also been observed (see Table 28.2). (× 38 000)

**Discussion:** Although the concentration of sustentacular cells varies greatly in paragangliomas, nerve fibres are rare. The overall frequency of neurosecretory granules in functional carotid body paragangliomas appears to correlate directly with the catecholamine content of the tumour tissue.[1889]

Megamitochondria, intermediate filaments and microtubules may also be seen.[1909] Crystalloidal structures similar to those seen in alveolar soft part sarcoma have been described in a case of malignant paraganglioma of the organ of Zuckerkandl,[30] but have not been recorded in other paragangliomas.[2186] Ultrastructural analysis of a malignant carotid body paraganglioma associated with von Hippel-Lindau disease revealed only chief cells, with cytoplasmic processes and NSG measuring 120 ± 28.5 nm in diameter.[1897]

References: 30, 395, 433, 578, 827, 1645, 1882–1914

# 14 Pancreatic islet tumours

The combination of immunohistology and EM has again amplified knowledge of the confused subject of the gastroenteropancreatic endocrine cells, which are listed in Table 14.1 according to the Lausanne classification.[1636,1638] A detailed account of these cells and related tumours is clearly beyond the scope of this work; however, the principal pancreatic endocrine cells and tumours are discussed in Table 14.2. Immunocytochemistry is indispensable to precise diagnosis of pancreatic islet neoplasms; as already foreshadowed in the general comments on endocrine tumours, the classical granule morphology in tumours secreting insulin, gastrin and glucagon appears to be diagnostic, but the value of EM is limited by the occurrence of tumours with non-specific granules, poorly granulated cytoplasm, or mixed populations of granules (Table 14.3).[928, 942, 952]

In an analysis of 125 pancreatic endocrine tumours, Heitz et al[942] found that 50 of 95 hormonally active tumours contained immunoreactive polypeptides without corresponding hormonal symptoms, and 15 of 30 clinically non-secretory tumours possessed multiple cell lines. The characteristic secretory granules of 2 to 3 cell types were found in 12 of 18 neoplasms examined by EM, and 11 also contained small non-diagnostic granules 110–150 nm in diameter. In this series most insulinomas and all 10 PP-omas were benign, whereas many of the gastrinomas, glucagonomas and VIP-omas were considered malignant on the basis of metastasis or invasion of peripancreatic structures.

**Table 14.1   Classification of gastroenteropancreatic endocrine cells***

| | Stomach | | Small intestine | | Large | Function proposed |
| Pancreas | Oxyntic | Pyloric | Upper | Lower | intestine | or ascertained |
|---|---|---|---|---|---|---|
| (P) | P | P | P | | | Bombesin? |
| EC | EC | EC | EC | EC | EC | 5HT + peptides |
| D₁ | D₁ | D₁ | D₁ | H | H | VIP or vipoid |
| F | (F) | F | (F) | F | F | PP or PP-like |
| D | D | D | D | | | Somatostatin |
| B | | | | | | Insulin |
| A | A | (A) | | | | Glucagon |
| (X) | X | (X) | | | | Unknown |
| | ECL | | | | | H or 5HT; peptide? |
| (G) | | G | (G) | | | Gastrin |
| | | | S | (S) | | Secretin |
| | | | I | I | | Cholecystokinin |
| | | | K | K | | GIP |
| | | | VL | VL | | IPH? |
| | | | | N | | Neurotensin |
| | | | L | L | L | GLI |

*Lausanne 1977 classification[1636,1638]

( ) = Only few cells or restricted to few species or to fetal life

(From Solcia et al.[1636] Reproduced by permission)

169

**Table 14.2  Pancreatic endocrine cells and tumours**

| Cell type[*] | Secretory product | Granule morphology | Granule size | Tumour[†] | Remarks |
|---|---|---|---|---|---|
| A | Glucagon | Rounded, with central or eccentric round dense area (double-core appearance) | $200 \pm 125$ nm[952] $252 \pm 65$ nm[925] $250 \pm 70$ nm[975] | Glucagonoma | Typically associated with necrolytic migratory erythema as part of the diabetes-dermatitis syndrome<br><br>See Fig 14.4 |
| B | Insulin | Pleomorphic, with crystalline forms | $250 \pm 59$ nm[952] $302 \pm 75$ nm[925] $200-250$ nm[950] $300 \pm 70$ nm[975] | Insulinoma | Akagi & Fujii[916] reported granule diameters of 140–470 nm (average 255 nm) in insulinomas. The crystalline granules are diagnostic, but smaller atypical and non-specific rounded granules may be present. See also Table 14.3 and Figs. 14.1–14.3 |
| D | Somatostatin | Rounded. Variable density, and often weakly osmiophilic. Granules have gastrin granule-like morphology, but most antral and duodenal antisera fail to label D cells | $220 \pm 48$ nm[952] $259 \pm 148$ nm[925] $300-350$ nm[950] $260 \pm 100$ nm[975] | Somatostatinoma | Clinical features in the reported cases have included a diabetic glucose tolerance curve, steatorrhoea, achlorhydria and cholelithiasis. May be clinically silent.<br><br>Granules in somatostatinomas generally 250–400 nm in diameter, with variable and often low electron-density. |
| PP (F, $D_2$) | Pancreatic polypeptide | Small, rounded or angulated | $110 \pm 23$ nm[952] $115 \pm 20$ nm[925] $100-150$ nm[950] $140 \pm 60$ nm[975] $149 \pm 28$ nm[942] | PP-oma. PP-like cells may be seen in different types of tumour, including insulinomas, glucagonomas, gastrinomas and tumours associated with the WDHA syndrome | ?WDHA syndrome. Presence of PP-like cells cannot be equated with a definite secretory product, but identifies the tumour as endocrine in type |
| $D_1$ | VIP-like polypeptide | Small, rounded | $135 \pm 28$ nm[952] $127 \pm 23$ nm[925] $130-180$ nm[975] | VIP-oma. $D_1$-like cells may be found in different types of endocrine tumours | WDHA syndrome. The role of VIP as a neurotransmitter has now been established; it stimulates cyclic AMP production in end-organ cells in a manner similar to cholera toxin<br><br>VIP or a VIP-like substance has been associated with a variety of tumours, including islet cell tumours, neuroblastoma, ganglioneuroma, phaeochromocytoma, medullary thyroid carcinoma and bronchogenic carcinoma |
| (G) | Gastrin | See remarks | See remarks | Gastrinoma | Most gastrinomas contain cells with diagnostic rounded granules, identical to those of antral G cells, with a mean diameter of $200 \pm 60$ nm to $290 \pm 50$ nm. The granules display variable osmiophilia and some may appear flocculent or empty. Most tumours also have cells with smaller, more pleomorphic and non-diagnostic granules with a mean diameter of about $125 \pm 30$ nm,[929,950] and some cases contain only non-specific granules (Fig. 14.6). Cells with granules like those of A, D and EC cells may also be seen.[929] Association with the Zollinger-Ellison syndrome. See Figs. 14.5 and 14.6 |
| Other | See remarks | See remarks | See remarks | See remarks | Other pancreatic endocrine tumours include carcinoid-islet tumours eliciting an atypical carcinoid syndrome, pancreatic corticotrophinomas producing Cushing's syndrome and parathyrinomas with an ectopic hypercalcaemia syndrome. Production of antidiuretic hormone, neurotensin and cholecystokinin has also been recorded[933] |

[*] Lausanne 1977 Classification[1636,1638]

[†] Since many pancreatic endocrine tumours produce multiple polypeptides,[950,953,954] their classification on the basis of a single secretory product is arguably undesirable, although clinical manifestations are usually related to one dominant hormone; the terms in this table have been used solely for brevity

References: 916, 919, 920, 922, 925, 927–930. 932–935, 937, 938, 941, 942, 947–950, 952–955, 958, 960, 961, 963–965, 967, 972, 974–977, 979–981, 987–990, 1623, 1636, 1638, 3145

**Table 14.3    Ultrastructural classes of pancreatic islet tumours,
based on granule morphology and frequency**

I    Tumours with homogeneous population of granules typical of
    corresponding normal cell type

I I    Tumours with mixed populations of typical and atypical granules

III    Tumours with atypical granules only

IV    Poorly granulated tumours

In a study of 28 insulinomas, Creutzfeldt et al[928] identified the following
ultrastructural classes and proportions of tumour: Type I – 46 per cent; Type
II – 25 per cent; Type III – 14 per cent; Type IV – virtually agranular
tumours – 14 per cent. Only Types I and II could be diagnosed
ultrastructurally, and 8 of the 28 cases could not be recognized as insulinomas
by EM alone.

References: 928, 929, 952

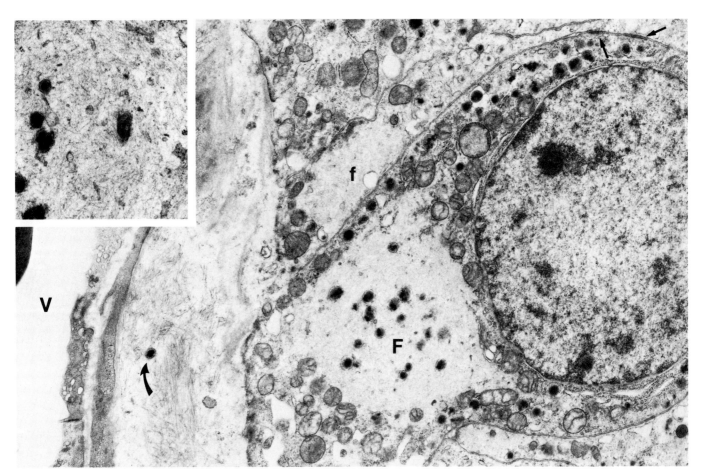

**Fig. 14.1  Insulin-secreting pancreatic islet tumour (insulinoma):
Fibrous bodies and granules**

Tumour from the pancreatic tail of a 38-year-old man who presented with
episodic syncope. Intermediate filaments in one cell form a prominent fibrous
body (F), in which secretory granules, including crystalline forms, are
enmeshed. An adjoining cell contains a smaller collection of filaments (f).
Intermediate junctions (straight arrows) are present, and the cell nest is
intermittently bordered by basal lamina. A secretory granule (curved arrow) is
evident within connective tissue between the B cells and the blood vessel (V),
possibly in transit to the vascular lumen, although persistence of the limiting
membrane suggests that it may be displaced artefactually. (× 16 100)

    **Inset:** Portion of a fibrous body at higher magnification; the component
filaments are approximately 10 nm in diameter (see Table 2.9). (× 21 400)

    References: 916, 918, 922, 925, 927, 928, 930, 932, 935, 950, 952, 958,
961, 965, 975, 979, 990

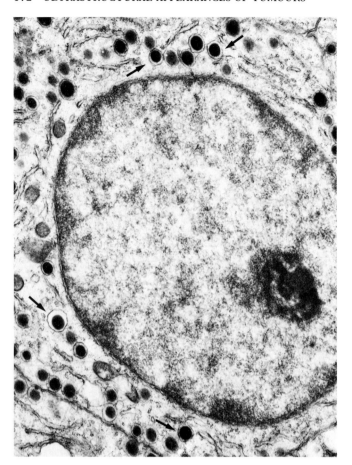

**Fig. 14.2 Insulin-secreting pancreatic islet tumour: Granule morphology I**

These neoplasms consist of tightly apposed cells containing distinct cytoplasmic granules which measure 200–300 nm (Tables 14.2 and 14.3). The granules are round to oval, but instead of the crystalline core characteristics of normal B cells, the granules in this case consist of large dense spherules separated from the limiting membrane by a distinct halo (arrows). The nuclei generally display smooth contours with moderate amounts of euchromatin, and possess prominent nucleoli. (× 20 000)

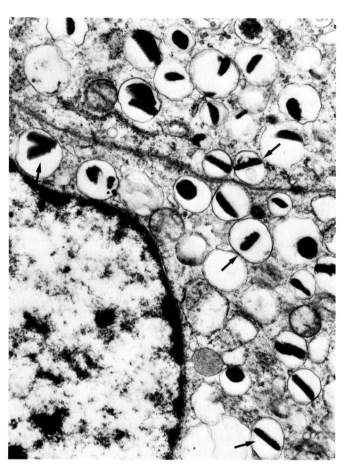

**Fig. 14.3 Insulin-secreting pancreatic islet tumour: Granule morphology II**

A crystalline body in the secretory granules (arrows) of these cells is fairly common. Although only a small fraction of the granules may contain typical crystalline cores, occasionally they predominate. The literature suggests that these characteristic granules occur in more than half of the cases of insulinoma examined by EM (Table 14.3). It is thought that the crystalline granules develop by condensation of spherical cores. In other cases the granules are not structurally specific, and to add to the problem, neoplasms with a mixture of cell types also exist. Ribosome-lamella complexes have also been described (see Table 28.2). (× 20 000)

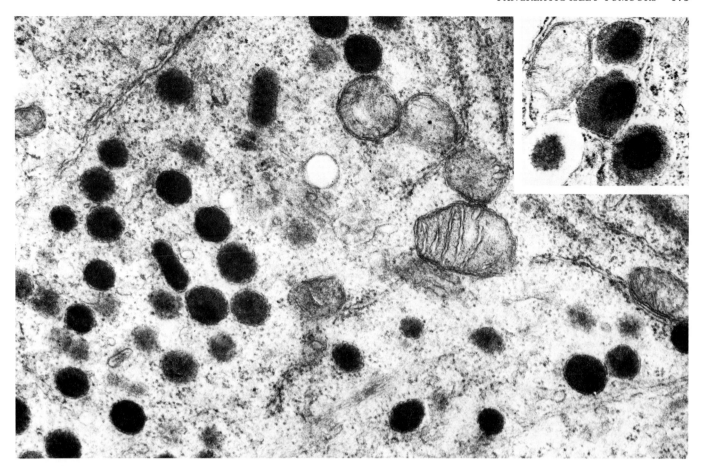

**Fig. 14.4 Glucagon-secreting pancreatic islet tumour (gluca-gonoma): Granule morphology**

Tumour from a 45-year-old man who presented with necrolytic migratory erythema. Nodules of closely apposed cells were seen, and the nuclei were slightly irregular with much euchromatin.

The glucagon-secreting neoplastic cell is characterized by the typical granules of the A cells of pancreatic islets. These granules are round to oval and measure approximately 200 ± 125 nm (Table 14.2). Only a small peripheral halo separates the electron-dense material of the granule from its limiting membrane. In some instances a core of exceptionally electron-dense material can be distinguished from the rest of the granule contents. In some reported glucagonomas, the classical ultrastructural characteristics of the granules were not detected (class III tumours; Table 14.3). (× 39 000)

**Inset:** This electron micrograph shows the electron-dense core of the secretory granules of a glucagonoma cell. (× 42 700)

**Discussion:** This double-core granule morphology is typically seen in A cells fixed with glutaraldehyde. In tissue initially fixed in osmium tetroxide, the outer medium-density component of the granule matrix is replaced by a lucent halo around the dense core, because of extraction of contents during osmium fixation.[45] It is unclear whether secretory granules possessing only the electron-dense core material represent another secretory product. There is abundant evidence that some pancreatic islet tumours can produce more than one hormone (Table 14.2).

References: 45, 919, 922, 925, 927, 935, 947, 948–950, 952, 960, 961, 972, 975, 977, 988

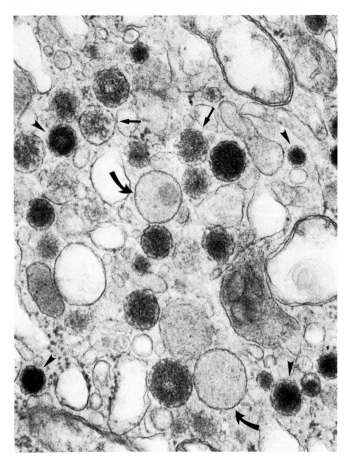

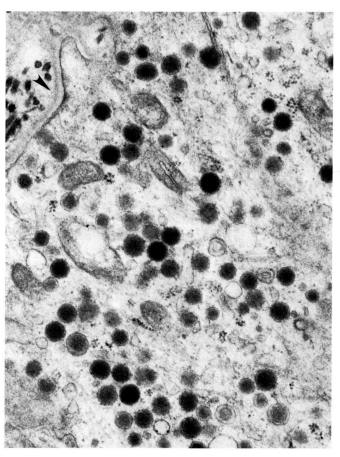

**Fig. 14.5   Pancreaticoduodenal islet cell tumour: Granule morphology: Gastrin-like granules**

Hormonally silent tumour from the duodenal wall of a middle-aged man. The tumour displayed moderate immunoreactivity for gastrin, with negative reactions for somatostatin and glucagon, despite the use of potent antisera. The large lucent granules (curved arrows) measure 330–375 nm in diameter; they resemble typical G-cell granules, although lacking a truly 'empty' appearance. Smaller granules with dense cores and diameters in the range of 140–260 nm are also present (arrowheads). In addition, there are intermediate forms with flocculent cores of medium density (straight arrows). Most granules in this case had dense cores; aggregates of intermediate filaments, prominent Golgi complexes, acinar spaces with rare collections of micropsammoma bodies (Fig. 14.7), and intracytoplasmic neolumina were other notable features. (× 44 900)

(Case contributed by Dr. A. E. Seymour)

**Fig. 14.6   Pancreatic islet tumour with hypergastrinaemia: Granule morphology: Non-specific granules**

Malignant pancreatic tumour associated with peptic ulceration, in a 36-year-old man. The serum gastrin assays were elevated, and continued to rise after total gastrectomy, in keeping with a diagnosis of Zollinger-Ellison syndrome.

As illustrated here, this tumour contained a population of round membrane-bound secretory granules, averaging 170 nm in diameter, with electron-dense cores. A few granules had cores of medium density and there were rare lucent granulo-vacuolar structures, but convincing G-cell granules could not be found. Note the adjacent basal lamina (arrowhead). (× 31 000)

**Discussion:** Although granules of this type may be found in gastrinomas (class III tumours; Table 14.3), they lack specificity and therefore cannot be equated with a definite secretory product. Their only diagnostic value lies in establishing the endocrine nature of a particular tumour.

Studies in the rat[940] have suggested that G-cell granules evolve from relatively small electron-dense progranules through intermediate forms to large electron-lucent mature granules. The dense progranules were 230 ± 44 nm in diameter and appeared to contain prohormone. The intermediate granules measured 275 ± 63 nm and probably corresponded to the conversion of prohormone to hormone, whereas the large lucent structures seemed to contain mainly hormone and were 310 ± 61 nm in diameter. The progranules constituted a greater proportion of the granule population in active than resting G cells and showed more intense immunoreactivity than the mature granules. It is therefore to be expected that some gastrinomas will predominantly contain immature small dense granules, reflecting uninhibited metabolic activity, with rapid gastrin synthesis, packaging and exocytosis.

See Table 14.2.

References: 922, 925, 927, 929, 938, 940, 952, 956, 961, 974, 975, 981, 990

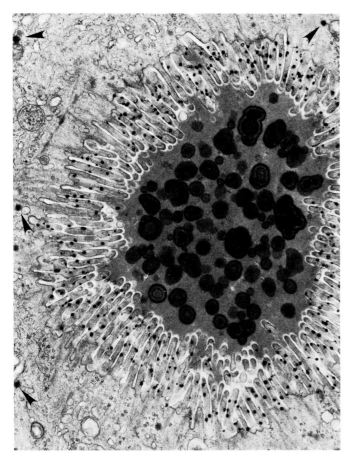

**Fig. 14.7   Pancreaticoduodenal islet cell tumour: Intracytoplasmic crypt with microcalcification**

Pancreaticoduodenal tumour with no clinical evidence of secretory activity. The crypt contains numerous laminated calcific concretions, some having a targetoid appearance.

Tiny electron-dense microspheres, presumably representing centres of calcification, are localized along the luminal microvilli. Some are situated on, or just beneath, the plasma membranes. Their distribution is probably a reflection of alkaline phosphatase activity. Alkaline phosphatase is frequently associated with mammalian cell membranes, and has been most intensively investigated in the brush border of intestinal epithelium, where it is located at the inner layer of the membrane covering the microvilli.[47]

A few round secretory granules (arrowheads) are evident in the cytoplasm. Note also the penetrating microvillous core rootlets, although glycocalyceal bodies are not present. (× 13 600)

Extracellular psammoma bodies in duodenal carcinoid-islet tumours are reported to be associated with the presence of somatostatin, but are not a feature of pancreatic somatostatinomas.[821] However, this tumour yielded a negative immunocytochemical reaction for somatostatin (same case as Fig. 14.5).

References: 47, 821

# 15 Juxtaglomerular cell tumour

Renin-producing juxtaglomerular cell tumours of the kidney represent an extremely rare cause of systemic hypertension. By LM they resemble haemangiopericytomas (see Table 23.1), but ultrastructural examination demonstrates cytoplasmic granules resembling those normally found in juxtaglomerular cells. The granule morphology includes mature spheroidal forms, and the characteristic rhomboidal renin protogranules (Figs. 15.1 and 15.2).[1023] These tumours may contain numerous mast cells,[1023] and neural tissue has also been reported.[993]

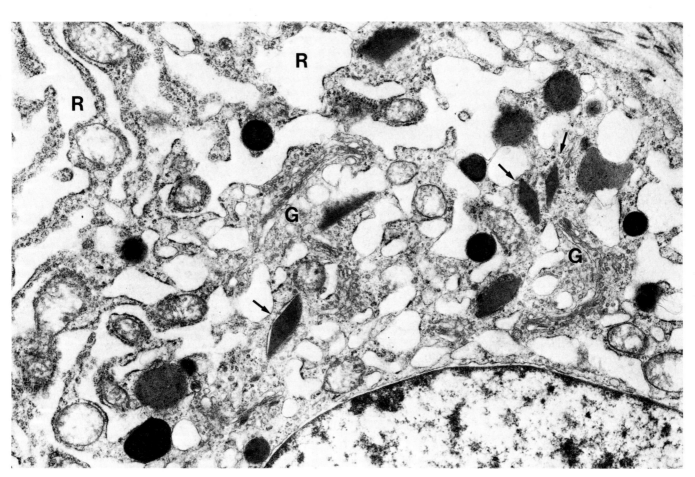

**Fig. 15.1  Juxtaglomerular cell tumour (reninoma): Cell detail**

Renal tumour from a hypertensive 13-year-old boy with documented hyperreninaemia. The granules include both rounded forms, and the diagnostic rhomboidal (renin) protogranules (arrows). The Golgi apparatus (G) is prominent, and the cisternae of the rough endoplasmic reticulum (R) are markedly dilated. In addition to juxtaglomerular cells, this tumour contained numerous stromal mast cells. (× 17 700)

(Case contributed by Drs. G. Phillips and T. M. Mukherjee.)
References: 993, 996, 1016, 1018, 1021, 1023, 1025

176

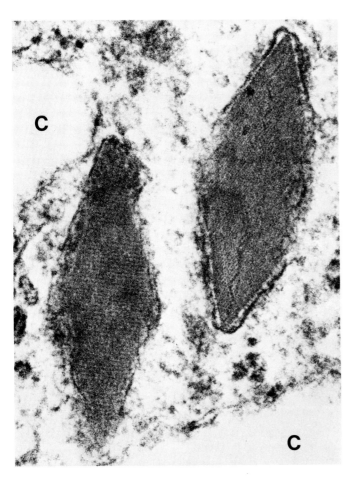

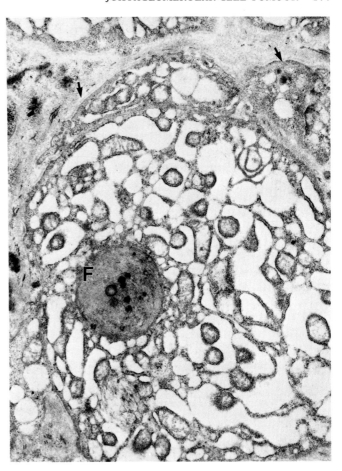

**Fig. 15.2 Juxtaglomerular cell tumour: Rhomboidal protogranules**

These membrane-bound rhomboidal protogranules have a crystalline substructure, with transverse and oblique patterns, and a centre-to-centre periodicity of approximately 6–10 nm. One protogranule also has a longitudinal 'zigzag' pattern, suggesting a fracture plane. Spheroidal granules in juxtaglomerular cell tumours are thought to evolve from these rhomboidal protogranules. Portions of dilated cisternae (C) of RER are also evident. (×120 600)

**Fig. 15.3 Juxtaglomerular cell tumour: Fibrous body and dilatation of RER**

The rough endoplasmic reticulum in the juxtaglomerular cell illustrated shows pronounced cisternal dilatation, occupying most of the cytoplasm. A fibrous body (F) is also evident, consisting of a collection of intermediate filaments with associated lipid and a few granules (see Table 2.9). External lamina can be seen in some regions (arrows). Same case as Figs. 15.1 and 15.2. (×9900)

# 16 Carcinoid tumours

Most of the general comments on endocrine tumours made earlier (Chapter 10) apply equally to carcinoid tumours. Characteristic differences in granule size, morphology and staining reactions may be found in tumours of fore-, mid- and hind-gut origin (Table 16.1),[1622] although it is emphasized that departures from the typical granule morphology occur; ultrastructural prediction of the anatomical origin of a particular tumour is therefore unreliable. A variety of neuroendocrine secretory products can be identified in gastrointestinal carcinoid tumours by immunocytochemistry; serotonin (5-HT) is present in most cases, but gastrin, somatostatin, neurotensin, motilin, glucagon and pancreatic polypeptide in differing combinations are detectable occasionally.[664]

Carcinoid tumours affecting various sites are listed in Table 16.2, and bronchopulmonary carcinoid tumours are classified in Table 16.3. Melanotic neuroendocrine carcinomas are discussed in Chapter 7.

**Table 16.2  Reported primary sites of carcinoid tumours**

Ear (bony portion of external auditory canal)
Larynx
Bronchus and lung
Thymus
Parotid gland
Gastrointestinal tract
Liver
Gall bladder
Pancreas
Skin*
Breast†
Kidney
Urinary bladder
Prostate
Testis
Uterine cervix
Endometrium§
Ovary (including strumal carcinoid tumour)

*Cutaneous neuroendocrine carcinoma; see text, Chapter 6

†See text, Chapter 5

§Mixed carcinoid tumour-adenocarcinoma[1173]

**Table 16.1  Classical enterochromaffin cell types and related carcinoid tumours***

| Characteristics | Foregut cells | Midgut cells | Hindgut cells |
|---|---|---|---|
| Anatomical sites | Bronchus, stomach, duodenum, pancreas | Jejunum, ileum, appendix, right hemicolon | Left hemicolon, rectum |
| Granule morphology | Rounded, uniform (see Figs. 16.3 and 16.4) | Pleomorphic, elliptical and angulated, similar to those shown in Fig. 7.1 | Rounded, uniform |

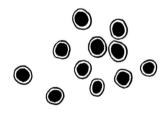 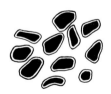 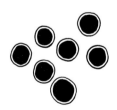

| | | | |
|---|---|---|---|
| Granule size in carcinoid tumours[1622] | Mean 185 nm, range 180–220 nm | Mean 230 nm, range 75–500 nm | Mean 190 nm, range 165–235 nm† |
| Argentaffinity | Negative | Positive | Negative |
| Argyrophilia | Positive | Positive | Negative |

*In carcinoid tumours, departures from the classical granule characteristics limit the value of this scheme; for example, bronchial carcinoid tumours are notoriously variable in their staining properties and they may contain granules of midgut type.[473] Nevertheless, the granule morphology may be of value in deciding on the order of investigations to identify the source of a metastatic carcinoid tumour; in addition, pleomorphic midgut-type granules are useful in excluding islet cell tumours, as these all contain rounded granules, with the exception of some insulinomas (see Chapter 14)

†The size differences between foregut and hindgut granules have been exaggerated in the above illustrations

**Table 16.3  Classification of bronchopulmonary carcinoids and related tumours**

| Tumour | Neurosecretory granules | | | Comments |
| --- | --- | --- | --- | --- |
| | Morphology | Frequency | Size | |
| *CLASSES ACCORDING TO DISTRIBUTION AND SIZE OF TUMOUR* | | | | |
| Central bronchial carcinoid tumour | Round, occasionally polymorphous | Numerous | 70–500 nm, generally in range 100–300 nm | Different types of bronchial carcinoid tumour have been proposed on the basis of granule size.[460] Tumours with small granules 140 nm in diameter are said to resemble pulmonary P cells, while those with larger granules have been likened to type 3 cells |
| Peripheral pulmonary carcinoid tumour | Round | Numerous | Average 110–140 nm | Ultrastructural appearances similar to centrally located tumours |
| Pulmonary tumourlets | Round | Numerous | 60–180 nm, average 90–100 nm | — |
| *CLASSES BASED ON CELL MORPHOLOGY* | | | | |
| Oncocytic bronchial carcinoid tumour | Round | Focally numerous only | 150–250 nm, average 220 nm | Marked mitochondrial hyperplasia. See Fig. 16.8 and Table 2.1 |
| Spindle cell carcinoid tumour | Round | Numerous | Approximately 50–240 nm, generally in range 110–150 nm | Pulmonary carcinoid tumours may show other configurations on LM, including trabecular, adenopapillary and clear cell patterns |
| Melanotic bronchial carcinoid tumour | Round | Apparently not numerous | 200–400 nm | Granular melanosomes but no striated (stage II) melanosomes were found by Grazer et al.[490] See Chapter 7 |
| Atypical carcinoid tumour | Round | Infrequent to numerous | 80–140 nm | Defined by nuclear atypia, mitotic activity and focal necrosis. Neurosecretory granules may be seen concentrated in cytoplasmic processes. See Figs. 16.5 and 16.7 |
| Medullary carcinoma-like tumour of lung | See comments | See comments | See comments | Amyloid-containing stroma.[487] Thyroid counterpart characterized by numerous round granules with diameters in range 150–250 nm. See Figs. 11.5–11.7, 16.1 and 16.2 |
| Small cell carcinoma, intermediate cell subtype | Round | Sparse | 80–150 nm | Aggressive carcinoma representing a 'large cell' variant of oat cell carcinoma |
| Small cell carcinoma (oat cell carcinoma) | Round | Sparse | 50–200 nm, usually in range 80–140 nm | See Chapter 6 |

References: 437, 447, 448, 453, 455, 456, 460, 462–464, 467, 471, 473, 483, 484, 486, 487, 489–491, 493, 495, 498, 506, 519, 533, 536, 540, 543, 547, 565, 566, 569, 572, 579, 589, 593

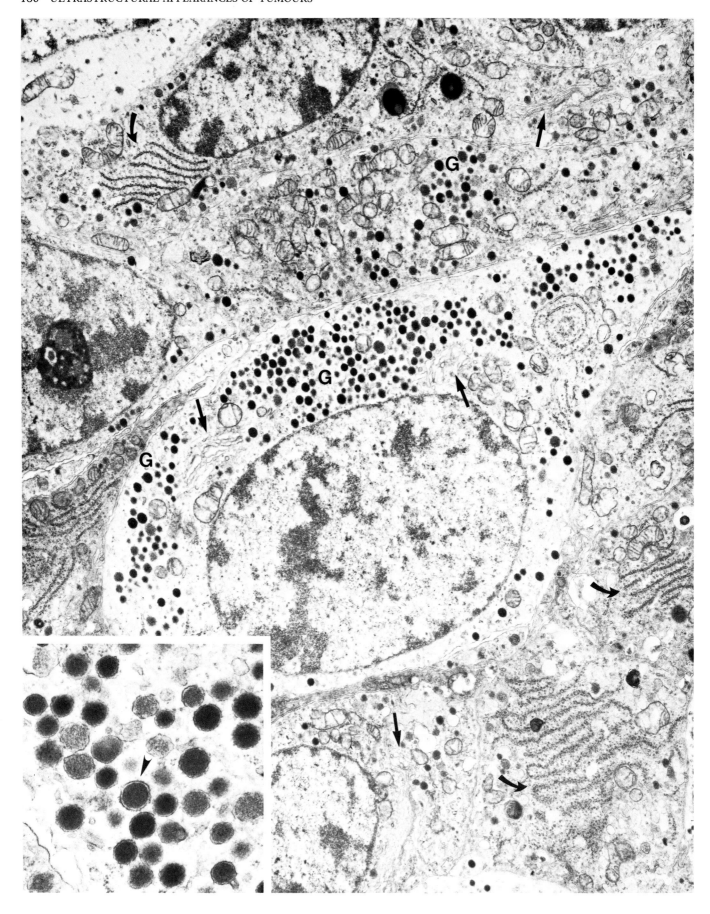

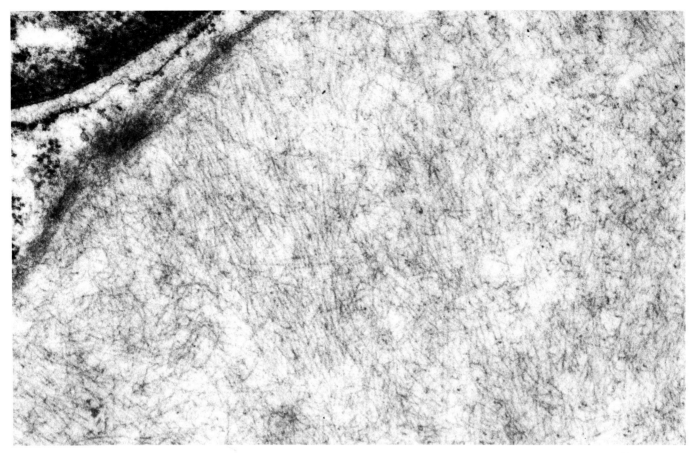

**Fig. 16.2  Neuroendocrine carcinoma: Stromal amyloid**

There are numerous, haphazardly distributed, non-branching amyloid fibrils, averaging 9–10 nm in diameter, in the intercellular space (see Table 3.3). Same case as Fig. 16.1. (× 64 700)

**Fig. 16.1** *(Facing page)* **Neuroendocrine carcinoma with stromal amyloid (medullary carcinoma-like tumour): Cell population and neurosecretory granules**

Surgical specimen of retroperitoneal lymph node metastasis from a malignant neuroendocrine (APUD) tumour, possibly of hepatic origin. The patient presented with Cushing's syndrome, and was found to have extreme elevations of serum ACTH, calcitonin and $\beta$-endorphin levels.

Both light and darker cells are apparent in this low-power micrograph, and both cell types contain dense membrane-bound secretory granules (G). Parallel stacks of RER (curved arrows) and prominent Golgi complexes (straight arrows) can be seen in some cells. Although closely apposed, the cells have few specialized intercellular junctions. (× 10 600)

**Inset:** These cytoplasmic granules have the typical features of membrane-bound dense-core neurosecretory granules. In some, a thin lucent halo between the core and the unit membrane can be delineated (arrowhead). The average diameter of the granules is 230 nm. (× 32 700)

References: 487, 662, 1622, 1640

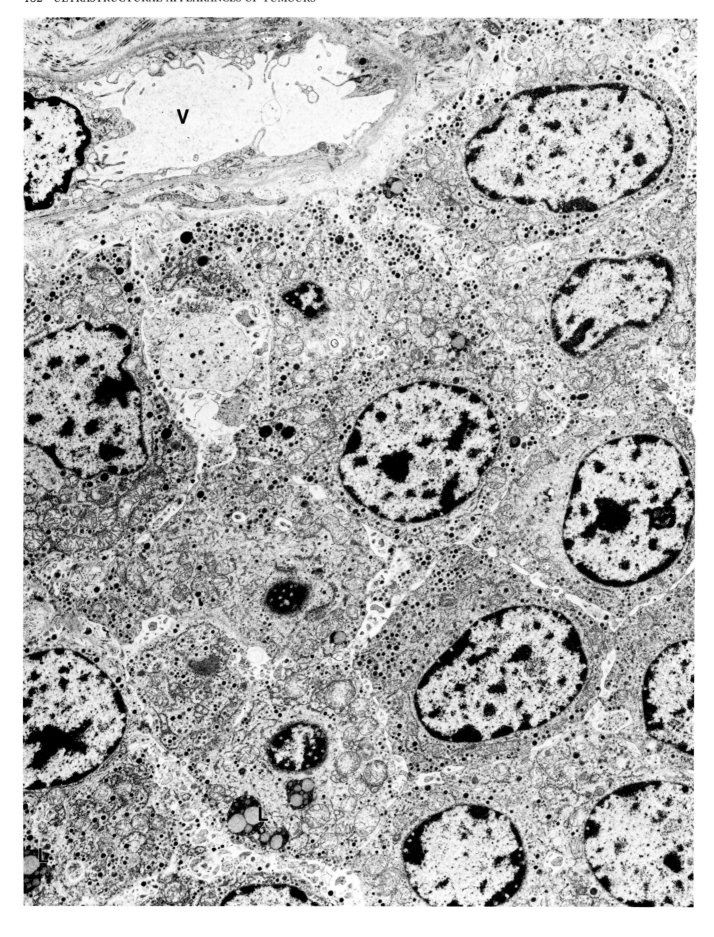

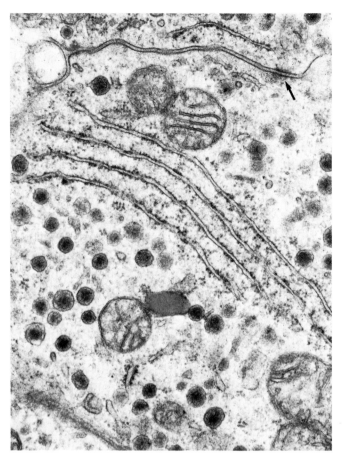

**Fig. 16.4  Bronchial carcinoid tumour: Neurosecretory granules and RER**

Central bronchial tumour from a 52-year-old man. These rounded neurosecretory granules average 180 nm in diameter, with a range of 125–225 nm. The haloes between the cores and the limiting membranes are poorly developed. Sporadic filamentous granules and large rounded granules exceeding 400 nm in diameter were also found in this case. The parallel strands of RER are a common feature of endocrine neoplasms. An intercellular junction (arrow) is also evident. (× 29 200)

**Discussion:** Subtypes of bronchial carcinoid tumours have been proposed,[460] based on granule size and morphology. Tumours with small dark granules averaging 150 nm in diameter are said to resemble pulmonary P cells (normal adult bronchial endocrine cells). On the other hand, larger more lucent granules with diameters averaging 470 nm are claimed to be similar to type 3 cells (normal fetal bronchial endocrine cells). Tumours with polymorphic, targetoid and extremely large granules (up to 1000 nm) have also been recorded.[540]

References: 455, 456, 460, 467, 471, 540, 565

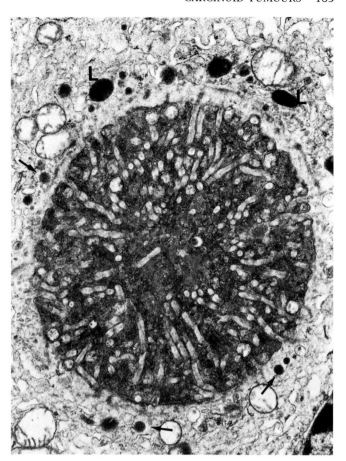

**Fig. 16.5  Atypical carcinoid tumour: Intracytoplasmic crypt**

Tumour of right lower lobar bronchus in a 24-year-old man; metastases were found in the superior bronchial lymph nodes. The crypt contains electron-dense material and is lined by microvilli. A few round neurosecretory granules (arrows) and larger, more pleomorphic lysosomes (L) are present in the surrounding cytoplasm. (× 18 000)

'Atypical' carcinoid tumours are so designated on the basis of cytological atypia by LM.

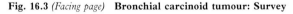

**Fig. 16.3** *(Facing page)*  **Bronchial carcinoid tumour: Survey**

Tumour of right lower lobar bronchus in a 30-year-old woman. The cells have relatively uniform ovoid nuclei with marginated heterochromatin, and they contain numerous cytoplasmic neurosecretory granules averaging 170 nm in diameter (Tables 16.1 and 16.3). Scattered lipofuscin bodies (L) can also be seen. Intercellular junctions are few. A stromal blood vessel (V) is evident. (× 7000)

References: 436, 438, 446, 448, 458, 460, 462, 473, 483, 484, 486, 487, 489–491, 495, 503, 516, 519, 533, 536, 540, 541, 543, 547, 566, 589

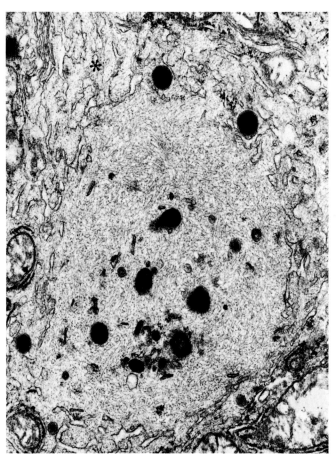

## Fig. 16.6   Carcinoid tumour: Filamentous body

A collection of intermediate cytoplasmic filaments averaging 10 nm in diameter is seen in this bronchial carcinoid tumour, together with neurosecretory granules and smooth endoplasmic reticulum (*). These appearances may reflect dysfunctional intracellular granule transport. (× 24 900)

See Table 2.9.

References: 436, 439, 489, 819, 2666

## Fig. 16.7   Atypical peripheral carcinoid tumour of lung: Acinar differentiation

Subpleural tumour of right middle lobe in a 70-year-old man. The cells lining the acinar space (A) have poorly developed microvilli and are joined by subluminal junctional complexes. Scattered desmosomes are present (arrowheads). The neurosecretory granules tend to be concentrated abluminally (arrows). (× 5400)

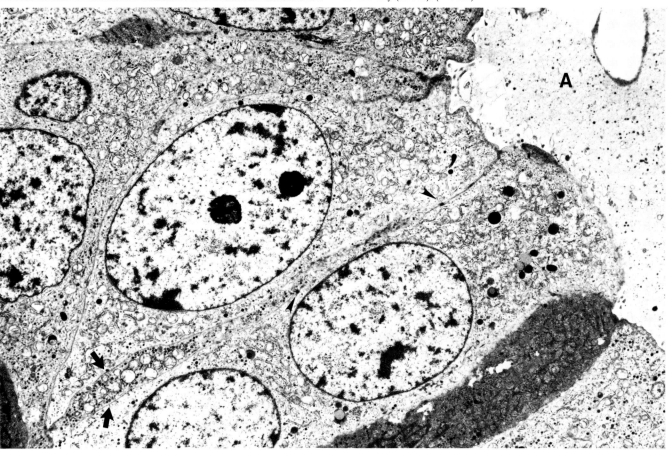

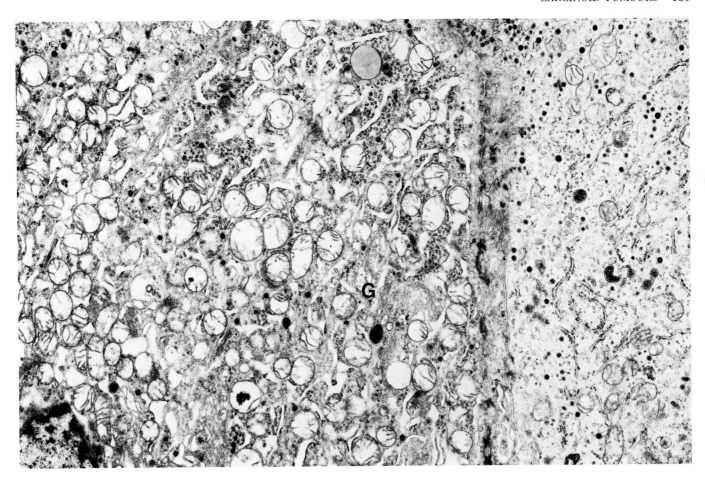

**Fig. 16.8    Peripheral pulmonary carcinoid tumour: Mitochondrial hyperplasia**

Portions of two adjoining tumour cells are illustrated; that on the left shows considerable mitochondrial hyperplasia and hypertrophy, corresponding to an oncocytic appearance on light microscopy. The mitochondria have generally clear matrices, with few densities. The Golgi complex (G) and RER can be seen, but most of the cytoplasm is occupied by the mitochondrial accumulation, and there are correspondingly few neurosecretory granules (NSG). In contrast, mitochondria are much less prominent in the cell on the right, and NSG are more frequent. (× 12 600)

Oncocytic carcinoid tumours consisting predominantly or entirely of oncocytic cells are partly distinguished from oxyphilic bronchial gland adenomas by the presence of NSG in the former. Oncocytic cells are also described in atypical and melanotic bronchopulmonary carcinoid tumours.

See Tables 2.1 and 16.3.

References: 437, 451, 452, 480, 490, 569, 571, 572, 579, 593

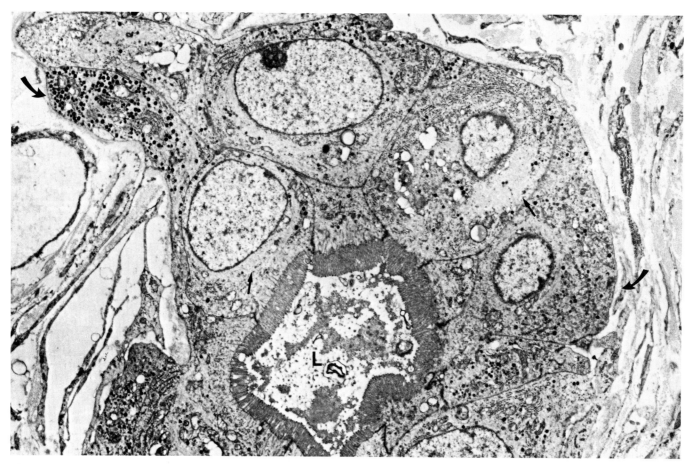

**Fig. 16.9  Appendiceal carcinoid tumour: Architecture with acinus formation**

This neoplasm consists of nodules of tightly adherent cells occasionally surrounding a luminal space (L), into which microvilli protrude. Paranuclear aggregates of filamentous material (straight arrows) and abluminal granules (curved arrows) characterize the cytoplasm. Desmosomes are present between adjoining cells and there is a basal lamina around the aggregate. (× 4300)

References: 659, 662, 664, 789, 791, 795, 826, 829–834, 850, 857, 1622, 1632

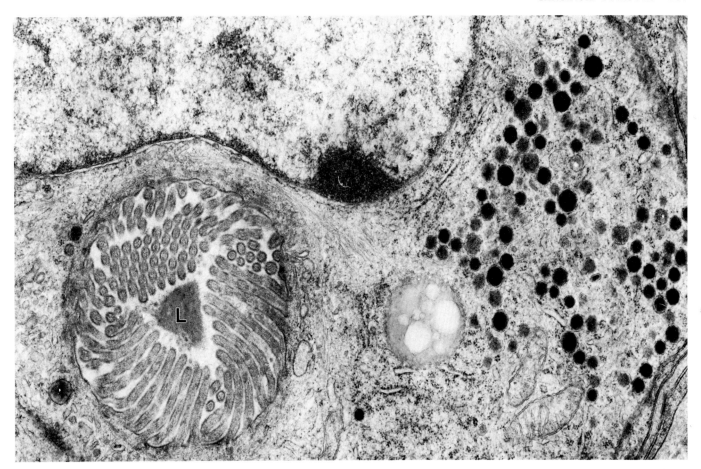

**Fig. 16.10 Appendiceal carcinoid tumour: Cell morphology**

A prominent collection of typical enterochromaffin granules is seen in the basal region of the cell. In addition to a lipid globule and small bundles of paranuclear filaments, there is a neolumen (L) lined by microvilli. In some carcinoid tumours, goblet cells are admixed with the enterochromaffin cells. The mucin in such cells appears as large and small vacuoles, or osmiophilic granules. Both mucin and neurosecretory granules have been found within the same cells by light- and electron-microscopy in a proportion of gastrointestinal and other carcinoid tumours, casting doubt on the possible neuroectodermal derivation of enterochromaffin cells (see Introduction and Chapter 7). (× 27 100)

# 17 Central neural tumours

## GLIAL AND NEURITIC TUMOURS

The morphological spectrum of central neural neoplasms has been greatly elucidated since the advent of electron microscopy and immunocytochemistry. Generally, cells showing either glial or neuritic differentiation are characterized in part by cytoplasmic processes. Cytoplasmic intermediate filaments are more profuse in glial cells (Figs. 17.5 and 17.8), whereas microtubules are a major feature of neuritic cells (see Figs. 13.8 and 17.2–17.4). However, microtubules also occupy the processes of immature astrocytes and small numbers are found occasionally in poorly differentiated astrocytomas; they may also occur in low-grade fibrillary astrocytomas. Intercellular junctions, primitive synaptic contacts, and in some instances recognizable synapses (Fig. 17.2), also characterize tumours of neuritic cells. In addition, specific structures such as dense-core granules are seen occasionally, strongly indicating neuritic differentiation and being typical of neuroblastoma (Fig. 13.7). Depending on the tumour type, the cells comprising neuritic tumours exhibit differing degrees of maturity; highly differentiated neuronal-ganglionic cells are seen in ganglioneuroma (Figs. 17.1 and 17.2), while the cell population in neuroblastoma and medulloblastoma consists of primitive neurites (see Figs. 13.7, 13.8, 17.3 and 17.4).

In *astrocytomas*, filaments are most abundant in low-grade fibrillary and pilocytic tumours, but may be few or absent in the blunt cytoplasmic processes found in protoplasmic astrocytoma;[2000] they are usually depleted in high-grade astrocytomas such as glioblastoma multiforme. Two types of intermediate filament have been identified in glial cells, including fetal and neoplastic astrocytes:

1. Vimentin.
2. Glial fibrillary acidic protein (GFAP), which represents a consistent and useful antigenic marker for astrocytes and ependymal cells.

Accordingly, GFAP can usually be demonstrated in astrocytomas, glioblastoma multiforme, ependymoma, subependymoma and in the astrocytic component of mixed gliomas. Conversely, neuronal cells, oligodendroglioma, most choroid plexus papillomas, meningiomas, and mesenchymal cells yield a negative reaction. For more detail, the recent review by Rubinstein[1997] on this subject is recommended.

Irregular electron-dense cytoplasmic conglomerates may also be seen in proliferative astrocytoses, corresponding to the presence of Rosenthal fibres by LM. They occur in cells with numerous filaments (Fig. 17.8), with which they appear to be continuous, and they are most often encountered in low-grade astrocytomas and reactive astrocytoses; in our opinion EM is useless in distinguishing between such reactive and neoplastic proliferations. The astrocytic cells in ganglioglioma have also been recorded to contain filaments 6.5–11.5 nm in diameter, and Rosenthal fibres.[1998]

Cystic degeneration in fibrillary astrocytomas is sometimes accompanied by the development of cytoplasmic hyaline droplets, which appear to represent autophagic vacuoles and cytosegrosomes.[2000] In gemistocytic astrocytomas the cytoplasm of the neoplastic astrocytes is populated with numerous glial filaments, autophagic vacuoles, mitochondria, polyribosomes and stacks of RER.[2000] Ultrastructural studies have also confirmed the astrocytic character of the monstrocellular glioblastoma.[1969] The nature of the subependymal giant cell astrocytoma classically associated with tuberous sclerosis is less certain. GFAP is detectable in some cases but others yield negative results, and a positive reaction for a neurone-specific protein is reported, raising the possibility of ganglionic differentiation. This problem has yet to be clarified, but Rubinstein[1997] suggests that subependymal giant cell astrocytoma may not be a uniform entity.

With the exceptions of ependymal and choroid plexus neoplasms, intercellular junctions in gliomas are rare. If present, they are poorly developed and may resemble those in the subpial astrocytic layer; astrocytes in this region may also have a distinct external lamina.

*Ependymomas* often contain cells which form distinct lumina with tight junctions between adjacent cells.[1991,2020] Microvilli and less commonly cilia protrude into the luminal region (Fig. 17.10), while a poorly formed basal lamina is sometimes evident; less differentiated glial cells may also be present, but their proportions vary from case to case. Similar ependymal features (including microvilli, desmosomes, basal lamina and cytofilaments) characterize myxopapillary ependymomas, although cilia are less frequent than in normal ependyma.[2007] The ultrastructural appearances of *choroid plexus papillomas* also have similarities to ependymal cells, the tumour cells being characterized by numerous apical microvilli but fewer cilia.[1982] Subluminal junctional complexes are also present, while the basal plasmalemma and its associated external lamina may form a highly elaborate infolded pattern.[1982] Haemosiderin-containing lysosomes and electron-dense apoptotic cells with elongated cytoplasmic processes are also recorded.[1982] The endothelium lining the stromal blood vessels is usually fenestrated in type.[1932]

In contrast, *oligodendrogliomas*[1933] are characterized by elaborate infolding of plasma membranes (Fig. 17.11), often producing concentric mesaxon-like structures analogous to the appearances seen with Schwannian differentiation, and autophagosomes are occasionally prominent (see Table 18.2).[2133] Finally, EM has demonstrated that the entity previously called *'microgliomatosis'* represents a malignant lymphoma (Figs. 17.12 and 17.13).

## MENINGIOMAS

The ultrastructure of these neoplasms reflects the architecture of the cells forming the pia and dura mater. The majority display a meningotheliomatous appearance, while a few have distinct fibroblastoid characteristics. Meningotheliomatous meningiomas consist of cells with elaborate cytoplasmic extensions (Figs. 17.14 and 17.15). The length, complexity, and degree of interdigitation of these varies, but distinct desmosomes occur between closely apposed plasma membranes. The density of cytoplasmic vimentin filaments is also variable, and is less prominent in so-called transitional meningiomas which also have relatively short blunt cell processes, with lesser interdigitation than the meningotheliomatous variety. Meningiomas with 'hyaline' inclusions (*'pseudopsammomatous' meningiomas*) have secretory features, as indicated by intracytoplasmic neolumina, lined with microvilli and possessing a distinct glycocalyx (Figs. 17.18 and 17.19).

The status of *angioblastic meningioma* has elicited considerable controversy among neuropathologists and electron microscopists, some believing it to represent a meningeal haemangiopericytoma.[2046] This view is based in part on the considerable ultrastructural differences from conventional meningotheliomatous meningioma; these include less elaborate intertwining of processes, smooth muscle-like features and foci of external laminal material in the extracellular compartment. Nevertheless, the cells in at least some cases differ from pericytes in that well defined desmosomes are present, while a pericellular external lamina is absent (Fig. 17.20). For these reasons we consider that a meningothelial form of 'angioblastic' meningioma is a recognizable entity by EM. It is likely that the category of angioblastic meningioma as defined by LM is non-uniform, and includes richly vascularized meningothelial meningiomas (Fig. 17.20), leptomeningeal haemangioblastomas (see Fig. 23.10), and meningeal haemangiopericytomas (see Figs. 23.8 and 23.9); in addition, transitions between haemangiopericytomas and 'conventional' types of meningioma are described.[2034] This topic is discussed in detail by Kepes[2034] and Rubinstein.[1997]

An inflammatory variant of meningioma is also recorded;[2040] this resembles a plasma cell granuloma by LM, but EM demonstrates varying proportions of meningothelial and inflammatory cells.

Focal deposits of external laminal material are sometimes seen in meningiomas, while spicules of calcium salts may occur on the surface of some cells or within others. Similarly, calcific material may also be present in the stroma of these neoplasms,[2042] where long-spacing collagen may also be found (see Table 3.4). Fenestrated endothelium sometimes lines the vasculature of meningiomas and there may be wide interendothelial spaces and numerous micropinocytotic vesicles, accounting for the lack of a blood-tumour barrier.

**Fig. 17.1** *(Facing page — top)* **Ganglioneuroma: Cell morphology**

This large cell closely resembles a mature ganglion cell. The nucleus (N) is slightly irregular and contains much euchromatin. Strands of RER and ribosomal rosettes are plentiful, and back-to-back lamellae can be discerned (arrows). Many mitochondria are evident, and the Golgi complex is well developed. Microtubules (arrowheads) and dense bodies are also present. Small dense-core vesicles are usually uncommon. (× 18 000)
References: 1960, 1998, 2025

**Fig. 17.2** *(Facing page — bottom)* **Ganglioneuroma: Synaptic junction**

Synaptic contacts (arrows) are usually rare in ganglioneuroma, but can be seen on the surface of the perikaryons of a few neoplastic cells or on their dendritic processes. Most nerve fibres in these tumours are unmyelinated. Satellite cells and Schwann cells may be found, while interstitial elements are typically abundant. Prominent microtubules (arrowheads) can also be seen in this field. (× 38 000)

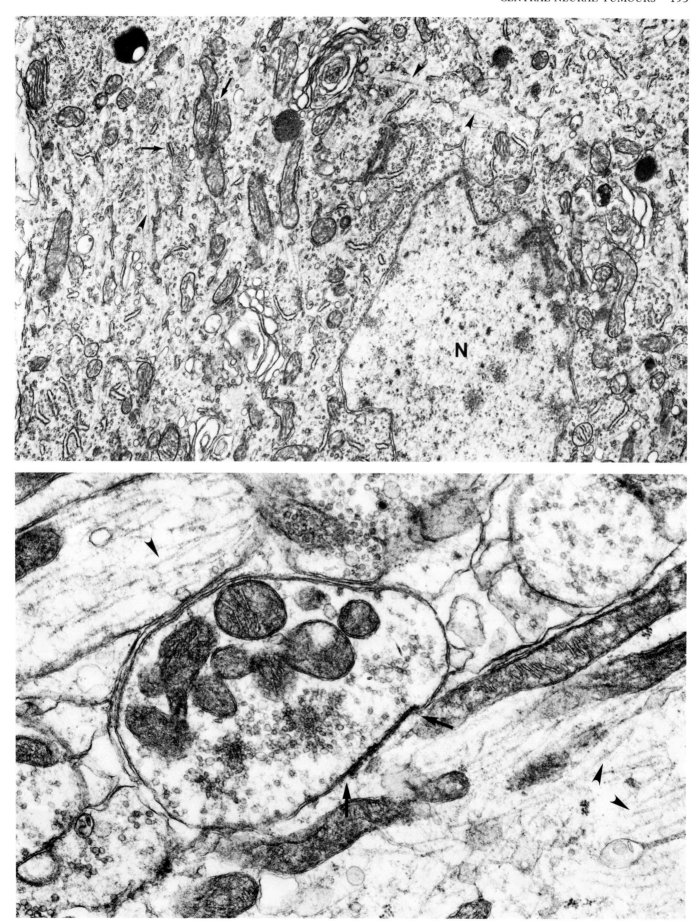

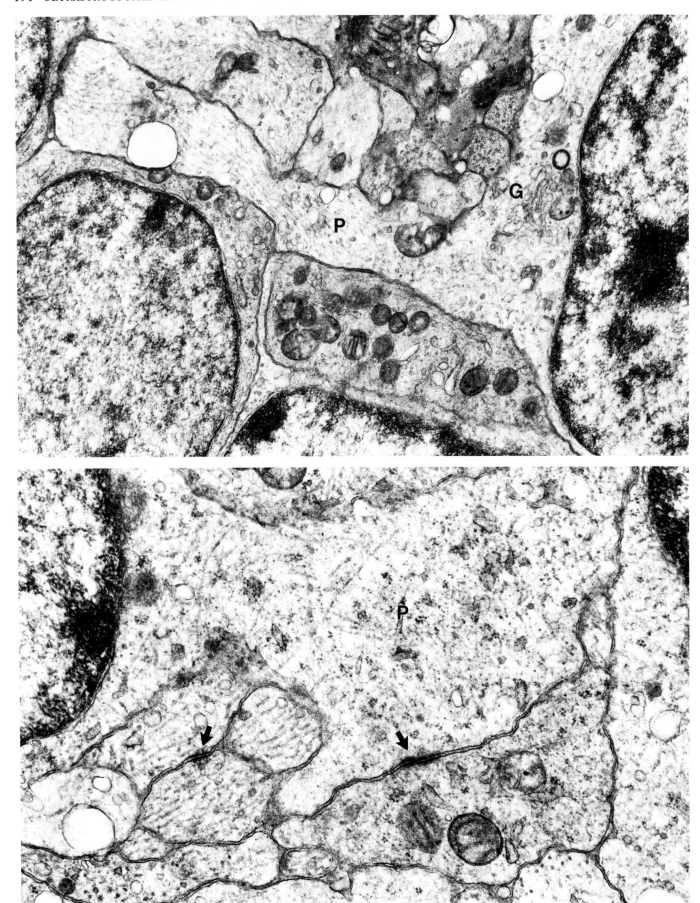

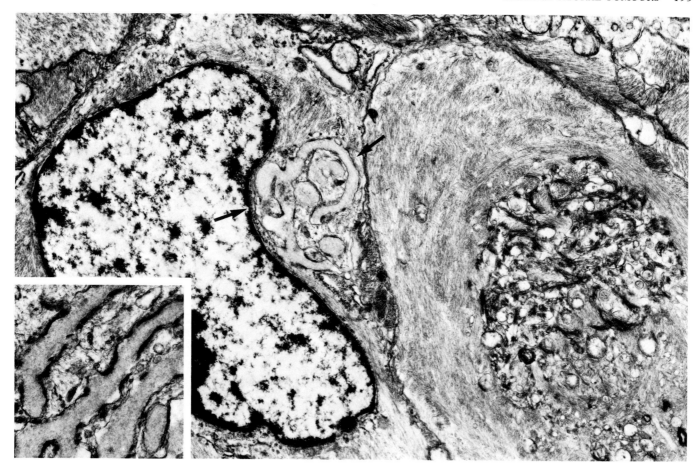

**Fig. 17.5 Cerebral astrocytoma: Cell topography, external lamina and glial filaments**

The main bodies of two neoplastic cells as well as several intertwining cytoplasmic processes can be seen. Cytoplasmic filaments are characteristic of these cells, occurring in both the perikaryon and in the cytoplasmic projections. Organelles are few, and the nucleus is slightly irregular. A thick external lamina (arrows) was seen on the surface of some of the neoplastic cells; it is emphasized that the presence of such laminal material in astrocytomas is highly unusual. (× 12 600)

**Inset:** There are hemidesmosomes between the neoplastic cells and the external lamina; the cells of such astrocytomas resemble those of the subpial astrocytic layer. (× 18 700)

References: 1928, 1929, 1935, 1938, 1940, 1941, 1954, 1974, 1991, 1997, 2000, 2001, 2008, 2010

**Fig. 17.3** *(Facing page — top)*  **Cerebellar medulloblastoma: Primitive dendritic processes and organelles**

The nuclear:cytoplasmic ratio of these neoplasms is high, but the cytoplasm is not always confined to a perinuclear rim, and may form short, blunt processes (P) which interdigitate with other cell bodies and processes. Microtubules are plentiful in both perikaryons and processes, and mitochondria are occasionally more numerous in the blunt processes. Small Golgi complexes (G) can sometimes be seen. Neurofilaments may also be plentiful, and in some spongy variants of medulloblastoma, the smooth endoplasmic reticulum is not only well developed, but is also dilated. Melanosomes have been described in pigmented tumours (melanotic medulloblastoma; see Table 8.1). Astrocytic differentiation is also seen in some medulloblastomas. (×20 600)

**Discussion:** Small poorly differentiated neurites similar to those seen in medulloblastoma, and including the presence of microtubules, have been described in pineoblastoma and pineocytoma; in one study the latter also contained larger neuronal cells with neurosecretory granules 50–120 nm in diameter. Astrocytic elements were also present in both of these tumour types.[1918]

References: 1925, 1931, 1968, 1979, 1986, 1999

**Fig. 17.4** *(Facing page — bottom)*  **Cerebellar medulloblastoma: Cell contacts and neurotubules**

Portion of the cell body of a neoplastic cell and an expanded cytoplasmic process (P) are shown in close juxtaposition with adjacent processes of varying size. Observe the many microtubules, especially in the cytoplasmic extensions — whereas major cytoplasmic organelles usually tend to be concentrated in the paranuclear region. Small intermediate junctions (arrows), consistent with primitive synaptic contacts, are seen between apposed processes, but true synapses are not present. (× 35 000)

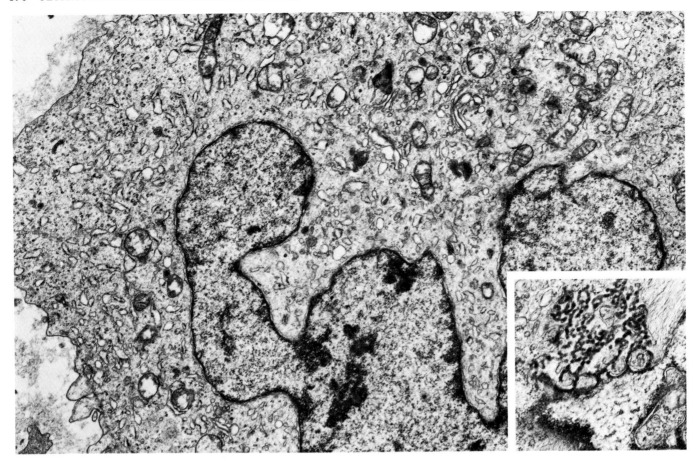

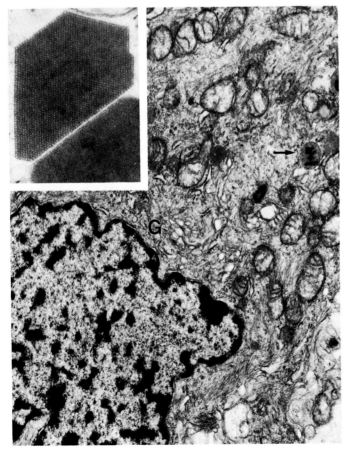

## Fig. 17.6 Cerebral glioblastoma multiforme: Cell morphology and heterochromatin bands

The cells of this neoplasm are irregular and have small surface projections. Surface membrane microprojections as well as coated vesicles are more frequently seen in these neoplasms than in low-grade astrocytomas. The nucleus is irregular and eccentric, and contains much euchromatin. Cytoplasmic organelles are prominent, but filaments are few. (× 12 700)

**Inset:** A web of thread-like heterochromatin strands projects from the nuclear periphery. (× 24 000)

References: 1938, 1941, 1949, 1954, 1956, 1964, 1969, 1972, 1991, 2013

## Fig. 17.7 Cerebral glioblastoma multiforme: Filaments and crystalloids

Sometimes cells in this neoplasm possess distinct cytoplasmic processes and contain large aggregates of cytoplasmic filaments both in the main cell body and in the projections. Detail of a cell body and the proximal portion of a broad process is shown here. In addition, observe the moderately well developed Golgi apparatus (G) and a crystalloid-containing dense body (arrow). (× 12 900)

**Inset:** Crystalline inclusions in a cell from a glioblastoma multiforme; these may represent abnormal peroxisomes. (× 39 700)

References: 1964, 2004

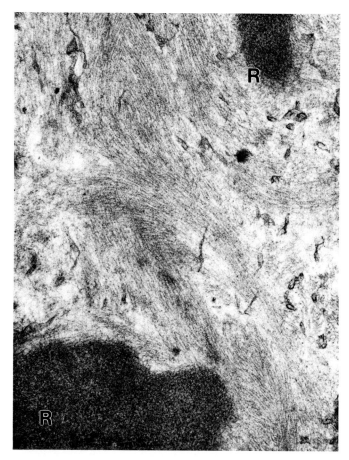

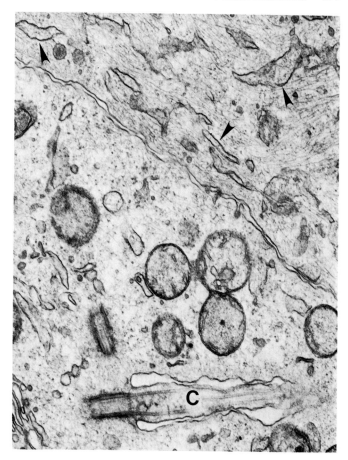

**Fig. 17.8   Glioblastoma multiforme: Glial filaments and Rosenthal fibres**

Highly anaplastic malignant astrocytoma of the cervical spinal cord of a 13-year-old girl with von Recklinghausen's neurofibromatosis. The astrocyte cytoplasm contains numerous glial filaments, approximately 10 nm in diameter, which merge with denser granular bodies (R) conforming to Rosenthal fibres. (× 36 400)

References: 1956, 1991, 1997, 1998, 2000

**Fig. 17.9   Cerebral glioblastoma multiforme: Cytoplasmic detail**

In this electron micrograph the cytoplasm of the neoplastic cells possesses only a few filaments. The smooth endoplasmic reticulum appears to be proliferated (arrowheads). In addition, a cilium (C) is present in one cell. Gap junctions can be demonstrated occasionally by freeze-fracture techniques. (× 31 300)

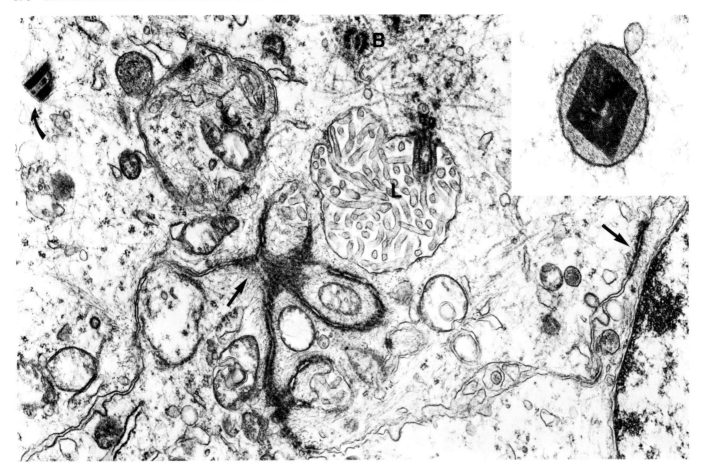

## Fig. 17.10 Cerebral ependymoma: Cell fine structure and crystalloid

This tumour is characterized by the formation of various junctions (straight arrows), including junctional complexes, between adjoining cells — as well as the production of lumina (L) into which cilia, and more frequently microvilli, project. Tight junctions have been demonstrated between such cells. Cytoplasmic filaments and microtubules are seen, together with a basal body (B). **Inset:** A secretory granule with a crystalline core is present (se also curved arrow). The nature of this granule is obscure. (×16 800. Inset: ×33 300)

References: 1967, 1991, 1993, 1998, 2007, 2020

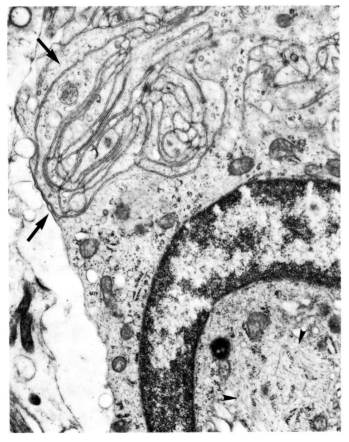

## Fig. 17.11 Glioma: Oligodendrocytic differentiation

The nucleus of the cell is invaginated by a portion of cytoplasm rich in microtubules (arrowheads). The peripheral cytoplasm is dissected by plasmalemmal inversions in the fashion of a mesaxon (arrows). In brain tumours such folded cytoplasmic processes are thought to be specific for oligodendrocytic differentiation. Mitochondria are usually numerous, and may be elongated and atypical. Cytoplasmic crystalline bodies may also be found. (× 20 000)

References: 1927, 1933, 1944, 1991, 2000, 2009, 2012, 2133

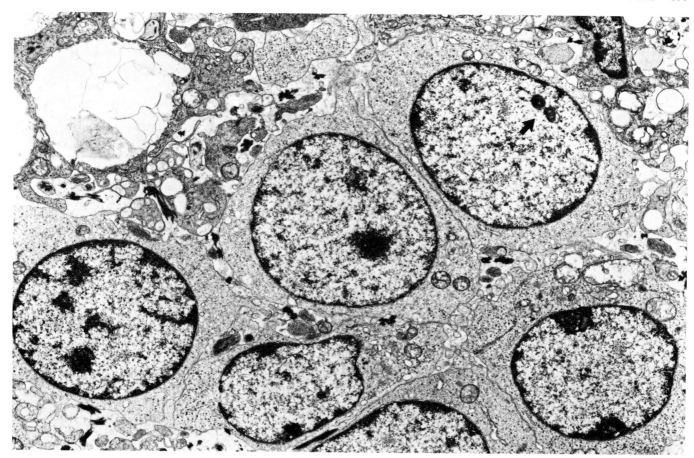

**Fig. 17.12 Cerebral 'microgliomatosis': Lymphocytoid cell population**

The neoplastic cells have a lymphocytoid appearance. Although cell contours are slightly irregular, the nuclei are rounded and have moderate amounts of euchromatin. Nucleoli, and nuclear bodies (arrow) are also evident. Apart from ribosomal rosettes, only a few organelles are present. (× 4700)

References: 216, 217, 1936, 1953, 1955, 1957–1959, 1989, 1991, 2016

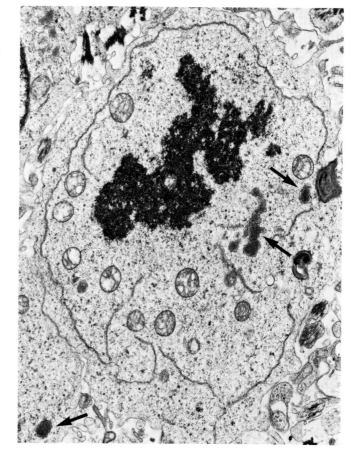

**Fig. 17.13 Cerebral 'microgliomatosis': Metaphase mitosis**

A cell in metaphase displays markedly elongated strands of RER. In addition, osmiophilic material has accumulated in dilated segments of the endoplasmic reticulum (arrows). Note the absence of filaments, tubules and intercellular junctions. (× 9500)

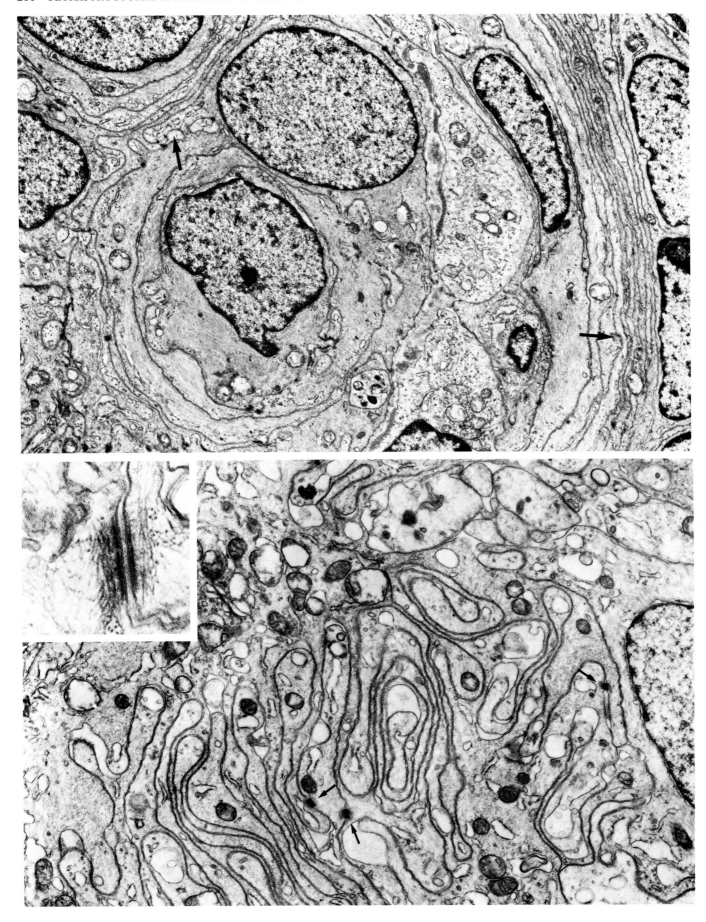

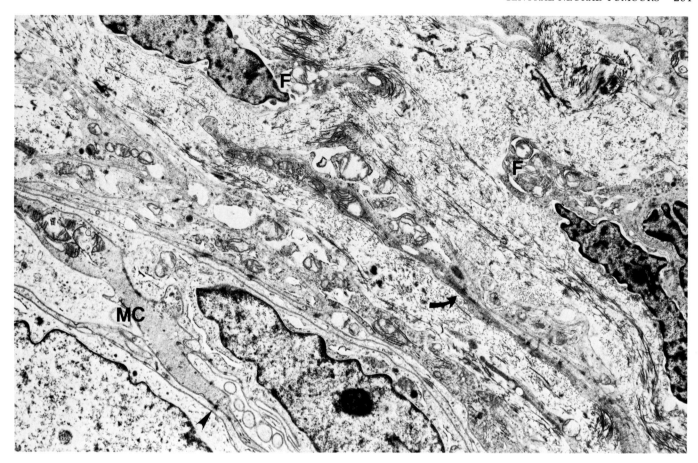

**Fig. 17.16 Meningioma: Transition from meningothelial to fibrous tissue**

In this micrograph there is a transition from the meningothelial cells (MC) with interlocking processes and desmosomal junctions (arrowhead) to a fibrous area where numerous collagen fibres occupy the extracellular matrix, with separation of individual fibroblastoid cells (F). A collection of elongated meningothelial processes (curved arrow) is still evident in the collagenous focus. The meningothelial cells in this field possess few cytofilaments. (× 9000)

**Fig. 17.14** *(Facing page — top)* **Meningotheliomatous meningioma: Cell morphology and processes**

In this variety of meningioma many cells are large and rounded, each containing a spherical nucleus with much euchromatin. In addition to the plump rounded cells, others are polygonal; still others are flattened or spindle-shaped, and have interdigitating or layered processes (arrows) as illustrated in this micrograph. Desmosomes occur between adjoining cells or their processes; gap junctions, tight junctions, and hemidesmosomes have also been reported. Intermediate (vimentin) filaments occupy most of the cytoplasm in all of these cell types, and a peculiar submembranous ribosomal-filamentous complex has been described; so too have osmiophilic granulofilamentous inclusions, associated with intermediate filaments and possibly representing the dense components of desmosomes.[2031] (× 7200)

References: 466, 517, 2027–2035, 2038–2042, 2044, 2045, 2047–2051

**Fig. 17.15** *(Facing page — bottom)* **Meningotheliomatous meningioma: Cell processes and desmosomes**

This electron micrograph depicts the interdigitating patterns of the processes of the neoplastic cells. Observe the desmosomes (arrows) between closely apposed membranes of interlocking cell processes. **Inset:** Detail of a desmosomal junction between adjacent processes. (× 9100. Inset: × 80 300)

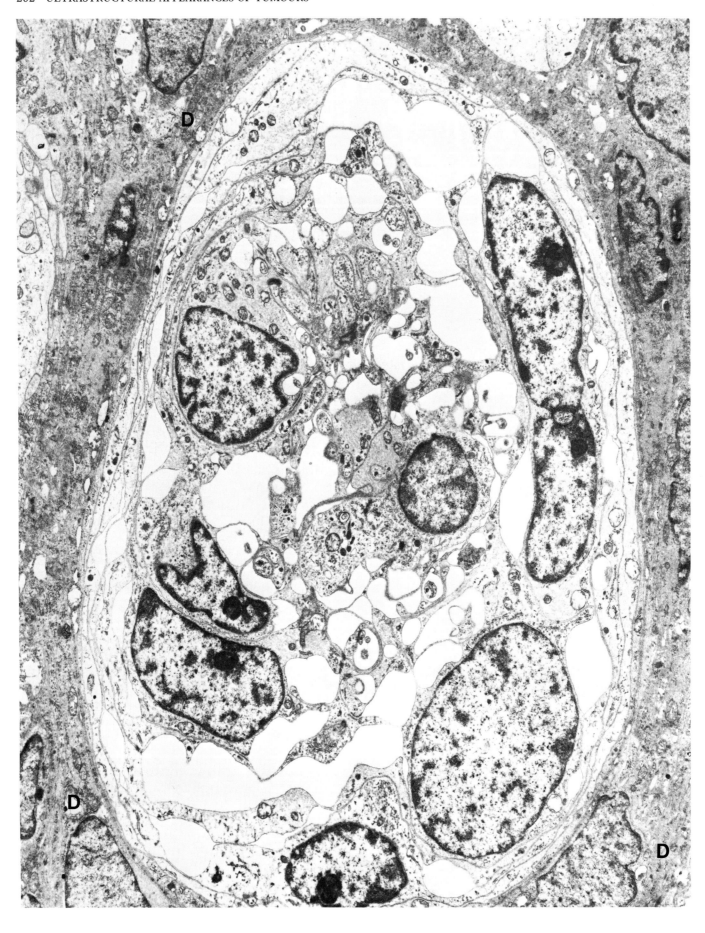

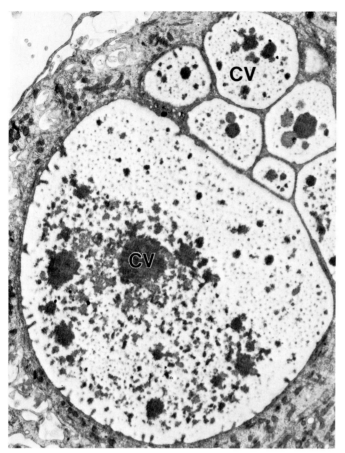

**Fig. 17.18  Pseudopsammomatous meningioma: Survey**

This neoplastic cell possesses large cytoplasmic vacuoles (CV) which contain flocculent electron-dense material. In addition, short, blunt microvilli project into the lumina. (× 5900)

**Discussion:** Intracytoplasmic crypts (neolumina), lined by microvilli with filamentous cores and a coating of glycocalyceal material have rarely been described in meningiomas.[2035] Enlargement and/or fusion of the crypts with an intraluminal accumulation of finely granular or lamellar material corresponds to the presence of hyaline inclusions (pseudopsammoma bodies) on LM. Budka[2027] has demonstrated immunoreactive IgM, IgA and secretory component within the inclusions, while a glycolipid component has also been detected.[2034] Distinct pericytic cells may also occur in this form of meningioma.[2039]

References: 2027, 2033, 2034, 2035, 2039

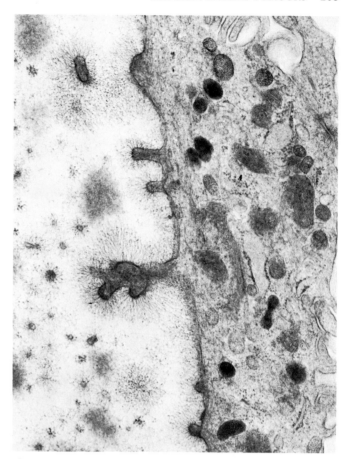

**Fig. 17.19  Pseudopsammomatous meningioma: Detail of vacuole**

The microvilli projecting into the cytoplasmic vacuoles are covered by fine antenullae. (× 32 600)

**Fig. 17.17** *(Facing page)*  **Meningioma: Meningothelial whorl and cell processes**

Within the pale, whorled collection of meningothelial cells there are numerous elongated cell processes, forming a complicated interdigitating pattern. Adjacent plasma membranes often show close apposition, with scattered desmosomes, but elsewhere there are wide cistern-like intercellular spaces, forming an 'open' pattern. The whorl is surrounded by electron-dense cells (D) and their processes. The appearances resemble normal arachnoidal fine structure. (× 7200)

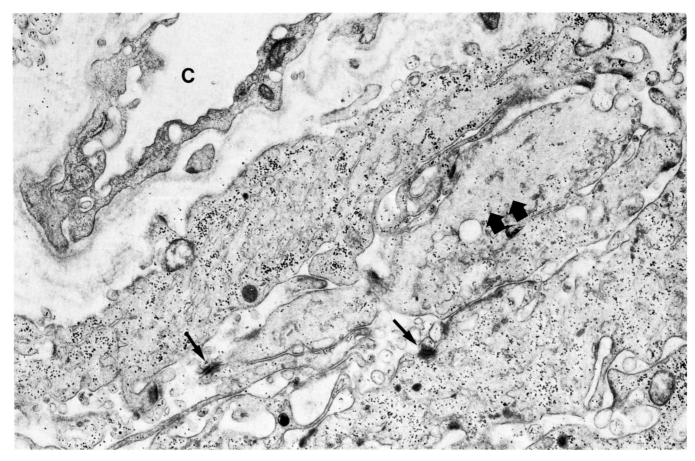

**Fig. 17.20  'Angioblastic' meningioma: Perivascular region**

The processes of the meningotheliomatous cells are closely packed around a capillary (C). Unlike pericytes they display desmosomes (arrows) between adjacent processes, and lack a circumferential external lamina. Intermediate filaments (bold arrows) and monogranular glycogen are present in the cytoplasm. (× 21 300)

References: 1997, 2034

**Fig. 17.21** *(Facing page)*  **Meningioma: Calcification**

**A:** There are spicules of electron-dense material on the surfaces of two adjoining cells; this is probably the earliest evidence of calcification. (× 19 800)

**B:** In other regions the surface layer of electron-dense material is extensive, and in addition spicules are present in both the nucleus and cytoplasm of some of the encased cells. Such cells maintain only faint outlines of the nuclear and cytoplasmic components. (× 7200)

**C:** Calcification in this portion of the neoplasm is much more pronounced, and the encased cells are barely discernible. (× 5400)

**D:** Here calcification is advanced, and electron-dense spicules surround the collagen fibres of the interstitium. (× 18 000)

References: 2034, 2042

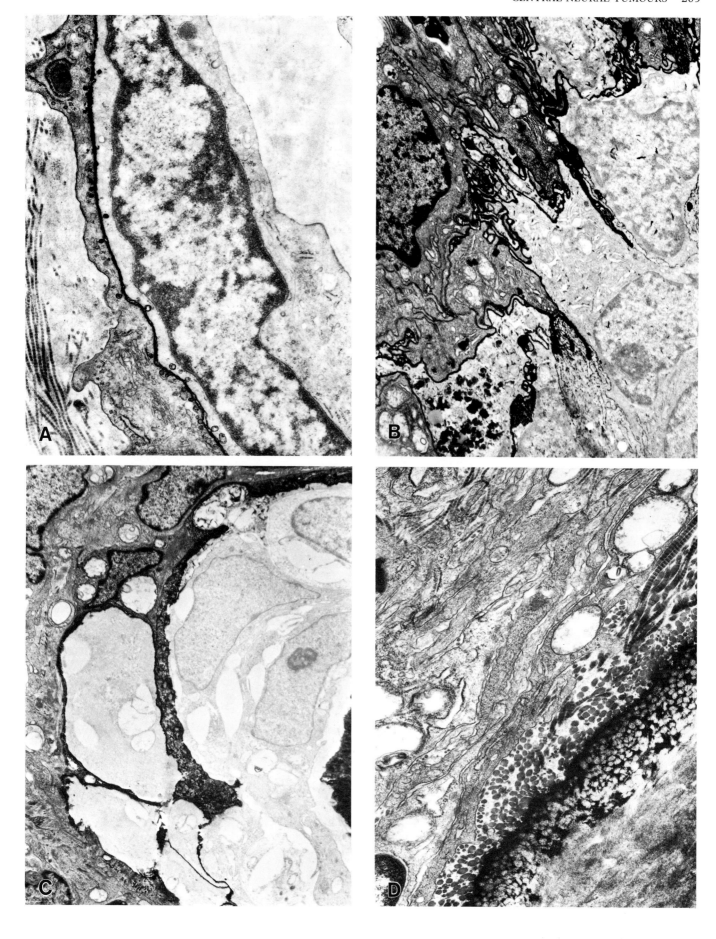

# 18 Peripheral neural tumours

## GENERAL REMARKS AND BENIGN NERVE SHEATH CELL TUMOURS: SCHWANNOMA, PERINEURIOMA AND NEUROFIBROMA

Although tumours of peripheral nerves may consist of an admixture of cells resembling Schwann cells, fibroblasts or perineurial cells, one type tends to predominate. EM may be the only definitive means of morphologically typing the predominant cell, and has led to the identification of perineurial cells in some tumours histologically resembling neurofibromas.[2061] The comparative ultrastructure of peripheral nerve tumours is considered in Table 18.1.

In *Schwannomas* the component cells have a distinct external lamina which is typically continuous and multilayered (Fig. 18.2). There are also cytoplasmic extensions of varying complexity, as well as infoldings of the plasmalemma, the latter presumably representing a mimicry of mesaxon formation. Cell junctions are rare and the π bodies of Reich[2110] are similarly infrequent. Melanosomes in all stages of evolution can be found within the Schwann cell cytoplasm in melanotic Schwannomas, indicating melanin synthesis by these cells and not simply passive transfer from other cells (see Table 8.1 and Fig. 18.5).

Glandular elements are rarely present in Schwannian neoplasms. Ultrastructural study of the glandular component of one such case[2103] revealed non-ciliated columnar and cuboidal epithelial cells which were characterized by surface microvilli with an associated glycocalyx, subluminal junctional complexes and a basal lamina. Penetrating microvillous core rootlets and apical cytoplasmic bodies thought to resemble R bodies were also present, suggesting intestinal epithelial differentiation. The spindle cell component was malignant by LM, and EM demonstrated Schwannian properties. The presence of neuroendocrine cells containing immunoreactive somatostatin has been described in the glandular component of another case.[2105]

A cellular variant of Schwannoma liable to be misinterpreted as a malignant tumour has recently been emphasized;[2112] this variant is characterized by hypercellularity, a storiform pattern, a low mitotic index (≤6 mitoses/40 high power fields), and, occasionally, moderate nuclear pleomorphism. Follow-up studies suggested a benign clinical course. The differential LM diagnosis included fibrous histiocytoma, leiomyoma, malignant nerve sheath cell tumour and unclassifiable sarcoma. EM revealed typical features of Schwannian differentiation, and Luse bodies were found in 2 of 14 cases.[2112]

In *perineurial tumours* the component cells have processes which often contain micropinocytotic vesicles, but the external lamina is fragmentary and concentrated along one side of the cells (Fig. 18.7). Infolding of the plasmalemma is infrequent, but intermediate junctions are easily seen. In addition, collagen bundles are readily found in the stroma. The controversy surrounding the identity of the perineurial cells is discussed in Table 18.1.

In *neurofibromas* the predominant cells usually resemble fibroblasts, lacking a distinct external lamina, junctional contacts, or infoldings of the cell membrane.[2065,2081,2110] Perineurial cells and intermediate perineurial-fibroblastoid forms are also described;[2061] the possible significance of these observations is considered in Table 18.1. Collagenous connective tissue is prominent.

'Luse' bodies,[45] consisting of fibrous long-spacing collagen (FLSC), although present in both Schwannomas and neurofibromas, are more frequently seen in the former (Fig. 18.2). In a given spindle cell neoplasm, a marked abundance of FLSC favours a *benign* nerve sheath cell tumour. Although described in malignant Schwannoma, FLSC is usually poorly developed, if detectable at all.[2101] It is also emphasized that FLSC occurs in non-neural tumours (see Table 3.4), but does not usually produce well formed Luse bodies.

## MALIGNANT SCHWANNOMA

Schwann cell morphology is depleted to varying degrees in malignant Schwannomas, but EM can nevertheless support the diagnosis by:

1. Excluding alternative diagnoses such as malignant fibrous histiocytoma[2072] and leiomyosarcoma (see Chapters 20 and 21).
2. Identifying abortive Schwannian differentiation by features such as slender overlapping cell processes, granular flocculent material parallel to the cells, and foci of external lamina (Figs. 18.6–18.8).[2057,2101]

These features are most evident in highly differentiated areas of tumours arising in continuity with a nerve trunk or in patients with von Recklinghausen's neurofibromatosis; they are less obvious in tumours lacking these features but resembling malignant Schwannoma by LM.[2101] Perineurial cells are sometimes recognizable (Fig. 18.7), while highly anaplastic nerve sheath cell tumours may consist only of undifferentiated cells devoid of processes, intercellular junctions and external laminae.

Foci of residual disarrayed Schwannian and/or perineurial cells incorporated into non-neural malignancies infiltrating

**Table 18.1  Comparative ultrastructure of benign peripheral nerve sheath tumours**

| | Schwannoma | Neurofibroma | Perineurioma |
|---|---|---|---|
| Cell shape | Bipolar in Antoni A tissue, stellate in Antoni B areas | Variable. Elongated, irregular, or rounded | Spindled and stellate |
| Cell processes | Elaborate long interleaving processes with infolding reminiscent of mesaxon formation, and enfolding of stroma with 'mesocollagen' (pseudomesaxon) formation. Cells in Antoni B areas have fewer processes than in Antoni A tissue, with less frequent interleaving; in addition, the processes tend to be more delicate and may produce a lacework pattern (Fig. 18.3) | Irregular fibroblastic extensions, elaborate Schwannian/perineurial processes, and scattered axonal processes | Long thin processes. Infoldings uncommon |
| Intercellular junctions | Inconspicuous | Inconspicuous | Frequent intermediate junctions |
| External lamina | Typically continuous, forming single or multiple layers | Present adjacent to Schwannian/ perineurial cells. May not be continuous in plane of section | External lamina is discontinuous and concentrated along one side of perineurial cells; although not present around individual cells, a continuous lamina may be seen at the periphery of cell groups |
| Micropinocytotic vesicles | Not conspicuous | Not conspicuous | Prominent |
| Rough endoplasmic reticulum | Inconspicuous | Prominent in fibroblastic cells | Inconspicuous |
| Extracellular matrix | Variable. Fibrous long-spacing collagen usually present. Abundant proteoglycan-rich matrix characterizes Antoni B tissue | Abundant, with wide separation of cells. Fibrous long-spacing collagen may be present, but is less common than in Schwannoma | Prominent collagenous matrix |
| Corresponding appearance by light microscopy | Schwannoma | Neurofibroma | Neurofibroma. Similar ultrastructural appearances have been described in Pacinian neurofibroma, and in neurofibroma with tactile corpuscle-like structures |
| Remarks | Component cells have Schwannian appearances. Rarely, melanosomes are present within the Schwann cells<br><br>See Figs. 18.1-18.5<br><br>Meningeal neoplasms occasionally enter into the differential diagnosis, but are distinguished by the presence of numerous desmosomes and cytoskeletal filaments | Neurofibromas are generally thought to contain neoplastic Schwann cells, but Erlandson & Woodruff[2061] described perineurial and fibroblastoid cells, and others intermediate between these two types. Perineurial cells proliferating in response to nerve injury may acquire fibroblastoid appearances, and the authors therefore suggested that the fibroblastoid component of neurofibromas consists of altered perineurial cells. However, modified perineurial cells usually retain their external laminae and this hypothesis has not been conclusively established. The fibroblastoid cells usually predominate<br><br>See Figs. 18.10 and 18.11 | Component cells similar to perineurial sheath cells of small cutaneous peripheral nerves<br><br>The distinction between Schwann cells and perineurial cells is controversial, and the latter are considered by some authors to represent structural-functional variants of Schwann cells, dependent on their position within the nerve sheath in normal circumstances and the pattern of differentiation in the case of tumours.[1998] Experimental malignant 'Schwannomas', for example, contain perineurial-type cells;[1998] irrespective of the histogenetic arguments, this observation tacitly accepts a recognizable pattern of perineurial cell differentiation, which may be encountered in some human nerve sheath cell tumours.[2061]<br><br>Whether neural tumours composed of perineurial cells should be accorded the separate ultrastructural status of 'perineurioma' instead of being included in the LM category of 'neurofibroma' will depend in part on individual nosological preferences. We are not in complete agreement on this issue; DWH and MC prefer to classify tumours composed of perineurial cells according to the appearances by LM, whereas JMP designates at least a proportion of these tumours as perineuriomas.<br><br>See Figs. 18.7 (malignant Schwannoma) and 18.9 ('perineurioma') |

References: 45, 109, 1996, 1998, 2032, 2034, 2061, 2065, 2072, 2084, 2107, 2108, 2110

nerve trunks are liable to be misinterpreted as evidence of neoplastic nerve sheath cell differentiation. In contrast, the diagnosis of *bona fide* malignant Schwannoma can be supported by the following procedures and observations:[1996]

1. Ensuring from semithin sections that representative areas of the neoplasm have been selected for examination.
2. Determining that nerve sheath cell properties persist throughout multiple tissue blocks.
3. Schwannian characteristics are often poorly developed in malignant Schwannomas, and Schwannian-axonal complexes are not seen. In contrast, incorporated non-neoplastic Schwann cells are highly differentiated, sometimes producing micro-organoid structures in the form of complexes with axons, which occasionally include myelin sheaths.
4. Malignant nerve sheath cell nuclei are usually atypical and pleomorphic, with irregular contours and prominent nucleoli (Fig. 18.6).

# GRANULAR CELL TUMOURS

The genesis of these neoplasms is obscure.[2131] The suggestion that they represent Schwannian tumours has been prompted by the presence of circumferential external laminae and resemblance of the angulate bodies to the inclusions sometimes seen in the cytoplasm of Schwann cells,[45,2132] while a relationship to perineurial cells has also been mooted.[2226] However, the granular inclusions are not specific by themselves and actually are nothing more than autophagosomes (Figs. 18.12 and 18.13). It is mainly their large number within individual neoplastic cells which has resulted in the delineation of this neoplasm as a morphological entity, although the basis for their massive accumulation is quite obscure.[47] However, granular cells characterized by prominent autophagosomes may be found in other circumstances, as shown in Table 18.2. Angulate bodies may represent the most distinctive feature of granular cell tumours (Figs. 18.12 and 18.13, and Table 18.2).[2131]

**Table 18.2  Granular cells characterized by autophagic vacuolar alteration in pathological tissues**

| Condition | Angulate bodies | Comments |
|---|---|---|
| Granular cell tumour (GCT) | + | Schwannian origin generally favoured, but myofilaments noted in one GCT affecting the urinary bladder.[2114] Typical granular cells and angulate body-containing cells have also been recorded in a benign dermal neurofibroma and in a metastasizing GCT from a patient with von Recklinghausen's neurofibomatosis[2064] |
| | | Compare with oncocytic neoplasms (Fig. 11.1) |
| Malignant GCT | ± | — |
| Granular cell epulis | + | Development from odontogenic epithelium has been proposed, but Lack et al[2121] described histiocytoid features in the granular cells and favoured a nesenchymal derivation |
| Granular cell pituicytoma of neurohypophysis | ? | — |
| Oligodendroglioma | – | Granules represent swollen lysosomes with dense mottling and myelin figures, and include morphologically diverse autophagic vacuoles.[2133] By LM, the granular cells in oligodoendrogliomas closely resemble astrocytic cells in mixed gliomas |
| Granular cell adamantinoma | – | — |
| Wilms' tumour | – | One case, in which autophagic vacuoles were similar to those of GCT, but appeared to be histochemically different, in that reactions for non-specific acid esterase and acid phosphatase were negative.[1015] ??relationship to finding of neural tissue in a case of Wilms' tumour |
| Vascular leiomyosarcoma | – | — |
| Bizarre leiomyoma of uterus | – | Myelin figures present. Lysosomes often contained mitochondria |
| Irradiated myometrium | – | Cytolysosomes in myocytes. Appearances similar to those seen in bizarre uterine leiomyoma |
| Appendiceal granular cell lesion | – | Granules reported to differ from those of GCT, being heterogeneous and including myelin figures |
| Reactive granular cells in sites of trauma | – | Granular cells are histiocytes with intracytoplasmic electron-dense material |

References: 45, 1015, 1240, 2064, 2113–2135

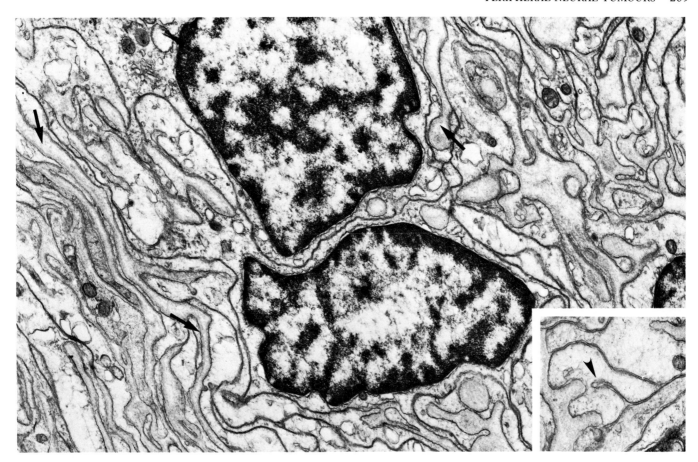

**Fig. 18.1 Schwannoma: Survey of Antoni A tissue**

The neoplastic cells have slightly irregular nuclei with a relatively thin sheet of surrounding cytoplasm, from which intertwining processes emanate. Intercellular junctions are not seen, but external laminae can be discerned (arrows), even at this magnification. Long-spacing collagen is detectable in the interstitium of many of these neoplasms, but $\pi$ (Reich) bodies are generally rare. (× 10 800)

**Inset:** In some profiles the cytoplasm of the cells is dissected by invagination of the plasmalemma (arrowhead). (× 24 300)

See Table 18.1.

References: 576, 805, 2055, 2058, 2061, 2062, 2065, 2068, 2076, 2077, 2079, 2083, 2085, 2087, 2088, 2094, 2096, 2097, 2100, 2110, 2112

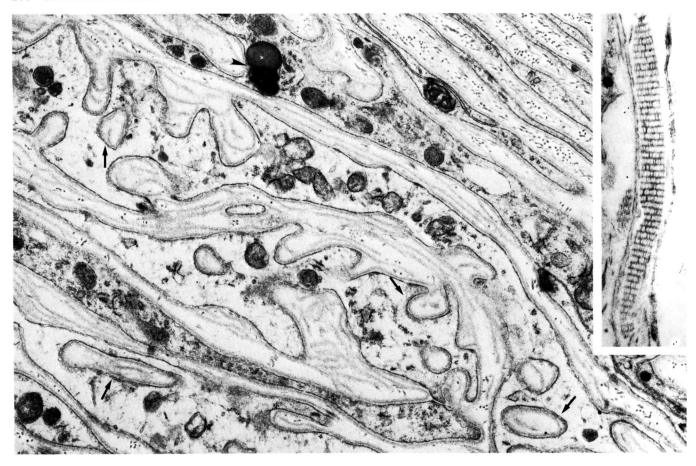

## Fig. 18.2 Schwannoma: External laminae and fibrous long-spacing collagen

Multiple and continuous layers of external laminal material lie adjacent to the cell processes which tend to isolate small stromal pockets (arrows). One cell contains a lipofuscin body (arrowhead). (Formalin fixation, × 20 900)

**Inset:** Circumscribed elongated aggregate of fibrous long-spacing collagen (Luse body) in an acoustic Schwannoma. (Formalin fixation, × 12 000)

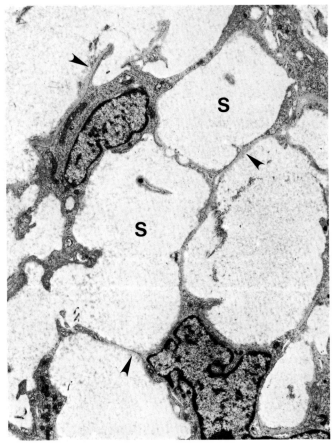

## Fig. 18.3 Schwannoma: Antoni B tissue

Needle biopsy of a spindle cell tumour in the neck of a 19-year-old man. Delicate processes emanate from the cell bodies, forming a simple reticular pattern. There is an abundant intervening stroma (S), whose delicate flocculent appearance reflects an abundance of proteoglycans. The processes have an associated external lamina in some areas (arrowheads). (× 5900)

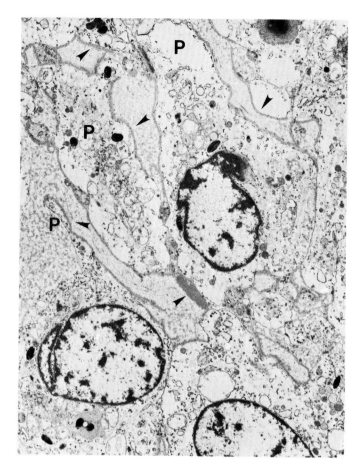

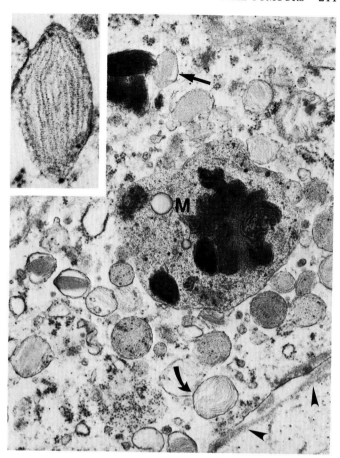

**Fig. 18.4 Melanotic Schwannoma: Survey**

Pigmented intramural tumour of stomach, from a 52-year-old woman. Despite a locally infiltrative growth pattern, there was no evidence of recurrence or metastasis on post-operative follow-up.

Cytoplasmic processes (P) and external lamina (arrowheads) characterize these Schwannian cells, while electron-dense melanosomes are present in the processes and cell bodies. The melanosomes and absence of myofilaments aid in excluding a smooth muscle neoplasm. (× 4600)

Although rare, melanotic Schwannomas are convincingly recorded in the literature.[2089] Most occur along the neuraxis, and the location of the tumour in this case appears to be exceptional. Ultrastructural examination of melanotic Schwannomas reveals the typical appearances of Schwann cells,[2089] which also contain melanosomes at all stages of development, indicating in situ synthesis (see Table 8.1).

(Specimen contributed by Drs. D.K. Burns and F.G. Silva; details of this case are published elsewhere[790] ).

References: 790, 2060, 2071, 2086, 2089, 2106

**Fig. 18.5 Melanotic Schwannoma: Melanosomes**

Same case as Fig. 18.4. Detail of Schwann cell cytoplasm. Atypical melanosomes in various stages of maturation dominate this field. A large compound melanosome (M) is present, and portion of a heavily melanized melanosome lies near the top of the micrograph; only a few have the internal periodicity characteristic of stage II melanosomes (straight arrow). Others display deviant patterns, and some have a pleated coil configuration (curved arrow). Note also the adjacent external lamina (arrowheads). (× 24 800)

**Inset:** Detail of a stage II melanosome with a filamentous interior in the same tumour. (× 64 400)

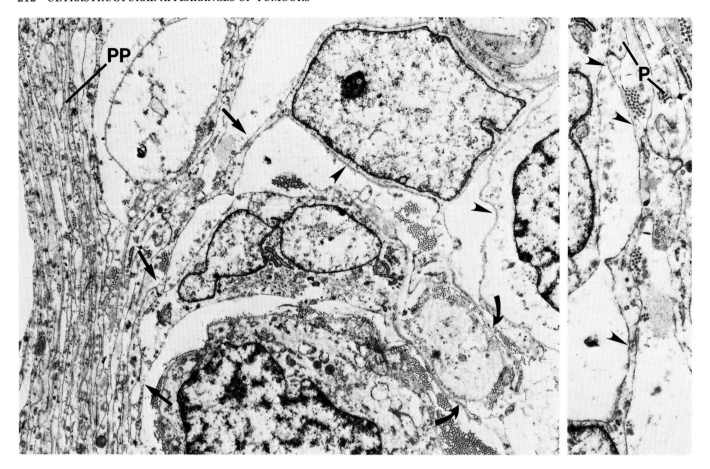

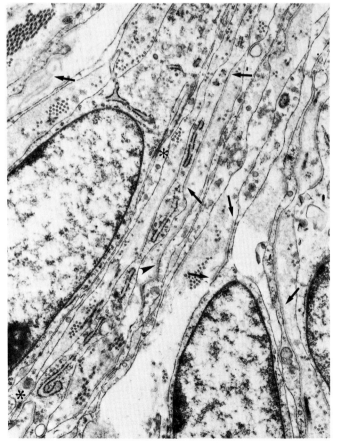

## Fig. 18.6 Malignant Schwannoma: Epithelioid and perineurial cells

Recurrent infiltrating tumour of the parotid-facial nerve region. Composed of both spindle and epithelioid cells, this Schwannoma also contained numerous small nerve trunk-like formations, consisting of central atypical epithelioid cells and a circumferential layer resembling perineurium. One such formation is illustrated here. The central epithelioid cells have pleomorphic nuclei and are invested by a delicate discontinuous external lamina (arrowheads). Slender processes emanate from the cell bodies; some (curved arrows) enfold both cells and the collagen-containing stroma, while others (straight arrows) merge with the layered perineurial processes (PP) on the left. Note that myelin sheaths and Schwannian-axonal complexes are not present. These appearances suggest that the perineurial processes may represent a pattern of neoplastic cell differentiation, rather than the residual perineurium of nerve trunks permeated by tumour. Nevertheless, the capacity of malignant Schwannoma to develop within, and infiltrate along, pre-existing nerve trunks is well recognized. (Formalin fixation, × 9500)

**Inset:** Epithelioid cell process (arrowheads) merging with perineurial-type processes (P), at higher magnification. (× 16 100)

(Figs. 18.6–18.8 — all from the same case — modified from Robertson et al[1996] and published by permission).

References: 362, 1996, 2052, 2054, 2056, 2057, 2060, 2072, 2073, 2095, 2101–2103, 2105, 2109

## Fig. 18.7 Malignant Schwannoma: Perineurial processes

Numerous layered perineurial processes traverse the field. Micropinocytotic vesicles can be discerned (arrowhead). Note the fragmentary external lamina concentrated along one side of the cells (arrows). Sporadic poorly developed intermediate junctions are present (*). One of the nuclei contains a moderately prominent nucleolus. (Formalin fixation, × 14 900)

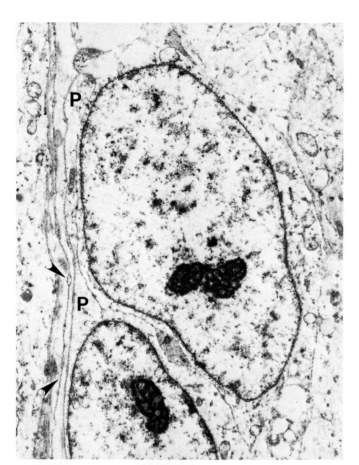

## Fig. 18.8 Malignant Schwannoma: Poorly differentiated area

These cells are characterized by a high nuclear:cytoplasmic ratio, and prominent nucleoli are evident. An elongated process (P) with accompanying external lamina emanates from one cell, while another extremely delicate process (arrowheads) subdivides the extracellular matrix. (Formalin fixation, × 7500)

## Fig. 18.9 Perineurioma: Cell processes and junctions

Observe the apposition of the membranes of adjacent plump cell bodies and cell processes. The external laminae (straight arrows) are fragmented; in addition, small intermediate junctions are present (curved arrows). Micropinocytotic vesicles are another feature of perineurial cells (Fig. 18.7); only a few vesicles (V) are present in this field. (× 24 700)

See Table 18.1.

References: 2061, 2084, 2107, 2108

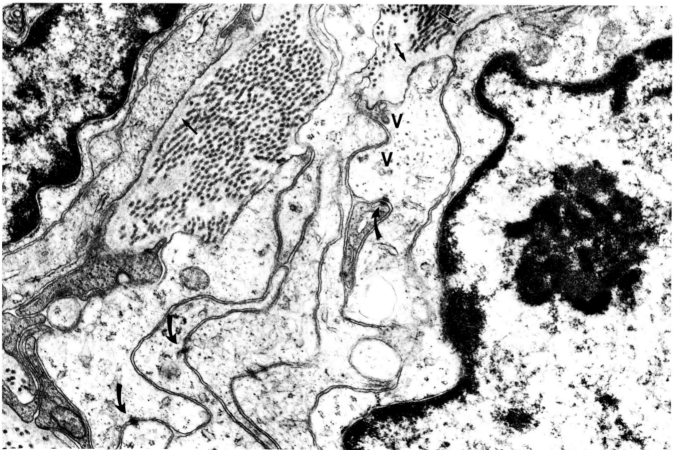

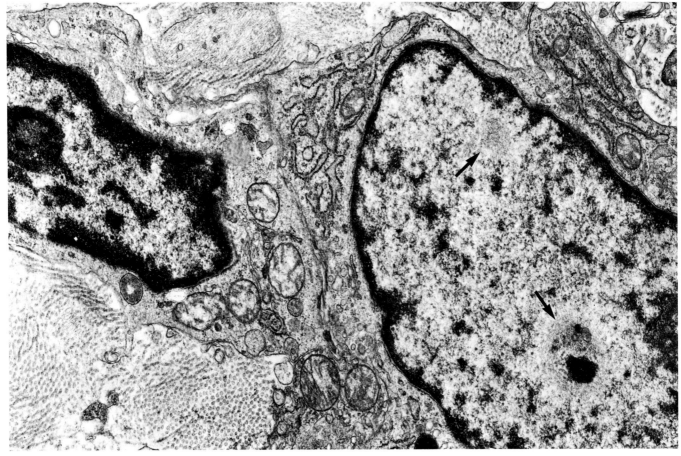

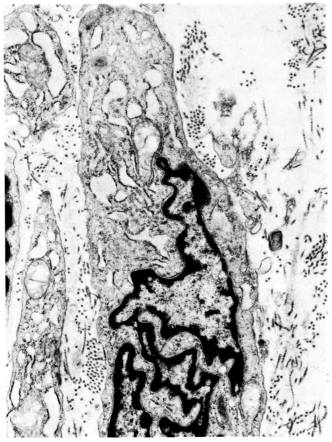

**Fig. 18.10** *(Above)* **Neurofibroma: Cell morphology**

The predominant cell is fibroblastoid (see Table 18.1), and lacks interlocking processes or cell junctions. In addition, there is abundant collagenous connective tissue. Nuclear bodies are also evident (arrows). Long-spacing collagen is sometimes observed, and mast cells may be frequent. (× 22 400)

Erlandson & Woodruff [2061] have suggested that such fibroblastoid cells may represent modifications of perineurial cells, which were also identified in their series of 10 neurofibromas (see Table 18.1).

References: 2061, 2064, 2065, 2075, 2083, 2098, 2107, 2108, 2110

**Fig. 18.11** *(Left)* **Neurofibroma: Fibroblastoid cell**

Fibroblastoid cell with an irregular nucleus in a neurofibroma. Some cisternae of the RER are dilated; there is much interstitial collagenous connective tissue in various stages of formation. (× 14 800)

**Fig. 18.12** *(Facing page)* **Granular cell tumour: Survey of granular and angulate-body cells**

Cutaneous tumour over iliac crest of a woman aged 48 years. The cytoplasm of the mature granular cells is packed with numerous pleomorphic lysosomal granules (G). Endoplasmic reticulum, mitochondria and Golgi complexes, which are said to be features of 'early' granular cells, are inconspicuous. The nucleus (N) contains little heterochromatin. An angulate-body cell (A) is also present, and in one area there is some interleaving of cell processes (P). There are numerous collagen fibres in the stroma; fibrous long-spacing collagen may also be seen (see Table 3.4). (× 10 600)

**Inset:** External lamina (arrowheads) adjacent to the granular cells. (× 20 000)

See also Table 18.2.

References: 332, 366, 2113–2135, 2226

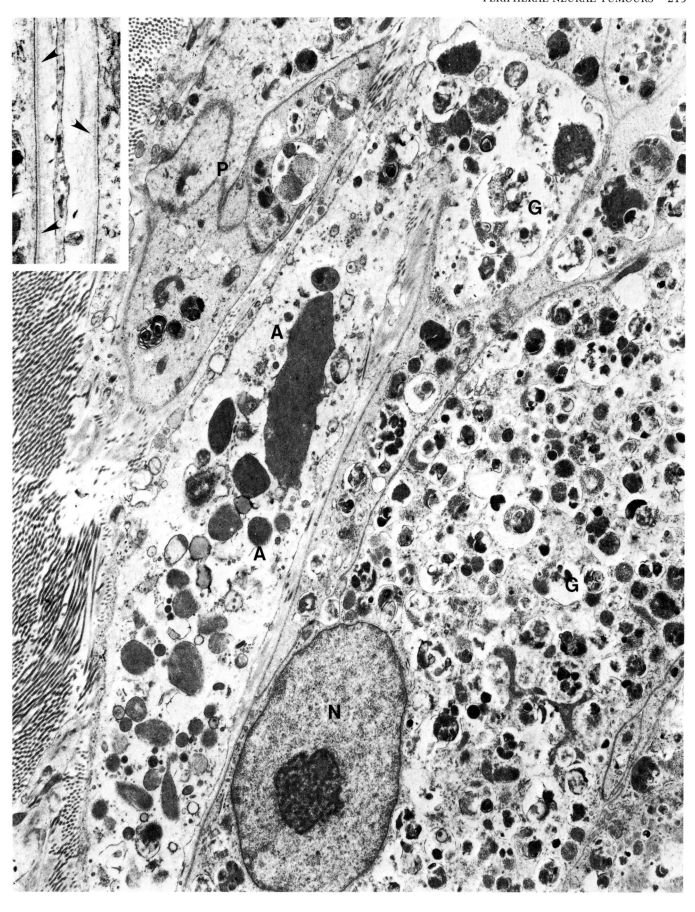

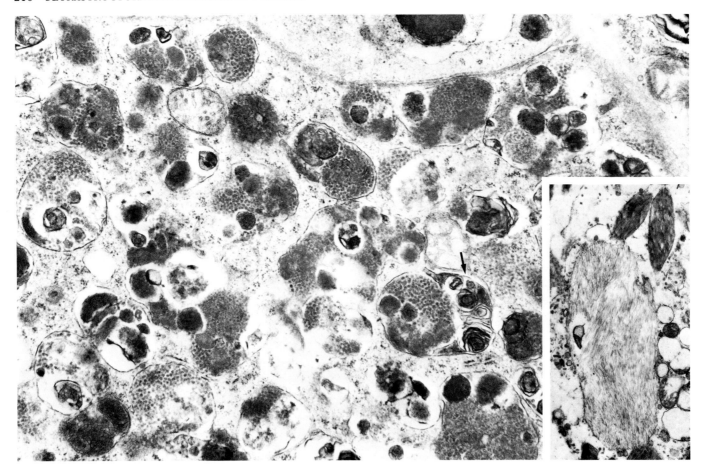

**Fig. 18.13 Granular cell tumour: Granules and angulate bodies**

The cytoplasmic lysosomal granules are shown here in detail. The granules with a vesicular internal substructure resemble multivesicular bodies, while membranes are apparent in other granules, occasionally forming myelinoid figures (arrow). **Inset:** Typical granules within an angulate body cell, showing the unit membrane and the fibrillar internal material of variable density. Angulate-body cells appear to correspond to the 'Gaucher-like' cells described by Bhawan et al.[2113] (× 26 300. Inset: × 10 300)

Similar ultrastructural appearances are described in malignant granular cell tumour.[2120]

References: 2113, 2120

# SECTION FOUR
# TUMOURS OF THE SOFT AND HARD SUPPORTING TISSUES

# 19 Lipogenic tumours

The fine structure of adipose tissue tumours is the subject of a notable recent review by Fu et al.[2337]

White adipose tissue develops from precursor cells ultrastructurally indistinguishable from fibroblasts. With the onset of lipoblastic differentiation, the cells evolve through a series of stages, arbitrarily designated as early, intermediate and late lipoblasts, with eventual development into mature lipocytes.[2229,2337] This line of differentiation is marked by a gradual increase in cytoplasmic lipid droplets (eventually producing monovacuolar late lipoblasts and lipocytes), together with increasing amounts of external lamina and both smooth-surfaced and micropinocytotic vesicles. As these changes evolve, there is a reciprocal diminution of RER and Golgi complexes, and the mitochondrial morphology alters from spherical to elongated and filamentous. Glycogen appears transiently in intermediate lipoblasts. This evolution also involves a change in cell shape from the elongated bipolar profiles of the fibroblastoid precursors, to ovoid late lipoblasts and lipocytes (Fig. 19.1).

In lipoblastomatosis the recorded ultrastructural appearances include fibroblastoid prelipoblasts, together with early and late lipoblasts and mature lipocytes.[2337]

In spindle cell lipoma,[2332] the cells are predominantly fibroblastoid and may contain few lipid droplets, but the presence of relatively mature monovacuolar fat cells with a well-developed continuous pericellular external lamina is also recorded.[2332,2335]

*Hibernoma* is characterized by rounded multivacuolar fat cells with an associated external lamina;[2338] in addition to the lipid, these lipocytes contain numerous pleomorphic mitochondria,[2345] while gap junctions and subplasmalemmal linear densities are also reported.[2226] In an ultrastructural study of three hibernomas, Gaffney et al[2338] reported an inverse relationship between lipid droplet size and mitochondrial frequency; they also described micropinocytotic vesicles, often associated with plasmalemmal invaginations, and a paucity of 'cytoplasmic membrane systems'.

*Liposarcomas* recapitulate the embryonal development of adipose tissue,[2226] and contain undifferentiated and fibroblastoid cells, as well as early, intermediate and late lipoblasts and mature lipocytes in varying proportions, depending on the tumour type and degree of differentiation. Myxoid liposarcoma is typified by intermediate lipoblasts, but late lipoblasts and fibrosarcoma-like areas may also be seen (Fig. 19.1).[2337] Poorly differentiated mesenchymal cells and cells containing abundant mitochondria and glycogen are found in round cell liposarcomas, while pleomorphic liposarcomas are composed of pleomorphic primitive cells and fibroblasts, with few lipoblasts.[2337]

*The presence of numerous lipid droplets is by itself insufficient to establish lipoblastic-lipocytic differentiation.* Varying numbers of lipid-laden cells can be found in disparate tumours as listed in Table 2.11. The ultrastructural identification of lipoblastic-lipocytic differentiation should therefore include other evidence, such as the features listed above (see also Fig. 19.1), together with absence of the patterns of differentiation seen in other lipid-containing but non-adipose tumours. The nature of most adipose tissue tumours is readily apparent by LM, but EM is occasionally claimed to be of value in detecting liposarcomatous features in small cell tumours.[86] Nevertheless, in inexperienced hands there is a risk of overdiagnosis of lipogenic neoplasms by this technique; we consider EM to have only a secondary role in the identification of this group of tumours, with LM remaining the mainstay of diagnosis.

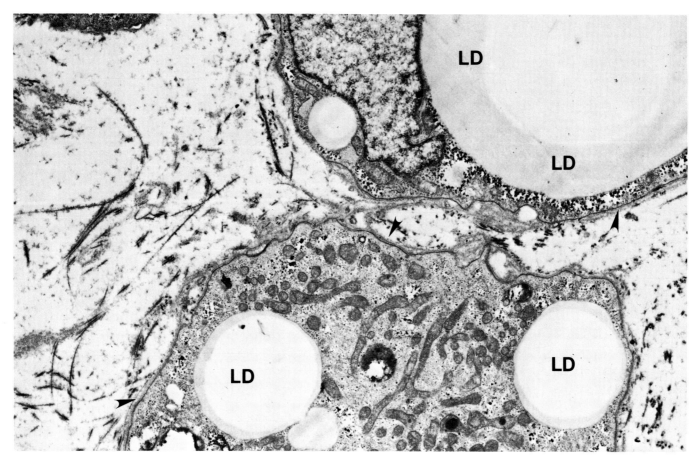

**Fig. 19.1 Myxoid liposarcoma: Survey**

Segments of two tumour cells are seen. The nucleus is eccentric while large lipid droplets (LD) are present in the cytoplasm. Note the filamentous mitochondria and the dense glycogen granules. An external lamina surrounds the cell surface (arrowheads). The appearances conform to those of late lipoblasts. The interstitium consists of a few scattered collagen fibres and wisps of osmiophilic proteoglycan-rich material. (× 11 000)

The *combination* of cell shape, lipid droplets, glycogen, elongated mitochondria, micropinocytosis and a discontinuous external lamina is useful in identifying lipoblastic differentiation in myxoid liposarcoma; in addition, this tumour lacks the cellular heterogeneity of the myxoid variant of malignant fibrous histiocytoma (see Chapter 20).[2234]

References: 2226, 2234, 2330, 2331, 2336, 2337, 2339, 2342, 2343, 2348

# 20 Fibrohistiocytic tumours

## MYOFIBROBLASTOSES AND FIBROSARCOMA

The description of the myofibroblast has been largely achieved by EM, initially in inflammatory processes with contracting fibrous repair, and later in apparently neoplastic fibroproliferations.[351] Superficially resembling fibroblasts, myofibroblasts are additionally characterized by bundles of thin (5–7 nm) cytoplasmic filaments with associated focal densities (see Figs. 3.14–3.16). The bundles are distributed longitudinally, and many are situated at the periphery of the cell body. Segments of external lamina lie adjacent to the plasmalemma, while the adjoining plasma membranes form intermediate junctions in areas of close apposition. Low-grade fibroproliferative disorders, notably the fibromatoses, appear to consist largely of myofibroblasts (see Table 3.5).[2299] A predominance of myofibroblasts in extensively sampled fibroproliferative disorders is considered by some authorities to suggest a benign or locally infiltrative process such as a fibromatosis.[347] However, fibrosarcomas containing abundant myofibroblasts are recorded (see Table 3.6), although fibroblasts usually constitute the principal cell type. It has also been suggested that fibrosarcomas containing numerous myofibroblasts may have a more favourable prognosis than those with only a few or none, but metastasizing myofibroblastic sarcomas are described.[2179]

## FIBROUS HISTIOCYTOMAS

Benign and malignant fibrous histiocytomas consist of mesenchymal cells with a spectrum of differentiation, including varying proportions of fibroblasts, myofibroblasts, histiocytes, fibrohistiocytes and undifferentiated mesenchymal cells.[2276] (Throughout this work we have used the term 'histiocyte' as a synonym for 'macrophage', while fibrohistiocytes combine the structural features of macrophages and fibroblasts). Xanthomatous and multinucleated giant cells are also frequent, and Langerhans' cell granules have been found rarely in the histiocytoid cells (see Table 28.3).[2315] By detecting this polymorphic cell population — in concert with both routine light microscopy and the immunocytochemical demonstration of $\alpha_1$-antiprotease ± muramidase (lysozyme) — EM can contribute to recognition of the fibrohistiocytic character of a particular tumour. However, it is of little use in evaluating behavioural properties, and *it is cautioned that sporadic stromal histiocytes are often present in other neoplasms, including various sarcomas.*

Cells with features of pericytes (see Chapter 23) have been reported in haemangiopericytic areas of malignant fibrous histiocytoma (MFH) of bone, with appearances claimed to be intermediate between undifferentiated mesenchymal cells and fibroblasts.[2651] Striated muscle cells are also described in an angiomatoid MFH,[2289] but the illustrations, which include sarcolemmal crenellations, strongly suggest atrophic myocytes (see Introduction). In contrast, Sun et al[2311] found endothelial and pericytic appearances, with atypical vasoformative structures and Weibel-Palade bodies, in two cases of angiomatoid MFH, presumably representing the vascular component (see Chapter 23).

The ultrastructural differential diagnosis of MFH includes rhabdomyosarcoma, fibrosarcoma,[2276] sclerosing liposarcoma, malignant Schwannoma[2072] and smooth muscle tumours. Apart from lacking the distinctive combinations of appearances characterizing these other neoplasms, MFH is composed of a far more variegated cell population with frequent histiocytoid elements.

The fine structure of MFH of bone is identical to the soft tissue counterpart. The differential diagnosis in this site includes osteosarcoma, fibrosarcoma, dedifferentiated chondrosarcoma, metastatic sarcomatoid renal carcinoma and perhaps giant cell tumour (see Chapter 25). Once again, LM is the mainstay of this exercise; the role of EM is secondary and often insignificant. Several cell lines also occur in osteosarcoma, but pleomorphic fibroblastoid-osteoblastoid cells with copious dilated RER often predominate, and chondrocytes and stromal hydroxyapatite crystals may be found (see Figs. 25.3–25.6). Histiocytic cells predominate in giant cell tumour, while epithelial features, including 'desmosomes', have been reported in the sarcomatoid variant of renal cell carcinoma;[1001] dedifferentiated chondrosarcoma is discussed in Chapter 25.

The fine structure of benign fibrous histiocytoma of bone resembles that of extra-osseous fibrohistiocytic tumours, and erythrophagocytosis has been recorded.[2305]

## OTHER FIBROHISTIOCYTOID TUMOURS

The giant cell tumour of tendon sheath[2535,2549] also represents a fibrohistiocytic lesion, some of the component cells having the ability to fuse and form syncytia. In addition, fibrohistiocytic differentiation is described in the few reported ultrastructural studies of so-called malignant giant cell tumour of soft parts,[2226,2242] indicating that it represents a giant cell variant of MFH (Figs. 20.12 and 20.13).[2188] Giant cell tumour of bone also has fibrohistiocytic properties but is discussed in Chapter 25, while the possible relationship of epithelioid sarcoma to the spectrum of fibrohistiocytic neoplasia is considered in Chapter 24.

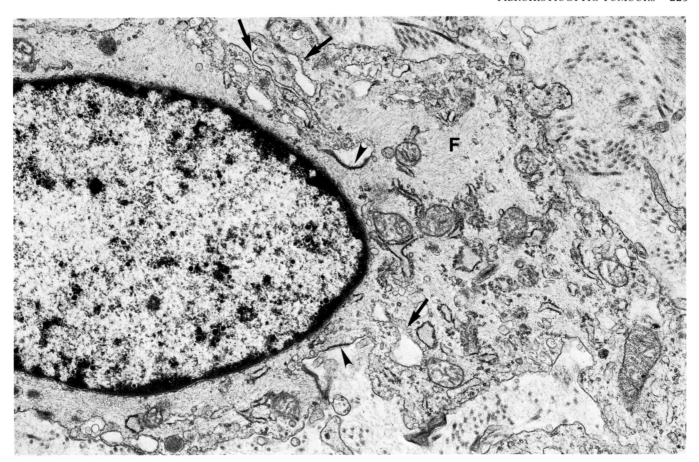

## Fig. 20.1 Nasopharyngeal angiofibroma: Cell morphology

The intervascular stromal cells in nasopharyngeal angiofibromas are said to resemble activated fibroblasts,[2229] but their appearances differ considerably from either classical fibroblasts or smooth muscle cells. A few mitochondria are evident in this case, but RER is sparse. Much of the cytoplasm is occupied by intermediate filaments (F) devoid of dense bodies and presumably representing vimentin. Subplasmalemmal linear densities with an associated external lamina (arrowheads) are present at the cell periphery, and there are numerous micropinocytotic vesicles, as well as caveola-like plasmalemmal invaginations (arrows). Occasional lysosomal bodies are also evident. Intranuclear spheroids are less conspicuous than in Fig. 20.2, more closely resembling conventional perichromatin granules. (Formalin fixation, × 14 800)

(Case contributed by Dr. A.E. Seymour).
References: 384, 426, 427, 429, 2229

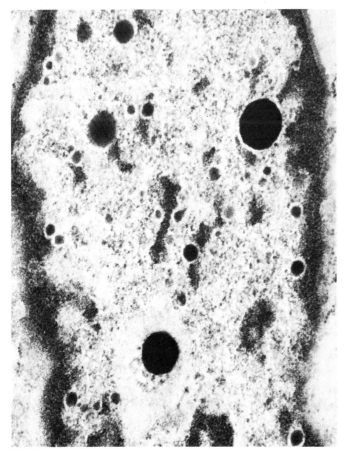

## Fig. 20.2 Nasopharyngeal angiofibroma: Nuclear particles

Tumour of middle turbinate in a 16-year-old youth. This fibroblast nucleus contains many rounded particles of variable size and electron-opacity. The largest are extremely dense and measure up to 335 nm in diameter, while the smallest particles are more lucent and have diameters in the vicinity of 60 nm. Each spheroid is surrounded by a lucent halo approximately 11–17 nm in width. The morphology of these particles suggests that they may represent giant perichromatin granules. (Formalin fixation, × 41 700)

In recurrent tumours these distinctive nuclear particles have been recorded to diminish in both size and number, increasingly resembling perichromatin granules and eventually disappearing.[2229]

(Case contributed by Dr. A.E. Seymour).

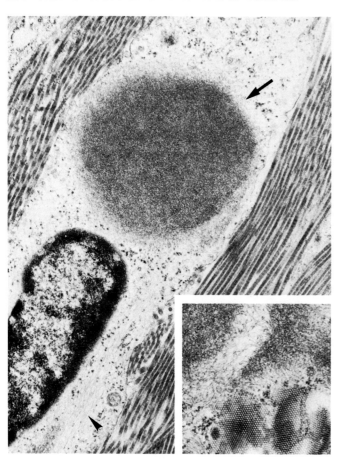

### Fig. 20.3 Infantile digital fibroma: Cytoplasmic inclusion and crystalloids

A large paranuclear inclusion (arrow) is evident in this cell. Note the intermediate filaments (arrowhead). In some cases the inclusions are continuous with microfilaments containing dense bodies. (× 17 600)

**Inset:** Portion of an inclusion showing a fibrillary substructure. The nearby crystalloids are composed of tightly packed hexagons; such crystalloids are infrequent in digital fibromas. (× 30 300)

(Case contributed by Prof. J.F.R. Kerr).

References: 2206, 2226, 2229, 2245, 2248, 2250, 2264, 2279, 2298, 2306

### Fig. 20.4 Fibrosarcoma: Survey

These neoplasms consist of irregular spindle-shaped or stellate fibroblastoid cells with large irregular nuclei (arrows) containing much euchromatin. Thin cytoplasmic extensions intrude into the collagenous interstitium. Myofibroblasts are frequently found in low-grade fibrosarcomas (see Table 3.6). (× 8200)

References: 2226, 2229, 2254, 2258, 2259, 2272, 2273, 2281, 2285, 2300, 2308, 2318, 2569, 2647

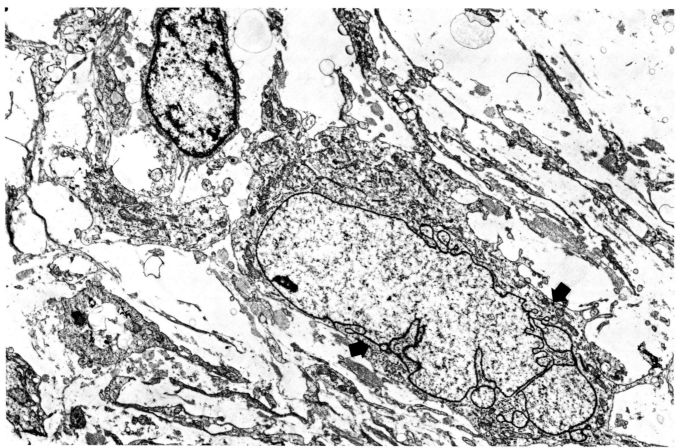

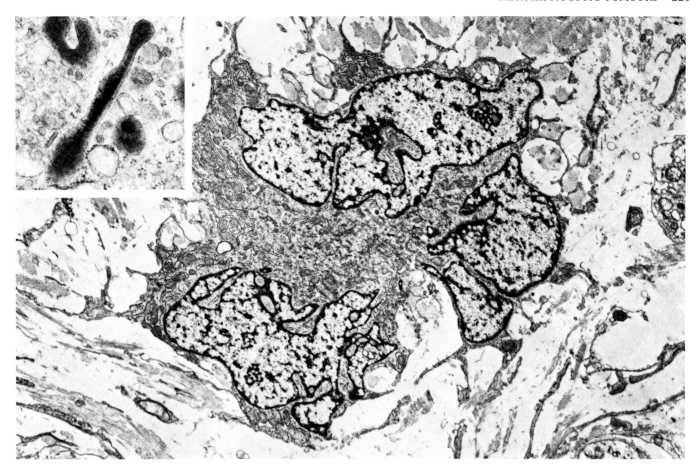

**Fig. 20.5 Fibrosarcoma: Multinucleated cell**

Multinucleated cells are sometimes seen; the nuclear contours are again irregular and the cytoplasmic features resemble those of fibroblasts. Loose interstitial collagenous tissue is present. (× 5500)

**Inset:** Membrane-bound collagen fibres are occasionally found within the neoplastic cells (see also Fig. 3.19). (× 34 700)

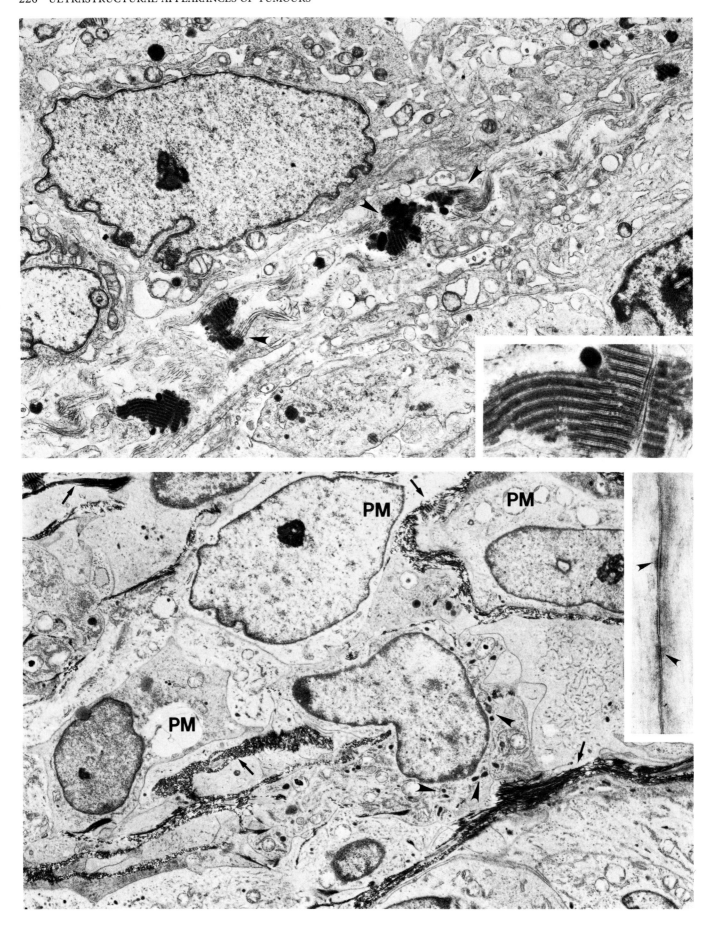

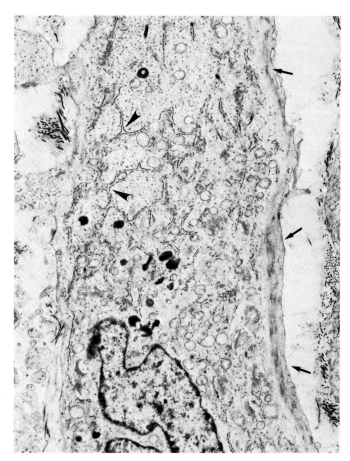

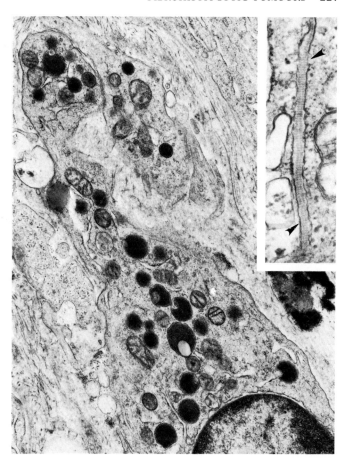

**Fig. 20.8 Malignant fibrous histiocytoma: Myofibroblast**

Tumour of deep soft tissues of the thigh, from a 70-year-old man. The cell illustrated represents a myofibroblast; in addition to moderate quantities of branching lamellae of RER (arrowheads) and scattered lysosomes, there are bundles of peripheral longitudinally-arranged fine filaments — which cannot be individually resolved at this power — with focal densities (arrows). Thick branching lamellae of RER are a characteristic feature of fibroblastoid cells. (× 7000)

Fibroblasts and myofibroblasts sometimes predominate in malignant fibrous histiocytomas — including cases with a storiform or myxoid pattern by LM; when they do so in the absence of histiocytoid cells with malignant features, one can argue that such tumours are better classified as fibrosarcomas.[2277]

See also Tables 3.5 and 3.6.
References: 2254, 2277

**Fig. 20.9 Malignant fibrous histiocytoma: Histiocytoid cell with lysosomes, and banded inclusion in RER**

The cell illustrated contains numerous membrane-bound electron-dense lysosomes whose diameters range from 250–750 nm. (× 13 500)

**Inset:** A strand of cross-banded fibrous material has accumulated within a cisterna of the RER (arrowheads). The nature of the material is uncertain, but its periodicity is approximately 15 nm, and it may represent a collagen precursor. Crystalloidal inclusions may also develop within such dilated cisternae. (× 31 000)

Reference: 2313

**Fig. 20.6** *(Facing page — top)* **Malignant fibrous histiocytoma: Cell types**

Tumour from the lower limb of a 57-year-old woman. These fibroblastoid cells have slightly irregular nuclear profiles. Nuclear bodies and complex nuclear projections were prominent in other areas. The cisternae of the RER are mildly dilated, whereas lysosomes are infrequent. Intercellular junctions and external lamina are not present. In addition to native collagen fibres, the extracellular matrix contains sharply circumscribed electron-dense collections of collagen with regular periodicity; these are continuous with collagen fibres in some areas (arrowheads) and may be allied to fibrous long-spacing collagen. (× 8600)

**Inset:** Collagen aggregate showing complex banded periodicity of 100–105 nm. (× 28 300)

References: 444, 520, 546, 562, 696, 2221, 2226, 2229, 2234, 2246, 2249, 2251, 2254, 2255, 2267, 2274–2277, 2280, 2283, 2284, 2288, 2289, 2291, 2293, 2295–2297, 2301, 2307, 2312–2315, 2323, 2583, 2591, 2594, 2612, 2616, 2620, 2632, 2640, 2647, 2651

**Fig. 20.7** *(Facing page — bottom)* **Malignant fibrous histiocytoma: Architecture and intercellular junctions**

These poorly differentiated mesenchymal cells (PM) form interlocking processes, with close apposition of plasma membranes, but small amounts of intervening collagenous matrix are often present (arrows). One cell contains a few lysosomes (arrowheads). (× 5500)

**Inset:** Intercellular junctions (arrowheads) are occasionally found between apposed plasma membranes. Such junctions lack the classical morphology of desmosomes and should not be misconstrued as evidence of epithelial differentiation. (× 32 400)

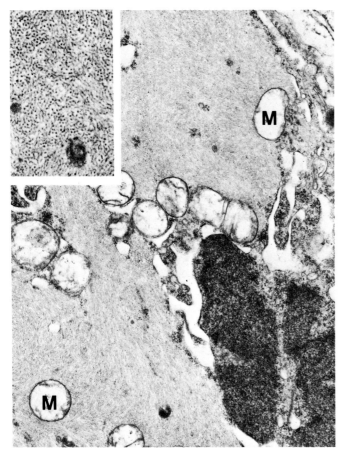

**Fig. 20.10 Malignant fibrous histiocytoma: Intermediate filaments**

A mass of chromatin representing a metaphase mitosis occupies the lower right corner of this field. Apart from ballooned mitochondria (M) and dilated RER, most of the cytoplasmic constituents in this cell are replaced by a feltwork of 10 nm filaments. Morphologically different from actin microfilaments, these filaments lack dense bodies and correspond to the presence of immunoreactive vimentin (see Table 2.8). They are usually found in a paranuclear position. Intranuclear 'barreloid' inclusions composed of undulating fibrils 18–23 nm in diameter have also been reported.[2313] (× 14 900)

**Inset:** The intermediate filaments are shown here in transverse section. (× 49 000)

Reference: 2313

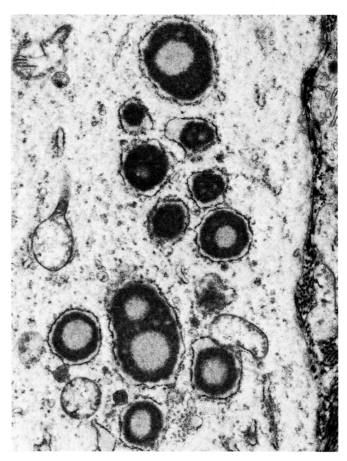

**Fig. 20.11 Malignant fibrous histiocytoma: Dilatation of RER with intracisternal material**

Tumour from the neck of a 77-year-old man. Flocculent electron-dense material has accumulated within the cisternae of the RER; some of the intracisternal globules have central rounded lucent areas, producing a doughnut-shaped configuration. Such globules may correspond to the presence of immunoreactive $\alpha_1$-antitrypsin ($\alpha_1$-antiprotease). (× 12 300)

**Fig. 20.12** *(Facing page)* **Malignant fibrous histiocytoma, giant cell type (malignant giant cell tumour of soft parts): Giant cell and paracrystalline inclusion**

There are multiple nuclear profiles within this fibrohistiocytic giant cell, including apparent micronuclei. In one area the nuclear envelope appears to have ruptured, with extrusion of chromatin (arrow). The cytoplasm contains pleomorphic lysosomes (L), abundant RER with dilated cisternae (E), and peripheral fine filaments (arrowheads), which cannot be individually resolved at this magnification. The interstitium (IS) contains a few bundles of collagen fibres. Intracytoplasmic collagen fibres similar to those depicted in Fig. 3.19 were also found in this case. (× 7000)

**Inset:** A paracrystalline structure in the cytoplasm of a tumour cell is shown here at high magnification; a longitudinal linear substructure is evident near each end (arrows). (× 50 300)

References: 2188, 2226, 2242, 2244, 2317

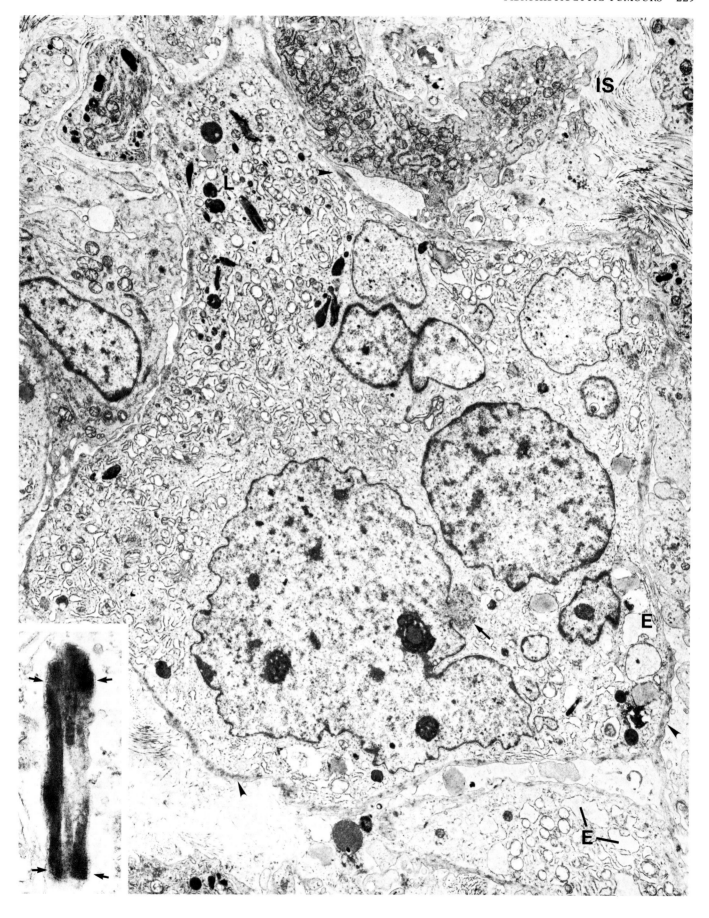

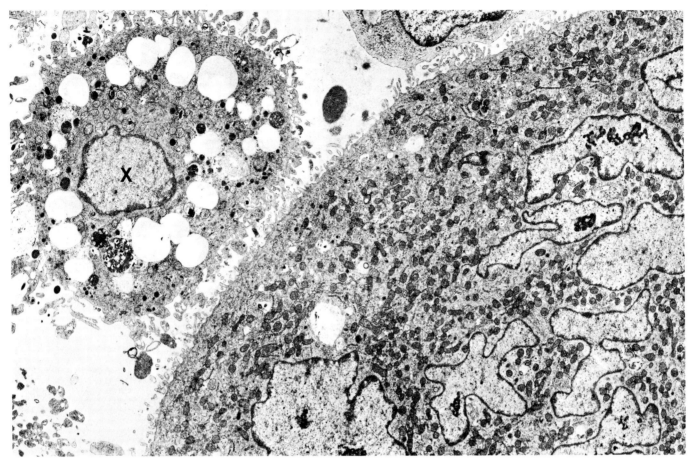

**Fig. 20.13 Malignant fibrous histiocytoma, giant cell type: Giant and xanthoma cells**

Multiple nuclear profiles are conspicious in this polykaryon, which also contains innumerable mitochondria. There are frequent cytoplasmic ruffles on both the giant cell and the adjacent xanthomatous cell (X) in which pale lipid droplets are plentiful. (× 5600)

# 21 Smooth muscle tumours

The component cells of these neoplasms resemble normal smooth muscle cells to varying degrees, as indicated by the presence of longitudinally orientated thin (5–7 nm) cytoplasmic filaments with focal densities along the course of the filamentous aggregates. Intermediate (10 nm) and thick (15 nm) myofilaments are sometimes visible in normal mammalian smooth muscle (Table 21.1); thick filaments have also been recorded in a case of leiomyomatosis peritonealis disseminata associated with endometriosis,[2376] a glomus tumour[2359] and a leiomyosarcoma of bone,[2402] but are not usually detectable in smooth muscle tumours. A few strands of RER may be present (in contrast to their frequency in myofibroblasts), while micropinocytotic vesicles are readily found; however, scattered myofibroblasts are often present in addition to the predominant smooth muscle cells in both benign and malignant tumours, emphasizing the morphological continuum between fibroblasts and smooth muscle at the fine-structural level.[2254,2362] Subplasmalemmal dense plaques (attachment zones), intercellular junctions and external laminae are also seen, the laminal material being most prominent adjacent to highly differentiated myoid cells. Filaments are typically numerous in well differentiated benign neoplasms, but their numbers are variable and may be extremely low in epithelioid smooth muscle tumours (leiomyoblastomas) and leiomyosarcomas (Figs. 21.3, 21.4 and 21.8). External laminae are also poorly formed or absent in these latter tumours. The cytoplasmic clarity characteristic of the cells in epithelioid smooth muscle tumours by LM has been attributed both to an artefact of fixation and to the presence of light cells with electron-lucent cytoplasm.[805]

A distinctive malignant intramural gastric tumour has recently been reported in association with pulmonary chondroma and/or extra-adrenal paraganglioma (Carney's triad).[793] By LM this neoplasm resembles an epithelioid leiomyosarcoma. An ultrastructural study of three such tumours[815] revealed appearances similar to those of epithelioid smooth muscle tumours; the cytoplasm contained relatively few haphazardly distributed fine filaments, without dense bodies.[798,815]

Deletion of myoid characteristics in poorly differentiated smooth muscle neoplasms can render the ultrastructural diagnosis difficult and even impossible. *Minimal criteria for the recognition of smooth muscle differentiation* in mesenchymal cells include at least a few longitudinally orientated microfilaments associated with dense bodies, together with a paucity of RER. When microfilaments are present, other markers such as a fragmentary external lamina and sporadic intercellular junctions are usually also detectable. Weiss & Mackay[2403] analyzed the ultrastructure of 20 malignant gastrointestinal smooth muscle tumours, divided evenly into spindle cell and epithelioid neoplasms according to the predominant LM pattern. A morphological spectrum was observed, ranging from obvious smooth muscle differentiation, to the most anaplastic tumours with no trace of myoid properties. Only five cases, all spindle cell tumours, had definite smooth muscle features. The remaining cases were subdivided into two categories:

1. An intermediate group designated as poorly differentiated, in which occasional attachment plaques and foci of external lamina were seen, in the absence of myofilaments.

2. A 'mesenchymal' group whose morphology merged with the intermediate class, but in which myoid features were not seen.

In many cases the nature of poorly differentiated smooth muscle tumours can therefore only be suspected from the ultrastructural appearances, and a precise diagnosis is achieved by integration of the morphology on both LM and EM; the anatomical location may also be of diagnostic importance, but there is evidence that a proportion of gastric wall neoplasms represent nerve sheath cell tumours.[805]

**Table 21.1 Major ultrastructural features of normal and neoplastic smooth muscle**

| Cell component | Remarks |
| --- | --- |
| Actin-containing microfilaments | 5–7 nm in diameter. Arranged parallel to long axis of myocyte and associated with dense bodies which contain $\alpha$-actinin. As well as having contractile and locomotor functions, actin is thought to represent a cytoskeletal protein, and constitutes up to 10–15 per cent of the protein content of some non-myoid cells. Actin occurs in two physically distinct states — a polymerized filamentous form and a disaggregated gel state — and is associated with a number of other proteins. Profilin appears to promote actin polymerization and gelsolin is implicated in its depolymerization; cross-linking proteins (actin-binding protein, filamin) are also described. Brevin is thought to shorten actin filaments and may be similar to villin. For details of other microfilament-associated proteins, see the review by Weber & Osborn[296] |
| | Six tissue-specific forms of actin have been identified, embodying minor variations in the amino acid sequences; these different forms occur in skeletal and cardiac muscle, visceral and vascular smooth muscle, and non-myoid cells in which $\beta$- and $\gamma$-actin are found[297] |
| | See Figs. 21.1 and 21.6 |
| Intermediate filaments (decafilaments) | 10 nm in diameter. Contain desmin (M. Wt. 55 000 Daltons). Located near dense bodies. Morphologically identical to other intermediate filaments such as glial and vimentin filaments. See Table 2.8 and Fig. 21.7 |
| Thick myosin-containing filaments | 14–16 nm in diameter, with a reported range of 12–20 nm. Filaments have tapering ends and are said to differ from the myosin filaments of striated muscle in that they lack uniformity and have irregular transverse profiles;[2361] they are not demonstrated by freeze-fracture techniques. It has been suggested they represent a labile form of myosin;[2361] they are infrequently revealed by conventional preparative procedures and are best demonstrated by glycerination of smooth muscle at pH 6.0. Their preservation seems to require a balance of divalent cation and ATP concentrations, pH and osmolality. |
| | The ratio of thin:thick filaments in normal smooth muscle is at least 15:1 and *it is emphasized that myosin-like filaments are evident only rarely in smooth muscle tumours (see text, this chapter and Chapter 22)* |
| Dense bands (dense plaques, attachment zones, 'hemidesmosomes') | Located at the plasma membrane and elongated in the long axis of the cell. Structure differs from true hemidesmosomes. Thin filaments insert into the dense bands which are often associated with intermediate filaments and vinculin. |
| | See Figs. 21.1, 21.4 and 21.6 |
| | The dense plaques closely resemble subplasmalemmal linear densities (SPLD), which are said to be a marker of mesenchymal cells.[2214] However, the external lamina usually associated with SPLD is by definition fragmentary and restricted to the region of the densities. Because smooth muscle, striated muscle, pericytic and Schwann cells are invested by a continuous external lamina under normal circumstances, their dense plaques are not classified as SPLD. Nevertheless, external lamina is often depleted in tumours differentiating as these cell types, especially when poorly differentiated, and their dense plaques may then fulfill the criteria for designation as SPLD.[2214] Such observations suggest that a distinction between dense plaques and SPLD is essentially artificial |
| Intermediate-like junctions | — |
| Micropinocytotic vesicles | Grouped in rows along plasma membrane. Flask-shaped, measuring about 120 nm in depth and 70 nm in diameter, the neck being 35 nm across. Significance uncertain. See Figs. 21.1 and 21.6 |
| Sarcoplasmic reticulum | SER present, and may be prominent. RER inconspicuous in mature smooth muscle (distinguishing these cells from myofibroblasts), but is often abundant in developing smooth muscle. In tumours, radial cisternae are predominantly found in leiomyosarcoma. See Figs. 21.2 and 21.8 |
| External lamina | Normally about 20 nm in thickness and separated from the plasmalemma by a thin lucent zone. See Figs. 21.1 and 21.5–21.7 |
| Other | Mitochondria, microtubules, occasional lysosomes and multivesicular bodies, and gap junctions are also described |

References: 39, 47, 180, 278, 296, 297, 2214, 2361, 2376, 2402

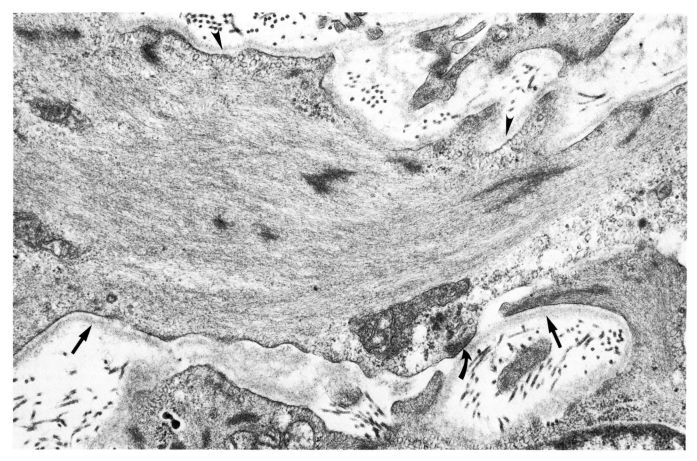

**Fig. 21.1  Glomus tumour: Detail of smooth muscle differentiation**

Recurrent subungual glomus tumour of finger. This electron micrograph is included for two reasons:

1. To illustrate the fine structure of highly differentiated smooth muscle cells.
2. To emphasize that the intervascular glomus cells characteristic of these tumours have smooth muscle (not pericytic) properties.

The cell morphology in this field strikingly resembles normal smooth muscle, but the cells in glomus tumours often have rounded contours. Many microfilaments with associated dense bodies occupy the cytoplasm. RER is conspicuously absent. Subplasmalemmal arrays of micropinocytotic vesicles are evident (arrowheads), as are a few attachment plaques (so-called hemidesmosomes), one of which is indicated by the curved arrow. A well developed external lamina (straight arrows) surrounds the cells. (× 28 200)

**Discussion:** Immunocytochemical analysis of glomus tumours also supports the smooth muscle nature of the intervascular cells, with absence of endothelial markers and a strongly positive reaction for myosin.[2381] Miettinen et al[2381] report that the intermediate filaments appear to consist of vimentin without desmin, as described in some normal vascular smooth muscle cells.

Junctions are often seen between closely apposed cells in smooth muscle tumours and myofibroblasts can also be detected between the more obvious smooth muscle cells.

References: 592, 800, 824, 995, 2226, 2229, 2349, 2354, 2359, 2360, 2368–2370, 2380–2382, 2397, 2398, 2400, 2503, 2526

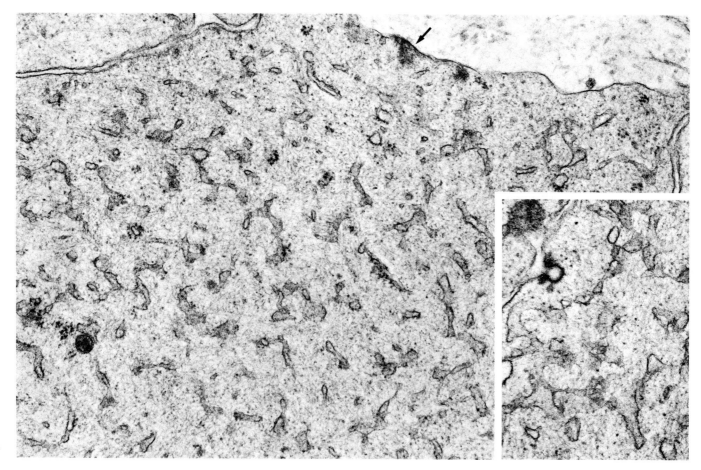

**Fig. 21.2  Duodenal smooth muscle tumour: Endoplasmic reticulum and depleted myofilaments**

Spindle cell tumour of duodenum in a 33-year-old man. The neoplasm had a maximal diameter of 40 mm, and mitoses numbered less than 1 per 10 high power fields.

The myofilamentous apparatus in this myocyte is poorly developed, and filaments are in disarray between the ramifying cisternae of the endoplasmic reticulum. External lamina is not present and there are no dense bodies (fusiform condensations) among the filaments, but an attachment zone can be seen (arrow). Compare with the more typical myocytic appearances in a glomus tumour (Fig. 21.1) and the myofilamentous component of the leiomyosarcomas shown in Figs. 21.7 and 21.8. **Inset:** Coated vesicle and ramifying endoplasmic reticulum in the same tumour. (× 32 600. Inset: × 35 700)

In seemingly benign smooth muscle tumours, a paucity of microfilaments is more characteristic of epithelioid smooth muscle tumours (Fig. 21.3). The prediction of biological behaviour in smooth muscle tumours is best made on the basis of LM and other clinicopathological features, but even then uncertainty may persist.

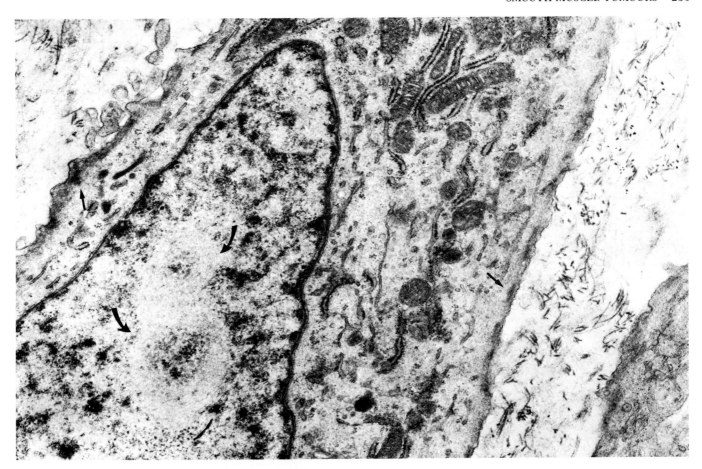

**Fig. 21.3 Gastric epithelioid smooth muscle tumour (leiomyoblastoma): Paucity of myofilaments**

This area of the neoplasm consists of cells with elongated nuclei possessing irregular contours and which typically contain large nuclear bodies (curved arrows). The concentration of cytoplasmic organelles is higher than in leiomyoma and cytoplasmic filaments with focal densities are less conspicuous (arrows). Similarly, external laminal material is rarely present. Loose interstitial collagenous tissue is seen. (× 18 200)

References: 796, 811, 814, 2226, 2355, 2357, 2386, 2403

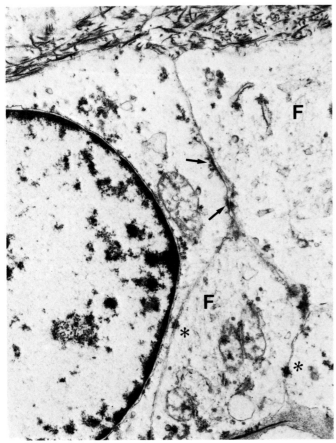

**Fig. 21.4 Epithelioid area of gastric smooth muscle tumour: Absence of microfilaments**

One of these epithelioid cells contains a rounded nucleus. Actin-like microfilaments and dense bodies are conspicuous by their absence. Small numbers of intermediate filaments (F) are present in two areas. Attachment plaques (arrows) and intermediate junctions (*) can also be discerned. (Formalin fixation, × 14 400)

A paucity of myofilaments is typical of epithelioid smooth muscle tumours and in many instances they cannot be found.

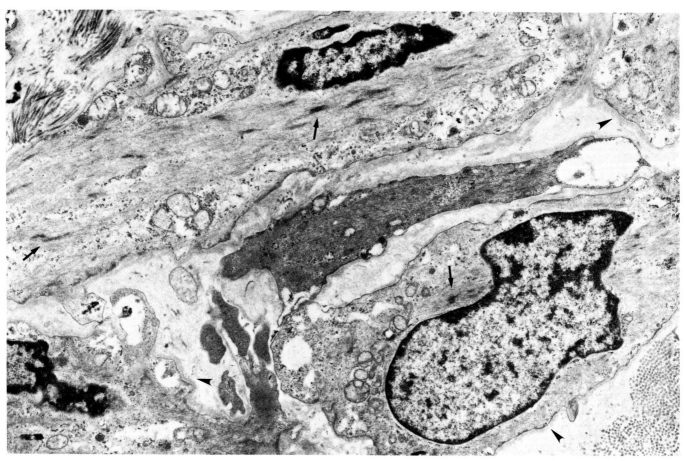

**Fig. 21.5  Leiomyosarcoma: Myoid cells**

Tumour of inferior vena cava in a man aged 22 years. In this view the nuclei
are not crenellated. There is a paucity of RER, but numerous fine cytoplasmic
filaments with dense bodies (arrows) are evident. Peripheral attachment zones
are prevalent, and a mantle of external lamina (arrowheads) surrounds the
cells. (× 13 000)

References: 597, 793, 798, 814, 2226, 2229, 2350–2353, 2356, 2358, 2360,
2362–2368, 2371, 2372, 2374, 2375, 2379, 2383, 2385, 2387, 2389, 2390,
2392, 2393, 2399, 2401–2404

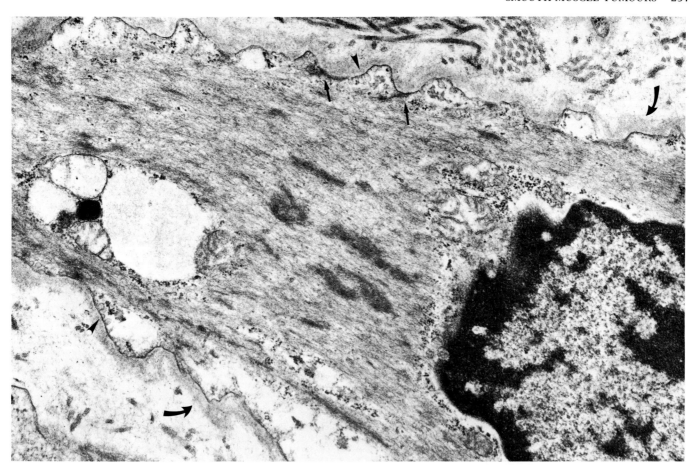

## Fig. 21.6  Leiomyosarcoma: Cell detail

The cytoplasm contains numerous elongated microfilaments averaging approximately 6 nm in diameter; they are aligned longitudinally and have associated dense bodies. Peripheral attachment zones (straight arrows) are occasionally seen in relation to the plasma membrane, beneath which there are foci of micropinocytotic vesicles (arrowheads). A mantle of external laminal material (curved arrows) lies next to the plasma membrane. (× 27 500)

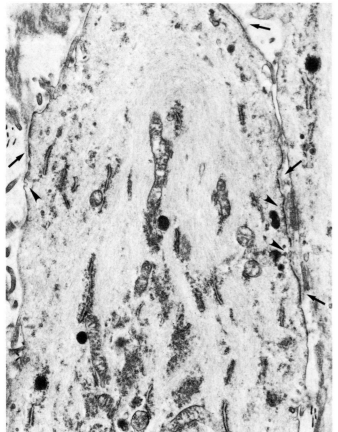

## Fig. 21.7  Probable poorly differentiated leiomyosarcoma: Myoid cell

Non-epithelial spindle cell tumour from the lower lip of a 70-year-old man. The possibility of an atypical fibroxanthoma was entertained because of the anatomical location, but the tumour cells were devoid of $\alpha_1$-antiprotease and lysozyme. In addition, the multiplicity of mesenchymal cell types expected in a fibrohistiocytic tumour was not evident by EM. Instead, the majority of the neoplastic cells resembled that depicted here.

The cytoplasm contains a feltwork of intermediate filaments (presumably representing desmin and/or vimentin), and a few strands of RER. Microfilaments with dense bodies are not present. Nevertheless, subplasmalemmal linear densities with a fragmentary external lamina (arrows), micropinocytotic vesicles (arrowheads) and absence of the processes typical of nerve sheath cells suggest the smooth muscle nature of the cell. (Formalin fixation, × 8300)

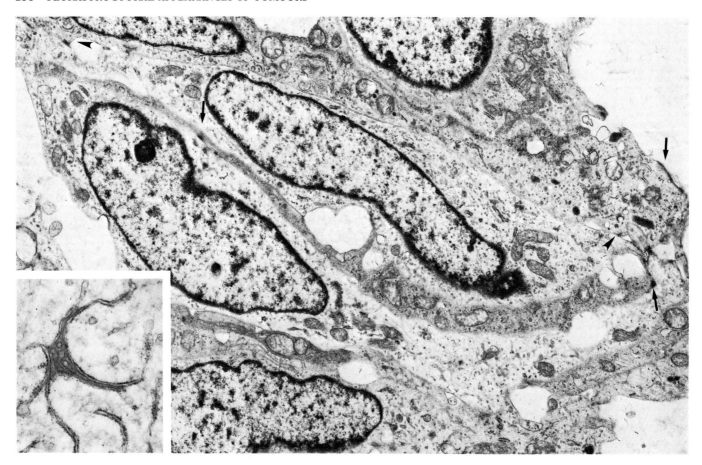

**Fig. 21.8 Poorly differentiated leiomyosarcoma: Paucity of myofilaments**

Tumour of the small intestine in a 64-year-old woman. In this field the malignant cells are poorly differentiated, with scanty peripheral myofilaments and few attachment zones (arrows). Infrequent small intermediate junctions are present (arrowheads), but external lamina cannot be delineated. There is realtively little RER, but in primitive areas like this the paucity of the myofibrillary apparatus may make the distinction between smooth muscle and other poorly differentiated mesenchymal cells difficult, and at times impossible. (×8400)

**Inset:** 'Star'-shaped configuration of RER. Such profiles are claimed to be a characteristic of the neoplastic cells in leiomyosarcoma. (× 26 200)

# 22  Striated muscle tumours

## MINIMAL CRITERIA FOR THE RECOGNITION OF STRIATED MUSCLE DIFFERENTIATION BY ELECTRON MICROSCOPY

Essential fine-structural criteria for the recognition of striated muscle differentiation in neoplasms include aggregates of elongated thick (15 nm) myosin-like filaments and non-specific thin (5 nm) actin-like filaments, with the formation of abortive sarcomeres (Figs. 22.6–22.8). Non-specific intermediate (10 nm) filaments, most representing desmin,[2435] may also be found (see Table 2.8.). Disaggregated myosin is present in many different cell types and tapering thick myofilaments have now been identified in normal and neoplastic mammalian smooth muscle (see Chapter 21);[2361] such myosin filaments are seen only rarely in smooth muscle and the reasons for their lability are not entirely clear. Therefore, on theoretical grounds, the simple presence of thin and thick filaments (although hitherto often used for the detection of normal fetal myogenesis and rhabdomyoblastic differentiation in tumours)[2425] is inadequate for the unequivocal attribution of striated muscle properties; ideally, organization into sarcomeric structures should also be sought. However, the thick myosin filaments rarely found in smooth muscle tumours do not form banded clusters with the thin filaments; moreover, smooth muscle tumours are in most instances readily distinguishable from embryonal and alveolar rhabdomyosarcomas by LM. Thus, the finding of aggregated parallel thin and thick filaments in *the small round cell tumours* indicates rhabdomyoblastic differentiation, even in the absence of definite sarcomeric arrangements.

In an exhaustive literature review on the ultrastructure of rhabdomyosarcoma, Bundtzen & Norback[2410] proposed that specific sarcomeric markers such as Z-lines are indicators of striated muscle differentiation. However, great caution must be exercised in accepting Z-lines in the absence of thick filaments as being diagnostic. We have encountered sarcomeric caricatures composed of thin filaments with dense Z-line-like bodies in myofibroblasts, and similar structures can occur in smooth muscle and myoepithelial cells. The Z-lines must therefore be sufficiently well developed to be distinguishable from the dense bodies of smooth muscle-like cells, as indicated by a rectangular non-fusiform profile, with the long axis perpendicular to the inserting filaments.

Depending on the extent of cell organization, tumours differentiating as striated muscle often contain other components of the myofilamentous apparatus, including A-, I-, M- or H-bands. In transverse section a regular hexagonal spacing of thin filaments around myosin filaments may be seen.[39,45] These features are developed to the greatest degree in benign myoid tumours such as adult or fetal rhabdomyomas (Figs. 22.1 and 22.2).[2451]

## RHABDOMYOMAS

The fine structure of adult rhabdomyoma may mimic that seen in non-neoplastic disorders of voluntary muscle, and disarrayed sarcomeres and triads, sarcolemmal inversion, and tubular honeycomb structures may be found. Nemaline bodies, similar to those characteristic of nemaline myopathy,[2441] have been consistently recorded in the published ultrastructural studies of adult rhabdomyoma (Figs. 22.3 and 22.4), and are also described in the fetal type.[2432] The accumulation of peripheral lakes of glycogen within the myocytes corresponds to the 'spider web' appearance of some of the cells seen on LM (Fig. 22.1). Fetal rhabdomyomas contain myocytes with a range of differentiation; the filamentous apparatus may be disorganized and mitochondria sparse.[2433] Konrad et al[2433] have also recognized a third type of extracardiac rhabdomyoma — namely that occurring in the female genital tract — in which they described an abundant stroma and an orderly arrangement of myofilaments producing well defined sarcomeres; cytoplasmic bodies similar to those of infantile digital fibroma were also found.

So-called cardiac rhabdomyomas are also characterized by massive intracellular accumulation of glycogen and a myofilamentous content similar to extracardiac rhabdomyomas, but are distinguished by the presence of zebra bodies and both desmosomes and nexus junctions between cells.[2417,2418,2449,2450,2454]

## RHABDOMYOSARCOMA

In rhabdomyosarcomas the number of myofilaments in the malignant cells varies greatly (Figs. 22.6–22.8), even within the same tumour. Some cells may display highly developed transversely aligned sarcomeres, while others contain only non-specific thin filaments.[2438] The identification of elongated thick filaments sometimes requires a prolonged search, and in poorly differentiated tumours lacking cross-striations by LM,

EM will allow a definitive diagnosis in approximately half the cases examined.[45] The immunocytochemical demonstration of cytoplasmic myoglobin, the MM isoenzyme of creatine kinase,[2429] or desmin may also be of value, especially in malignancies resembling rhabdomyosarcoma in other respects, but lacking myosin-like myofilaments. Unfortunately, immunoreactive myoglobin is most readily demonstrable in well differentiated rhabdomyosarcomas, but is undetectable in a significant proportion of the problem group of poorly differentiated rhabdomyosarcoma-like tumours — even in some containing diagnostic myofilaments by EM. Such poorly differentiated tumours lacking either myoglobin or myosin-like filaments can otherwise be classified simply as embryonal sarcomas, as their possible myogenic nature remains unproven; however, their biological behaviour and prognosis conform to those of rhabdomyosarcoma and they are best treated as such.

In neoplasms infiltrating voluntary muscle, degenerating muscle fibres incorporated into the advancing edge of the tumour may show considerable disorganization of myofilaments and simulate rhabdomyoblastic differentiation.[64,2226] This potential source of error can be overcome by:

1. Sampling the neoplasm from sites normally devoid of striated muscle.
2. Ensuring from semithin sections that the tissue sampled is truly representative.
3. Recognizing atrophic myocytes by their sarcolemmal crenellations and continuous pericellular external lamina, often with retraction of the plasma membrane away from redundant folds of lamina (Figs. 0.5–0.8).
4. Identifying diagnostic myofilaments in cells devoid of external lamina.

Finally, other neoplasms which may also show rhabdomyoblastic differentiation must be excluded (Table 22.1).

**Table 22.1 Neoplasms consistently or rarely showing rhabdomyoblastic differentiation**

Fetal rhabdomyoma
Rhabdomyosarcoma (embryonal and alveolar)*

Carcinosarcomas with heterologous elements, including malignant mixed Müllerian tumours
So-called cystosarcoma phyllodes
Sertoli-Leydig cell tumour of ovary with teratomatous-rhabdomyosarcomatous differentiation
Wilms' tumour†
Pulmonary blastoma
Medulloblastoma (medullomyoblastoma)
Malignant intra-ocular medulloepithelioma
Malignant Schwannoma (Triton tumour)
Ganglioneuroblastoma-malignant mesenchymoma
Malignant mesenchymoma
Ectomesenchymoma

*Although rhabdomyoblastic cells have been reported in so-called pleomorphic rhabdomyosarcoma, some of the ultrastructural features illustrated suggest atrophic myocytes (Figs. 0.5–0.9) incorporated into sarcomas as a result of invasion, rather than malignant rhabdomyoblasts; most tumours formerly classified as pleomorphic rhabdomyosarcoma appear to represent malignant fibrous histiocytomas

†See text, Chapter 30

References: 45, 64, 73, 1026, 1213, 1295, 1325, 1427, 2056, 2111, 2163, 2178, 2196, 2221, 2411, 2425, 2427, 2440, 2453, 2687

**Fig. 22.1** *(Facing page)* **Adult-type rhabdomyoma: Survey view and tubular honeycomb array**

Cervical tumour from a 64-year-old man with multicentric rhabdomyomas of the palate and neck, initially interpreted by LM as multiple extrasalivary oncocytomas. The myocyte in this low power electron micrograph contains peripheral lakes of particulate glycogen (G), while the sarcoplasm elsewhere displays many osmiophilic pleomorphic Z-lines (arrows), which are sometimes transversely aligned. (× 5000)

**Inset:** This honeycomb array consists of a regular network of branching tubules averaging 35 nm in diameter. The tubules are continuous with surrounding membranes, consistent with their formation by proliferation of T-tubular membranes. The development of such arrays is a non-specific occurrence, having been described in a number of disorders of striated muscle, including neurogenic atrophy, muscular dystrophies and polymyositis, as well as in rhabdomyomas. (× 34 300)

See also Fig. 0.8.

References: 2229, 2405, 2408, 2413, 2415, 2431–2433, 2435, 2439, 2446, 2448

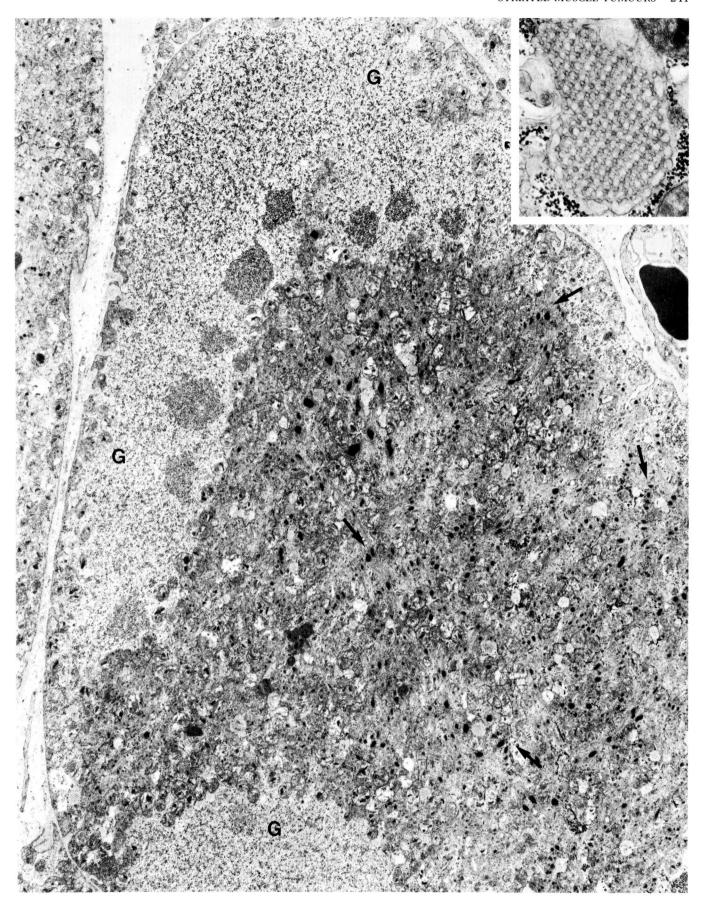

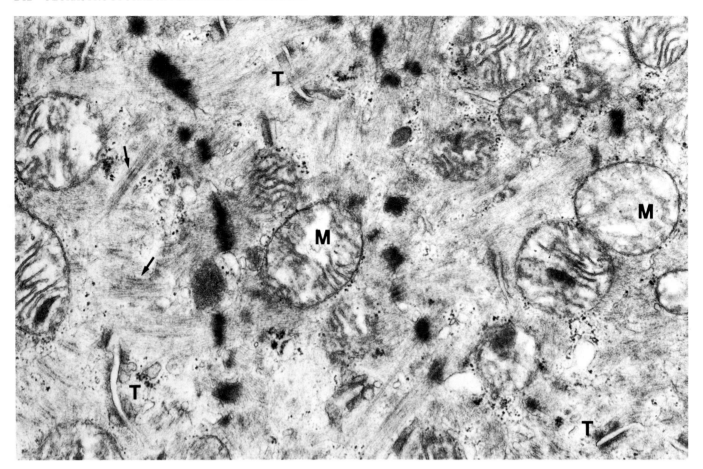

**Fig. 22.2   Adult-type rhabdomyoma: Myofilaments**

In this field there are numerous disarrayed aggregates of fine myofilaments
5–6 nm in diameter, together with smaller numbers of elongated thick myosin-
like myofilaments averaging 15 nm in diameter (arrows). The fine filaments
are often continuous with pleomorphic Z-lines, forming sarcomeric
caricatures, although other bands are not evident. There are also many
disorientated triads (T), whose normal relationship to A–I junctions has been
lost. The mitochondria (M) are prominent; as shown in Fig. 2.5 they
sometimes contain lamellar crystalline inclusions. (× 30 900)

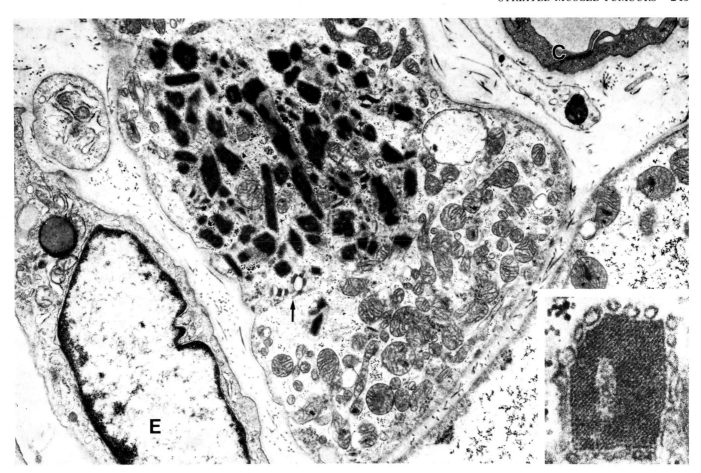

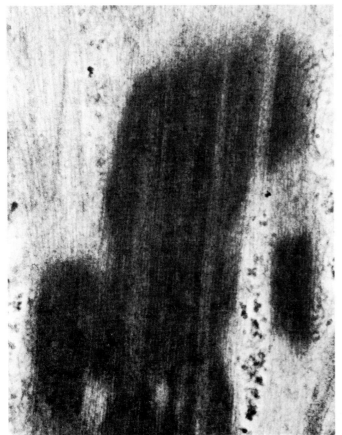

**Fig. 22.3  Adult-type rhabdomyoma: Nemaline bodies I**

A group of elongated osmiophilic nemaline bodies is apparent within the myocyte, together with triads (arrow) and surrounding mitochondria. Portion of a capillary (C) is present at the upper right, and an endothelial cell (E) can be seen at the opposite corner. At higher magnification (inset), a transversely sectioned nemaline body shows a latticed pattern of thin filaments spaced at intervals of about 10 nm and is intimately surrounded by a wreath of small vesicles. (× 12 500. Inset: × 91 100)

**Fig. 22.4  Adult-type rhabdomyoma: Nemaline bodies II**

At high magnification nemaline bodies are seen to consist of parallel fine filaments orientated in the long axis, and there is also a transverse periodicity of 15–17 nm. Note the continuity with fine myofilaments. That nemaline bodies represent modified Z-bands is supported by apparent transitions from Z-lines to these structures, their continuity with thin myofilaments, and their quadratic latticework configuration in transverse section (Fig. 22.3, inset). Although nemaline bodies have consistently been reported in the few fine-structural studies of rhabdomyomas published so far, they have also been described in other muscular disorders, most notably in so-called nemaline myopathy,[2441] but also in polymyositis and centronuclear myopathy. (× 74 100)

See also Fig. 0.9.

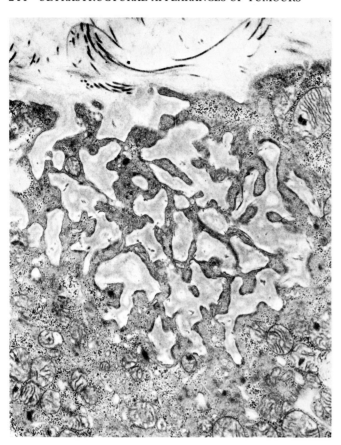

### Fig. 22.5 Adult-type rhabdomyoma: Sarcolemmal inversion

The sarcolemma and its associated external lamina form a complex pattern of inversion into the myocyte, reminiscent of T-tubule development. (× 12 700)

### Fig. 22.6 Rhabdomyosarcoma: Myofilaments and sarcomere formation

Aggregates of thick and thin filaments forming sarcomeric structures are basic diagnostic features; in highly differentiated cases, micro-organoid formations closely resembling normal sarcomeres are found. In this illustration, parallel arrays of both microfilaments and thick filaments (arrowheads) can be seen, the former inserting into Z-disc-like material (arrows). Ribosomes are closely associated with individual myofilaments. (× 24 500)

Primitive cells devoid of differentiating features predominate in poorly differentiated cases and the identification of diagnostic myofilaments may require prolonged scrutiny. Lipid-rich cells simulating lipoblasts have also been reported.[2434]

References: 39, 45, 2226, 2229, 2406, 2407, 2410–2412, 2414, 2420, 2421, 2425, 2426–2430, 2434, 2437, 2438, 2440, 2443–2445, 2447, 2452, 2453, 2455–2458

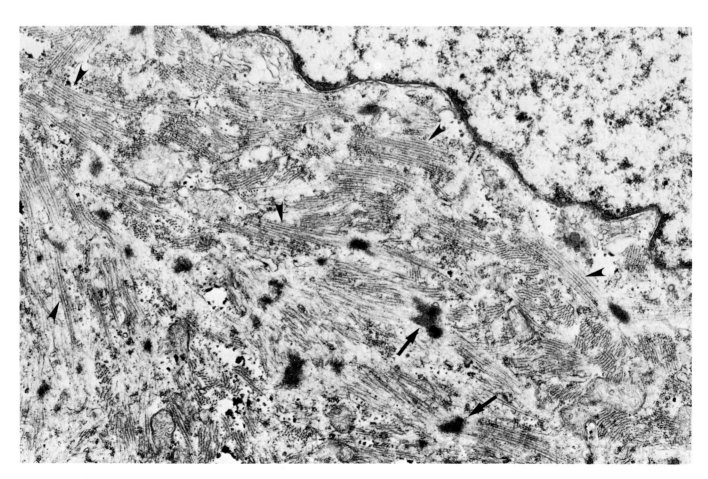

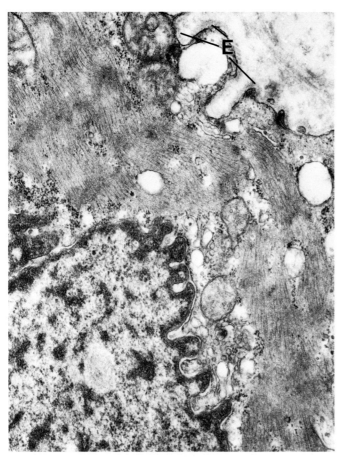

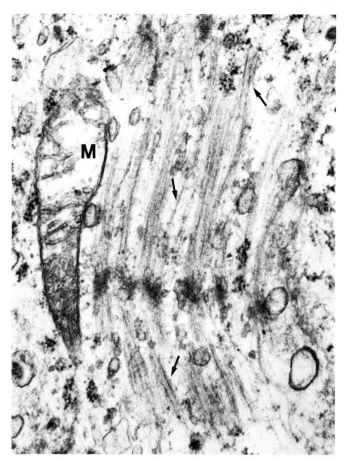

**Fig. 22.7   Rhabdomyosarcoma: Myofilaments**

In this micrograph, striated muscle differentiation is indicated by the roughly parallel arrays of thick filaments and electron-dense zones reminiscent of abortive Z-lines. A mantle of fragmented external lamina (E) borders the cell. In highly differentiated rhabdomyosarcomas the lamina may form a continuous layer which is usually smooth and non-redundant, but in other cases it is fragmentary, if present at all. (× 26 400)

Reference: 2410

**Fig. 22.8   Rhabdomyosarcoma: Myofilaments**

Polypoidal alveolar rhabdomyosarcoma of the nasal cavity, in a 26-year-old woman. These sarcomeric caricatures consist of transversely aligned aggregates of microfilaments averaging 5 nm in diameter, together with fewer thick myofilaments about 15 nm in diameter (arrows) and osmiophilic Z-line-like areas. A swollen mitochondrion (M) is also evident. (Formalin fixation, × 45 500)

The family history in this case is of interest, in that a sister had died of an osteosarcoma at the age of 12 years. Both parents had worked in a uranium reprocessing plant for 9 years.

# 23　Vasoformative tumours

Vasoformative tumours may contain elements resembling endothelial cells, pericytes, or smooth muscle cells, one of which usually predominates.

## ANGIOSARCOMAS: THE RECOGNITION OF ENDOTHELIAL DIFFERENTIATION BY ELECTRON MICROSCOPY

The ultrastructural appearances of angiosarcomas are quite variable. Pericytic, myoid and undifferentiated cells, as well as sporadic extravascular fibroblasts and histiocytes are often present in addition to the predominant neoplastic endothelium.[2471] The diagnosis hinges on the detection of abortive vasoformative structures (Fig. 23.1), but the lumina of the neoplastic vessels are often small in poorly differentiated tumours; the vascular channels may be undetectable by LM — especially in the solid dendritic cell angiosarcoma, which resembles Ewing's tumour by LM[2475] — and are sometimes difficult to visualize by EM (Figs. 23.2 and 23.3). The endothelium is plump, with large irregular nuclei; the cytoplasm is usually plentiful and non-fenestrated, but intraluminal protrusions and discontinuities resembling fenestrae are occasionally seen. Large cytoplasmic vacuoles may also occur, and conceivably represent intracellular microlumina,[2516] as indicated by associated micropinocytotic vesicles and cytoplasmic flaps; they can therefore be considered analogous to the intracytoplasmic crypts of glandular epithelial neoplasms. Intermediate cytofilaments are generally found, while micropinocytotic vesicles are often depleted in comparison to normal endothelium, and junctions are poorly formed. The development of the external laminae is often abortive and fragmentary, but multilayering can occur. Nevertheless, the presence of a basal lamina investing cell clusters is a valuable aid in the detection of small vessels lacking obvious luminal spaces and erythrocytes, while a compressed slit-like lumen and subluminal intercellular junctions are confirmatory findings (Fig. 23.3).

Weibel-Palade bodies are rare,[2516] but should be carefully sought, as they are pathognomonic of endothelial differentiation (see Figs. 3.4, 3.5, 23.3 and 23.5).[39] However, cytoplasmic granules resembling Weibel-Palade bodies warrant careful scrutiny before designation as such, to avoid misidentification of other granular cytoplasmic constituents such as lysosomes. Evidence of the tubular substructure should be present, either in the form of longitudinal periodicity, or circular profiles in transverse section (see Fig. 3.5). It is equally important to ensure that these bodies are present within the neoplastic cells before attributing vasoformative properties to a tumour; in non-endothelial neoplasms, poorly formed stromal blood vessels with swollen endothelium can sometimes be misinterpreted as part of the neoplastic cell population, probably explaining the occasional reports of these granules in tumours such as malignant fibrous histiocytoma.

Endothelial alkaline phosphatase and adenosine triphosphatase activity can be demonstrated in well-formed blood vessels, but are weak or inapparent in solid spindle cell areas.[2471] The immunocytochemical identification of factor VIII-related antigen (VIII-RAG) is a valuable guide to the diagnosis.

## KAPOSI'S SARCOMA

Kaposi's sarcoma continues to be a tantalizing enigma among tumours, because of both its uncertain nature and the possible aetiological implications of its geographic distribution. The recent recognition of this sarcoma as part of the acquired immunodeficiency syndrome (AIDS), suggests a viral aetiology for the tumour, but viral particles are only rarely detectable in the sarcoma cells by EM of biopsy tissue.

The ultrastructural appearances include vascular spaces lined by endothelial cells (Figs. 23.4), often with slit-like lumina and interendothelial gaps.[2500] Pericytic cells may be present near the vascular channels, but a deficiency of pericapillary dendritic pericytes is described, perhaps accounting for areas of telangiectasia.[2500] The stroma is characterized by extravasated erythrocytes, and fibroblastoid cells whose derivation is unclear; the fibroblasts may show avid phagocytic activity[2529] and myoid cells are also reported.[2492] The presence of an endothelial component correlates with the demonstration of factor VIII-RAG in a variable number of tumour cells, and the multiplicity of cell types is perhaps explicable by multidirectional mesenchymal differentiation.

AIDS-related Kaposi's sarcomas are more aggressive than those lacking this association. McNutt et al[2500] report that these aggressive tumours share the ultrastructural appearances of Kaposi's sarcoma unrelated to AIDS, but they additionally exhibit necrosis of individual endothelial cells and entrapment of collagen fibres by prominent cytoplasmic processes.

246

We have also observed a self-limited Kaposiform dermal vasoproliferative reaction in *orf* (infectious pustular dermatosis), a cutaneous poxvirus infection endemic in Australian sheep shearers. In one such case EM easily demonstrated myriads of poxvirus particles, in keeping with orf virus,[140] within the overlying vacuolated keratinocytes.

## SO-CALLED INTRAVASCULAR BRONCHIOLO-ALVEOLAR TUMOUR (IVBAT) AND RELATED LESIONS

IVBAT is a rare distinctive pulmonary tumour whose formerly enigmatic nature has been dramatically clarified in recent times by EM and immunocytochemistry. In a pioneering ultrastructural study, Corrin et al[474] found no indication of bronchiolo-alveolar epithelial differentiation; type II alveolar cell proliferation, presumably reactive, was seen only at the periphery. Instead, the tumour cells displayed endothelial differentiation, including tubulated cytoplasmic granules conforming to Weibel-Palade bodies (Fig. 23.5), and myofilaments were also present. Subsequent studies[441,450,596] confirm these observations — although Weibel-Palade bodies are not always detectable;[441] they are reinforced by the immunohistological demonstration of factor VIII-RAG in many of the tumour cells.[450,475]

The natural history of IVBAT has long been uncertain, but its malignant character has recently been confirmed by extra-thoracic spread and hepatic metastasis.[450,596] It can therefore be regarded as an indolent epithelioid angiosarcoma of lung[450] and has a number of morphological features in common with a group of extra-pulmonary epithelioid endothelioses including epithelioid haemangioendothelioma,[2530] endovascular papillary angioendothelioma of the skin[2480] and 'leiomyosarcomatosis possibly arising from hamartomas of the liver'.[2482] These conditions are characterized by stromal sclerosis, a low rate of metastatic spread and a prolonged natural history.[450]

By virtue of its propensity to extend along vascular channels, IVBAT also has similarities to malignant angioendotheliomatosis (MA). EM has demonstrated Weibel-Palade bodies in the incohesive intravascular cells of MA, but sclerosis is not seen and the clinical course is rapid.[2512,2531,2711] However, the exact status of MA is unclear, and some cases appear to represent angiotropic lymphomas.

## HAEMANGIOPERICYTOMA

The neoplastic cells of haemangiopericytomas are arranged concentrically around blood vessels.[2474] The layers of the component cells vary from tightly packed to loosely arranged patterns. The cells have processes of varying length, some of which form sporadic intermediate junctions with others of their kind, and junctions are occasionally numerous (Figs. 23.8 and 23.9). The external laminae at the abluminal aspect of the cells are often poorly formed, but loosely packed external lamina-like material sometimes accumulates between adjoining

cells. A few actin-like microfilaments are often present, particularly at the luminal aspect of the cells. Similarly, micropinocytotic vesicles are preferentially distributed within the subluminal cytoplasm. In addition, multidirectional differentiation in the form of smooth muscle, fibroblastoid cells, myofibroblasts, phagocytes and possibly endothelium, is recorded.[39,2474]

The role of EM in the evaluation of haemangiopericytomas is limited by two factors:

1. The characteristic architectural features are frequently lost in poorly differentiated tumours, where the relationship of the neoplastic cells to blood vessels is inapparent.
2. An haemangiopericytoma-like pattern may be found in a variety of tumours by LM, as listed in Table 23.1

The diagnosis is therefore dependent on the demonstration of a pure and typical haemangiopericytic pattern by LM, with EM playing only a secondary role in selected cases (see footnote to Table 23.1).

**Table 23.1  Some tumours and tumour-like lesions which may show an haemangiopericytoma-like pattern***

Haemangiopericytoma

Granuloma pyogenicum
Lymphangiomyoma
Congenital generalized and localized fibromatosis (infantile myofibromatosis)
Infantile fibrosarcoma
Congenital/infantile haemangiopericytoma
So-called minute pulmonary chemodectoma
Angioblastic meningioma†
Cerebellar haemangioblastoma
Fibrous histiocytoma of soft tissues
Glomus tumour
Epithelioid smooth muscle tumours (leiomyoblastoma)
Leiomyosarcoma
Dedifferentiated liposarcoma
Synovial sarcoma
Mesenchymal chondrosarcoma§
Endometrial stromal nodules and sarcomas
Phaeochromocytoma
Juxtaglomerular cell tumour
Mesothelioma
Thymoma
Carcinoid tumour
Primitive neuroectodermal tumour[2196]

*As assessed by light microscopy; in this table the description 'haemangiopericytoma-like' is used in its broadest sense

†See text, Chapter 17

§Although a pericytic pattern is seen consistently in mesenchymal chondrosarcoma, the neoplastic cells have little resemblance to either normal pericytes or those comprising haemangiopericytomas (see Chapter 25).[2579] Similarly, the pericyte-like areas of thymomas consist of epithelial cells,[2670] and the fine structure of some of the other tumours listed above (such as phaeochromocytoma and juxtaglomerular cell tumour) is quite distinctive. In contrast, the haemangiopericytoma-like areas in malignant fibrous histiocytoma[2651] and synovial sarcoma have pericytic ultrastructural features; we have also found foci of haemangiopericytic differentiation in a pleomorphic sarcoma of bone complicating Paget's disease.

## HAEMANGIOBLASTOMA

Usually affecting the cerebellum, this tumour has haemangiopericytoma-like appearances on EM and consists of vascular channels, lined by fenestrated endothelium[2529] and surrounded by pericytes and stromal cells. The stromal cells are the most distinctive component (Fig. 23.10), and contain varying numbers of intermediate filaments, together with lipid droplets, whorled collections of SER and micropinocytotic vesicles. Hirano bodies are also recorded and there is an adjacent fragmentary external lamina.[2529]

## OTHER VASCULAR TUMOURS, GLOMUS TUMOUR AND SCLEROSING HAEMANGIOMA OF LUNG

Apart from a paucity or absence of Weibel-Palade bodies, endothelial fine structure in *haemangiomas* does not usually deviate greatly from normal; benign angiomatous lesions are not considered further, because they pose no diagnostic dilemmas on LM.

Ultrastructural studies have also demonstrated that *glomus tumours* consist almost entirely of smooth muscle cells,[2359,2400] rather than endothelial cells or pericytes as postulated earlier (see Fig. 21.1).

The nature of the *so-called sclerosing haemangioma of lung* continues to arouse controversy, with conflicting ultra-structural interpretations. Some investigators[494,515] describe endothelial characteristics, while the majority favour epithelial differentiation.[503,504,518,561] Mixed epithelial and mesenchymal features are also reported.[558] Katzenstein and associates[514] recently documented nine cases in which they found evidence of mesothelial differentiation. Factor VIII-RAG and muramidase were undetectable in the six tumours examined by immunocytochemistry, and Weibel-Palade bodies could not be found in the seven cases studied by EM, thereby virtually excluding endothelial differentiation. The cells possessed prominent interdigitating cytoplasmic processes and a discontinuous external lamina, and were linked by intermediate-type junctions. True desmosomes with convergent tonofilaments were not seen. In five instances the tumour cells formed acinar-cystic spaces, and in two of these the lining microvilli resembled those usually seen in mesotheliomas. Electrophoresis of two cases revealed a strong band of hyaluronic acid characteristic of mesothelioma.

The fine structure of cardiac myxoma is discussed in Chapter 24.

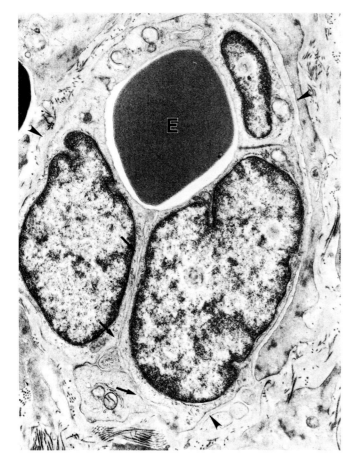

**Fig. 23.1 Angiosarcoma: Endothelial cells forming blood vessel I**

Angiosarcoma of spleen from a 60-year-old woman. Figs. 23.1–23.3 are all from this case and form a tripartite sequence of diminishing vasoformative properties.

Haemangioendothelial differentiation is shown clearly in this field; the neoplastic endothelium surrounds a small channel containing an erythrocyte (E). Elsewhere the lumen forms a slit-like space (arrows). Basal lamina (arrowheads) surrounds the vessel. (× 11 400)

Closed endothelial fenestrations are uncommon in angiosarcomas; if present, they are usually confined to highly differentiated areas. Discontinuities and spaces resembling fenestrae are seen occasionally. Large intracytoplasmic vacuoles are also reported, and are thought to represent abortive subcellular vascular lumina.

References: 765, 1396, 2226, 2229, 2475, 2479, 2493, 2499, 2502, 2507, 2509, 2516, 2517, 2533

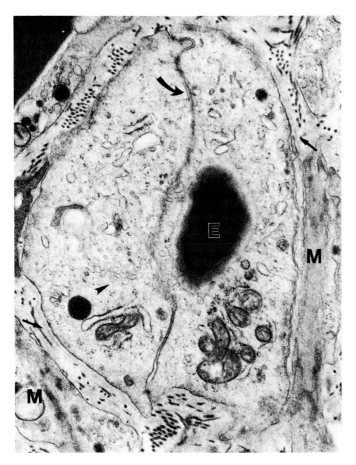

**Fig. 23.2 Angiosarcoma: Endothelial cells forming blood vessel II**

Small vascular spaces lined by plump endothelial cells usually predominate in angiosarcomas, but the vasoformative character of the tumour may not be immediately obvious because the lumina are often reduced to slit-like spaces (curved arrow). Because of obliquity of sectioning, the luminal erythrocyte (E) appears to be situated outside the compressed lumen. Micropinocytotic vesicles (arrowhead) are concentrated around the lumen, but are also present at the abluminal aspect of the endothelium. The vessel is partly surrounded by a poorly formed basal lamina (straight arrows). Two of the perivascular cells have the features of smooth muscle (M). (× 19 900)

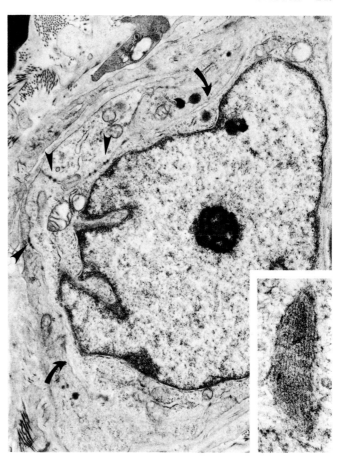

**Fig. 23.3 Angiosarcoma: Endothelial cells forming blood vessel III, and Weibel-Palade body**

The vascular lumen is represented by a slit-like channel (curved arrows), while the interendothelial spaces are punctuated by poorly developed junctions (arrowheads). The cytoplasm is scanty in proportion to the irregular nucleus, which contains much euchromatin and a moderately prominent nucleolus. (× 10 800)

**Inset:** Weibel-Palade bodies with the typical periodicity are rarely found in the malignant endothelial cells. (× 55 400)

**Discussion:** Two criteria must be fulfilled before granules resembling Weibel-Palade bodies assume diagnostic significance in a suspected vasoformative tumour:

1.  It must be established that the granules represent *bona fide* Weibel-Palade bodies by their characteristic rod-shaped tubular fine structure.
2.  It must be proven that the cells containing these structures represent neoplastic cells rather than the stromal microvasculature.

See also Figs. 3.4 and 3.5.
Reference: 2478

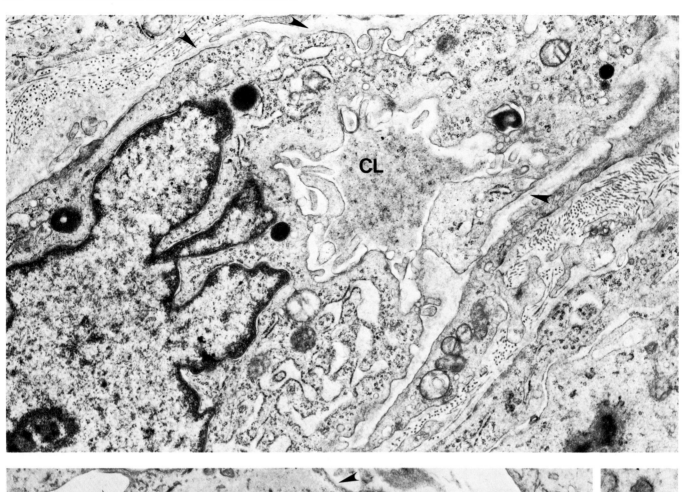

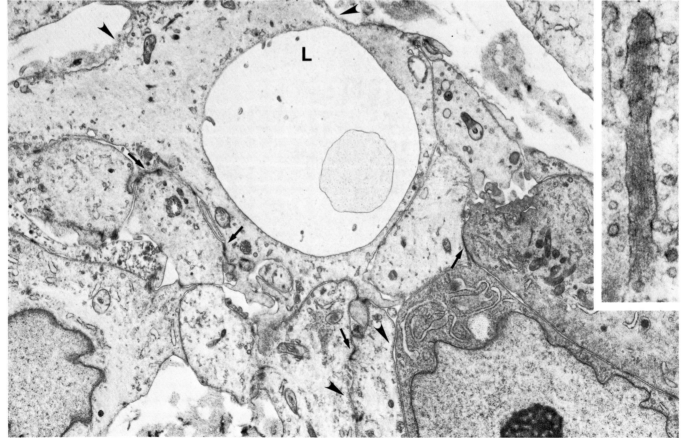

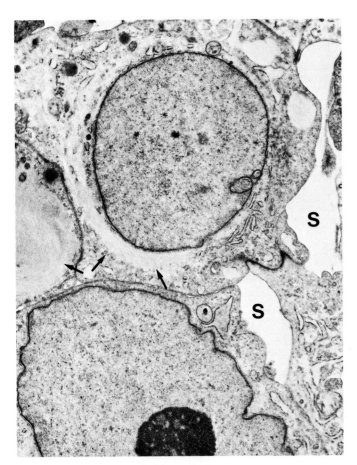

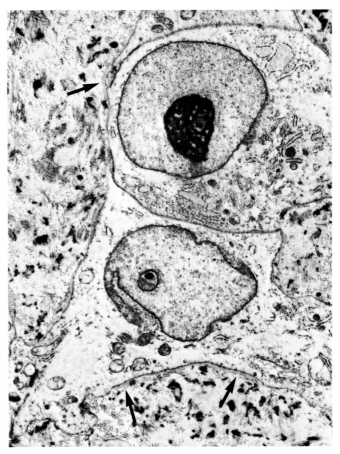

**Fig. 23.6 IVBAT: Endothelial features II**

Micropinocytotic vesicles and intercellular junctions are again depicted. The extracellular space (S) is focally expanded, in keeping with an abortive vascular lumen. Intermediate filaments are prominent within the cytoplasm (arrows). Focal densities resembling those of smooth muscle cells were occasionally associated with the filaments elsewhere. In addition to the predominant endothelial differentiation, smooth muscle-pericytic features have previously been described. (× 10 400)

**Fig. 23.7 IVBAT: Sclerotic area**

Here the tumour cells are surrounded by an abundant matrix containing collagen and elastin fibres. Note the fragmentary external lamina (arrows) investing the cell group. (× 8300)

Figs. 23.5–23.7 are all from the same case and are pathognomonic of endothelial differentiation.

**Fig. 23.4** *(Facing page — top)* **Kaposi's sarcoma: Survey**

Tumour from a 2-year-old child born in Sardinia. The neoplastic cells form a small capillary-like lumen (CL). The nucleus is large and irregular, and contains a moderately prominent nucleolus. External lamina (arrowheads) surrounds the vascular structure, while pericytic processes in turn surround the lamina. (× 17 500)

Cross-banded linear structures similar to those illustrated in malignant fibrous histiocytoma (see Fig. 20.9) may ocupy the cisternae of the RER;[2529] erythrophagocytosis by endothelial cells is evident occasionally[2529] and there is an encompassing variably developed external lamina.

References: 2226, 2229, 2476, 2492, 2500, 2529

**Fig. 23.5** *(Facing page — bottom)* **So-called intravascular bronchiolo-alveolar tumour (IVBAT): Endothelial features I, including Weibel-Palade body**

One slightly irregular nucleus contains much euchromatin and a prominent central nucleolus. Micropinocytotic vesicles are aligned along the closely apposed plasma membranes (arrowheads) and there are diminutive intercellular junctions (arrows). One of the cells contains a prominent rounded intracytoplasmic lumen (L) bordered by micropinocytotic vesicles, consistent with a subcellular vascular channel. (× 9300)

**Inset:** Classical Weibel-Palade bodies were found in a few cells in this case. (× 61 600)

(Case contributed by Prof. B. Corrin).

References: 441, 450, 474, 475, 596

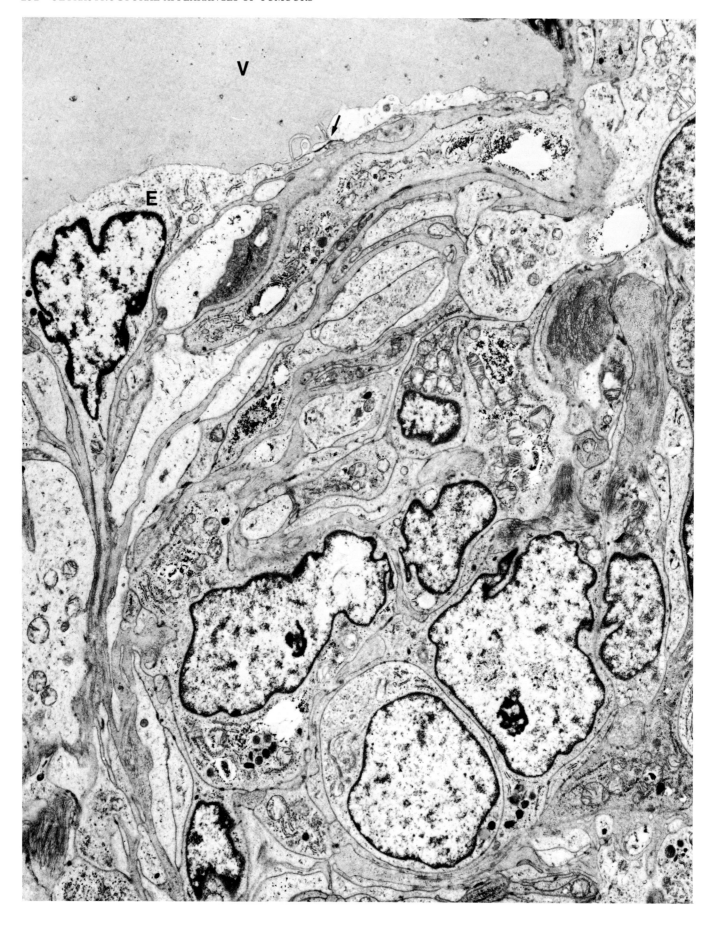

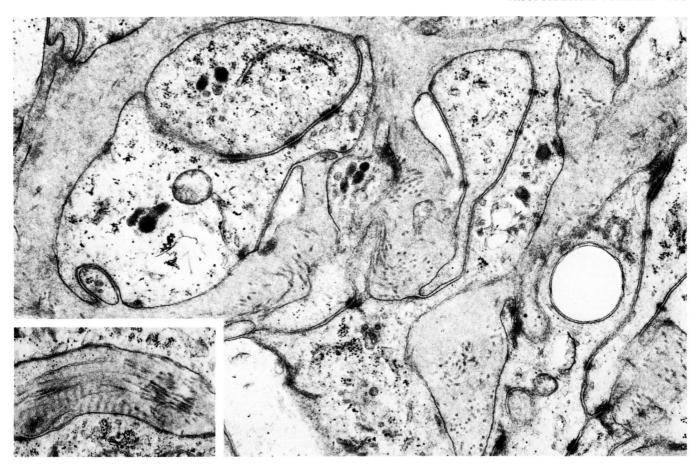

**Fig. 23.9 Haemangiopericytoma: Cell processes and fibrous long-spacing collagen**

The cell processes often enfold each other, and there is an unusually high concentration of intermediate junctions. Small plasma membrane-associated dense plaques are also present. **Inset:** Intercellular long-spacing collagen in the same tumour (Table 3.4). (× 28 400. Inset: × 25 200)

**Fig. 23.8** *(Facing page)* **(Malignant) haemangiopericytoma: Low power survey**

Presacral haemangiopericytoma in a 61-year-old man. One of the endothelial cells (E) lining the vascular space (V) appears to delve deeply into the perivascular area. Interendothelial junctions are present (arrow). Most of the field is occupied by pericytes which have complex interdigitating cytoplasmic processes. These are partly surrounded by external lamina, with small amounts of intervening collagen. (× 7100)

Eleven months after resection of the primary tumour, the patient underwent removal of an apparently solitary pulmonary metastasis. LM revealed a sclerosing extensively dedifferentiated haemangiopericytoma, but the cells were no longer recognizable as pericytes by EM. Instead, they resembled modified fibroblasts, albeit with sporadic foci of external lamina, groups of cytoplasmic 10 nm filaments and scattered intermediate junctions; interlocking cell processes and grouping of cells around blood vessels were no longer discernible. A transition to endothelial cells is also recorded in the literature.[2474]

EM is of no value in predicting the biological behaviour of haemangiopericytomas, the exercise being difficult and often impossible by LM.

References: 772, 1252, 2226, 2474, 2484, 2490, 2495, 2501, 2503, 2505, 2506, 2508, 2511, 2514, 2515, 2523, 2529

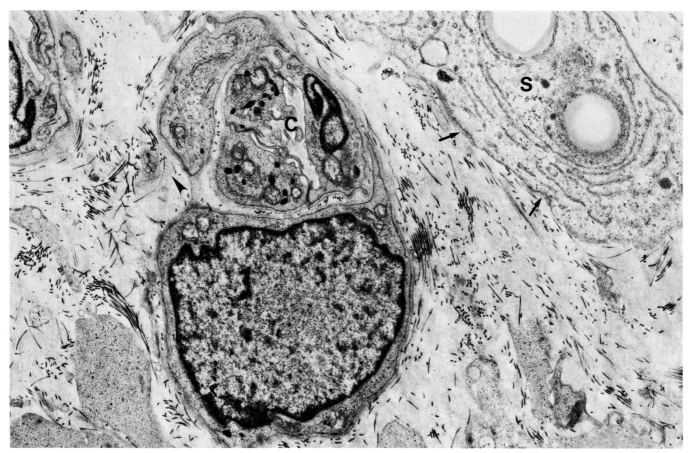

**Fig. 23.10 Cerebellar haemangioblastoma: Survey**

A small capillary (C) surrounded by a prominent pericyte traverses an interstitium consisting of a few small poorly packed collagen bundles, together with amorphous osmiophilic material and 100 nm collagen (arrowhead). Portion of a lipid-containing stromal cell (S) with a fragmentary external lamina (arrows) is also present. (× 10 200)

References: 1934, 1961, 2003, 2005, 2472, 2477, 2483, 2522

# 24 Miscellaneous soft tissue tumours

Miscellaneous tumours of mesenchymal soft tissues are considered in this chapter. The nature of some is obscure, but the ultrastructural appearances may nevertheless be of diagnostic value, notably in alveolar soft part sarcoma. In other cases such as synovial sarcoma and cardiac myxoma, EM is of considerable conceptual interest, but has little diagnostic value.

## CARDIAC MYXOMA

The notion that cardiac myxomas might simply be organized thrombi was laid to rest long ago and they are now generally regarded as neoplasms, a concept strongly supported by a case complicated by 'embolic' phenomena in the choroid plexus and bone, with continued growth of the 'emboli' over a decade.[2469] Nevertheless, the nature of these tumours has remained elusive. Various cell types have been reported, including myxoid, endothelial and smooth muscle cells, as well as fibroblasts, myofibroblasts and macrophages. An origin from multipotent mesenchymal cells,[2463] endocardium, endothelium, vasoformative reserve cells and myofibroblasts has been variously proposed. Feldman et al[2462] could not identify multiple distinct cell classes and thought that the cells shared features of smooth muscle and fibroblasts (myofibroblasts); chondroid features have also been described.[2459] However, the endothelial-endocardial nature of cardiac myxoma is supported by the immunocytochemical demonstration of factor VIII-related antigen in the constituent cells.[2468]

## ALVEOLAR SOFT PART SARCOMA (ASPS)

The nature of this strange tumour is disputed.[2186,2215] The fine structure is typified by cytoplasmic aggregates of membrane-bound crystalloidal material with a periodicity of 10 nm, and numerous mitochondria (Figs. 24.1 and 24.2).

A resemblance between the crystalloids and the material in Z-lines and nemaline bodies has been claimed as evidence of myoid differentiation.[2190] However, neither Z-line material nor nemaline bodies become membrane-bound during myogenesis, and filaments are not usually seen in alveolar soft part sarcoma.[2186] Paraganglionic differentiation has been proposed,[2239] and similar crystalloids are described in a malignant paraganglioma.[30] Nevertheless, virtually identical crystalloids have also been reported in other seemingly unrelated situations, including a Schwannoma (see Table 2.6).

DeSchryver-Kecskemeti et al[2182] have proposed that ASPS represents a 'malignant angioreninoma', based on the demonstration of immunoreactive renin in the neoplastic cells, a suggested fine-structural resemblance of the cytoplasmic crystalloids to renin protogranules, and the crystalloidal zinc content on X-ray microanalysis. They also describe ultrastructural evidence of smooth muscle differentiation in the form of focal external lamina, membrane-associated dense plaques, micropinocytotic vesicles and longitudinally orientated fine filaments with dense bodies, leading to the postulate that the 'cell of origin' is a modified smooth muscle cell. Nevertheless, these observations need to be evaluated with considerable reservations:

1. The renin protogranules of juxtaglomerular (JG) cells are characterized by transverse periodicity instead of the longitudinal linear pattern typifying the crystalloids of ASPS (Fig. 24.2B1).
2. The crystalloids of ASPS show greater morphological diversity than JG granules.
3. As a general consideration, the identification of an antigenic secretory product in a neoplasm is not *necessarily* pathognomonic of a particular cell lineage in the absence of other corresponding differentiating properties.
4. The cytoplasmic architecture in the case of ASPS illustrated in this atlas (Fig. 24.1) bears a resemblance to endocrine epithelium, with no evidence of smooth muscle differentiation. However, immunoreactive desmin and vimentin have been detected in ASPS,[2183] suggesting smooth muscle properties.
5. Unlike JG cell tumour of the kidney, ASPS is unassociated with systemic hypertension.

These reservations are reinforced further by the report of Mukai et al[2215] who were unable to detect renin, tropomyosin, neurone-specific enolase, S-100 protein or myelin proteins by immunohistochemistry in any of their three cases of ASPS. Extracts of tumour tissue did not contain significant levels of renin on biochemical analysis, the activity being far less than in normal kidney (approximately 0.15–1.0 per cent), while inactive renin was undetectable. These authors raise serious doubts as to the specificity of the antibody used by DeSchryver-Kecskemeti et al[2182] and conclude that the nature of ASPS remains an open question — a view with which we are in complete agreement.

## SO-CALLED SYNOVIAL SARCOMA

The derivation of synovial sarcoma is also contentious,[2188,2559] and may be quite unrelated to synovial membranes; although often developing in juxta-articular locations, these tumours are usually anatomically separate from either synovial membranes or tendon sheaths, and occurrence within joint cavities is exceptional.[2188,2538]

Fibroblastoid cells, mast cells and collagenous connective tissue are seen in the stromal component (Fig. 24.4). The tubular component in *biphasic synovial sarcoma* strikingly resembles glandular epithelium and consists of cuboidal cells resting on a basal lamina (Fig. 24.3); microvilli and occasional cilia project into the luminal space, and junctional complexes occur between adjoining cells. Although the stromal fibroblastoid cells are similar to synovial B cells, they are devoid of specificity, and the tubular elements bear little resemblance to either normal or hyperplastic synovium.

Synovial membranes are normally lined by two cell types,[2548] namely type A cells resembling macrophages (with prominent Golgi complexes and pinocytotic vesicles, but little RER) and fibroblastoid type B cells (with plentiful RER, but a relative paucity of vesicles and Golgi complexes). Intermediate forms combining these features occur (type C cells) and several authorities believe that type A and B cells simply represent structural-functional modulations of a single cell line,[189,2546,2559] although there is evidence that type A cells originate from bone marrow whereas type B cells do not.[2541]

Intercellular junctions are usually inapparent in routinely processed human synovium;[2559] junctions may become obvious in hyperplastic synovial disorders such as rheumatoid arthritis, but there is little similarity to the junctional complexes bordering gland-like spaces in bimorphic synovial sarcoma. Furthermore, the interface between the lining cells and the subsynovium in normal synovial tissue is indistinct, lacking a basal lamina, in stark contrast to the tubular component of synovial sarcoma.

The very existence of an embryologically distinct synovial lining is questionable.[2541] In the absence of movement, synovium does not develop in the embryo;[2541] conversely, synovial membranes with the characteristic lining cells can form in pseudoarthroses.[2559] Edwards et al[2541] have accordingly proposed that *'synovial lining is simply an accretion of macrophages and fibroblasts stimulated by mechanical cavitation of connective tissue.'* Any neoplasm differentiating as synovium would therefore be expected to have a fibrohistiocytic morphology.

Glandular differentiation in soft tissue tumours is not unique to synovial sarcoma and occurs rarely in Schwannomas,[2103] for which a synovial 'histogenesis' has never been seriously proposed (see text of Chapter 18). The epithelial character of the tubular component of synovial sarcoma is further supported by immunohistochemical studies; the epithelium-like cells contain cytokeratins, but are devoid of vimentin, whereas the spindle cells contain vimentin without cytokeratins.[2537,2555]

The term 'synovial sarcoma' should therefore be viewed as one of diagnostic and prognostic convenience rather than a reflection of histogenetic reality; *'adenosarcoma of soft tissues'* would seem a more accurate designation, the tubular elements perhaps explicable by a process of epithelial metaplasia developing in a mesenchymal malignancy.

The identity of a *monophasic fibrous synovial sarcoma* (MFSS) is no less controversial than the nature of the biphasic form. Ghadially[2559] dismisses the concept as *'. . . absurd. If it is not biphasic then it is not a synovial sarcoma'.* Others believe that a monophasic form exists and is distinguishable from fibrosarcoma and other sarcomas by LM, on the basis of a characteristic spindle cell pattern with tight cellular whorls, haemangiopericytic areas, a paucity of collagenization, and often an admixture of numerous mast cells.[2188, 2552] It is also known that the tubular foci of biphasic tumours may be exceedingly sparse and subtle in appearance, and are easily missed unless a large number of tissue blocks is subjected to meticulous examination.[2552] Krall et al[2552] reported abortive tubular properties in an ultrastructural analysis of three monophasic tumours. Schmidt & Mackay[2559] found that the cells comprising MFSS were identical to the spindle cell component of biphasic tumours; in addition, they claimed distinctive features for the cells of MFSS, including bland rounded nuclei, close apposition of cells, thickening of adjacent plasma membranes and fewer cytoplasmic organelles than fibroblasts. Mickelson et al[2554] studied four MFSS by EM; they detected occasional intermediate junctions together with a relative lack of collagen synthesis, and considered the findings distinct from both the biphasic form and fibrosarcoma. Cytokeratin-positive cells are also recorded in apparently pure MFSS.[3148] The balance of these observations would favour the existence of a monophasic fibrous variant of the tubulofibroblastoid malignancy we have been discussing above, but the 'synovial' appellation is no more appropriate, if no less entrenched.

In an ultrastructural study, Cooney and associates[2177] have supported a previously proposed common synovial histogenesis for epithelioid sarcoma, so-called chordoid sarcoma and MFSS.[2196] This support is based in part on the identification of pseudoacinar spaces with 'microvilli or filopodia' and 'related tight junctions', as well as condensation of extracellular matrix into external lamina-like material. The accompanying electron micrographs are unfortunately inconclusive; the junctions have a distinct intermembranous space, resemble intermediate rather than 'tight' junctions and are not subluminal in location. Such membrane specializations lack discriminant value, and we have already noted that mesenchymal cells such as myofibroblasts and smooth muscle possess both intermediate-type junctions and external lamina without implying 'synovial' properties. The pseudoacinar spaces, some of which contain collagen fibres, can be alternatively interpreted as focal micro-expansions of the intercellular matrix or dilatation of invaginating vacuolar membranes accompanying oligociliogenesis. The microvillous projections appear to lack filamentous cores and more closely resemble plasmalemmal flaps. Assigning synovial characteristics on the basis of such non-specific findings because of a vague similarity to bimorphic synovial sarcoma — which in any case is morphologically quite different to normal synovium — has beclouded the literature. This type of histogenetic fantasy arguably finds its ultimate codification in the concept of 'tendosynovial sarcoma',[2196] which gathers biphasic and monophasic synovial sarcoma, epithelioid sarcoma, so-called chordoid sarcoma and clear cell sarcoma into a single nosological conglomerate.

The entire situation can therefore be summarized:

1. *Normal synovial lining cells have fibroblastoid-histiocytoid characteristics.*
2. *Neoplasms differentiating as synovium would predictably exhibit genealogically non-distinctive fibrohistiocytic properties, of the type seen in giant cell tumour and fibroma of tendon sheath, pigmented villonodular synovitis and fibrous histiocytomas.*
3. *The glandular component of bimorphic synovial sarcoma has epithelial features dissimilar to normal synovial membranes.*
4. *Claims of 'synovial histogenesis' for other sarcomas based on a resemblance to biphasic synovial sarcoma are therefore specious.*

## CLEAR CELL SARCOMA OF TENDONS AND APONEUROSES

The nature of clear cell sarcoma (CCS) is disputable.[2226,2542] Melanin pigment is seen in some cases, and typical melanosomes within the clusters of closely apposed epithelioid cells have been identified on ultrastructural examination (Figs. 24.6 and 24.7).[2170,2173,2198] However, a proposed division into 'synovial' and melanocytic subtypes[2232] is tenuous (see preceding discussion). CCS is perhaps most appropriately viewed as a malignant blue naevus, a malignant melanotic nerve sheath cell tumour, or a malignant melanoma[2176] of soft tissues.

## EPITHELIOID SARCOMA

Ultrastructural studies of epithelioid sarcoma have been largely preocupied with the vexed question of 'histogenesis', but have not conclusively established its nature. The epithelioid cells vary from polygonal to spindled, and possess distorted nuclei and plentiful cytoplasm.[2189,2193] The cell peripheries sometimes form elaborate processes, described as filopodial, microvillous or interdigitating.[2189,2193,2205,2211]

A proportion of the cells contain abundant intermediate filaments,[2206] which are the most characteristic cytoplasmic component, often being concentrated in the perinuclear territory (Fig. 24.5), and with finger-print-like condensations in one case.[2205] Presumably responsible for the cytoplasmic eosinophilia by LM, these 10 nm filaments resemble those seen in fibrous histiocytomas (see Fig. 20.10), but this class of filament lacks morphological specificity. Immunocytochemical

analysis of an epithelioid sarcoma has disclosed vimentin in the absence of both cytokeratins and desmin.[2211] However, in a more recent study Chase et al[3146] have reported the presence of immunoreactive cytokeratins within the epithelioid cells in 24 of 32 cases (vimentin and other intermediate filaments were not investigated in this series). Sporadic intercellular junctions (variously designated as 'tight junctions',[2211] 'true desmosomes'[2193] and 'desmosome-like'[2205]) occur between closely apposed plasma membranes of the epithelioid cells.

Cystic or pseudoacinar spaces are also described[2193] and these sometimes contain amorphous matter, fine fibrils and collagen fibres. Miettinen et al[2211] report gland-like spaces, but the accompanying electron micrograph is not convincing.

A resemblance to synovial sarcoma, nodular synovitis[2218] and normal synovium has been claimed, because of the acinus-like spaces, cell processes and intercellular junctions, and a 'synovial' histogenesis accordingly invoked.[2193,2205,2211] However, conclusive glandular organization of these features and typical junctional complexes have not been illustrated to our knowledge, and the epithelioid cells lack an external lamina.[2205,2218] For these reasons and those already discussed we find the arguments for a relationship to bimorphic synovial sarcoma — much less a 'synovial' derivation — inconclusive. We do not find the reported presence of cytokeratins decisive by itself, since we have identified cytokeratins within mesenchymal cells on one occasion, and there are considerable differences between epithelioid and synovial sarcoma in both LM appearances and anatomical distribution — including the predilection of epithelioid sarcoma for the skin and subcutis. Fibrocytic properties have been alternatively proposed,[2189] and it is noteworthy that the surface flaps of macrophages may assume elaborate patterns resembling microvilli; myofibroblasts are also recorded in this tumour.[2205] On the basis of current knowledge we consider that epithelioid sarcoma cannot be accurately classified.

## EXTRASKELETAL EWING'S TUMOUR, CHONDROSARCOMAS AND OSTEOSARCOMA

The ultrastructural appearances of these extraskeletal tumours are essentially identical to their osseous analogues and they are therefore not considered here (see Chapter 25). An extraskeletal small cell tumour resembling atypical Ewing's sarcoma is illustrated in this atlas, but the electron micrographs appear in Chapter 25 to emphasize the morphological spectrum of the tumour (see Fig. 25.9).

## UNCLASSIFIABLE SARCOMAS

Some sarcomas are so poorly differentiated that no identifying features can be detected by either LM or EM. In such instances histochemical or immunocytochemical procedures may prove useful, as well as ultrastructural evaluation of tumour maintained in tissue culture or transplanted into nude mice,[193] but a small percentage will always remain unclassifiable.

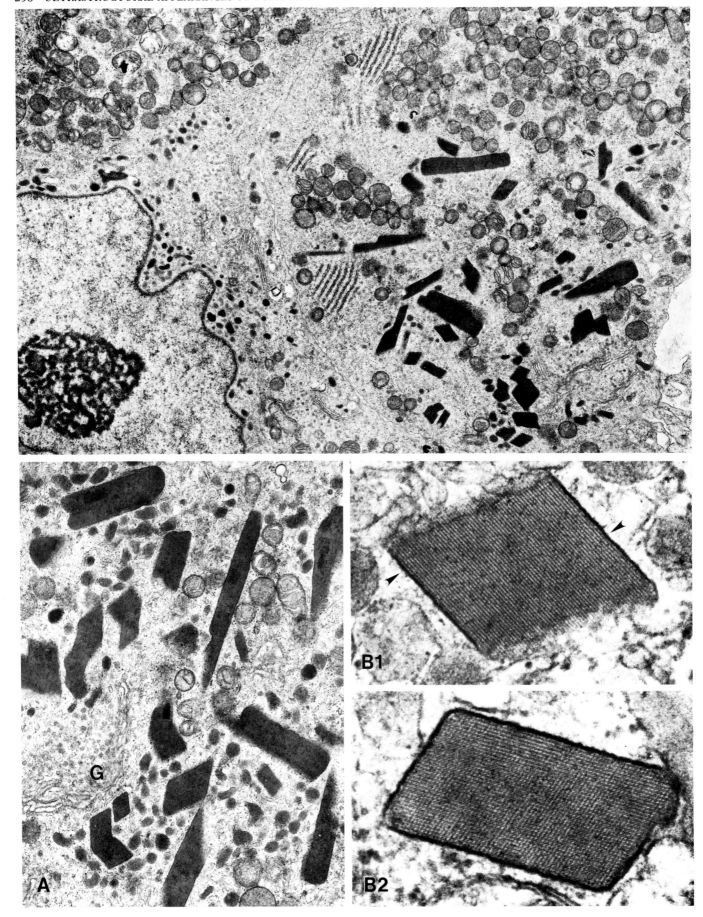

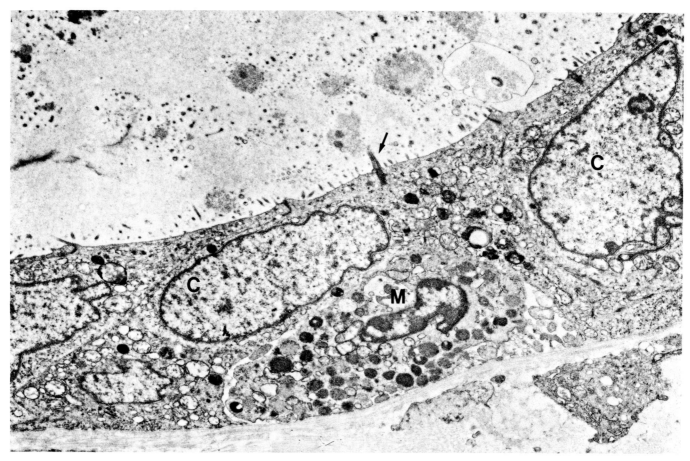

**Fig. 24.3  Synovial sarcoma: Tubular component**

The tubular component of this neoplasm consists of cuboidal cells (C) with large irregular nuclei. The cytoplasm contains lipofuscin granules. Microvilli and cilia (arrow) project into the lumen of the tubule which also contains flocculent electron-dense material. The cells rest on a thin basal lamina; mast cells (M) are present between adjoining cuboidal cells. (× 8000)
References: 362, 2226, 2538, 2539, 2544, 2545, 2547, 2551, 2553, 2556, 2557, 2559

**Fig. 24.2** *(Facing page — bottom)* **Alveolar soft part sarcoma: Crystalloids and granules**

**A:** The Golgi complex (G) with associated small vesicles can be seen, and there are numerous rounded and elliptical membrane-bound granules in the adjacent cytoplasm. The crystalloids shown here are thought to evolve from the granules, and their outlines encompass needle-like, rhomboidal and irregular shapes. (× 14 500)
**B1:** The crystalloid detailed here in longitudinal section has a regular linear paracrystalline substructure, spaced at intervals of approximately 10 nm. Membranes are closely applied to two parallel sides of this rhomboidal profile (arrowheads). (× 100 100)
**B2:** A regular cross-hatched configuration is evident in this transverse plane through another crystalloid. The point-to-point spacing again approximates 10 nm. Note the membrane closely investing all sides of this profile. Compare with the nemaline bodies shown in Figs. 22.3 and 22.4. (× 120 600)

Although highly characteristic, these crystalloids may only be present in about one-third of alveolar soft part sarcomas and Erlandson[39] could not find them in six consecutive cases; however, the ultrastructural diagnosis is problematical in their absence.
Figs. 24.1 and 24.2 are from the same case.
Reference: 39

**Fig. 24.1** *(Facing page — top)* **Alveolar soft part sarcoma: Cell morphology**

Tumour of leg in a 22-year-old man. The nucleus is slightly irregular and contains abundant euchromatin. The nucleolonema forms a skein-like pattern. Numerous mitochondria are evident in the cytoplasm, as are stacked lamellae of RER and prominent Golgi complexes. Rounded and elliptical granules are concentrated in the juxtanuclear region of one cell, while the cytoplasm of the adjoining cell contains numerous crystalloids including elongated and rhomboidal forms. Cytoplasmic filaments are conspicuous by their absence. (× 8800)

The organellar complement and cell organization resemble the pattern seen in endocrine tissues, and a paraganglionic derivation has been proposed, but no monoamines were detected in this case by formaldehyde-induced fluorescence.[2186]

(Case contributed by Dr. T. O. Ekfors).
References: 39, 45, 2182, 2186, 2190, 2191, 2215, 2226, 2229, 2235, 2239

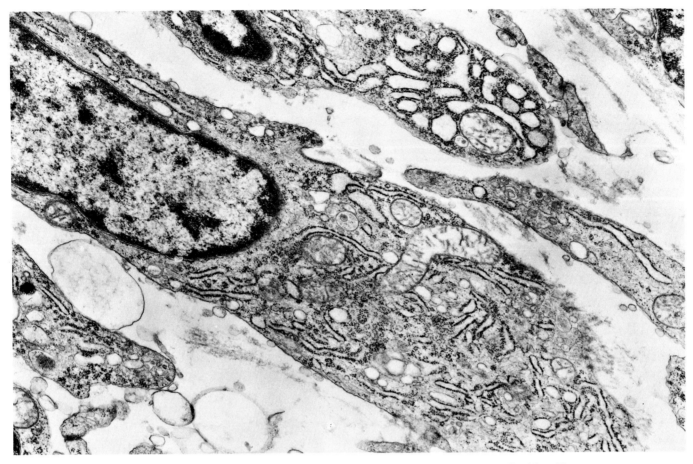

**Fig. 24.4  Synovial sarcoma: Fibroblastoid component**

The spindle cell component surrounding the tubular structures (Fig. 24.3) has obvious fibroblastic features; scattered collagen fibres are interspersed between adjoining cells. Intermediate junctions may be encountered between the spindle cells in this neoplasm. (× 17 000)

**Fig. 24.5  Epithelioid sarcoma: Cytoplasmic detail**

Intermediate filaments occupy much of the cytoplasm of this cell and are seen in both longitudinal and transverse section, the latter being indicated by the arrowheads. Although the most characteristic cytoplasmic feature of epithelioid sarcoma, prominent collections of intermediate filaments are not specific for this neoplasm; compare with Fig. 20.10 (malignant fibrous histiocytoma). Micropinocytotic vesicles are arrayed along the closely apposed plasma membranes. (× 36 900)

**Inset:** Small intermediate junctions between adjoining cells have been documented repeatedly in epithelioid sarcoma. Compare with Figs. 3.16 and 20.7 (intermediate junctions between myofibroblasts and in malignant fibrous histiocytoma), and with Figs. 4.3 and 5.3 (desmosomes in squamous and adeno-carcinomas). (× 19 900)

References: 2189, 2193, 2205, 2206, 2211, 2218, 2226, 2233

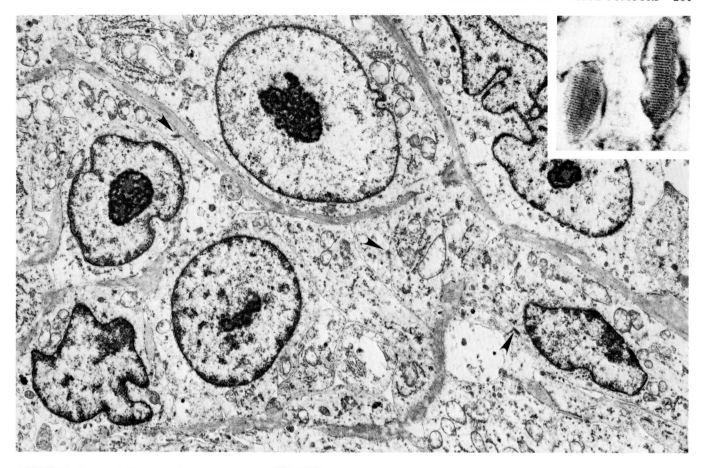

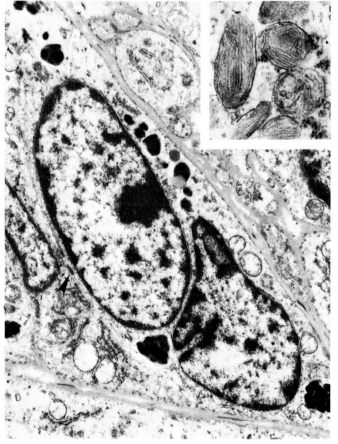

## Fig. 24.6 Clear cell sarcoma of tendons and aponeuroses: Architecture and melanosomes

Tumour from the sole of foot of a 32-year-old woman. The lump had been present for 'several years'.

Nucleoli are typically prominent. A thick external lamina invests cell groups and individual cells; in other cases laminal material may be inconspicuous or absent. Electron-dense melanosomes are quite inconspicuous in this poorly melanized area. The cytoplasm contains moderate numbers of mitochondria and a few strands of RER. Mitochondria, glycogen particles and Golgi complexes are prominent in some cases. A few intercellular junctions can be discerned (arrowheads). (Formalin fixation, × 8600)

**Inset:** Melanin is detectable in many cases of clear cell sarcoma. In this instance, stage II melanosomes were easily identified, even in areas which were amelanotic by LM. (Formalin fixation, × 89 900)

References: 2170, 2172, 2173, 2176, 2198, 2200, 2202, 2217, 2226, 2232, 2542

## Fig. 24.7 Clear cell sarcoma of tendons and aponeuroses: Melanosomes

Melanotic area of the tumour shown in Fig. 24.6. Electron-dense stage III-IV melanosomes are evident in the cytoplasm. External lamina and poorly developed intercellular junctions (arrowhead) are also present. (Formalin fixation, × 9900)

**Inset:** Atypical stage I–II melanosomes with a pleated coil configuration in the same case. (Formalin fixation, × 37 500)

# 25 Tumours of cartilage and bone

The ultrastructural pathology of bone tumours has been reviewed recently by Roessner & Grundmann,[2631] and Steiner.[2647]

## STROMAL CHARACTERISTICS OF CHONDROID AND OSTEOBLASTIC TUMOURS

In addition to the fine structure of the component cells, the stromal morphology of chondroid and osteoblastic tumours is of diagnostic value (see also Chapter 3). Cartilaginous matrix is typified by a loose pattern of proteoglycan granules together with collagen fibres and filaments (Figs. 25.1–25.3), and giant collagen fibres (amianthoid fibres) are found occasionally.[47,2581]

In contrast, the stroma of osteogenic sarcoma is characterized by focal hydroxyapatite deposition.[2602,2659] The hydroxyapatite crystals appear as dense spicules closely apposed to collagen fibres (Fig. 25.6), and their chemical characteristics can be elucidated by elemental X-ray microanalysis. The pattern of stromal mineralization has similarities to that seen in normally calcifying tissues and healing fractures. So-called extracellular matrix vesicles (EMV) and calcifying nodules have been reported in addition to hydroxyapatite and the haphazardly dispersed collagen fibres.[2638] The matrix vesicles represent membrane-bound structures 50–450 nm in diameter and are claimed to be the initial sites of calcification.[2638] In osteosarcomas they are associated with high levels of alkaline phosphatase, pyrophosphatase and ATPase, which promote mineralization by antagonizing the inhibitory effects of ATP and pyrophosphate on calcification. The resultant accretion of hydroxyapatite spicules is followed by rupture of the vesicle membrane and the formation of calcospherites. Nevertheless, the status of EMV as distinctive centres of calcification is open to serious doubt and others, notably Ghadially,[47] regard them as cell debris on which calcium may be preferentially precipitated. In accordance with this view, stereological analysis of normal epiphyseal growth plates demonstrates that EMV are concentrated in resting zones remote from sites of calcification.[2628] It seems likely that they are derived from degenerating chondrocytes, even though their content of phospholipid, electrolytes and possibly enzymes is said to differ from that of the plasmalemmal regions of chondrocytes. The unmineralized osteoid matrix consists of collagen fibres associated with finely granular material.[2647]

## CHONDROID NEOPLASMS

With the exceptions of chondroblastoma,[2603] dedifferentiated chondrosarcoma,[2593] and mesenchymal chondrosarcoma,[2579,2649] the architecture of chondroid neoplasms often closely simulates normal cartilage; the matrix is plentiful, and pericellular depletion of filaments (Fig. 25.3) corresponds to the lacunae seen by LM. The neoplastic cells have scalloped margins, with small processes protruding into the interstitium (Fig. 25.1). Glycogen is often abundant, particularly in clear cell and myxoid tumours.[2579,2601] Lipidic globules vary in both number and size, and are not usually prominent. The amount of RER also varies, but the Golgi apparatus is moderately developed.

Roessner & Grundmann[2631] claim to have identified ultrastructural differences between benign and malignant chondroid cells. Benign cartilaginous tumours are characterized by a low nuclear:cytoplasmic ratio and abundant organelles including small mitochondria, as well as glycogen rosettes and perinuclear intermediate filaments. On the other hand, the chondroid cells of highly malignant chondrosarcomas have irregular and atypical nuclei, an elevated nuclear:cytoplasmic ratio and poorly developed surface projections; there is also depletion of organelles such as mitochondria, as well as filaments, and glycogen (except in clear cell chondrosarcomas). Nevertheless, these nuclear alterations are evident by LM, which is still the mainstay of diagnosis, along with the clinical features, anatomical localization and x-ray findings. An ultrastructural prediction of biological behaviour in conflict with these findings would seem adventurous indeed.[2647]

*Benign epiphyseal chondroblastoma* is composed of large polyhedral cells with irregular and often multilobate nuclei, microvillous cytoplasmic protrusions, a perinuclear Golgi complex, small mitochondria and intermediate filaments.[2631] The nuclear fibrous lamina is often thickened,[2647] a phenomenon also observed in chondromyxoid fibroma[2647] (see Fig. 1.4). The extracellular matrix is sparse.

*Dedifferentiating foci of chondrosarcoma* are said to contain mesenchymal cells embedded in a sparse matrix, resembling the cellular areas of mesenchymal chondrosarcoma[2593] and with intermediate junctions between cells. The chondroid areas of one such dedifferentiating tumour were composed of chondrocytic cells with the typical intervening granulo-filamentous matrix.

The well differentiated areas of *mesenchymal chondro-sarcoma*[2579,2649] contain relatively mature chondrocytic cells. In contrast, the cellular areas are composed of undifferentiated polygonal cells with smooth plasma membranes, and numerous free ribosomes and polyribosomes. These cells resemble Ewing's sarcoma cells,[2647] but contain little or no glycogen; they surround vascular spaces where there are few associated pericytes, and impart the haemangiopericytoma-like morphology seen by LM. The extracellular matrix is sparse. Elongated closely apposed fibroblastoid cells with intermediate junctions are also present, and transitional zones combining these patterns are described.[2649]

The malignant cells in *extraskeletal myxoid chondrosarcoma* (EMCS) show a fine-structural continuum, ranging from chondroblasts with peripheral cytoplasmic processes to undifferentiated mesenchymal cells.[2231] So-called 'chordoid' sarcoma has similar cartilaginous properties and can be considered to represent a form of EMCS;[2209,2231,2238] the report of Cooney and associates[2177] purporting to show synovial features can be discounted (see Chapter 24).

## CHORDOMA AND CHONDROID CHORDOMA

In contrast to the chondroid appearances discussed above, 'conventional' chordomas consist of aggregates of cells with desmosomal junctions and interdigitating cytoplasmic processes. Microvilli, pinocytotic vesicles and glycogen particles are usually present. The processes enclose rounded extracellular spaces corresponding in part to the physaliferous configuration on LM,[2631] while other vacuoles appear to be sequestered within the cytoplasm. In addition, small cytoplasmic vacuoles are produced by dilatation of the endoplasmic reticulum.

Distinctive mitochondria-RER complexes have also been described in the vacuolated physaliferous cells; they consist of flattened filamentous mitochondria alternating with single cisternae of the RER (Fig. 25.10).[39] Their significance is unclear.

To the best of our knowledge there is only one report documenting the ultrastructure of chondroid chordoma.[2655] The chordoid areas consisted of cells with chordoma-like features, including desmosomes, tonofilaments, short cytoplasmic processes, and mitochondria-RER complexes as illustrated in Fig. 25.10; in addition, intracisternal coated parallel tubules (see Fig. 8.5) were observed. In contrast, the cells comprising the chondrosarcoma-like regions had chondrocytic appearances.

## OSTEOGENIC SARCOMA

Osteosarcomas contain pleomorphic fibroblastoid cells with copious RER (seen as elongated and dilated cisternae, and vacuoles of varying size), but other classes of mesenchymal cells can also be identified. Depending on the pattern of appearances, Garbe et al[2580] divided the constituent cells into three types: atypical tumour osteoblasts, osteoblasts with varying degrees of maturity, and chondrocytic cells. On the other hand, Grundmann et al[2585] defined seven cell categories; undifferentiated and osteoblastic cells, osteocytes (surrounded by mineralized matrix), fibroblasts and myofibroblasts, chondroblasts and angioblasts. Similar findings were reported by Aho & Aho[2560] who recognized six cell types (fibroblastic, myofibroblastic, chondroblastic, osteoblastic, histiocytic and unclassified).

Even more recently, Martínez-Tello & Navas-Palacios[2614] have published a detailed ultrastructural study of 27 osteogenic sarcomas (18 'conventional', one associated with Paget's disease, two metastatic, five parosteal and one periosteal). They described the basic cells as osteoblast-like and also found chondrocytic, fibroblastic, myofibroblastic, histiocytoid and osteoclast-like cells, as well as multinucleated osteoblastoid cells, primitive cells, endothelium and pericytes. Malignant-appearing cells with plentiful dilated RER (Figs. 25.4 and 25.5) and a collagenous stroma with hydroxyapatite crystals (see above) were thought to be most characteristic of osteosarcoma. In an ultrastructural study of 10 cases of 'conventional' osteosarcoma, Shapiro[2641] reported the distinctive features to include malignant osteoblasts with abundant dilated RER, poorly differentiated osteoblasts with sparse RER in annular or lamellar arrangements, and undifferentiated cells; nuclear irregularity, marginated chromatin, multiple nucleoli and intracellular filaments were also typical. However, the appearances cannot always be distinguished from osteoid osteoma and osteoblastoma. Similarly, the fibroblastic, chondroid and fibrohistiocytic areas are morphologically indistinguishable from fibrosarcoma, chondrosarcoma and malignant fibrous histiocytoma respectively. Myofibroblasts, although rare in conventional osteogenic sarcoma, are numerous in parosteal osteosarcoma and they sometimes have conspicuously thickened nuclear fibrous laminae.[2614]

A small cell (microcellular) variant of osteosarcoma liable to be mistaken for atypical Ewing's sarcoma has recently been recognized.[2605,2629] EM in one such case revealed irregular nuclei and sparse cytoplasm containing moderate amounts of focally dilated RER. Glycogen was inconspicuous and the interstitium contained both collagen and amorphous material; hydroxyapatite was not detected,[2629] but Llombart-Bosch et al[2605] mentioned the presence of intercellular osteoid.

## GIANT CELL TUMOUR (GCT) OF BONE

The nature of the stromal cells in GCT as seen by routine LM is unclear,[2631] but ultrastructural examination reveals fibro-histiocytic properties, with multiple cell types. The dominant stromal cell is an ovoid to bipolar fibroblastoid cell with abundant RER (stromal cell type I).[2564,2631] The next most frequent cell is histiocytic, with rich acid phosphatase activity and a well developed Golgi apparatus (stromal cell type II). A third stromal cell has lymphocytoid appearances.[2631]

The giant cells resemble multinucleated histiocytic giant cells (see Fig. 20.13), containing up to 20 nuclear profiles per cell. The RER is abundant, and there are numerous mitochondria and sporadic lysosomes; intranuclear filaments are also described. The periphery of the giant cells may form short microvillous processes. The ruffled borders typical of osteoclasts are generally absent; if present, they tend to be sporadic and are unassociated with mineralized bone matrix.[2647]

## FIBROSARCOMA, MALIGNANT FIBROUS HISTIOCYTOMA, LEIOMYOSARCOMA AND ANGIOSARCOMA OF BONE

The ultrastructural appearances of these bone tumours are identical to their soft tissue counterparts as discussed in Chapters 20, 21 and 23.

## EWING'S SARCOMA

Although illustrated here, the fine structure of this perplexing tumour is compared with that of other small round cell tumours in Chapter 29 (see Table 29.1).

The nature of Ewing's sarcoma has remained an engima ever since its original description, and has not been solved by EM; endothelium, pericytes, smooth muscle, neuroblasts, mesenchymal cells, plasma cells and myeloblasts have been variously proposed as a potential cell of origin.[2184] Llombart-Bosch et al[2605,2609] recognize an angiogenic variant, while Schmidt et al[2637] claim to have detected sporadic neuritic features in Ewing's sarcoma of bone (Rupert Willis[2660] reversed rather than revisited!; see text, Chapter 29).

In contrast, Berthold et al[2171] intensively studied an extraskeletal Ewing's tumour and found negative reactions for specific and non-specific acetylcholinesterase, and catecholamine histofluorescence by the glyoxylic acid technique. Cultured tumour cells were exposed to a number of factors favouring the expression of neuronal properties in neuroblastoma cells, without any such morphological differentiation. Explanted Ewing's sarcoma cells have also been shown to produce simultaneously types I, III and IV collagen, perhaps favouring extremely primitive mesenchymal differentiation.[2184,2185]

## ADAMANTINOMA OF LONG BONES

Although endothelial properties have been ascribed to this type of adamantinoma,[2607] other studies convincingly illustrate epithelial features with well-developed desmosome-tonofilament complexes, indicating squamous differentiation.[2599,2622,2635] Immunoreactive cytokeratins have also been identified in the neoplastic cells, whereas factor VIII-related antigen was undetectable.[2599]

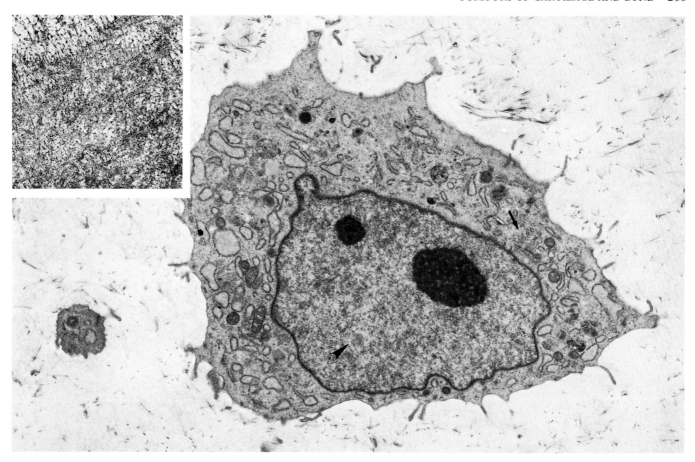

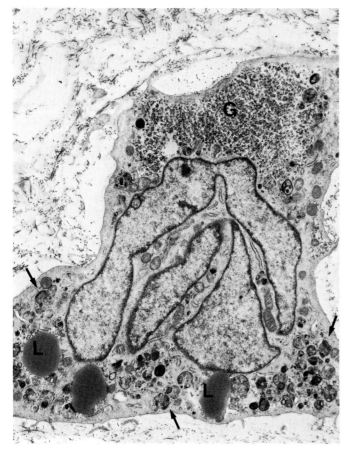

**Fig. 25.1   Chondrosarcoma and chondroma: Malignant chondrocyte morphology I, and extracellular matrix**

Highly differentiated chondrosarcoma of rib. The nucleus is characterized by slight irregularity, nucleolar prominence, and abundance of euchromatin; a nuclear body is also evident (arrowhead). Dilated cisternae of RER inhabit the cytoplasm. Although inconspicuous in this cell, the Golgi apparatus (arrow) was prominent in others. The characteristically scalloped periphery of chondrocytes is maintained, with flaps and spikes protruding into the interstitium. Pericellular depletion of collagen fibres is not evident (Fig. 25.3). Proteoglycan granules and so-called matrix vesicles were prominent elsewhere. (× 8500)

**Inset:** Chondroma. The chondroid nature of such neoplasms is indicated by the arrangement of the matrical components, including a lattice of filaments and granules within the cartilaginous matrix. (× 44 000)

In mesenchymal tumours the essential ultrastructural features of chondrocytic differentiation include numerous dilated strands of RER (sometimes containing finely granular intracisternal material resembling the extracellular matrix), as well as lipid droplets and glycogen rosettes.[2181]

References: 2175, 2181, 2225, 2230, 2231, 2238, 2562, 2568, 2575, 2576, 2579, 2581, 2593, 2601, 2615, 2621, 2631, 2646, 2647

**Fig. 25.2   Chondrosarcoma: Chondrocyte morphology II**

Marked nuclear irregularity is an obvious feature of this cell, and aggregated glycogen granules (G) are apparent. The cytoplasm also contains lipid droplets (L) and numerous lysosomes (arrows), possibly representing degenerative alterations. There are fewer cytoplasmic protrusions than in the chondrocyte shown in Fig. 25.1, but collagen fibres are more plentiful in the extracellular matrix. Same case as Fig. 25.1. (× 6700)

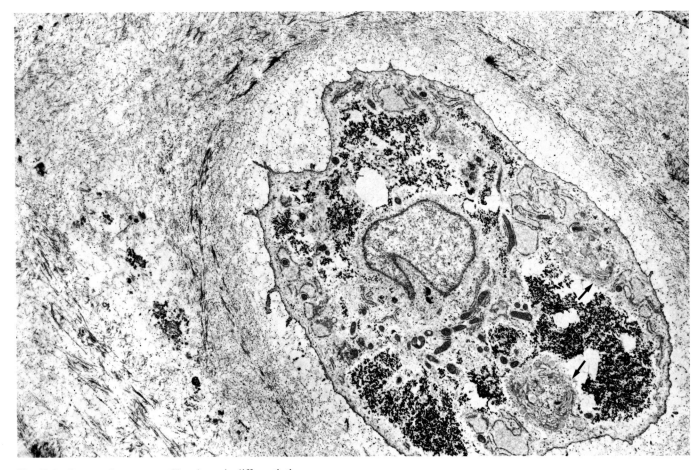

**Fig. 25.3   Osteogenic sarcoma: Chondrocytic differentiation**

Lower femoral tumour in a girl aged 16 years. The cell pictured here has the typical features of chondrocytic differentiation; nuclear chromatin is evenly distributed, the Golgi apparatus (arrows) and dilated RER are evident, and there are considerable quantities of particulate glycogen. The plasma membrane is unevenly scalloped, while the surrounding cartilaginous matrix contains a network of delicate fibrils and granules. There is a pericellular capsule in which the fibrils are inconspicuous, coresponding to the lacunae seen by LM. (× 5700)

The appearances in this field are indistinguishable from well differentiated chondrosarcoma.

**Fig. 25.4** *(Facing page)*   **Osteogenic sarcoma: Neoplastic cells**

Several mesenchymal cell types can be recognized in osteosarcomas (see text), the predominant cell usually being described as fibroblastoid or osteoblastic, and characterized by plentiful RER.

These sarcomatous cells have highly irregular nuclear profiles. The plasma membranes are also irregular, often forming ruffles, while abundant, focally dilated RER is apparent. The RER sometimes contains flocculent material of medium density; intracisternal coated parallel tubules resembling those described in malignant melanoma (see Fig. 8.5) are rarely present.[2613] Collagen bundles inhabit the stroma (S), but hydroxyapatite crystals are not evident in this field. (× 5100)

**Discussion:** Mitochondria are occasionally numerous and may contain calcific inclusions. Cytoplasmic lipid droplets and glycogen are recorded, as are perinuclear filaments, intracytoplasmic collagen[2647] and primitive intercellular junctions.[2580]

Steiner[2647] described two types of multinucleated giant cells in osteosarcomas; one contained abundant RER, while the other had osteoclast-like features, with numerous mitochondria, but lacked a ruffled periphery. In contrast, the giant cells in the 10 cases reported by Shapiro[2641] did not resemble osteoclasts; thought to develop by fusion of mononuclear tumour cells, they were characterized either by plentiful dilated RER, or by cytoplasm with only scattered mitochondria and flattened cisternae of RER.

References: 305, 391, 1216, 2036, 2237, 2560, 2573, 2577, 2580, 2582, 2585, 2595, 2596, 2602, 2613, 2614, 2626, 2627, 2629, 2632, 2639, 2641, 2647, 2659

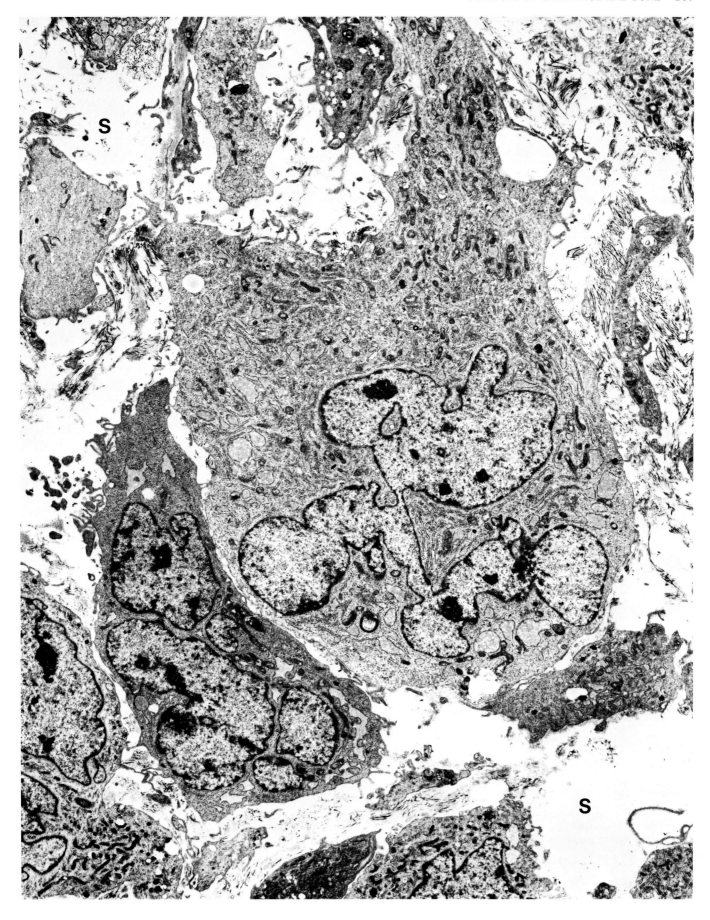

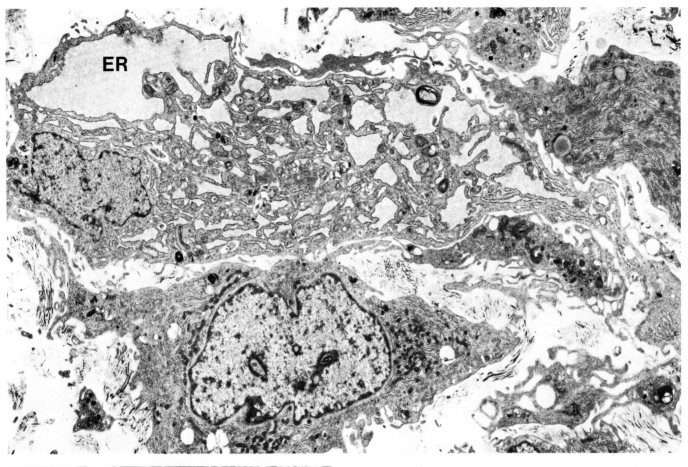

**Fig. 25.5 Osteogenic sarcoma: Neoplastic cells and dilated rough endoplasmic reticulum**

The RER (ER) in one of these cells is markedly dilated, and there are prominent peripheral cytoplasmic flaps. (× 6200)

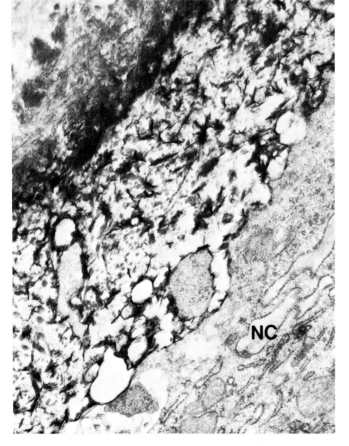

**Fig. 25.6 Osteogenic sarcoma: Hydroxyapatite deposition**

Calcification has occurred in this area of the sarcoma. Spicules of hydroxyapatite are present on the surface of the neoplastic cell (NC), and they surround collagen fibres in the interstitium. X-ray microanalysis of one such area revealed both calcium and phosphorus peaks. (× 22 800)

References: 2602, 2639, 2659

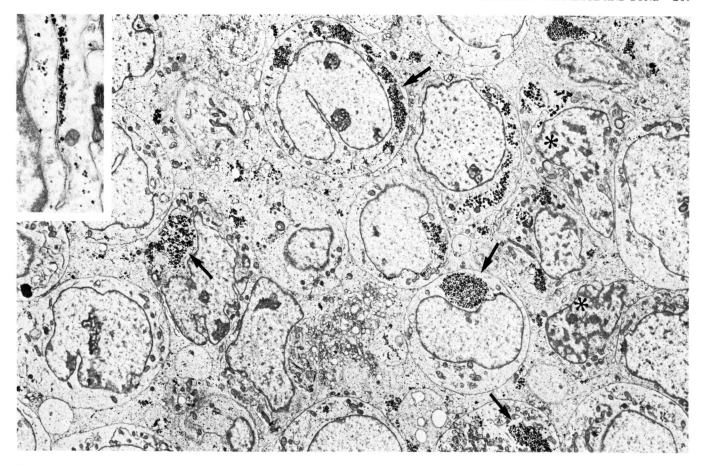

**Fig. 25.7  Ewing's sarcoma: Survey**

Close apposition of the rounded tumour cells is characteristic. The nuclei are mildly irregular and possess small nucleoli. Intermediate cells (*) with irregular nuclei and condensed chromatin are also evident (Fig. 25.9). Large aggregates of glycogen rosettes are present in the cytoplasm (arrows). (× 3700)

**Inset:** In some cells a close association is observed between glycogen particles and cisternae of the endoplasmic reticulum; the glycogen may also be spatially related to lipid droplets (Fig. 25.9C). (× 17 500)

**Discussion:** Pseudopod-like cell processes have been reported, but microtubules and mitochondria are rare within them. Glycogen granules may lie free in the interstitium; typically, there is little stroma between the neoplastic cells, and intracellular collagen is not present.

SEM of both typical and atypical forms of Ewing's sarcoma reveals rounded to polygonal cells with smooth contours; devoid of ruffles, the surface is interrupted by only sporadic groups of stubby microvillous processes and isolated cilia.[2608]

See Table 29.1.

References: 45, 2184, 2570, 2578, 2588, 2592, 2605, 2606, 2608, 2609, 2611, 2623, 2631, 2634, 2637, 2647, 2650

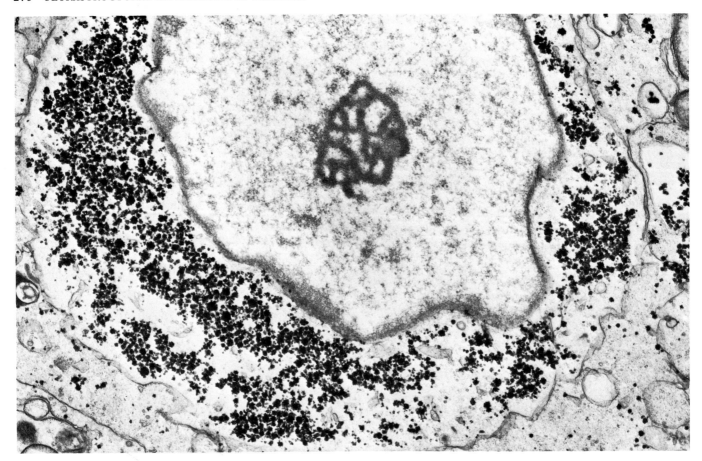

**Fig. 25.8 Ewing's sarcoma: Cell detail**

Large lakes of glycogen rosettes are seen. Some authors have described small intercellular junctions, but these are generally not prominent. Variable quantities of glycogen, cytoplasmic filaments, mitochondria, and profiles of endoplasmic reticulum have been reported in atypical cases (Fig. 25.9). (× 12 400)

**Discussion:** Ultrastructural assessment of cases of suspected Ewing's sarcoma may be facilitated by ensuring optimal preservation of glycogen. It is notable that *en bloc* staining with uranyl salts results in considerable extraction of glycogen. Lead staining is mandatory, and fixation with Karnovsky's osmium tetroxide-potassium ferricyanide fixative enhances glycogen preservation and demonstration.[156,2611] Although glycogen accumulation characterizes many neoplasms (see Table 2.10 and Fig. 2.16), it typically occurs as rosettes in Ewing's tumour; in other small round cell tumours (see Chapter 29) it is often seen in monoparticulate form, although rosettes have been detected, for example, in rhabdomyosarcoma.[47]

References: 47, 156, 2611

**Fig. 25.9** *(Facing page)* **Extraskeletal small cell tumour resembling atypical Ewing's sarcoma: Topography and cell detail**

Intramuscular tumour of the axillary region, in an 11-year-old girl. The neoplasm was not related to a nerve trunk, there was no paresis after its removal, and immunocytochemical studies for cytoplasmic myoglobin were negative.

**A:** The cell population shown in this field includes rounded pale cells, a smooth-contoured darker cell, and apparently degenerate cells with clumped heterochromatin, conforming respectively to the primary (P), intermediary (I) and secondary (S) cells which have been described in Ewing's sarcoma. The nuclei of the primary cells are occasionally grooved, and have little heterochromatin. Nucleolar margination is evident. There are scattered mitochondria and a few profiles of RER but cytoplasmic organelles are poorly represented. (× 5600)

**B:** The nucleus of this primary cell shows a shallow indentation, and the cytoplasm contains a few lysosomes and short profiles of RER; glycogen particles are infrequent. Blunt cell processes, microtubules, and dense-core granules were not evident (see Table 29.1). **Inset:** A few intercellular junctions were found, as shown here. (× 10 300. Inset: × 80 900)

**C:** Glycogen rosettes were generally not conspicuous; this electron micrograph depicts one of the few aggregates which were found, closely associated with lipid droplets. **Inset:** Bundles of cytofilaments have been recorded in atypical cases of Ewing's sarcoma, but myofilaments are not seen. (× 27 000. Inset: × 34 700)

References: 2171, 2184, 2185, 2194, 2207, 2219, 2224, 2240

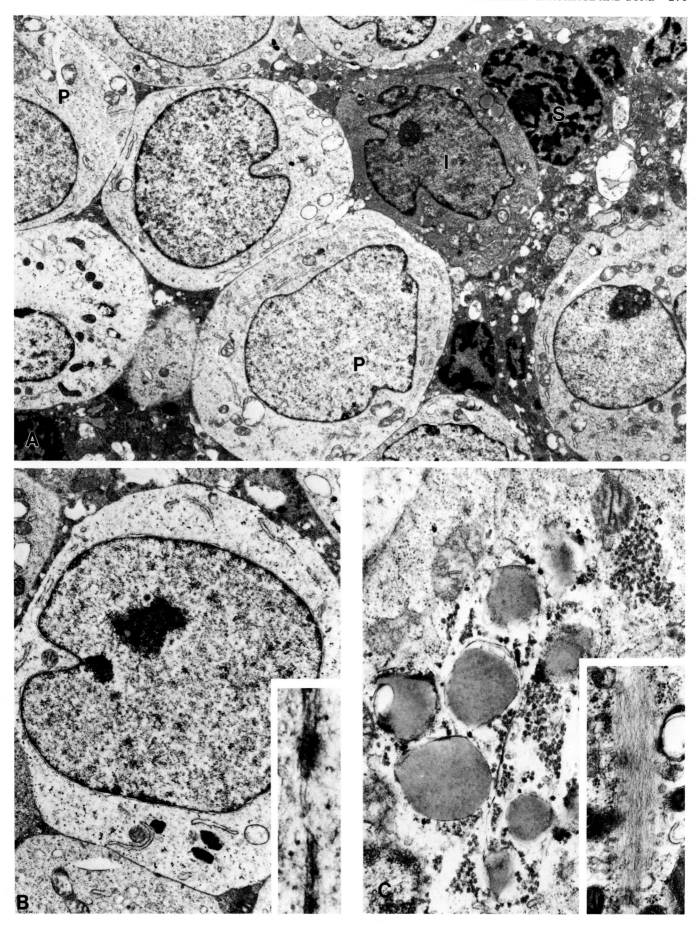

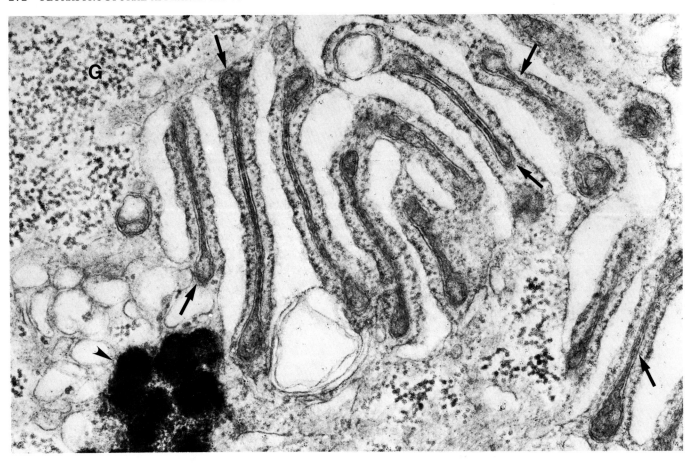

**Fig. 25.10  Chordoma: Mitochondria-RER complex**

In the cells of this neoplasm, a close association between alternating lamellae of RER and compressed, attenuated mitochondria (arrows) is often observed. These complexes can be found in most chordomas, but not all. A similar complex has been recorded in a parathyroid chief cell adenoma,[39] and we have once observed these formations in a malignant pleural mesothelioma. Glycogen particles (G) and portion of a siderosome (arrowhead) are also present. (× 63 900)

References: 39, 2226, 2597, 2618, 2621, 2631, 2655

# 26 Thymic tumours

## THYMOMA AND THYMIC CARCINOMA

Although often containing a variable admixture of lymphocytes, thymomas are ultrastructurally characterized by the presence of epithelial cells with cytoplasmic tonofilaments, prominent cell processes, numerous desmosomes, and basal lamina at the epithelio-stromal interface (Figs. 26.1–26.5). Intraepithelial microcysts largely replacing individual cells occur in up to 10 per cent of thymomas and acinus-like spaces are found in about 20 per cent.[2670] The haemangiopericytic pattern sometimes evident by LM has been shown by EM to be composed of epithelial cells (Table 23.1).[2670] Myoid cells are seen on rare occasions.[2670]

In lymphocyte-rich thymomas, the epithelial component may be obscured by the intensity of the lymphocytic infiltrate, producing a similarity to lymphocytic lymphoma by LM, but even in these cases the epithelial component is readily apparent on ultrastructural examination (Fig. 26.1). Most of the lymphocytes have smooth nuclear contours with abundant heterochromatin, and little cytoplasm. Lymphocytes with hyperconvoluted nuclei are seen occasionally,[64] and it is suggested that this appearance indicates a subpopulation of T-cells (see Tables 27.1 and 27.2); immunocytochemical analysis of a malignant thymoma using monoclonal antibodies indicates that these cells represent thymocytes rather than peripheral T-lymphocytes.[2681]

In *non-teratoid thymic carcinomas,* Wick et al[2693] detected composite squamous and neuroendocrine differentiation in two of 10 cases studied by EM, while four were classified as squamous cell carcinomas and the remaining four were neuroendocrine neoplasms. The basis for the cytoplasmic clarity characteristic of the extremely rare clear cell carcinoma of thymus is uncertain; Wolfe et al[2694] report both glycogen and lipid to be absent on ultrastructural examination and raise the possibility of 'hydropic degeneration'. The findings otherwise described in this tumour include tonofilaments, desmosomes, numerous mitochondria and abundant RER.[2694]

The fine-structural differential diagnosis of anterior mediastinal tumours, including thymoma, thymic carcinoid tumour, lymphocytic lymphoma and germinoma, is summarized in Table 26.1.

**Table 26.1**  Comparative ultrastructure of anterior mediastinal neoplasms

| | Thymoma | Lymphocytic lymphoma | Hodgkin's disease | Germinoma (seminoma) | Thymic carcinoid tumour | Oat cell carcinoma |
|---|---|---|---|---|---|---|
| External lamina | Prominent, often multilayered | Absent | Absent | Absent | Present, focal | Inconspicuous |
| Cell processes | Prominent, interleaving | Inconspicuous | Not conspicuous | Inconspicuous | Inconspicuous | Present |
| Desmosomes | Numerous, well developed | Absent | Absent | Infrequent | Occasional | Infrequent |
| Tonofilaments | Prominent, often aggregated into bundles | Absent | Absent | Absent | Inconspicuous. See remarks | Inconspicuous |
| Neurosecretory granules | Absent | Absent | Absent | Absent | Numerous. Granule diameters vary from 110–500 nm | Sporadic, found in cell body or processes. Diameter of granules in range 80–200 nm |
| Glycogen | May be present, but generally not prominent | Inconspicuous | Inconspicuous | Typically prominent | Not prominent | Not prominent |
| Nuclear projections | Inconspicuous | Frequent | Occasional | Inconspicuous | Inconspicuous | Present |
| Nucleoli | Not prominent | Not prominent | Prominent | Prominent; nucleolonema typically forms ribbons | Not prominent | Not prominent |
| Remarks | Variable and frequently dense admixture of lymphocytes See Figs. 26.1–26.5 The features listed above also characterize spindle cell thymoma and readily exclude other lesions entering into the differential diagnosis by LM, including nerve sheath cell tumours, smooth muscle neoplasms, mesothelioma, malignant fibrous histiocytoma and haemangiopericytoma | See Figs. 27.10–27.20 The nucleoli in immunoblastic lymphoma are typically large, central and non-filamentous. However, a filamentous pattern similar to that characterizing germinomas was present in one of our cases. Markedly elongated strands of RER are a useful guide to the diagnosis of lymphoma (see Fig. 27.17), while absence of glycogen, annulate lamellae and intercellular junctions are additional distinguishing features | Mixed cell population, sometimes with mononuclear phagocytic reaction See Figs. 27.1–27.5 | Stromal lymphocytic reaction, often with mononuclear phagocytes See Fig. 30.3 | Prominent Golgi complexes. Whorling filaments about 10 nm in diameter, forming so-called fibrous bodies, are described in various carcinoid tumours (Fig. 16.6; see also Table 2.9) Lymphocytes sparse or absent Approximately one-third of cases have ectopic ACTH production with Cushing's syndrome See Figs. 16.3–16.6 | Most cases are metastatic from lung, but some may be primary within the mediastinum See Figs. 6.1 and 6.2 |

(After Rosai & Levine[2683])

References: 447, 498, 2663, 2669, 2670, 2673, 2683, 2684, 2688, 2692

**Fig. 26.1** *(Facing page)* **Lymphocyte-rich thymoma: Survey of epithelial and lymphocytic components**

Locally invasive thymoma associated with myasthenia gravis. In this field there are numerous lymphocytes with prominent chromatin, a high nuclear:cytoplasmic ratio, and a paucity of cytoplasmic organelles. Pale epithelial cells (E) are scattered among the lymphocytes. Only a single epithelial nucleus (EN) can be identified, and this contains evenly distributed chromatin and two small nucleoli. The epithelial cytoplasm is relatively abundant and forms irregular prominent processes, but contains few tonofilaments in this area. Adjacent epithelial cells are attached by well developed desmosomes, some of which are indicated (arrows). (× 4700)

See Table 26.1.

References: 2662, 2663, 2665, 2670, 2671, 2673–2679, 2681, 2683, 2685–2688, 2690, 2691

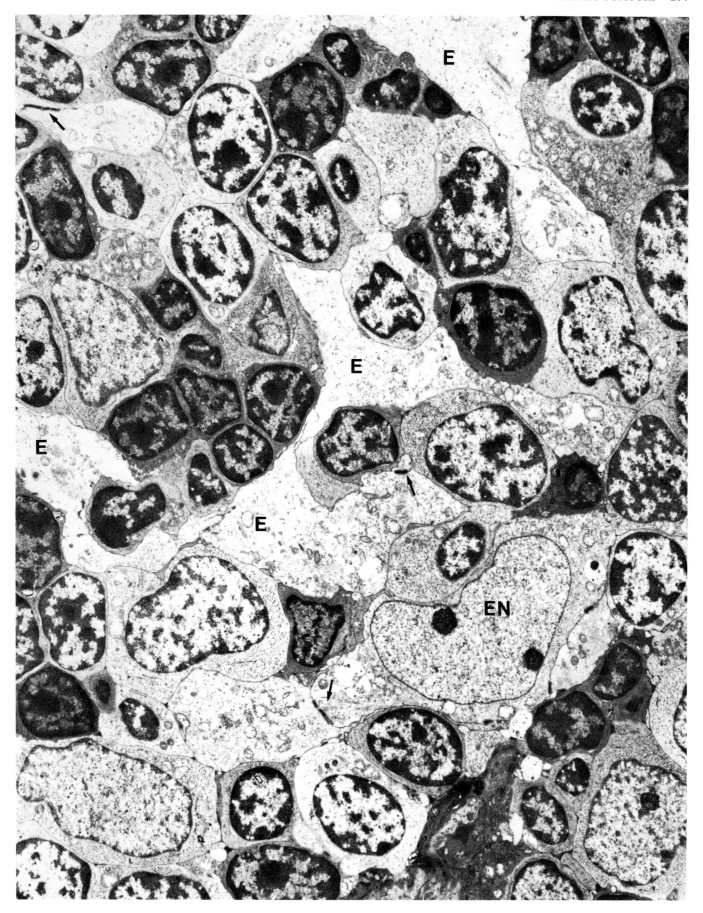

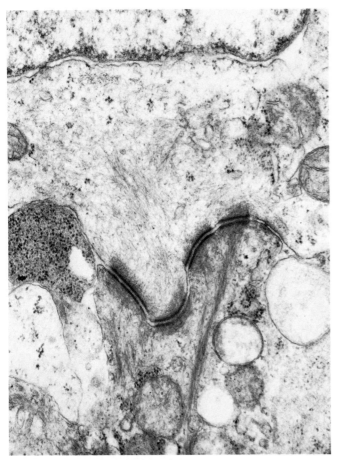

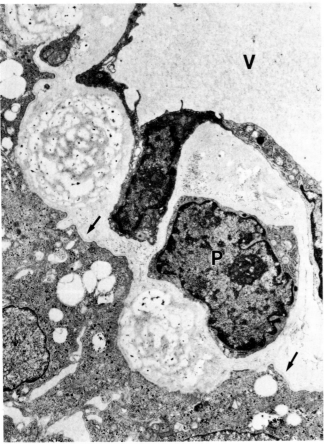

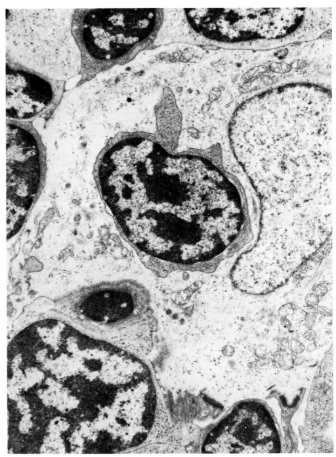

**Fig. 26.2** *(Top — left)* **Thymoma: Desmosomes and tonofilaments**

Two adjacent epithelial cells are attached by typical desmosomes. Tonofilaments are evident in the cytoplasm, aggregating into tonofibrillar bundles and converging onto the desmosomes. (× 30 200)

**Fig. 26.3** *(Top — right)* **Lymphocyte-rich thymoma: Lympho-epithelial interaction**

Thymoma associated with myasthenia gravis. Pale cytoplasm of an epithelial cell appears to completely surround a small lymphocyte, with extremely close apposition of their plasma membranes. The localization of the lymphocyte and the irregular profile of the epithelial-lymphocytic apposition are consistent with emperipolesis. However, it has been suggested that seemingly intracellular sequestration of this type may represent a bidimensional false impression created by oblique sectioning of epithelial processes incompletely enfolding an adjacent extracellular lymphocyte, rather than than true 'internal wandering'. The significance of this epithelial-lymphocytic interaction in thymomas is uncertain, but many of the cases in which it has been described have been myasthenic. (× 6800)
References: 2675, 2676

**Fig. 26.4** *(Bottom — left)* **Thymoma: Epithelial cells and basal laminae**

A group of epithelial cells is bordered at the epithelio-vascular interface by basal lamina (arrows) with nodular aggregates between the epithelial cells and the endothelium of the adjacent blood vessel (V). A pericyte (P) is also evident. (× 5700)
Reference: 358

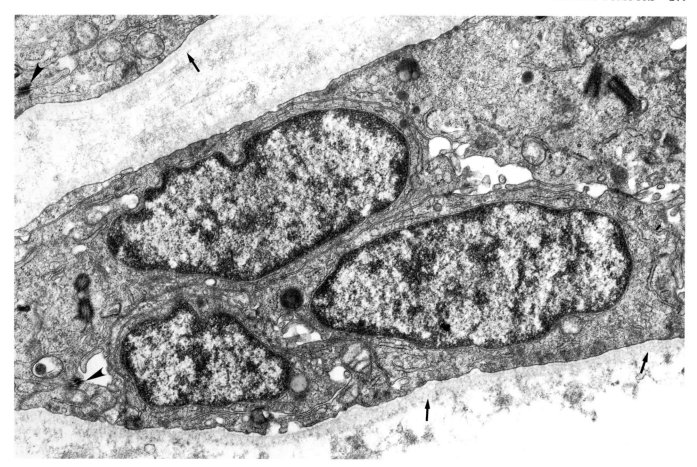

**Fig. 26.5   Thymoma: Epithelial predominance**

In this case the lymphocyte population was sparse, the neoplasm consisting of aggregates of epithelial cells surrounded by a distinct external lamina (arrows). Each has a slightly irregular nucleus; lysosomes and lipofuscin granules are readily found in the cytoplasm, although cytoplasmic filaments are inconspicuous. Desmosomes are present (arrowheads). (× 18 700)

# 27 Lymphoid and plasmacytic tumours

## THE NON-HODGKIN'S LYMPHOMAS AND HODGKIN'S DISEASE

In their ultrastructure the lymphomas are largely characterized by a deficiency of specific features other than an overall 'lymphocytoid' appearance of the participating cells, and the diagnosis is usually established by LM. However, there may be difficulty in determining whether a particular malignancy is a diffuse lymphoma or an anaplastic carcinoma. In these circumstances the diagnosis of lymphoma can be established on ultrastructural examination by absence of the indicators of epithelial differentiation, such as intercellular junctions, basal lamina, acinus formation, and cytoplasmic tonofilaments (see Table 0.2). The major ultrastructural features of lymphocytic lymphomas are contrasted with other small round cell tumours in Tables 29.1 and 29.2, and the distinction from other neoplasms affecting the anterior mediastinum is considered in Table 26.1.

Ultrastructural examination may facilitate both subtyping of lymphoplasmacytic neoplasms and assessment of the maturity of the component cells. Nuclear contours are easily evaluated, and the cleaved nuclei of some B-cell lymphomas can be recognized and distinguished from the more irregular nuclei of some T-cell tumours (Table 27.1).[2797,2925] Complex indentations of lymphocyte nuclei producing serpentine (cerebriform) profiles may be a specific — but inconstant — marker for T-lymphocytes; their presence characterizes both mycosis fungoides and the Sézary syndrome, but is not in itself diagnostic (Table 27.2). The distribution of nuclear heterochromatin may also be important in the subtyping of lymphomas, as a marginated 'clock-face' pattern hints at B-cell properties.

The ribosomal mass, and the number and length of the cisternae of the RER may be significant; when assessed in conjunction with nuclear morphology, cytoplasmic granules and maturity of the Golgi apparatus, they point to the degree of lymphocyte activation and to possible T- or B-cell properties (Table 27.1).[2797] For example, long parallel cisternae in association with a moderately developed Golgi complex suggest B-lymphocytes, whereas irregular nuclei, small foci of lysosomal dense bodies and a uropod indicate T-cell properties. The surface morphology of the lymphocytic cells may also be significant, and profuse microvilli suggest B-cells.[2697,2715] The electron-cytochemical demonstration of acid phosphatase is also of value in the diagnosis of T-lymphoblastic lymphoma and leukaemia, between 70 and 100 per cent of the lymphoblasts showing focal reaction product in the Golgi cisternae and lysosomes.[2777]

Inclusions within nuclei and the RER may occur in lymphocytic lymphomas; the intracisternal inclusions contain immunoglobulin, and may assume fibrillary and paracrystalline patterns (Fig. 27.14). Rarely, accumulation of intracisternal material displaces nuclei to the periphery of the cells, resulting in one form of so-called signet-ring cell lymphoma (Figs. 27.13–27.16).[2806] Large secretory granules are seen in some B-cell lymphomas, and lipid globules are a regular feature of Burkitt's lymphoma (Fig. 27.18); in the latter, the nuclei are only slightly indented, while the mitochondria, although few, are large and are often polarized to one side of the cell.

Reed-Sternberg cells in *Hodgkin's disease* have been the subject of close scrutiny, but there is no specific ultrastructural feature by which their nature can be determined (Fig. 27.1).[2849] On the other hand, the electron-dense dendritic cells of some lymphomas are indicative of follicular centre cell lymphomas.

In *plasmacytoma-myelomatosis* the participating cells are characterized by abundant RER, which sometimes contains intracisternal proteinaceous material or even crystalline inclusions (Fig. 27.29). The marginated nuclear heterochromatin pattern is depleted to varying degrees, and asynchronous nuclear-cytoplasmic development is usually evident.[2854] Intranuclear inclusions and pseudoinclusions may also occur (Figs. 27.27 and 27.29). Scanning EM shows the plasma membrane to be thrown into many microvillous projections,[3108,3124,3126] — a feature much less obvious on transmission EM (but see Fig. 27.28).

Some of the stromal components may be of diagnostic significance, namely intercellular amyloid fibrils in some plasmacytic tumours, and a prominent vascular reaction in immunoblastic lymphadenopathy.[2769,2778] Infiltration of vessel walls by malignant cells may be seen in the leukaemic phase of some lymphomas.

**Table 27.1  Comparative ultrastructure of lymphocytes in adult T-cell lymphoma-leukaemia and B-cell lymphomas***

| Feature | T-lymphocytes | B-lymphocytes |
|---|---|---|
| *NUCLEUS* | | |
| Shape | Irregular, convoluted, multilobate or cerebriform, but smooth contours also occur | Rounded or cleaved |
| Chromatin | Often speckled. Heterochromatin abundant in T-CLL,† but depleted in T-PLL† | Vesicular. Marginated heterochromatin may be seen in plasmacytoid cells, depending on the level of cell maturity and the degree of nuclear-cytoplasmic asynchrony |
| Nucleoli | Vary from inconspicuous to large | More prominent than in T-cells |
| Nuclear blebs | Often present | Often present |
| *CYTOPLASM* | | |
| Endoplasmic reticulum | Smooth (SER), forms vesicles | Rough (RER), more abundant than in T-cells, producing elongated strands and concentric patterns |
| Lysosomes and multivesicular bodies | More frequent than in B-cells | Usually few and aggregated |
| Inclusions and arrays | Parallel tubular arrays reported in T-CLL | May contain intracisternal fibrillary or crystalline inclusions (Fig. 27.14), in which immunoglobulin can be demonstrated by immunocytochemistry |
| Glycogen | More abundant than in B-cells | Usually sparse |
| Cell surface — scanning EM | Microvillous processes less numerous than on classical B-lymphocytes and surface may be relatively smooth | Abundant microvillous processes may be seen by scanning EM; compare Figs. 28.8 and 28.9. Cytoplasmic processes may also be evident by transmission EM; see Fig. 27.25 |
| *REMARKS* | Nuclear irregularity ± multilobation is the most useful ultrastructural indicator of T-cell properties | Abundance of RER, characteristically forming elongated strands, is the most valuable cytoplasmic indicator of B-cell differentiation on transmission EM |
| | Huhn and associates[2904] recognize 5 subtypes of T-CLL, including T-PLL and 4 subsets of T-CLL, partly based on the number of nuclear indentations, the heterochromatin pattern, nucleolar prominence, and the quantity and granule content of the cytoplasm | See Figs. 17.13, 27.10-27.17, 27.20, 27.24-27.29 and 28.6-28.8 |
| | See Figs. 27.6-27.9, 28.9 and 28.10, and Table 27.2 | |

*The ultrastructural features listed in this table are only intended to be a general guide; EM cannot replace accurate immunological marker studies in the identification of T- and B-cell properties. For example, T-lymphocytes can have plasmacytoid features on rare occasions

†T-CLL = T-cell chronic lymphocytic leukaemia; T-PLL = T-cell prolymphocytic leukaemia

(Modified from Eimoto et al[2736])

References: 2736, 2812, 2893, 2894, 2904, 2925

**Table 27.2  Lymphocytes with cerebriform nuclei in human tissues**

| Occurrence | Remarks |
|---|---|
| *NORMAL CELLS* | |
| Apparently normal spleen | Occasional cells |
| Blood of healthy subjects | In peripheral and umbilical cord blood. All of these cells have T-cell membrane characteristics.[2774] The proportion of cerebriform cells varies according to the extent of nuclear indentation required to designate them as cerebriform |
| Apparently normal skin | — |
| *LYMPHOID AND CUTANEOUS DISORDERS* | |
| Sézary syndrome | In cutaneous lesions and blood. Not all cerebriform lymphocytic cells in the Sézary syndrome and mycosis fungoides have T-cell characteristics as detected by E-rosette formation.[2774] |
| Mycosis fungoides (MF) | In cutaneous, lymph nodal and visceral infiltrates (Figs. 27.6–27.9). Distinction of MF from benign cutaneous lymphoid infiltrates *may* be facilitated by comparative assessment of nuclear contour index (NCI) values, defined as the nuclear perimeter per square root of nuclear area, and by determining the proportion of cells with a high NCI.[2772] McNutt & Crain[2772] reported mean NCI values of 4.6–5.4±0.1 for benign cutaneous lymphoid infiltrates, as opposed to 6.1±0.1 for MF. NCI values $\geq$ 6 were claimed to be specific for MF, but were not always found. The combination of a mean NCI $\geq$ 6.1 with 6 per cent of lymphocytes having values of $\geq$ 9 led to a false positive diagnosis in 3 per cent, but 50 per cent false negatives for 'early' MF |
| | In MF and the Sézary syndrome the lymphocyte populations with their characteristic cerebriform nuclei appear to correspond to a peripheral mature T-cell compartment carrying the T1 or T3 antigens (or both), probably representing Tμ(T-helper) cells. In contrast, T-lymphocytic lymphomas lacking this nuclear morphology mimic an earlier phase of T-cell development, corresponding to the thymic compartment |
| Some T-lymphocytic lymphomas | — |
| Prolymphocytic leukaemia | Occasional cells.[2906] T-cell prolymphocytic leukaemia may represent an accumulation of Tμ cells, whereas T-cell chronic lymphocytic leukaemia may consist of Tγ (T-suppressor) cells |
| Parapsoriasis en plaques | — |
| Contact dermatitis | — |
| Discoid lupus erythematosus | — |
| Psoriasis | — |
| Cutaneous vasculitis | — |
| Pityriasis lichenoides et varioliformis acuta | — |
| Pityriasic dermatitis | Case of self-limited dermatitis histologically simulating MF[2742] |
| Lichen planus | In subepidermal inflammatory infiltrate |
| Lymphomatoid papulosis | — |
| Solar keratosis | In dermal inflammatory infiltrate |
| Basal cell carcinoma | Within inflammatory infiltrate around tumour nodules |
| *OTHER TISSUES AND DISORDERS* | |
| Reactive lymph nodes | Occasional cells |
| Synovium in rheumatoid arthritis | — |
| Lymphocyte-rich thymoma | — |

References: 2697, 2723, 2724, 2732, 2739, 2740, 2742, 2767, 2772, 2774, 2795, 2822, 2906, 2925

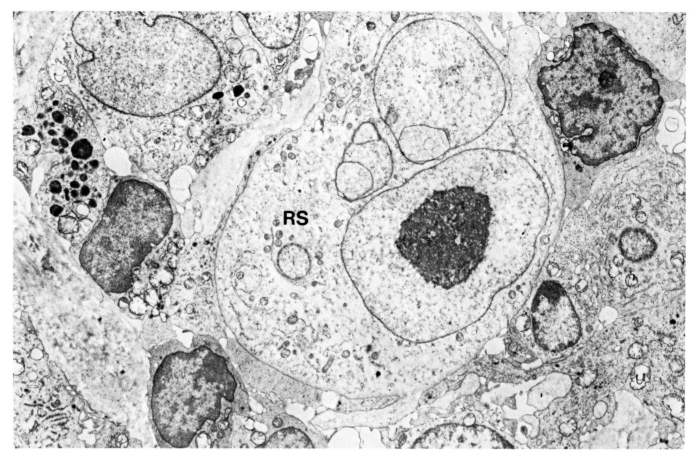

**Fig. 27.1   Hodgkin's disease: Survey**

A characteristic Reed-Sternberg cell (RS) is obvious in this low power electron micrograph. The classical binuclear appearance and nucleolar prominence are evident; however, some investigators have shown that profiles of this type may represent a bidimensional projection of a single bilobate nucleus. Lymphocytes in various stages of activation are seen surrounding the cell. Scanning EM of Reed-Sternberg cells reveals lamellar surface projections. (× 6000)

See Table 26.1.

**Discussion:** Some investigators have found a paucity of organelles in RS cells (as in this instance) and likened them to transformed lymphocytes. Others have described abundant cytoplasmic components, and a similarity to mononuclear phagocytes has been invoked. In addition to the characteristic macronucleoli, Peiper & Kahn[2704] recorded numerous organelles in the plentiful cytoplasm. The organelles had a tendency to localize in the paranuclear region (in contrast to their dispersal in the associated reactive mononuclear phagocytes), and they included mitochondria, lysosomes, hyperplastic Golgi complexes, short segments of RER, and variable numbers of polyribosomes and filaments.

References: 315, 2698, 2703, 2704, 2727, 2826–2830, 2834, 2835, 2839, 2844, 2845

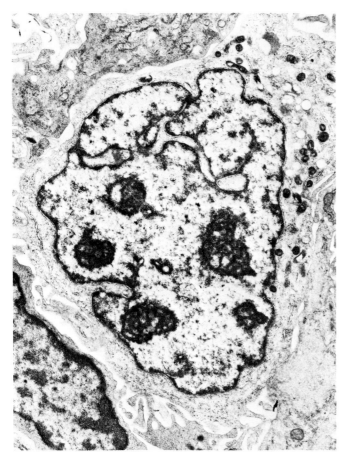

**Fig. 27.2  Nodular sclerosing Hodgkin's disease: Lacunar cell**

A lacunar cell occupies most of the field. Its nuclear contours are irregular and
its nucleoli prominent (but not as large as those of classical Reed-Sternberg
cells). Ribosomal rosettes and a few strands of RER are present in the
cytoplasm, together with scattered mitochondria and elements of the Golgi
complex. Lacunar cells are thought to be related to Reed-Sternberg cells;
shrinkage due to formalin fixation (± the presence of lipid globules) explains
their lacunar appearance under the light microscope. (× 8300)

**Discussion:** Classical lacunar cells are characterized by their size,
hyperlobate nuclei, and pale cytoplasm containing few organelles. They
appear to be weakly positive for acid phosphatase and non-specific esterase.[2832]
Bitypic reactions for λ and ϰ chains and IgG have also been found, suggesting
non-specific uptake. Hansmann & Kaiserling[2832] have proposed that lacunar
cells are related to interdigitating reticulum cells.

References: 2824, 2832

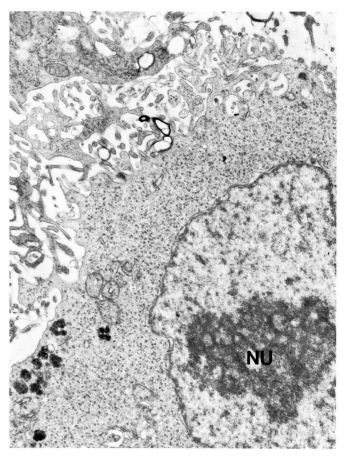

**Fig. 27.3  Hodgkin's disease: Large primitive cell with microvillous
projections**

This cell displays a mildly irregular nucleus with a very prominent nucleolus
(NU). Many ribosomal rosettes are present in the cytoplasm, together with a
few small mitochondria, a poorly developed Golgi complex and an aggregate
of lysosomes. The surface of the cell is highly irregular, with many flaps and
projections. (× 9600)

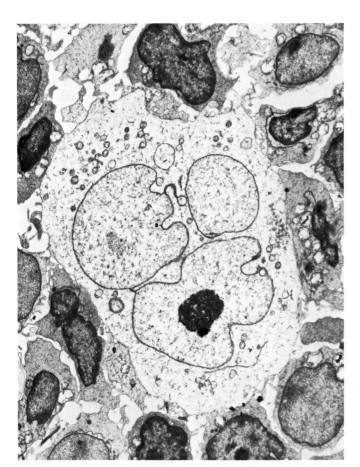

### Fig. 27.4  Hodgkin's disease: Lymphocyte rosette

Lymphocytes are closely apposed to the periphery of this Reed-Sternberg cell, which has lucent cytoplasm with few organelles. (× 4100)

**Discussion:** Some investigators correlate tightness of the lymphocytic apposition with cytotoxic changes in the Reed-Sternberg cells, which may have some prognostic significance.[2825]

Polymorphonuclear leukocytes, especially eosinophils, as well as plasma cells, activated lymphocytes, histiocytes and scattered fibroblasts are cells frequently found in lymph nodes affected by Hodgkin's disease. Mast cells have also been described.

Fibrin deposits are sometimes seen in Hodgkin's disease and occur in three locations:

1. Intercellular fibrin tactoids associated with apparently non-neoplastic lymphoid cells.
2. In close association with fibrous long-spacing collagen.
3. In areas of necrosis.

Such deposits may also be present in non-Hodgkin's lymphomas, albeit less often.

References: 2825, 2833, 2842, 2848

### Fig. 27.5   Hodgkin's disease: Mononuclear phagocytes

A large mononuclear phagocyte (M) shows many irregular phagolysosomal bodies and cytoplasmic processes (P). It is closely apposed to activated lymphocytes (L), while long-spacing collagen (curved arrow) is seen in the interstitium. (× 8000)

Such reactive mononuclear phagocytic cells can in part be distinguished from RS cells by their small nucleoli and less irregular nuclear profiles. Compare with Fig. 27.1.

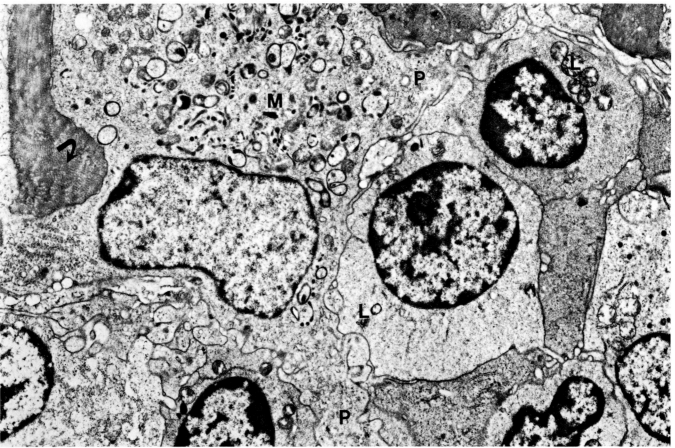

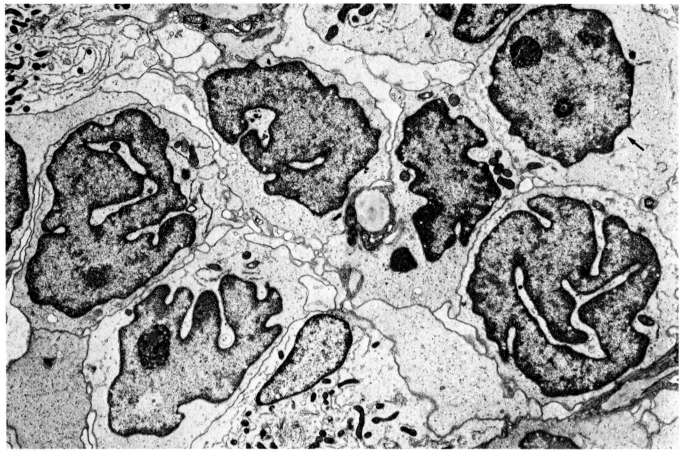

**Fig. 27.6  Mycosis fungoides: Lymphocytes with cerebriform nuclei**

Lymph node biopsy from a 63-year-old woman with a 4-year history of mycosis fungoides (MF). The outstanding characteristic of the lymphocytic cells illustrated here is marked nuclear indentation producing highly irregular 'cerebriform' contours. Note, however, that not all of the nuclei have this morphology and one (arrow) has a comparatively smooth outline. (× 6500)

Lymphoblastoid cells, lymphocytes and Langerhans' histiocytes are also recorded in the cutaneous lesions, in addition to the characteristic MF cells. According to Caorsi et al,[2726] lymphoid cells predominate in a ratio of approximately 20:1 and there may be close contacts between the lymphoid and Langerhans' cells.

(Case contributed by Prof. R.L. Kempson).

References: 2717, 2719–2724, 2726, 2729, 2730, 2734, 2735, 2739, 2740, 2744, 2747, 2766, 2767, 2773, 2794, 2795, 2805, 2808, 2811, 2815, 2822, 2823

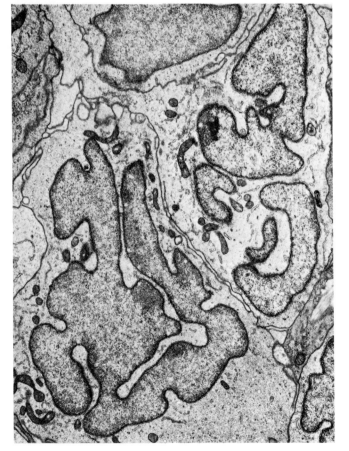

**Fig. 27.7  Mycosis fungoides: Lymphocytes with serpentine nuclear profiles**

Extreme nuclear irregularity characterizes these lymphocytic cells. Although this nuclear morphology is typical of mycosis fungoides and the Sézary syndrome it is by no means restricted to these conditions (Table 27.2). (× 7400)

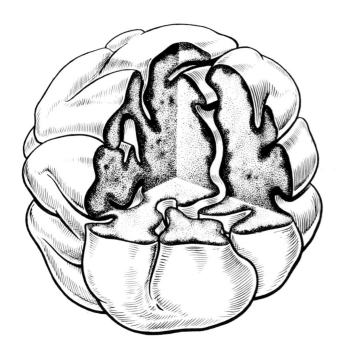

### Fig. 27.8  Cerebriform nucleus

A tridimensional reconstruction of a cerebriform nucleus is depicted here. A segment of the nuclear 'brain' has been cut away to show the typical serpentine profile as visualized by transmission EM.

These nuclear appearances were designated as cerebriform by light microscopy on the basis of shape and the presence of convolutions. The identification of serpentine nuclear profiles in routine paraffin-embedded sections may be difficult. By LM they are more easily detected in semithin resin-embedded sections, while electron microscopy most dramatically reveals the complexity of their indentations. Pronounced nuclear irregularity may indicate a T-cell lymphoma, but the hyperconvoluted contours characteristic of mycosis fungoides and the Sézary syndrome are uncommon in other T-cell lymphomas (see also Figs. 28.9 and 28.10). (Modified from Lutzner et al [2767])

### Fig. 27.9  Mycosis fungoides: T-cell epidermotropism

Preferential T-lymphocytic infiltration of the epidermis is a typical finding in mycosis fungoides and the Sézary syndrome, and the neoplastic lymphocytes may aggregate within the epidermis, forming Pautrier microabscesses. Although characteristic of these conditions, selective lymphocytic infiltration of the epidermis may also occur with systemic T-lymphocytic lymphomas.

In this micrograph, lymphocytes (L) with irregular nuclei are evident within the epidermis, separating the squamous cells (S). The nuclear contour indices of the lymphocytes range from 5.4 to 10.8, with an average of 7.6 (see Table 27.2). Basal lamina (arrowheads) is present at the dermo-epidermal interface. (× 5600)

References: 2734, 2764, 2772

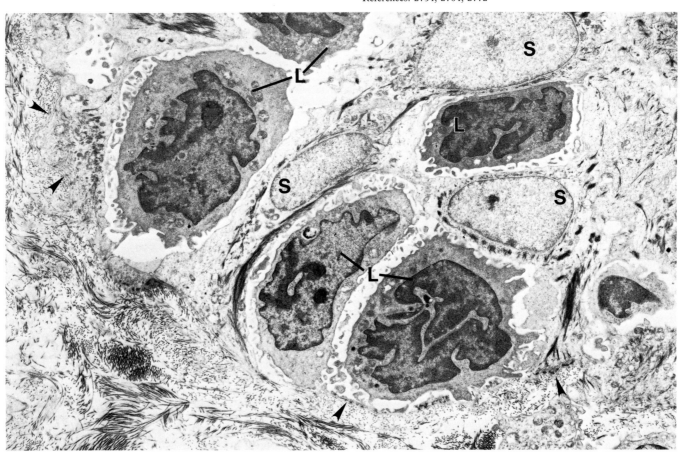

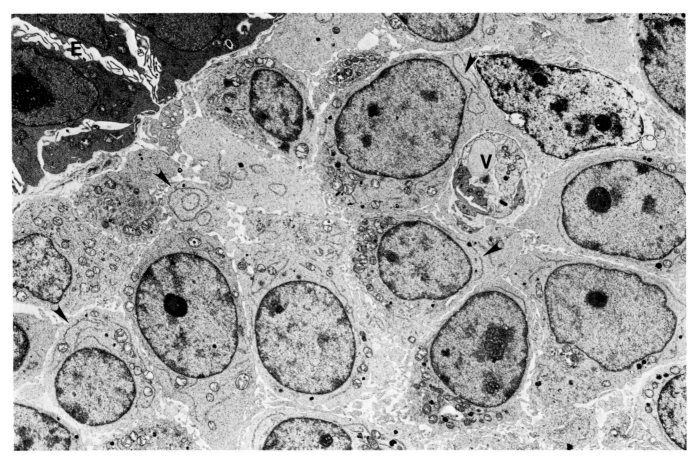

**Fig. 27.10  Small cell lymphocytic lymphoma: Survey**

Endoscopic gastric mucosal biopsy from a 77-year-old woman. The
differential diagnosis by LM on an earlier fibreoptic gastric biopsy included
malignant lymphoma and undifferentiated small cell carcinoma.

Most of this field is occupied by neoplastic lymphocytes. Observe the
smooth nuclear contours of this B-lymphocytic neoplasm. The nuclear
euchromatin content is considerably increased in comparison to normal, and
nucleoli are prominent. Long strands of RER (arrowheads) are present in
many of the cells, indicating B-cell properties; free ribosomes, which are not
resolved at this magnification, are more frequent. Mucosal epithelial cells (E)
inhabit the upper left corner, and a small vessel (V) can also be discerned.
(× 6000)

See Tables 26.1 and 29.2.

References: 2698, 2703, 2748–2750, 2756, 2797

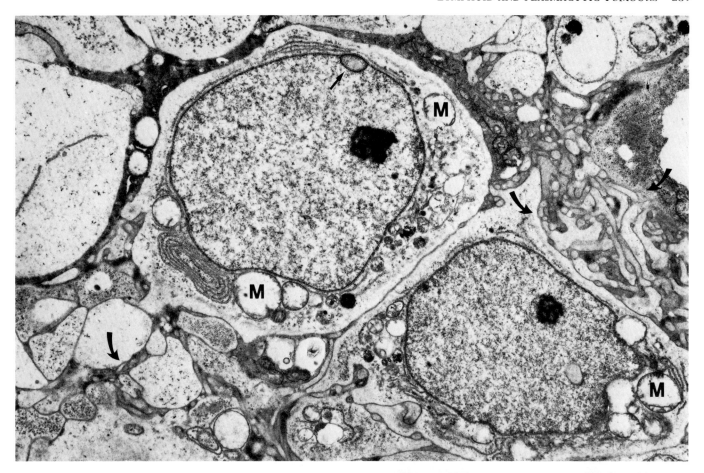

**Fig. 27.11 Follicular centre cell lymphoma (centroblastic lymphoma): Cell processes and plasmablastic differentiation**

The large lymphoid cells illustrated here are devoid of intercellular junctions, but electron-dense dendritic processes can be seen and there is an extremely complex interweaving of cytoplasmic processes (curved arrows). Nuclear chromatin is evenly dispersed and small nucleoli are apparent. A nuclear pocket (straight arrow) can be seen, and the same cell contains parallel and concentric lamellae of RER, suggesting plasmablastic differentiation. The mitochondria (M) exhibit hydropic changes. (× 3600)

References: 2698, 2703, 2743, 2756, 2761, 2763, 2765, 2770, 2792, 2796, 2797

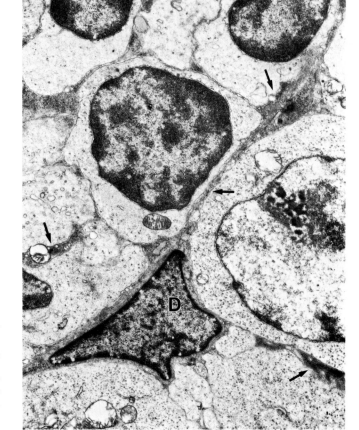

**Fig. 27.12 Follicular centre cell lymphoma: Dendritic cell and lymphocytes**

A thin electron-dense dendritic 'reticular' cell (D), whose processes (arrows) extend between the surrounding activated lymphocytes, is shown. Desmosomal junctions between adjacent dendritic cells may be seen in some cases. Observe the polygonal outline of the nucleus and the paucity of the cytoplasmic organelles. In comparison to normal and reactive germinal centres, dendritic cells are depleted in follicular lymphomas. (× 5400)

References: 2737, 2765, 2792

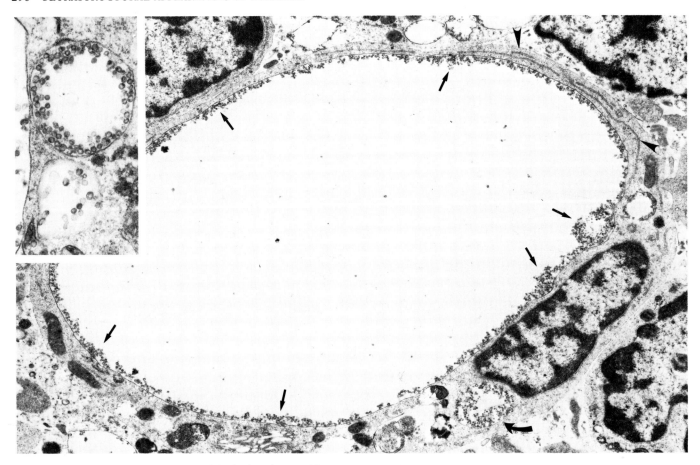

**Fig. 27.13 Follicular centre cell (centroblastic) lymphoma with so-called signet-ring cell features: Cytoplasmic vacuole**

Recurrent lymphoma from a 65-year-old man. He presented initially with a centrocytic-centroblastic lymphoma devoid of intracellular vacuoles. Remission followed treatment with combination chemotherapy, but the lymphoma recurred five years later and was then classified as predominantly centroblastic; by LM, moderate numbers of the lymphoid cells were seen to contain cytoplasmic vacuoles, with peripheral displacement of nuclei. Immunocytochemical studies demonstrated IgG-IgM/$\varkappa$ in some of the lymphoid cells.

This cell has the typical ultrastructural appearances of a so-called signet-ring cell lymphoma (see also caption to Fig. 27.14). A large vacuole with a smooth delimiting membrane occupies most of the cytoplasm, the eccentric nucleus being located near the plasma membrane. The centre of the vacuole appears empty, but there is a thin wreath of microvesicles (straight arrows) at its periphery. The microvesicles are packed more closely in a smaller neighbouring vacuole (curved arrow). Resembling multivesicular bodies (MVB), small vacuoles of this type often lie adjacent to the large vacuoles and it is possible that they develop into the clear vacuoles by progressive vesiculation (giant MVB)[2746] or by coalescence. Elongated membranous intravacuolar profiles may also be seen. Note the long strands of RER (arrowheads); the cells comprising this type of lymphoma usually have the features of centrocytes. (× 13 000)

**Inset:** Detail of microvesicles in small vacuoles. The vesicles usually range in size from about 30–60 nm. (× 31 000)

References: 2746, 2752, 2760, 2788, 2806, 2816

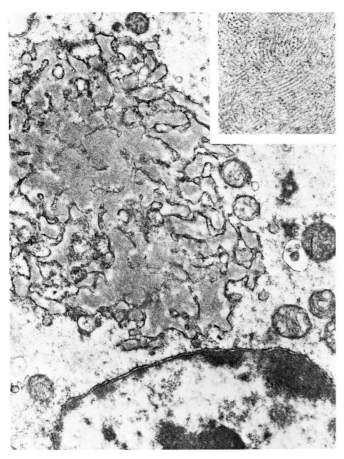

**Fig. 27.14** *(Top)* **Follicular centre cell (centrocytic-centroblastic) lymphoma: Russell body-like cytoplasmic inclusion**

The eccentric nucleus contains peripheral clumps of heterochromatin. In the cytoplasm the dilated cisternae of RER have coalesced and a finely fibrillary osmiophilic conglomerate is present in their lumina. ($\times$ 18 700)

**Inset:** The fibrillary substructure of the intracisternal contents is readily apparent. ($\times$ 33 000)

**Discussion:** Both intranuclear and intracytoplasmic inclusions are well documented in reactive and neoplastic plasmacytic proliferations (see Fig. 27.29), and in both Waldenström's macroglobulinaemia and chronic lymphocytic leukaemia. They are uncommon in nodular lymphomas and immunoblastic sarcoma, occurring in about 1 per cent of centrocytic-centroblastic lymphomas and occasionally in centroblastic lymphomas. Spagnolo et al[2806] have recently reviewed the occurrence of immunoglobulin-containing inclusions in nodular lymphomas, dividing them into three classes:

1. Intracisternal inclusions distending the RER and composed of filaments distributed both randomly and in parallel, producing a Russell body-like appearance by LM (see Fig. 3.8). These inclusions most often contain IgM/$\varkappa$, while IgG/$\varkappa$ is somewhat less frequent.
2. Rectangular to needle-shaped membrane-bound inclusions (Fig. 27.15) composed of parallel filaments 10.5–16 nm in thickness and with a spacing of 26.5–32 nm.
3. Membrane-bound vacuolar inclusions containing few to many microvesicles 30–62 nm in diameter (Fig. 27.13), to which may be added a fourth category:
4. Intracytoplasmic filamentous aggregates without investing membranes (Fig. 27.16).

We see little merit in using 'signet-ring cell lymphoma' as a general diagnostic appellation for lymphomas with such cytoplasmic inclusions; this expression fails to acknowledge their follicular centre cell (FCC) character and lacks precision in view of the varied appearances of the inclusions. It seems preferable to describe these cases as FCC lymphomas with vacuolar inclusions, Russell body-like inclusions and so forth. If the term is used, it is best restricted to a supplementary designation for FCC lymphomas with vacuolar inclusions, since the cells may closely resemble those of signet-ring cell carcinomas by LM; the differences are obvious by EM (compare Figs. 27.13 and 5.10).

A Gaucher-like appearance of lymphomatous cells when viewed by LM has also resulted from the accumulation of intracisternal crystalline inclusions containing IgM/$\varkappa$.[2784] Extracellular and intravascular immunoglobulin deposits are also described.[2783]

References: 2738, 2783, 2784, 2806, 2816

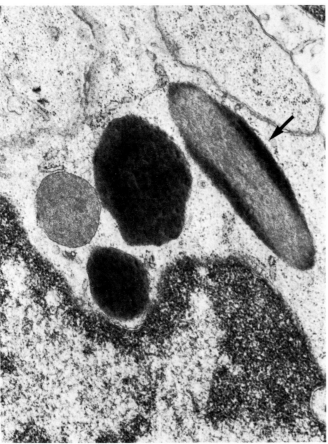

**Fig. 27.15** *(Bottom)* **Follicular centre cell (centrocytic) lymphoma: Cytoplasmic inclusions**

Electron-dense bodies are present in the cytoplasm of this lymphocytic cell; some are roughly spherical while one is needle-shaped (arrow), and their electron-density is non-uniform. ($\times$ 23 500)

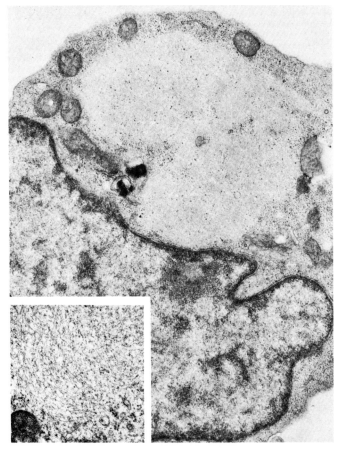

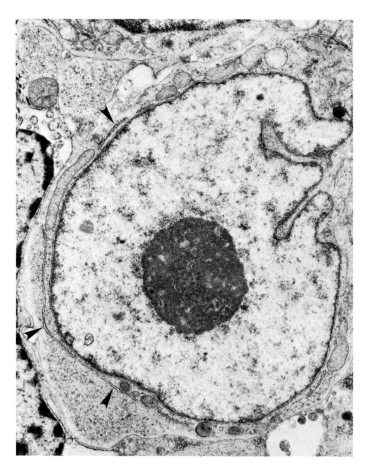

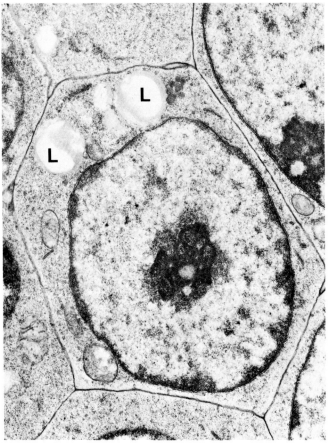

**Fig. 27.16** *(Top — left)* **Follicular centre cell lymphoma: Filamentous aggregate**

The nucleus is indented by a large aggregate of cytofilaments — not resolved at this magnification — occupying much of the cytoplasm and displacing most of the organelles. (× 19 200)

**Inset:** The filamentous nature of the paranuclear inclusion is evident at high magnification, the filaments possibly representing vimentin and/or immunoglobulin in filamentous form. Immunocytochemical studies demonstrated monoclonal IgM within the cytoplasm of some of the cells. (× 34 200)

**Fig. 27.17** *(Top — right)* **Immunoblastic lymphoma: Immunoblast**

The segmentally irregular nucleus contains a prominent central nucleolus. Ribosomes abound in the cytoplasm, where mitochondria and a few elongated strands of RER (arrowheads) are also evident. (× 10 100)

References: 2707, 2756, 2775, 2776, 2783, 2786, 2798

**Fig. 27.18** *(Bottom — left)* **Burkitt's lymphoma: Survey**

This tumour consists of closely apposed polygonal cells, characteristically showing monotonous nuclear uniformity. The nucleus contains a moderately prominent nucleolus while lipid globules (L) are frequent in the cytoplasm. (× 10 700)

References: 2698, 2756, 2759, 2800, 2802

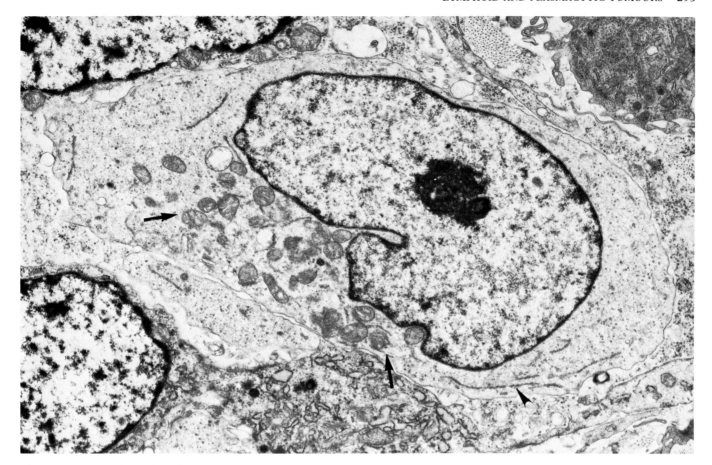

**Fig. 27.19  Large cell lymphocytic lymphoma: Lymphocytoid cell**

Most of the lymphocytes in these neoplasms are uniformly large; the nuclei are large and moderately irregular with much euchromatin and prominent nucleoli. Ribosomal rosettes and a few long strands of RER (arrowhead) are seen. Most of the mitochondria localize in one portion of the cytoplasm (arrows). (× 8900)

See Table 29.2.

References: 2698, 2703, 2712, 2741, 2748–2750, 2756, 2807

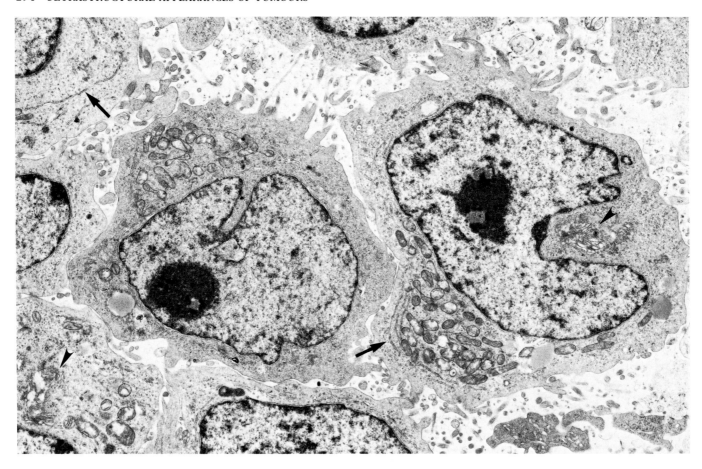

**Fig. 27.20  Large cell lymphocytic lymphoma: Lymphocytoid cells with microvillous processes**

Malignant lymphoma from a 42-year-old man with widespread lymphadenopathy and destructive osseous lesions. Histiocytic cells labelling for both $\alpha_1$-antiprotease and lysozyme were present, but were confined to the periphery of the lymphomatous infiltrates.

Rarely, the lymphocytoid cells comprising large cell lymphomas possess numerous microvillous processes, inviting ultrastructural misdiagnosis as adenocarcinoma. Note, however, that intercellular junctions are not present. In addition, the microvilli in these cases generally lack microfilamentous cores. The cleaved nuclei, strands of RER (arrows) and Golgi complexes (arrowheads) indicate B-cell properties. The nucleoli are prominent. With the exception of the cytoplasmic projections, the appearances conform to those usually seen in large cell lymphomas. (× 8200)

Reference: 2782

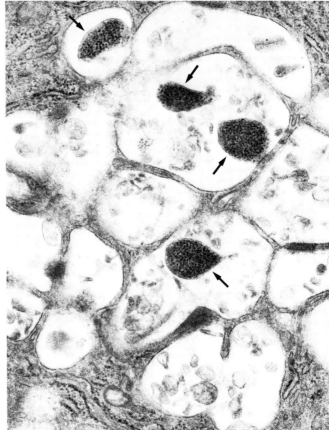

**Fig. 27.21  Large cell lymphocytic lymphoma: Mycoplasma-like profiles in histiocytes**

Large cell lymphocytic lymphoma with numerous histiocytes. In some lymphomas the vacuoles of a few histiocytes contain cytoplasmic fragments (arrows) which resemble Mycoplasma; we have never found nucleoid strands in these structures. (× 38 400)

Reference: 2841

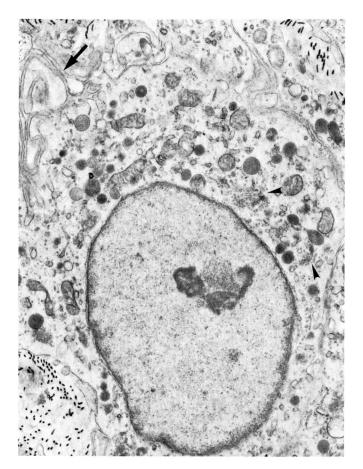

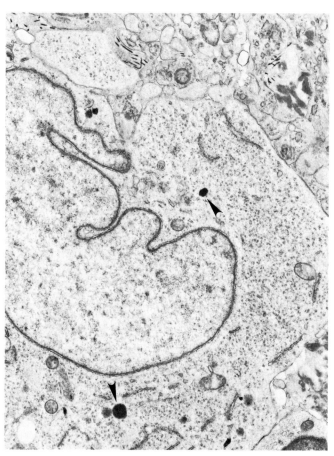

**Fig. 27.22  True histiocytic lymphoma: Cell detail I**

This cell has the features of a mononuclear phagocyte, possessing a central nucleus with a prominent nucleolus, while many lysosomes are present in the cytoplasm. The Golgi apparatus (arrowheads) is moderately developed and cytoplasmic flaps (arrow) project from the cell surface. (× 9800)

**Discussion:** The ultrastructural identification of histiocytic cells in true histiocytic lymphomas (as elsewhere) is largely based on the presence of lysosomes, phagocytic activity and cytoplasmic flaps, and absence of intercellular junctions in most instances. Other identifying features include the immunological detection of C3 and Fcγ receptors, as well as cytoplasmic $\alpha_1$-antiprotease and lysozyme. Acid phosphatase, α-naphthyl acetate esterase and 2-naphthyl thiol acetate esterase are additional cytochemical markers. It is likely that such enzyme-cytochemical procedures will be supplanted by use of monoclonal antibodies directed against components of macrophage membranes; these antibodies include FMC32, 63D3, PHM2, OKM1, 4F2 and HTF1.

References: 2698, 2753, 2756, 2814, 2820, 3069

**Fig. 27.23  True histiocytic lymphoma: Cell detail II**

Same case as Fig. 27.22. This cell has the features of promonocytes and monoblasts, with an eccentric, segmentally irregular nucleus, as well as many ribosomal rosettes in the cytoplasm. A few scattered lysosomal granules are also seen (arrowheads). (× 8800)

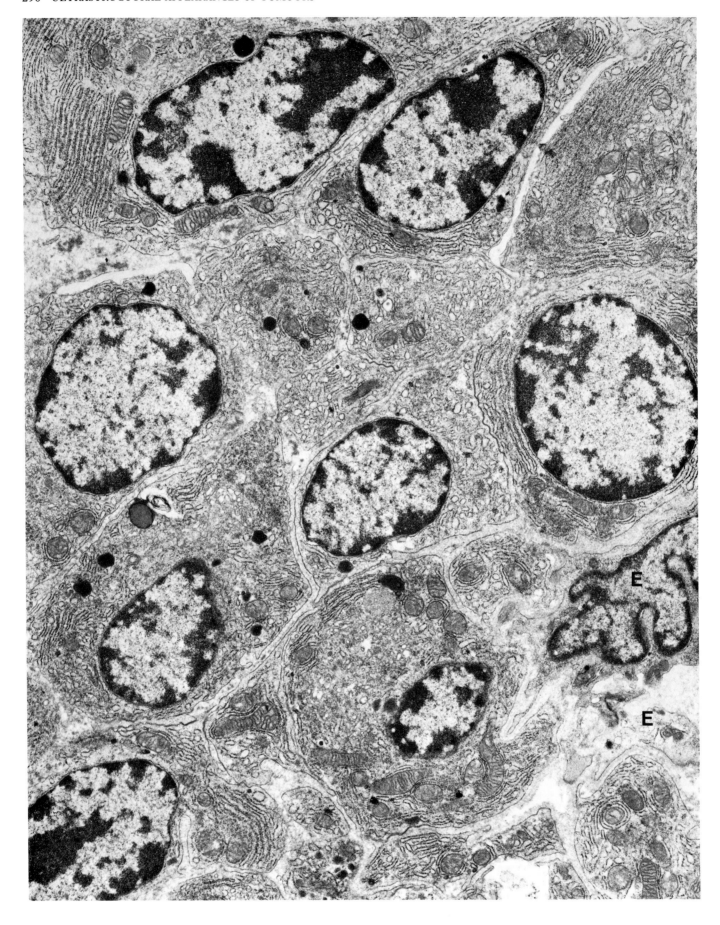

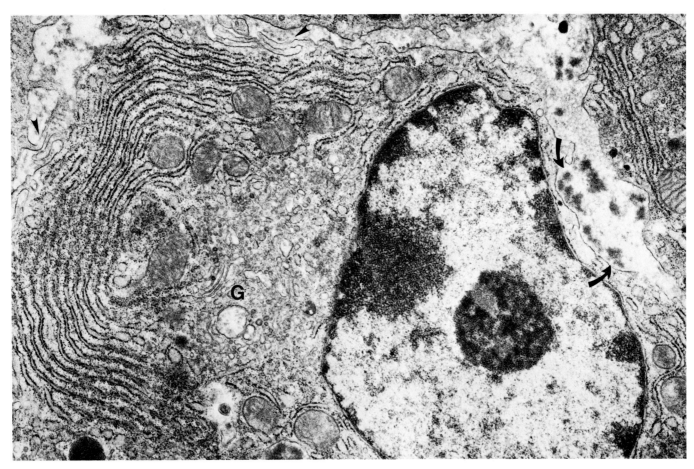

**Fig. 27.25   Lymph node plasmacytoma: Cell detail**

The cytoplasm contains prominent parallel arrays of RER, and the paranuclear Golgi apparatus (G) is moderately developed. In contrast, nuclear heterochromatin is depleted and the nucleolus is enlarged. Note the peripheral cytoplasmic flaps (arrowheads) and the flocculent material in the interstitium (curved arrows). (× 17 800)

**Fig. 27.24** *(Facing page)* **Lymph node plasmacytoma: Survey of plasmacytoid cells**

Apparently solitary plasmacytoma of submandibular lymph node in a woman aged 76 years; clinical investigations revealed no evidence of skeletal lesions or paraproteinaemia. In this field there is a uniform population of plasmacytoid cells with moderate amounts of marginated heterochromatin and abundant RER. The Golgi complex is prominent in some of the cells. Portion of a blood vessel with its lining endothelium (E) is included in the field. (× 10 800)

References: 2756, 3095, 3103, 3106, 3111, 3113, 3123, 3129, 3131, 3134

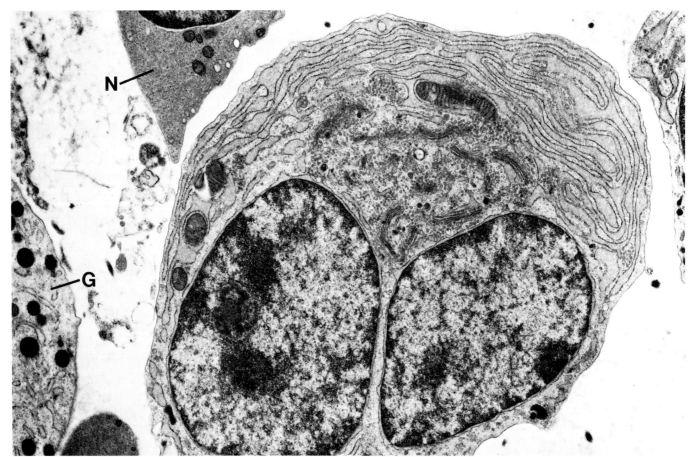

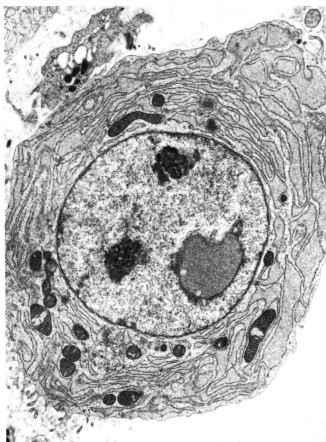

### Fig. 27.26  Multiple myeloma: Atypical plasma cell

Bone marrow biopsy from a 64-year-old woman with dimeric IgA myeloma, presenting as a non-cryoglobulinaemic glomerulonephritis with para-crystalline deposits. Two nuclear profiles are apparent in this myeloma cell. There are moderate quantities of dilated RER, and the Golgi apparatus is highly developed (corresponding to the paranuclear 'Hof' seen on LM). However, the nuclear heterochromatin is in comparison poorly formed, reflecting nuclear-cytoplasmic asynchrony ('maturation anarchy'). Portions of a normoblast (N) and a granulocyte precursor (G) are included in the field. (× 13 100)

**Discussion:** The constituent cells of so-called Waldenström's macro-globulinaemia are lymphocytoid in type, similar to those seen in chronic lymphocytic leukaemia but containing more numerous cytoplasmic organelles; these include stacked lamellae of RER, imparting a plasmacytoid appearance.[2698] Cytoplasmic inclusions may occur, and unusual globulo-fibrillary inclusions within expanded cisternae of the RER are described.[3128] Ribosome-lamella complexes have also been recorded (see Table 28.2). Membrane-bound intranuclear pseudoinclusions are sometimes seen, probably resulting from endonuclear herniation of immunoglobulin material accumulating in the perinuclear cistern, and blebs may project from the nuclear periphery.[3104]

References: 192, 1699, 2698, 2756, 2853, 3094, 3096, 3098–3100, 3102, 3105, 3107–3109, 3112, 3114–3122, 3124–3128, 3130, 3133, 3135–3138, 3140–3143

### Fig. 27.27  Multiple myeloma: Atypical plasma cell

The cytoplasm contains abundant dilated RER, but the nuclear euchromatin content is disproportionately increased. Pronounced dilatation of the RER with amorphous intracisternal contents corresponds to the presence of 'flaming' plasma cells (saurocytes) on LM. A membrane-bound intranuclear pseudoinclusion is evident, as are two nucleolar profiles. Same case as Fig. 27.26. (× 6700)

References: 3104, 3109, 3134, 3136

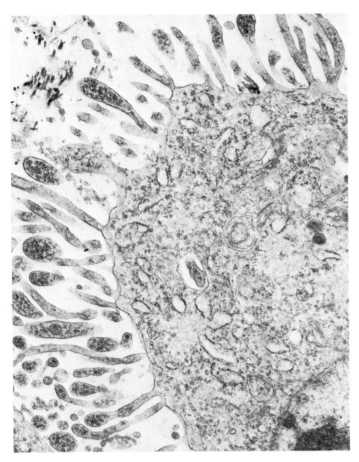

**Fig. 27.28   Multiple myeloma: Filopodial specializations (zeiosis)**

In a few instances many filopodial processes project from the cell surface; these possess bulbous ends which contain aggregates of ribosomal rosettes. A few processes are obviously branched (arrows). (× 21 300)

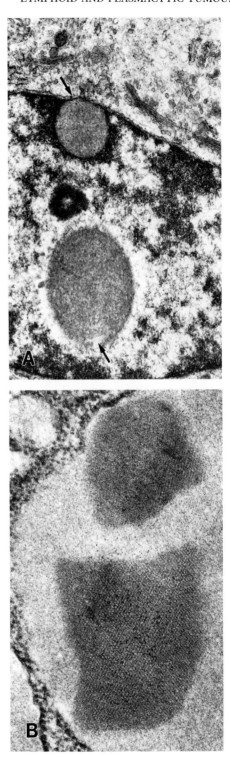

**Fig. 27.29   Multiple myeloma: Nuclear and cytoplasmic inclusions**

**A:** Myeloma cells generally have larger nuclei and more prominent nucleoli than normal plasma cells; large globular electron-dense inclusions (arrows) may accumulate within the nuclear envelope and distort the nuclear contours. The euchromatin is prominent. (× 9300)

**B:** The RER sometimes shows considerable dilatation, and crystalline material is rarely found within the dilated cisternae, as depicted here. Disorganized Golgi complexes, paranuclear filaments, multiple centrioles, swollen mitochondria and spherules are also reported. (× 112 800)

References: 2642, 3094, 3095, 3109, 3111, 3115, 3121, 3136

# 28 Leukaemias and histiocytoses

## THE LEUKAEMIAS

The diagnosis of most leukaemias, particularly the chronic forms, is readily established by light microscopy. However, difficulties are occasionally encountered in typing poorly differentiated blast cell leukaemias, and in these cases EM can sometimes assist in identifying the pattern of differentiation as granulocytic, lymphocytic or monocytic.[2865] Assessment is largely based on the presence or absence of cytoplasmic granules and their appearances, while nuclear morphology is more important than in most neoplasms (Table 28.1). Buffy coat preparations of blood are usually adequate,[2860] and if available are sometimes preferable to bone marrow tissue, where other haemopoietic precursor cells may complicate interpretation.

*Leukaemic lymphocytes* generally have the same fine-structural features as the malignant lymphoid cells comprising the lymphomas (see Chapter 27). Again, the degree of nuclear and cytoplasmic activation varies, being more marked in acute lymphoblastic leukaemia (ALL) than in chronic lymphocytic leukaemia (CLL). Nuclear irregularity when pronounced may be indicative of T-cell leukaemia[2912] and is most obvious in the Sézary syndrome.[2724] In so-called prolymphocytic leukaemia,[2899,2906,3011] clumps of nuclear heterochromatin are less obvious than in CLL, nucleoli are more prominent, and there is greater cytoplasmic development; the appearances are intermediate between CLL and ALL.

Scanning EM may also be useful in detecting the large flaps and clustered microvilli of hairy cell leukaemia (Fig. 28.14). In this condition the nucleus is indented and ribosome-lamella complexes are frequently present within the cytoplasm (see below).

Cytoplasmic granules characterize the *granulocytic leukaemias* (Figs. 28.1–28.3). Varying numbers of uniformly electron-dense primary granules occur in the cells of acute granulocytic leukaemia (AGL), while secondary and even tertiary granules appear in chronic granulocytic leukaemia (CGL). Elongated Auer bodies (rods) strongly indicate acute granulocytic or promyelocytic leukaemia,[2860,2947] but are unfortunately uncommon in AGL, and must be distinguished from the crystalline bodies sometimes seen in lympho-proliferative disorders (see Figs. 28.4 and 28.7). Nuclear morphology also varies according to the extent of differentiation; abundant euchromatin and multiple shallow indentations typify AGL, whereas heterochromatin is plentiful

and identations are fewer and deeper in CGL. Varying numbers of eosinophilic and basophilic granulocyte precursors may also be seen in the granulocytic leukaemias and on rare occasions they are prominent; basophils and eosinophils are usually seen in CGL, but a subtype of AGL with an excess of eosinophils is also recognized.

In *monocytic leukaemia* scanning EM reveals many cytoplasmic flaps on the cell surface.[2695,2992] Transmission EM shows an eccentric reniform nucleus. Small slightly pleomorphic granules, round to oval in shape and varying in electron-density, are scattered throughout the cytoplasm (Fig. 28.12).

Peroxidase electron-cytochemistry may be useful in the diagnosis of leukaemia (Table 28.1).[2855] The primary granules of granulocytic leukaemia demonstrate peroxidase activity and the reaction product may also be produced in the nuclear envelope and cisternae of RER. Similarly, peroxidase activity is found in the nuclear envelope and RER of monoblasts,[2994] but in the later stages of development this is confined to a few of the small granules of monocytoid cells. Poorly differentiated *megakaryocytic leukaemia* may also be detected by peroxidase electron-cytochemistry, as the reaction product is limited to the nuclear envelope and the endoplasmic reticulum (Fig. 28.18).[2856]

## HAIRY CELL LEUKAEMIA (HCL)

This unique form of leukaemia derives its name from the highly characteristic elaborate cytoplasmic flaps and processes of the leukaemic cells. These processes are easily detected by TEM, and are even more dramatically revealed by SEM (Fig. 28.14); they are most effectively demonstrated on circulating hairy cells, and buffy coat preparations are usually entirely satisfactory.

In splenic tissue the processes are less easily delineated because of close apposition of cells;[3009] complex interlocking processes can often be appreciated, but sometimes even these are inapparent. Adherence to splenic sinusoidal endothelium, with insinuation of processes between endothelial cells, and occlusive intrasinusoidal aggregates of hairy cells are also recorded.[3040]

Ribosome-lamella (lamella-particle) complexes are present in about half the cases — occurring in 20–100 per cent of the cells — but are not restricted to HCL (Table 28.2). Engulfment of

**Table 28.1 Comparative ultrastructure of acute leukaemias**

| | Acute lymphoblastic leukaemia (ALL) | Acute granulocytic leukaemia (AGL) | Acute myelomonocytic leukaemia (AMML)* | Erythroleukaemia (EL) |
|---|---|---|---|---|
| Nuclear morphology | Rounded to irregular, with folds, indentations, and sometimes multiple profiles | Large, rounded or lobulated | Large nucleus, more irregular than normal monocytic cells. Folding and indentations more prominent with increasing cell maturity | Irregular to rounded with increasing maturity |
| Nuclear projections and pockets | Generally prominent | Often present | Not conspicuous | Not conspicuous |
| Chromatin | Variable marginal condensation, less prominent than in normal lymphocytes | Dispersed, with peripheral condensation in more mature cells | Variable marginal condensation | Dispersed in proerythroblasts. Peripheral condensation with increasing cell maturity |
| Nucleoli | Small to prominent. Generally one profile only. Less numerous than in AGL and AMML | Large, generally marginated | Large, with prominent nucleolonema | Large, often multiple |
| Cytoplasm – volume and processes | High nuclear:cytoplasmic ratio | High nuclear:cytoplasmic ratio | Pseudopodial extensions | Abundant |
| Cytoplasmic granules | Typically absent. A few primary lysosomal granules may be present in Golgi region | Present, rounded or oblong. Larger than granules of monocytoid cells | Present, smaller and more pleomorphic than those in AGL | Agranular, or may have a few small lysosomal granules |
| Auer rods | Absent | Auer rods are present only occasionally in AGL but are numerous in acute promyelocytic leukaemia. See Fig. 28.4 | Auer rods may be found in granulocytic cells or unclassifiable primitive cells | Absent |
| Organelles | Sparse | Dilated segments of RER; mitochondria | Mitochondria, Golgi complexes, RER | Mitochondria may contain ferruginous micelles |
| Filaments | Often present in perinuclear region. Approximately 9 nm in diameter. Less prominent than in AGL and AMML | Often present | Monocytoid cells often have conspicuous filaments, 6–10 nm in diameter, in perinuclear region | Usually absent |
| Pinocytosis and phagocytic vacuoles | Not conspicuous | Not conspicuous | Monocytoid cells may show prominent phagocytic vacuoles | Pinocytotic vesicles typically prominent |
| Glycogen | Occasionally prominent | Not conspicuous | Not conspicuous | Often abundant |
| Peroxidase reaction | Negative | Positive | Granulocytic cells positive; monocytoid cells negative | Negative |
| Remarks | Abnormal lymphocytic cells show considerable morphological diversity, resemble lymphocytes to varying degrees. Rieder cells may be present, and also occur less often in AGL and AMML. Show microtubules in region of nuclear identation (see Fig. 1.5) See Fig. 28.5 | Presence of granules distinguishes AGL from ALL. Granules are larger and more evenly rounded than those of monocytoid cells. As in other malignancies, the cells show a range of differentiation, from myelocytes and promyelocytes to unclassifiable cells devoid of granules; myeloblasts constitute the most numerous cell type. Agranular primitive cells cannot be distinguished from lymphoblasts See Figs. 28.1–28.4 | *Descriptions in this section refer to monocytoid cells unless stated otherwise AMML shows continuous spectrum from predominantly AGL with monocytoid features, to almost pure monocytic leukaemia. Most cells are promonocytic; relatively few blasts See Figs. 28.12 and 28.13 | Concomitant variable proliferation of granulocytic and megakaryocytic precursors |

References: 2851, 2854, 2857, 2860, 2865, 2880

autologous erythrocytes and platelets by hairy cells is recorded, but is exceptional.[3027]

Despite numerous studies with a variety of techniques, including enzyme- and immuno-cytochemistry, the nature of hairy cells has long remained both elusive and controversial,[3014,3028] but current evidence suggests that they represent B-lymphocytes.[3029]

## PROLIFERATIVE HISTIOCYTOSES

The proliferative histiocytoses represent a heterogeneous collection of conditions characterized by abnormal cells whose ultrastructural appearances resemble to varying degrees those of either phagocytic mononuclear cells, or Langerhans' histiocytes.

### 1. Malignant histiocytosis

In malignant histiocytosis the participating cells display characteristics of mononuclear phagocytes (Figs. 28.19 and 28.20). Typically there is evidence of phagocytic activity, particularly erythrophagocytosis, many phagosomes containing red blood cells in various stages of degradation. Langerhans' cell (Birbeck) granules have been found only rarely in malignant histiocytosis (Table 28.3).[3062,3068]

The ultrastructural demonstration of 2-naphthyl thiol acetate esterase has recently been applied to the diagnosis of histiomonocytic neoplasia.[3069] Kim et al[3069] suggest three major diagnostic applications for this procedure:

1. The diagnosis of malignant histiocytosis, even in the absence of phagocytic activity and cytoplasmic processes.
2. The distinction between 'true' histiocytic lymphoma and large cell lymphocytic lymphoma.
3. The identification of monoblastic differentiation in otherwise unclassifiable leukaemias.

### 2. Histiocytosis X

In contrast, all of the components of the histiocytosis X group (eosinophilic granuloma, and the so-called Hand-Schüller-Christian and Letterer-Siwe syndromes) are characterized by infiltration of various tissues by cells whose morphology closely resembles the Langerhans' histiocyte (Fig. 28.21). The presence of Langerhans' cell granules appears to be specific for this type of histiocyte (Fig. 28.22); when found in the appropriate cellular environment such granules represent a valuable confirmatory finding in histiocytosis X, but are not restricted to this group of disorders (Table 28.3).[3087,3090]

**Table 28.2  Ribosome-lamella complexes in tumours**

| Tumour | Remarks |
|---|---|
| *LYMPHOHAEMOPOIETIC MALIGNANCIES* | |
| Hairy cell leukaemia | Ribosome-lamella complexes (R-LC) found in approximately 50 per cent of cases;[39] when present, occur in about 20–100 per cent of the hairy cells.[2699] See Figs. 28.15–28.17 |
| Monoblastic leukaemia | — |
| Acute lymphoblastic leukaemia | — |
| Chronic lymphocytic leukaemia | Described in 6–15 per cent of cases, in about 1–50 per cent of the lymphocytes.[2914] Coexistence and apparent continuity with annulate lamellae in the same cells noted in one case (?related to previous chemotherapy)[2914] |
| Sézary syndrome | — |
| Large cell lymphoma | Retroperitoneal tumour. R-LC present in about 15 per cent of cells[2787] |
| Lymphosarcoma cell leukaemia | — |
| Waldenström's macroglobulinaemia | — |
| Multiple myeloma | — |
| *OTHER BENIGN AND MALIGNANT NEOPLASMS* | |
| Parathyroid adenoma | — |
| Adrenal cortical adenoma | — |
| Paraganglioma | — |
| Insulinoma | In 20 per cent of cells in one case[965] |
| Sertoli cell tumour of testis | Calcifying tumour. R-LC in 10 per cent of cells, which contained up to 20 complexes[1126] |
| Meningioma | — |
| Cerebellar haemangioblastoma | — |
| Adenocarcinoma of lung | — |
| Oesophageal squamous cell carcinoma | — |

References: 39, 47, 64, 274, 783, 961, 965, 1126, 1806, 1905, 2699, 2787, 2793, 2858, 2870, 2879, 2914, 2943, 3009, 3032, 3043

**Table 28.3  Occurrence of Langerhans' cell granules (LCG) in pathological tissues***

| Disorder | Remarks |
| --- | --- |
| *HISTIOCYTOSES AND REACTIVE HISTIOCYTIC DISORDERS* | |
| Histiocytosis X | Characteristic of all components of the histiocytosis X complex, namely eosinophilic granuloma, so-called Letterer-Siwe disease, and the so-called Hand Schüller-Christian syndrome. Found in cutaneous, osseous, lymph nodal, pulmonary, neural and other visceral lesions. See Figs. 28.21 and 28.22 |
| Hyperplastic lymph nodes | — |
| Dermatopathic lymphadenitis | In Langerhans' cells in paracortical regions |
| Toxoplasmic lymphadenitis | — |
| Pulmonary sarcoidosis | — |
| Self-healing reticulohistiocytosis | — |
| Malignant histiocytosis | Most cases of malignant histiocytosis lack LCG |
| Malignant histiocytosis with eosinophilia | One case[3062] |
| *FIBROHISTIOCYTIC TUMOURS* | |
| Fibroxanthosarcoma of bone | One case[2620] |
| Malignant fibrous histiocytoma | Includes one case of post-irradiation sarcoma[2314] |
| Atypical fibroxanthoma of skin | McLay et al[2293] have also described LCG in a 'malignant fibrous histiocytoma' of skin |
| *EPITHELIAL TUMOURS OF SKIN* | |
| Syringoma | In dermal histiocytic cells |
| Cylindroma | In dermal/stromal histiocytic cells |
| Eccrine spiradenoma | In Langerhans' histiocytes |
| Syringocystadenoma papilliferum | In dermal histiocytic cells |
| Trichoepithelioma | — |
| Basal cell carcinoma of skin | In admixed Langerhans' cells |
| *MISCELLANEOUS NEOPLASMS* | |
| Squamous cell carcinoma | Pigmented squamous carcinoma of cornea and conjunctiva. LCG found in dendritic Langerhans' cells[2152] |
| Ameloblastoma | Within Langerhans' histiocytes in epithelial follicles |
| Pleomorphic salivary adenoma | Submandibular gland tumour[712] |
| Benign cystic ovarian teratoma | In Langerhans' cells within epidermal component |
| Yolk sac carcinoma | Suprasellar tumour. LCG found in admixed histiocytes[1151] |
| Metastatic adenocarcinoma in lymph node | — |
| Mesenchymal chondrosarcoma | Extraskeletal tumour. LCG observed in macrophages in perivascular regions[2579] |
| Thymoma | In histiocytic cells |
| Mycosis fungoides | In associated Langerhans' cells |
| Adult T-cell leukaemia in Japan | In dermal lesions[2933] |
| 'Reticulum cell sarcoma' | Cutaneous infiltrate. LCG in dermal histiocytic cells[3087] |
| *OTHER SKIN DISORDERS WITH HISTIOCYTIC INFILTRATION* | |
|  | Include pigmented progessive purpura, lichen planus, lichen nitidus, eruptive histiocytoma, actinic reticuloid, infantile papular acrodermatitis and the Ehlers-Danlos syndrome |

*LCG are regarded as specific for histiocytes of a particular lineage (Langerhans' cells); in all of the non-histiocytic conditions listed in this table, LCG have been observed only in associated/stromal histiocytoid cells

References: 64, 91, 442, 496, 712, 724, 1151, 1285, 1454, 1461, 1497, 2152, 2293, 2314, 2579, 2620, 2686, 2726, 2933, 3050–3053, 3056, 3059, 3061, 3062, 3067, 3072, 3073, 3075, 3078, 3081, 3086, 3087, 3090, 3093

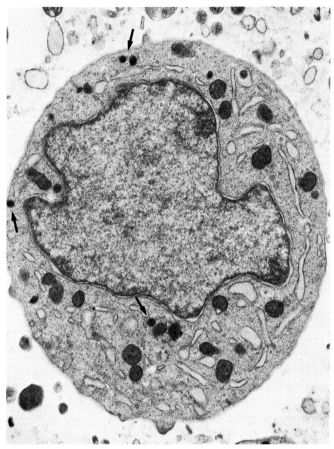

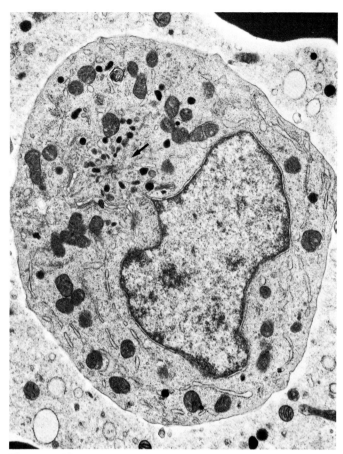

**Fig. 28.1** *(Above — left)* **Granulocytic leukaemia I: Myeloblast**

Figs. 28.1–28.3 are all from the same case, an example of predominantly promyelocyic leukaemia in a 76-year-old man; he was thought on clinical grounds to have an acute myeloblastic transformation of chronic granulocytic leukaemia (fine needle aspiration biopsy of a granulocytic sarcoma in the chest wall). The cells are arranged in a tripartite sequence of increasing maturity to illustrate the granulocyte precursors predominating in acute and chronic granulocytic leukaemias.

As depicted here, myeloblastic cells predominate in *acute myeloblastic leukaemia*. Immature granulocytes and myelocytes similar to (and often more mature than) the cell shown in Fig. 28.3 are dominant in *chronic granulocytic leukaemia*; myeloblasts are often also seen in CGL, but in smaller numbers, their frequency being partly dependent on the nature of the specimen. For example, more myeloblasts are encountered in bone marrow or buffy coat preparations than in peripheral blood.

This myeloblast has a slightly irregular nucleus with abundant euchromatin; nucleoli are often prominent in these cells, but are not included in this plane of section. The cytoplasm is dominated by numerous free ribosomes, strands of RER and mitochondria; there are only a few scattered uniformly dense primary granules (arrows). Secondary granules are uncommon in acute granulocytic leukaemia, as are Auer bodies. Irregularly shaped mitochondria, giant lysosome-like structures, and bundles of intermediate filaments are also described; so too are unusual configurations of the endoplasmic reticulum, including multilaminar and complex stellate arrangements. (× 12 600)

The number of granules varies greatly in leukaemic cells; mature neutrophilic granules are generally diminished, while immature granues are proportionately increased. In some cases of acute leukaemia it is not possible to determine whether agranular blast cells represent myeloblasts or lymphoblasts. The appearances of the granules may also be abnormal, with an unusually large or small size distribution.

References: 2851, 2852, 2854, 2855, 2857, 2860, 2863, 2865, 2866, 2876, 2878, 2883, 2944–2988

**Fig. 28.2** *(Above — right)* **Granulocytic leukaemia II: Early pro-myelocytic cell**

This cell has a distinct centrosome (arrow) adjacent to the nucleus, with granulogenesis in relation to the Golgi apparatus. Few granules are present in the remainder of the cytoplasm, which contains free ribosomes, RER and mitochondria. There is less heterochromatin than in normal promyelocytes. (× 11 700)

**Fig. 28.4** *(Facing page — bottom)* **Acute promyelocytic leukaemia: Auer bodies**

There are several rod-shaped and rhomboidal Auer bodies in the cytoplasm of this leukaemic promyelocyte. Some show evidence of an organized internal substructure, but this is more clearly depicted in the inset at left, where longitudinal periodicity of about 8 nm can be seen, the narrow spacing probably reflecting an oblique plane of section. In addition, some of the primary granules display internal periodicity spaced at intervals of 17 nm (arrows and inset at lower right), indicating an early phase of Auer body formation. (× 32 200. Inset, left: × 40 800. Inset, lower right: × 101 900)

(Case contributed by Dr T.M. Mukherjee).

**Discussion:** Auer rods are characteristic of granulocytic leukaemias, being described in acute granulocytic leukaemia (AGL), the myeloid cells of myelomonocytic leukaemia and acute promyelocytic leukaemia (APML). They are rarely seen in AGL (approximately 5 per cent of cases), and then only in a small proportion of cells, usually 1–5 per cent according to Bessis.[2854] They occur in greatest profusion in APML, where transverse sections reveal that they are formed by hexagonal arrays of tubules 5.5 nm in diameter.[2947] Their periodicity in APML typically varies from 17–25 nm, whereas narrower spacing of 6–13.5 nm is found in AGL.[2947] Thought to develop from primary granules, Auer rods likewise contain peroxidase, although the intensity of reactivity varies.

References: 2854, 2857, 2947, 2952, 2957, 2985

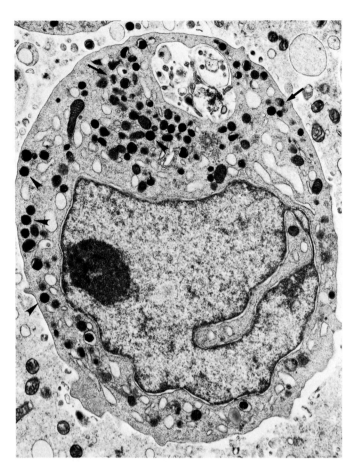

### Fig. 28.3 *(Left)* Granulocytic leukaemia III: Primitive granulocytic cell (promyelocyte-myelocyte)

Concentrated to one side of the cell, numerous granules inhabit the cytoplasm. They include round uniformly dense primary granules (arrowheads), and a few smaller secondary neutrophilic granules (arrows), some of which exhibit submembranous lucent areas; the contents of secondary granules may be extracted to varying degrees in glutaraldehyde-fixed material, with resultant electron-lucency.[45] Dumbbell-shaped (bacilliform) tertiary granules are not evident. Numerous free ribosomes and dilated cisternae of RER are still present in the cytoplasm.

The nuclear morphology is not commensurate with the cytoplasmic appearances (nucleocytoplasmic asynchrony), and is bizarre in its own right. An area of indentation enclosed by a nuclear bridge indicates early lobulation, yet a prominent marginated nucleolus and a nuclear body can be seen. In addition, there is no more heterochromatin than in the preceding two cells. (× 10 100)

Deviant granule and nuclear morphology, together with nucleocytoplasmic asynchrony, sometimes makes it difficult, and perhaps meaningless, to determine the exact stage of maturation of leukaemic granulocyte precursor cells. In other cases, mature segmented nuclei are found in hypogranular neutrophils, again reflecting aberrant maturation in leukaemic granulocytes.

References: 45, 2854, 2860

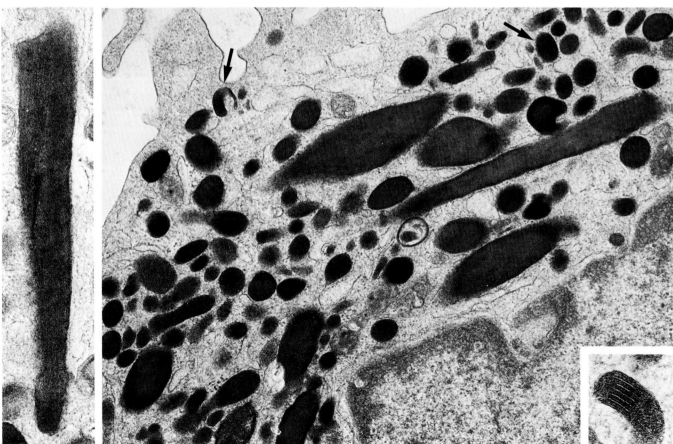

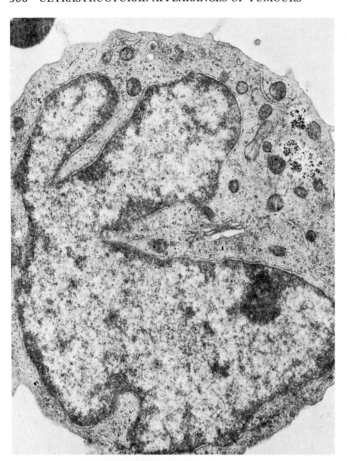

**Fig. 28.5 Acute lymphoblastic leukaemia: Cell morphology**

The nucleus is irregular and a small nucleolus is present. There are no specific features in the almost agranular cytoplasm. The Golgi apparatus is moderately developed and small aggregates of glycogen particles are present in the peripheral cytoplasm. (× 16 000)

References: 2854, 2857, 2860, 2865, 2883, 2888, 2889, 2912, 2916, 2919, 2922, 2925, 2926, 2929, 2930, 2935, 2936, 2940

**Fig. 28.6 B-lymphocytic leukaemia: Lymphocytes with cytoplasmic processes**

Buffy coat preparation. The cells have the characteristics of slightly activated lymphocytes, with round nuclei containing prominent marginated chromatin, and frequent single moderately developed nucleoli (arrows). The presence of large central nucleoli is often used as a guide to the diagnosis of prolymphocytic leukaemia. The cytoplasm contains numerous free ribosomes, small numbers of mitochondria, and a few strands of RER. The cell membranes often form delicate processes, but these are not as numerous, irregular or elongated as those seen in hairy cell leukaemia (see Fig. 28.15). (× 8500)

References: 2854, 2857, 2860, 2883, 2886, 2887, 2890, 2891, 2901, 2905, 2911, 2914, 2917, 2918, 2920, 2921, 2924, 2925, 2927, 2931, 2943

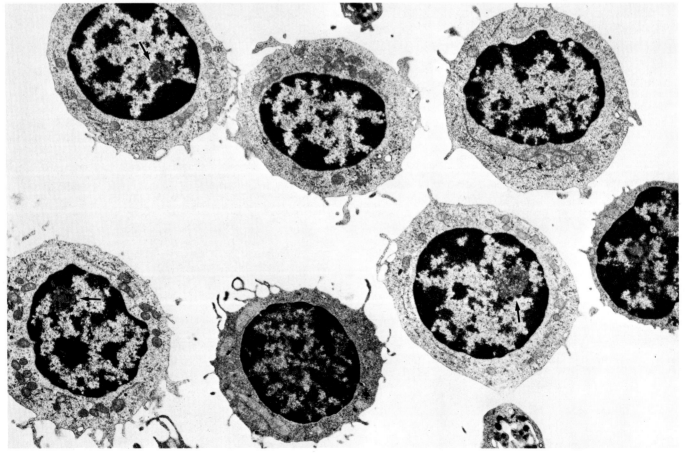

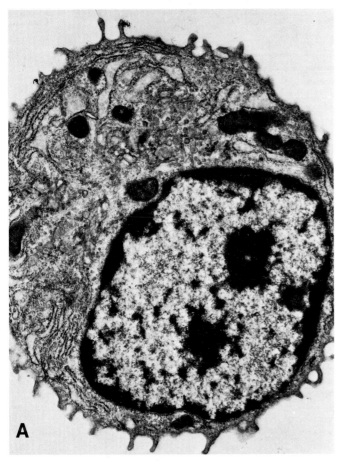

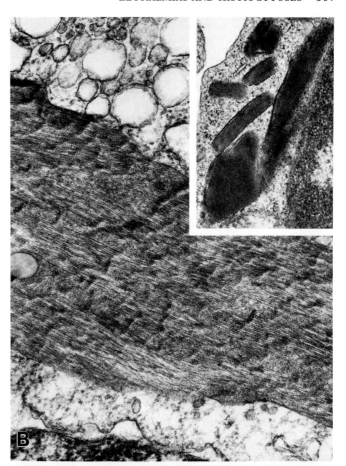

**Fig. 28.7** *(Above — left and right)* **Lymphocytic leukaemia (B-cell type): Plasmacytoid differentiation and crystalline inclusions**

**A:** Immunological studies on the leukaemic cells were characteristic of B-lymphocytes. The nucleus is rounded and has a prominent nucleolus. Long strands of RER occur in the cytoplasm; an abundance of RER is the most useful cytoplasmic predictor of B-lymphocytic properties.[2907,2925] Again, there are flaps and microvilli at the periphery of the cell. (× 12 600)

**B:** Crystalline material sometimes appears in the cytoplasm of these cells; here it is membrane-bound. Evidence suggests that it consists of immunoglobulin products. (× 52 000)

**Inset:** Crystalline structures resembling Auer rods, in chronic lymphocytic leukaemia. Membrane-bound inclusions of this type have occasionally been described in various lymphoproliferative disorders, including prolymphocytic leukaemia[2906] and chronic lymphocytic leukaemia.[2854,2860] In contrast to Auer bodies they are found in lymphocytic cells instead of myeloblasts; they are rod-shaped rather than needle-shaped, and are non-azurophilic.[2854] They have been shown to contain immunoglobulin products, whereas Auer bodies are characterized by the presence of peroxidase and acid phosphatase.[2854,2860] Immunofluorescence studies on this case demonstrated IgM within the inclusions, which usually contain IgM/λ,[2921] although IgA is also recorded (see also discussion to Fig. 27.14). (× 26 300)

References: 2854, 2860, 2890, 2891, 2906, 2907, 2911, 2925

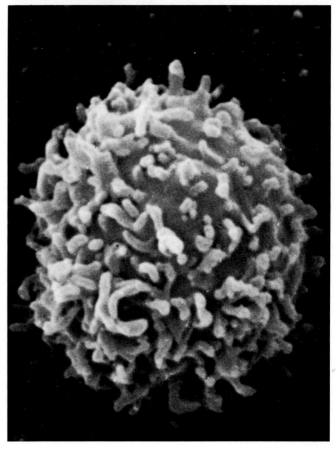

**Fig. 28.8 Chronic lymphocytic leukaemia (B-cell type): Surface morphology**

Scanning electron micrograph of chronic lymphocytic leukaemia. This cell displays many surface microvillous processes — a characteristic of B-lymphocytes. (× 17 000)

References: 2695, 2705, 2873–2876, 2898, 2920

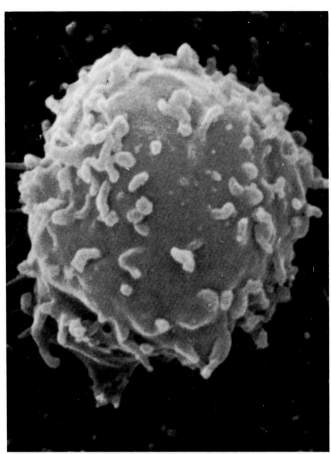

**Fig. 28.9 Lymphocytic leukaemia (T-cell type): Surface morphology**

This scanning electron micrograph shows that the surface microvillous processes of leukaemic lymphocytes of T-cell type are not as plentiful as those on the surface of B-lymphocytes (compare with Fig. 28.8). Most of the cell surface is relatively smooth. (× 17 000)
References: See Fig. 28.8

**Fig. 28.10 Lymphocytic leukaemia (T-cell type): Cell morphology**

Immunological testing indicated that these leukaemic cells were T-lymphocytes. Irregular nuclei, moderate amounts of heterochromatin and nucleolar prominence are evident. There are a few surface flaps and microvilli, while most of the organelles are concentrated in the uropod. (× 5200)

**Discussion:** As with some T-cell lymphomas, nuclear irregularity ± multilobation is the single most important morphological indicator of a T-lymphocytic leukaemia[2925] (see Table 27.1). Other findings in adult T-cell leukaemia-lymphoma include a speckled chromatin pattern, prominent cytoplasmic lysosomes, lipid droplets and glycogen. Cytoplasmic parallel tubular arrays have also been described in T-cell CLL, and Costello et al[2894] suggested that they may be characteristic of the T-suppressor subset of T-lymphocytes.

On the other hand, in classical hand-mirror cell leukaemia the perinuclear cytoplasm is reduced to a thin rim. The uropod ('handle') is slender and elongated, with surface microspikes.[2935,2936] The cells have neither B- nor T-lymphocytic characteristics.[2936] Hand-mirror cells are also recorded in acute granulocytic leukaemia.[2954]

References: 2728, 2780, 2809, 2812, 2894, 2907, 2912, 2925, 2934–2936, 2954

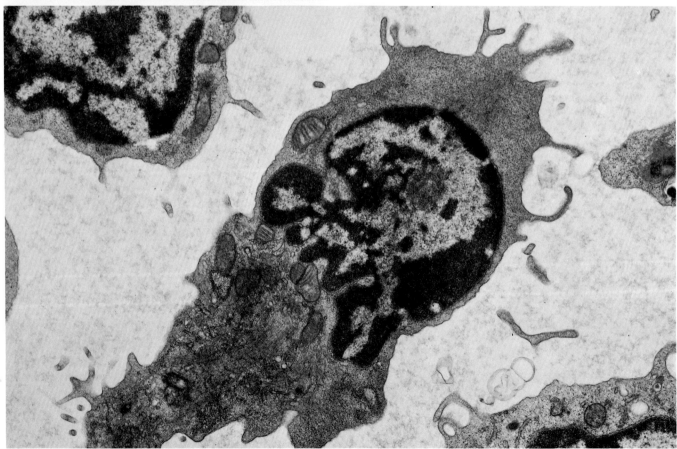

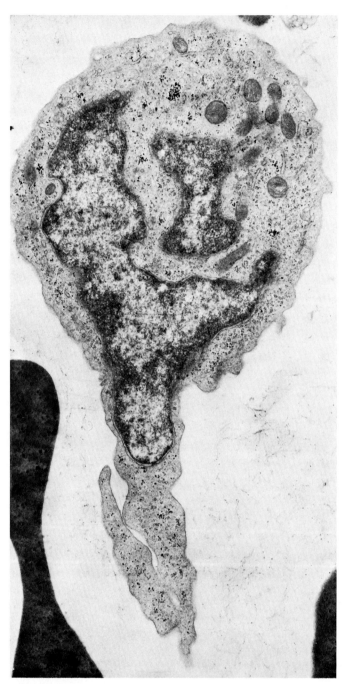

**Fig. 28.11 'Hand-mirror cell' leukaemia: Cell morphology**

This leukaemic cell displays a prominent uropod-like structure. The nucleus is irregular and glycogen granules are scattered in the thin rim of cytoplasm. (× 15 400)

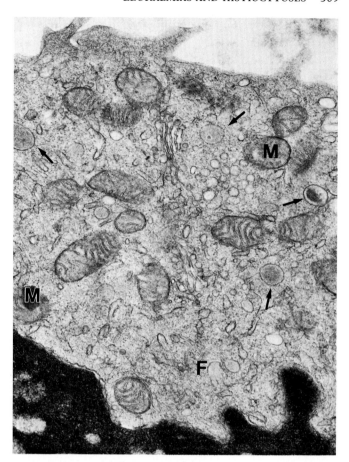

**Fig. 28.12 Monocytic leukaemia: Cell detail**

This leukaemic cell has an eccentric, irregular nucleus. Sometimes nuclear convolutions are more definite, and chromatin bridges may occur. There is a moderately well developed centrosphere in the paranuclear zone, and a few scattered pleomorphic lysosomal granules (arrows) are seen in the cytoplasm; these are less dense than primary granules of the granulocyte series. RER is sparse. Scattered cytoplasmic projections are seen at the cell periphery. Bundles of cytoplasmic filaments (F) are generally prominent in these leukaemias, and there are moderate numbers of mitochondria (M). (× 27 200)

See Table 28.1.

References: 229, 287, 2854, 2857, 2860, 2865, 2883, 2989–2994, 2996–3004

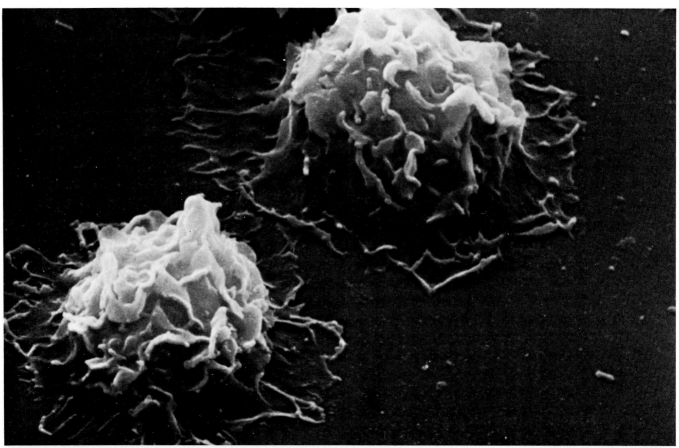

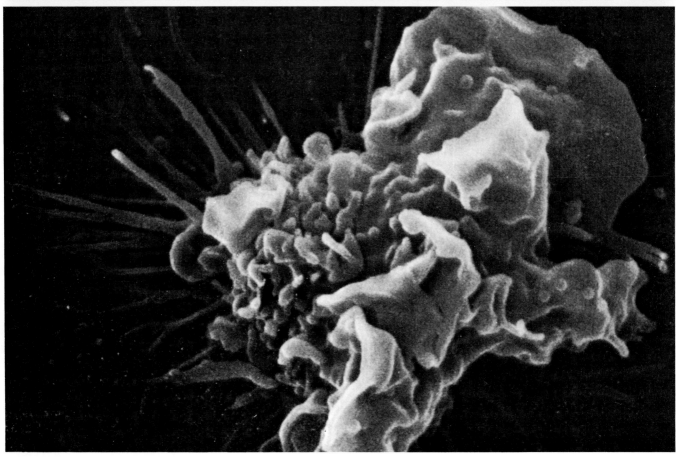

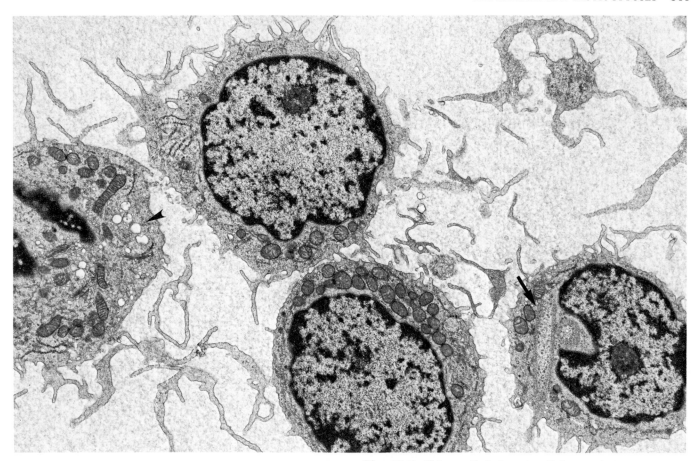

**Fig. 28.15 Hairy cell leukaemia: Cell morphology, including cytoplasmic processes**

Transmission EM of hairy cell leukaemia. Elaborate cytoplasmic processes constitute the outstanding feature of these 'hairy' cells. The nuclei are slightly irregular, and two contain moderately prominent nucleoli. Vesicles (arrowhead) and ribosome-lamella complexes (arrow) are also evident, even at this low magnification. (× 8600)

**Discussion:** Apart from ribosome-lamella complexes, the cytoplasmic contents of hairy cells include prominent mitochondria (sometimes with a cross-hatched internal pattern), small to moderately developed Golgi complexes, ribosomes, strands of RER and centrioles with associated microtubules. Vacuoles and vesicles, as well as lysosomes, are also reported; so too are aggregates of glycogen particles and fibrillary inclusions composed of filaments approximately 9 nm in diameter.[3014] Microfilaments are often present in the paranuclear region and can sometimes be seen entering the microvilli. Pentalaminar 'zipper-like' intercellular junctions resembling those of Langerhans' histiocytes have also been recorded.[3014,3027] Cawley et al[3014] have additionally found elongated inclusions related to the RER, while Hammar et al[3027] reported parallel tubular arrays.

References: 3005–3049

**Fig. 28.13** *(Facing page — top)* **Monocytic leukaemia: Surface morphology**

Scanning EM of the abnormal cells of monocytic leukaemia shows them to form many large, broad-faced, ruffled, cytoplasmic surface flaps. (× 4200)

References: 2876, 2992

**Fig. 28.14** *(Facing page — bottom)* **Hairy cell leukaemia: Surface morphology**

Scanning electron micrograph. The cell has many large, broad-based, cytoplasmic flaps protruding from its surface; in addition, there are clusters of stubby microvilli and slender filopodia. (× 17 300)

Reference: 3014

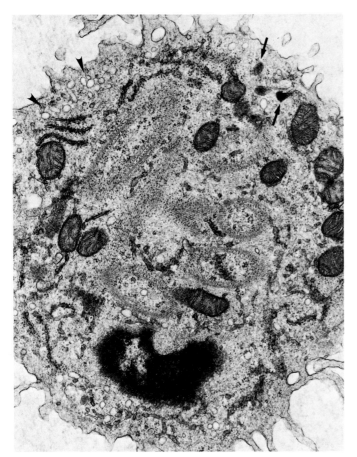

**Fig. 28.16 Hairy cell leukaemia: Cell morphology, including ribosome-lamella complexes**

Peripheral cytoplasmic processes are again evident. The cytoplasm contains several ribosome-lamella complexes in various planes of section. Note also the presence of mitochondria, strands of RER, vesicles (arrowheads) and a few small lysosomal bodies (arrows). (× 19 100)

There is evidence that cases of hairy cell leukaemia with frequent cytoplasmic inclusions have a less favourable prognosis than those with few or none. Similarly, cases with convoluted or indented nuclei seem to fare more poorly than those with ovoid nuclei.

Reference: 3006

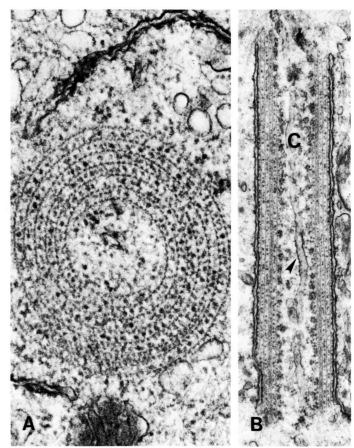

**Fig. 28.17 Hairy cell leukaemia: Ribosome-lamella complexes (R-LC)**

**A:** In transverse section, ribosome-lamella complexes are seen to consist of concentric lamellae alternating with ribosome-like particles. (× 72 500)

**B:** Case of hairy cell leukaemia in a 60-year-old man (splenectomy specimen). Longitudinal section of a ribosome-lamella complex. Lamellae of RER extend along the outer aspect of this structure, parallel to its long axis. Note the different appearance of the membranes of the RER in comparison to the lamellae of the R-LC. Characteristically, there is an inner core (C), continuous with the cytoplasm and devoid of lamellae. The core contents may include endoplasmic reticulum (arrowhead), occasionally in close apposition to the innermost lamellae; ribosomes and vesicles may also be seen in the cores, but mitochondria are consistently absent. (× 30 200)

**Discussion:** Detailed analysis of R-LC demonstrates that they are cylindrical structures approximately 2–4 μm in length.[3043] The internal diameter of about 400 nm appears to be constant, while the outer diameter varies from about 500–1300 nm. In high-resolution micrographs the lamellae appear to have a double tubular substructure and lack the trilaminar structure of the whorled membranous formations known as *Nebenkern* (see Fig. 2.7), from which they need to be distinguished — especially when the membranes are associated with glycogen particles (glycogen bodies; glycogen-membrane complexes). Illustrated in Fig. 2.17, such glycogen bodies are also recorded in leukaemia.[2859] The granules in R-LC contain RNA[2699] and are considered to be ribosomal.[47]

References: 47, 2699, 2859, 3014, 3043

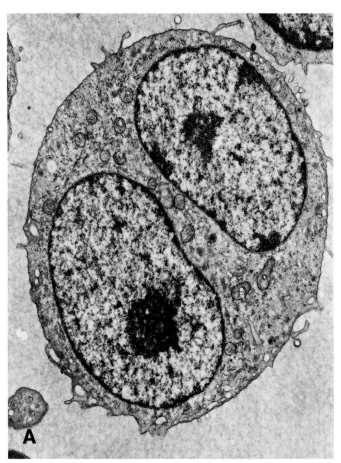

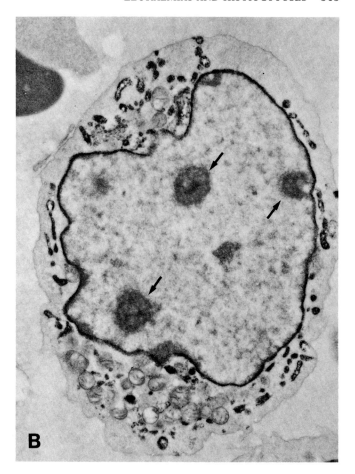

**Fig. 28.18 Megakaryoblastic leukaemia: Cell morphology and endogenous peroxidase activity**

**A:** A poorly differentiated binuclear cell is seen. This has a few peripheral cytoplasmic flaps, and apart from a few small granules, no specific cytoplasmic features are observed. (× 9300)

**B:** Peroxidase electron-cytochemistry reveals endogenous peroxidase activity, the reaction product being localized in the nuclear envelope and endoplasmic reticulum. The nucleus contains prominent nucleoli (arrows). (× 9600)

References: 2856, 2868

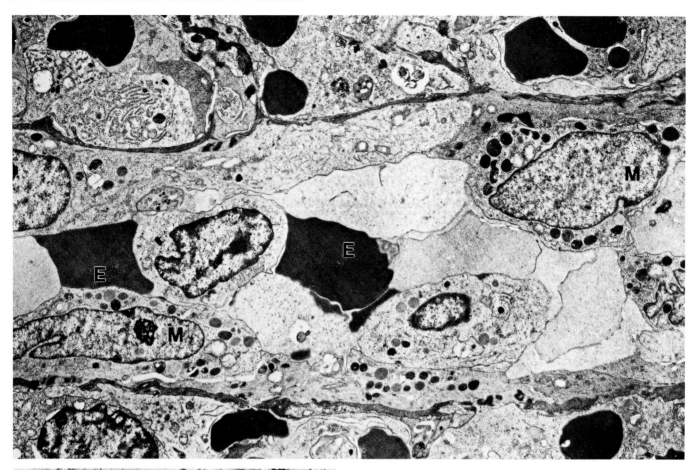

**Fig. 28.19 Spleen: Malignant histiocytosis: Survey**

Plump mononuclear phagocytes (M) containing many cytoplasmic phagosomes line the vascular channels in which erythrocytes (E) are apparent. Although the phagocytes are closely apposed, junctions are not seen. (× 4700)

References: 3052, 3060, 3062, 3063–3065, 3068, 3070, 3071, 3079, 3080, 3091

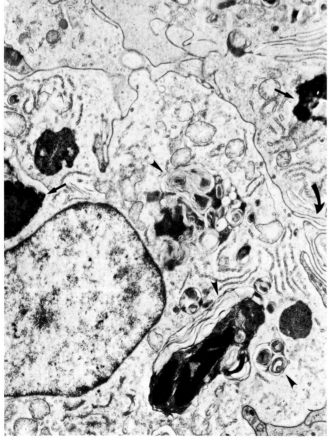

**Fig. 28.20 Spleen: Malignant histiocytosis: Histiocyte morphology**

The mononuclear phagocyte occupying most of this field has an irregular contour as a result of many flaps (curved arrow) interdigitating with those of adjoining phagocytes. Blebs and vermipodia are also described. There are large cytoplasmic phagosomes, some of which contain remnants of erythrocytes (straight arrows), while myelin bodies are evident in others (arrowheads). (× 7700)

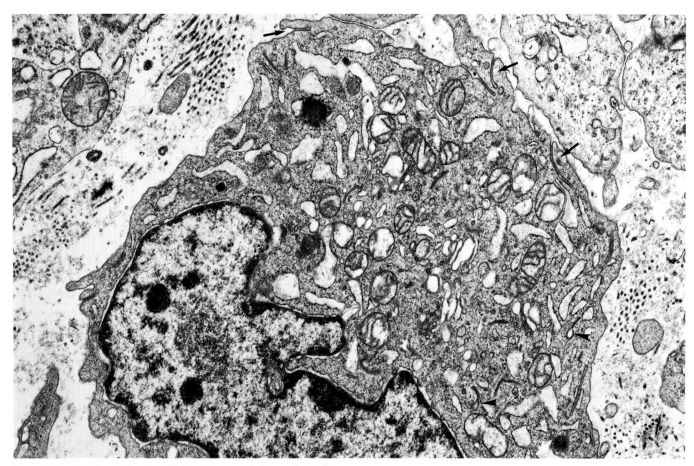

**Fig. 28.21 Histiocytosis X: Histiocyte morphology, including Langerhans' cell granules**

Solitary eosinophilic granuloma of frontal bone in a man aged 24 years. The histiocyte nucleus is irregular, and even at this relatively low magnification numerous Langerhans' cell granules (LCG) can be recognized; some of these are continuous with the cell membrane (arrows), while others have a fusiform expansion at one end (arrowheads), resulting in a 'tennis racquet' appearance. The endoplasmic reticulum is dilated. Lysosomes are not conspicuous in this cell. Mononuclear phagocyte-like cells with prominent lysosomes but no LCG may also be present.[3066] Highly contorted nuclear profiles are characteristic of Langerhans' histiocytes. (× 17 500)

See Table 28.3.

References: 3050–3053, 3055, 3059, 3066, 3067, 3072–3076, 3081, 3083, 3085, 3086, 3089, 3092, 3093

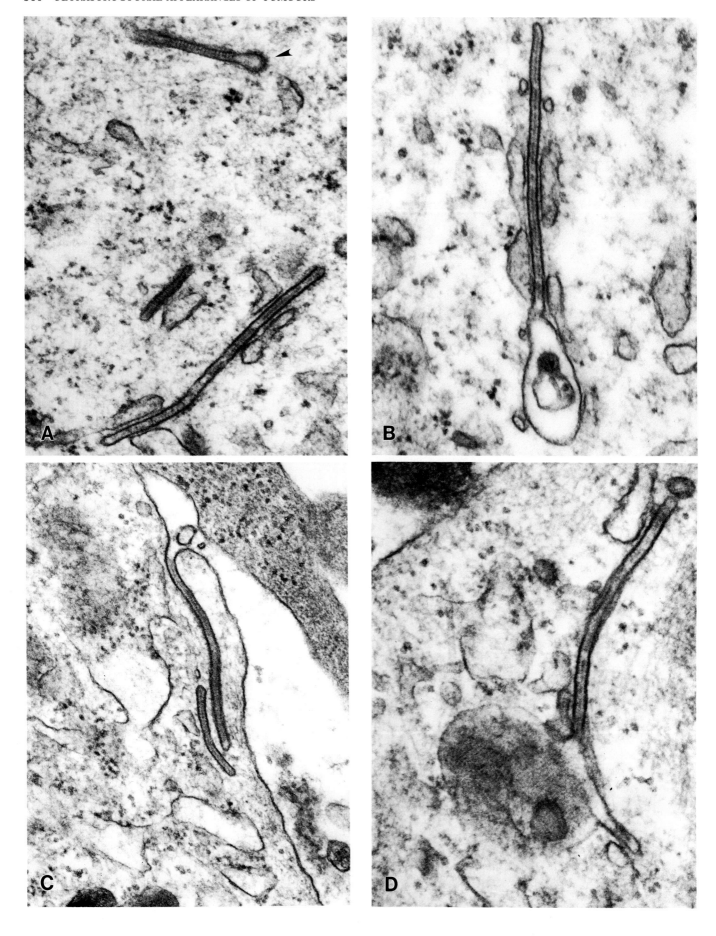

**Fig. 28.22** *(Facing page)* **Histiocytosis X: Langerhans' cell granules (Birbeck granules; X bodies)**

**A–D:** As shown in these illustrations, Langerhans' cell granules (LCG) represent elongated, straight or curved pentalaminar rod-shaped structures approximately 40 nm in thickness, with an outer limiting membrane and a central lamella. The granules may show transverse striations spaced at about 6–7 nm intervals (A), while a tangentially sectioned granule consists of a quadratic particulate latticework (D), the component particles being spaced approximately 5–6 nm apart. Terminal fusiform expansions are often present in the granules, resulting in the classical 'tennis racquet' profile; the expansion in A (arrowhead) resembles a coated vesicle. However, the expansion may be encountered anywhere along the granules (D). Birbeck granules may be seen in continuity with the plasma membrane (C), and it is highly likely that they are formed by a process of membrane infolding. Cylindrical cross-sectional profiles of the granules have never been reported, and serial sections indicate that they represent a population of discoid membranous structures with focal dilatations. The demonstration of LCG can be facilitated by zinc iodide-osmium incubation, as described by Rodriguez & Caorsi.[3082] (A: × 87 000. B: × 87 000. C: × 70 600. D: × 98 900)

References: 2726, 3082

# 29 The small round cell tumours

The differential diagnosis of the so-called malignant small round cell tumours by light microscopy constitutes a major problem in surgical pathology. A distinction between neuroblastoma, rhabdomyosarcoma, Ewing's tumour and malignant lymphoma is sometimes impossible, but ultrastructural examination of representative tissue will give a diagnosis in the majority of cases. Nevertheless, extremely poorly differentiated neuroblastomas and rhabdomyosarcomas may still pose a diagnostic dilemma, as their specific features are sporadic and poorly developed. Groups of microtubules or sheaves of non-specific filaments with focal densities may hint at the appropriate diagnosis, but a prolonged search may be necessary to demonstrate neuritic processes with neurosecretory granules, or myosin-like myofilaments (see Figs. 13.7, 13.8 and 22.6–22.8). In some instances a precise ultrastructural diagnosis cannot be made.

As more and more round cell tumours have been subjected to EM, atypical and 'hybrid' appearances have been reported. In a paper unfortunately lacking rigorous clinicopathological documentation, Schmidt et al[2637] have described four cases designated as Ewing's sarcoma of bone in which some cells had neuroblastoma-like properties — namely dendrite-like processes, neurosecretory granules less than 150 nm in diameter and microtubules — although the other ultrastructural findings were compatible with Ewing's tumour and included copious glycogen (but see Table 2.10). Alternatively, such ultrastructural appearances could also be interpreted as evidence of neuroblastoma. For example, Llombart-Bosch et al[2605] emphasize once again the similarity of Ewing's sarcoma and poorly differentiated neuroblastoma by LM (which may extend to the presence of glycogen deposits in both), and

mention the difficulty in distinguishing between them by EM. If on the other hand the diagnosis of primary osseous Ewing's tumour could be established beyond doubt, these observations might indicate that sporadic neuritic features are not necessarily restricted to neuroblastoma and allied tumours — including neuroendocrine carcinomas (see Fig. 13.6) — or that 'Ewing's tumour' as defined by LM may not be an entirely uniform entity. They emphasize yet again the importance of adopting a correlative clinicopathological approach to tumour diagnosis, of which EM is but one facet.

Many of these malignancies occur predominantly in infancy and childhood, but they are by no means so restricted. Oat-cell carcinomas are typically seen in adult life, and EM has facilitated the diagnosis of neuroblastoma in adults;[1852] however, the cutaneous tumours of the elderly, resembling neuroblastoma in their ultrastructure and previously reported as such,[1852] would now be classified as neuroendocrine (Merkel cell) carcinomas (see Chapter 6).[1535] The ultrastructural morphology of the small round cell tumours has been described and illustrated in preceding chapters (see Chapters 6, 13, 22, 25 and 27) and the major distinguishing ultrastructural appearances are summarized in Tables 29.1 and 29.2.

A similar problem exists with the differential diagnosis of small cell tumours affecting the nasal cavity and paranasal sinuses. in this instance the olfactory neuroblastoma (aesthesioneuroblastoma), whose fine structure is essentially similar to neuroblastoma in other sites, is one of several small cell malignancies affecting this region. These are listed in Table 29.3.

**Table 29.1 Comparative ultrastructure of malignant round cell tumours I: Small round cell tumours of infancy and childhood**

| | Neuroblastoma | Ewing's sarcoma | Rhabdomyosarcoma | Malignant small cell tumour of thoracopulmonary region[654] |
|---|---|---|---|---|
| Cell processes | Prominent, dendritic. Cells may be 'moulded' to each other. Cell surface is irregular. Adjacent plasma membranes may extend parallel to each other over prolonged distances | Inconspicuous | Inconspicuous | Present |
| External lamina | Usually not seen in poorly differentiated cases. If present, is restricted to 'differentiating neuroblastoma'[1875] in which neurosecretory granules are apt to be plentiful; differs morphologically from the fuzzy lamina-like material found in blastemal Wilms' tumours | Absent | May be prominent in highly differentiated tumours, but is usually fragmentary, and is sometimes absent in poorly differentiated examples | Absent |
| Intercellular junctions | Desmosomes, synaptic contacts and junctions | Infrequent small thickenings of apposed membranes | Generally inconspicuous, but desmosome-like junctions may be seen[2411] | Intermediate junctions |
| Filaments | Neurofilaments 8–12 nm in diameter | Typically absent, but occasional groups of filaments 8–10 nm in diameter are described in atypical Ewing's sarcomas | Present. Thin 5–7 nm microfilaments, with long thick myosin-like myofilaments 15 nm in diameter, forming abortive sarcomeres. Hexagonal spacing of thin filaments around thick myofilaments may be seen in transverse section. Dense Z-line-like structures usually evident, and A-, I-, H- and M-bands may be present | Absent |
| Microtubules | Prominent neurotubules 24–30 nm in diameter | Inconspicuous, but infrequent microtubules 20–27 nm in diameter have been found occasionally | Inconspicuous | Apparently inconspicuous |
| Granules | Neurosecretory granules (NSG) 90–240 nm in diameter, concentrated in cell processes | NSG characteristically absent. A few lysosomes may be present in some cases. | Infrequent small lysosomes only | Sporadic granules resembling NSG, 160–200 nm in diameter |

| | | | | |
|---|---|---|---|---|
| Glycogen | Usually inconspicuous, but considerable quantities may be seen in up to 10 per cent of cases | Classically present in copious amounts, forming 'lakes' and occurring as rosettes. However, glycogen is inconspicuous in some cases (see Table 2.10) | Often prominent, usually monoparticulate | Absent |
| Organelles | Sparse. Vesicles resembling synaptosomes are sometimes seen; these may or may not be polarized towards synaptic contacts | Sparse | Variable. Mitochondria may show tandem pattern. Sarcoplasmic reticulum present | Mitochondria, RER, Golgi complexes, and dense bodies 300–500 nm in diameter |
| Nuclear morphology* | Rounded or irregular | Rounded, occasionally indented | Irregular, often with multiple profiles | Rounded or irregular |
| Chromatin | Dispersed | Dispersed | Condensed, often marginated | Condensed |
| Nuclear blebs | Inconspicuous | Inconspicuous | Inconspicuous | Not conspicuous |
| Nucleoli | Small | Small. May be filamentous in atypical tumours | Prominent | 1–4 profiles |
| Remarks | Diagnosis rests on identification of NSG within dendritic processes, usually with microtubules and neurofilaments. See Figs. 13.7 and 13.8 | Diagnosis based on presence of copious glycogen (but see Table 2.10) and infrequent intercellular junctions, in absence of differentiating features seen in other small round cell tumours. Stroma between tumour cells is characteristically sparse and lacks collagen fibres, but may contain glycogen. Also needs to be distinguished from small cell osteosarcoma and the solid dendritic cell angiosarcoma of Bednár. See Figs. 25.7–25.9 and text, Chapter 25 | Diagnosis dependent on demonstration of long thick myosin-like filaments in addition to microfilaments, with the formation of abortive sarcomeres (but see text, Chapter 22). Proportion of cells with diagnostic filaments is highly variable. May contain poorly differentiated cells resembling those seen in Ewing's sarcoma. Intracellular collagen fibres may be present; these are not found in the other tumours listed in this table. See Figs. 22.6–22.8 | Resembles Ewing's tumour by LM, affects chest wall and peripheral regions of lung, but does not seem to be primarily a pulmonary neoplasm. Occurrence in childhood and adolescence. Neuroectodermal derivation suggested[654,656] |

*The nuclei of some of the tumours listed above and in Table 29.2 (for example, oat cell carcinoma of lung) may not be particularly 'small' when compared with other (non-small cell) neoplasms; in such instances the cell size is related to a paucity of cytoplasm, with close cellular (and nuclear) apposition

References: 39, 45, 64, 86, 498, 654–656, 1472, 1486, 1513, 1521–1523, 1527, 1538, 1628, 1629, 1852, 1871, 1875, 1876, 1880, 1882, 2207, 2410, 2411, 2425, 2438, 2440, 2475, 2570, 2588, 2605–2609, 2611, 2683, 2741, 2756.

**Table 29.2 Comparative ultrastructure of malignant round cell tumours II: Lymphomas and neuroendocrine carcinomas**

|  | Lymphocytic lymphoma | Large cell lymphoma[2741] | Oat cell carcinoma | Neuroendocrine (Merkel cell) carcinoma of skin |
|---|---|---|---|---|
| Cell processes | Inconspicuous | May show prominent complex filopodial extensions | Present | Present. Vary from sparse to plentiful. May be slender and intertwined, but generally less elaborate than neuritic processes of highly differentiated neuroblastomas. Sporadic clusters of microvillous processes may also be seen, but acini are not present |
| External lamina | Absent | Absent | Not conspicuous | Inconspicuous |
| Intercellular junctions | Absent | Absent | Scattered intermediate and desmosomal junctions | Sporadic intermediate junctions; rare desmosomes |
| Filaments | Typically absent | Typically absent | Occasional tonofilaments, but generally inconspicuous | Aggregates of intermediate filaments present in most cases, forming paranuclear fibrous bodies; appear to represent neurofilaments |
| Microtubules | Inconspicuous | Inconspicuous | Inconspicuous | Generally inconspicuous, but longitudinally-orientated microtubules within cytoplasmic processes are recorded,[1523] producing a dendrite-like appearance |
| Granules | Few lysosomes only | Few lysosomes only | Sporadic NSG 80–200 nm in diameter, in cell body and processes | Frequent NSG 80–200 nm in diameter, concentrated at cell periphery — forming linear subplasmalemmal arrays; also in dendrite-like processes if present |
| Glycogen | Inconspicuous | Generally inconspicuous | Inconspicuous | Inconspicuous |
| Organelles | Sparse. Ribosomes predominate | Sparse. Ribosomes predominate | Sparse. Confronting cisternae of endoplasmic reticulum often seen | Variable. Often sparse, with numerous free ribosomes, but mitochondria, Golgi complexes and strands of RER are sometimes present |
| Nuclear morphology | Rounded or cleaved | Rounded or cleaved | Rounded or irregular. High nuclear:cytoplasmic ratio | Uniform round nuclei; may contain nuclear bodies and/or fibrillary inclusions. High nuclear:cytoplasmic ratio |
| Chromatin | Condensed | Dispersed | Condensed | Abundant euchromatin with focal collections of heterochromatin |
| Nuclear blebs | Present | Present | Present | Inconspicuous |
| Nucleoli | Not prominent | Medium-sized to large | Not prominent | 1–3 nucleolar profiles |
| Remarks | See Fig. 27.10. See also Table 27.1 | See Figs. 27.19 and 27.20 | Most are primary in the respiratory tract, but identical carcinomas are described in other sites (Table 6.3)<br><br>See Figs. 6.1 and 6.2 | Frequency and distribution of NSG and presence of fibrous bodies in poorly cohesive polyhedral cells with little cytoplasm and uniform round nuclei are typical diagnostic features<br><br>Dendrite-like appearances may confer an ultrastructural resemblance to neuroblastoma in some cases; the distinction is facilitated by taking the associated clinicopathological background into account, including the patient's age (usually elderly) and the anatomical location (skin and subcutis ± regional lymph node metastases)<br><br>Melanosomes, neurone-specific enolase and polypeptides (somatostatin, calcitonin and ACTH) are also described in cutaneous neuroendocrine carcinomas<br><br>See Figs. 6.3 and 6.4, and text, Chapters 6 and 7 |

References: See Table 29.1

**Table 29.3    Possible differential diagnosis of small cell tumours of the nasal cavity and paranasal sinuses**

Primary neuroendocrine carcinomas
Small cell squamous carcinoma
Small cell adenocarcinoma
Classical neuroblastoma
Neuroblastoma with olfactory rosettes
Ganglioneuroblastoma
Retinoblastoma
Rhabdomyosarcoma
Ewing's sarcoma
Mesenchymal chondrosarcoma
Lymphocytic lymphomas
Burkitt's lymphoma
Granulocytic sarcoma
Metastatic small cell tumours

30. GONADAL, GERMINAL AND EMBRYONAL TUMOURS

# 30 Gonadal, germinal and embryonal tumours

## GYNAECOLOGICAL TUMOURS

Gynaecology was one of the first fields in which LM was used for tissue diagnosis,[2] and it is still the mainstay of the assessment of gynaecological neoplasms. In contrast, the contribution of EM has been more modest, although it may be of value in typing poorly differentiated carcinomas, particularly of the cervix and endometrium (see Chapters 4 and 5).[1152] Ovarian tumours in particular may display complex patterns of differentiation, the complexity often extending to the fine-structural level. EM has contributed to knowledge of the cell types present in several of these tumours, and multiple patterns of differentiation have been documented in some (see Chapter 7).

The major ultrastructural appearances of gynaecological neoplasms are summarized in Tables 30.1 and 30.2. Many of these have been illustrated in other sections of this atlas and therefore they are not extensively depicted here; for specific examples, see the Fig. numbers listed in Tables 30.1 and 30.2. In addition, the interested reader is referred to major reviews of these tumours.[1152-1155]

## TESTICULAR TUMOURS

EM has not played a major role in the differential diagnosis of testicular neoplasms, but it may be valuable in distinguishing between poorly differentiated primary germ cell tumours — notably seminoma — and some lymphoproliferative disorders. The neoplastic cells in seminomas are characterized by paucity of cytoplasmic organelles, prominent nucleolar spiremes, and few intercellular junctions (Fig. 30.3); annulate lamellae and glycogen are often evident in the cytoplasm. The fine structure of seminoma (germinoma) is compared with lymphocytic lymphoma in Table 26.1 (anterior mediastinal tumours); while the features of large cell lymphoma are listed in Table 29.2.

Embryonal carcinoma shows abortive tubuloacinar differentiation (Fig. 30.4). A similar pattern is also seen in endodermal sinus tumour,[1140-1151] whose ultrastructure resembles that of the yolk sac. Large amounts of secretory material within the RER and intercellular spaces also characterize endodermal sinus tumour (Fig. 30.7); although this material has been likened to basal lamina, it may in part be associated with the α-fetoprotein which is invariably present.[1140,1141,1143]

## WILMS' TUMOUR (NEPHROBLASTOMA) AND SO-CALLED MALIGNANT RHABDOID TUMOUR OF KIDNEY

The cell population of Wilms' tumour can be subdivided into four main compartments, arranged in highly variable combinations:[1026]

1. Blastema, closely resembling the cellular embryonic metanephric blastema (Figs. 30.8 and 30.9).
2. Tubular formations (Figs. 30.10 and 30.11).
3. Glomeruloid bodies (Fig. 30.13).
4. Stroma. Transitions between collections of blastema and incohesive stromal cells are often evident, and the spindled cells may retain blastemal features such as a layer of external lamina (Fig. 30.12). Fibroblastoid cells with copious RER occur in most cases. There may also be evidence of pluripotential differentiation in the form of smooth and striated muscle, cartilage, bone, adipose tissue and even ganglion cells.

Although most Wilms' tumours pose little diagnostic difficulty on LM, monomorphic blastemal nephroblastomas may enter into the differential diagnosis of the small round cell tumours.[86] A flocculent layer of external lamina-like material adjacent to the blastemal cells — similar to that depicted in Fig. 30.12 — is a useful diagnostic feature, as it does not occur in neuroblastoma (see Table 29.1).[1026] Monomorphic Wilms' tumours of this type have sometimes been termed 'renal sarcomas of childhood'[1007,1022] (and, even worse, 'bone metastasizing renal tumours'), but the blastemal appearances in Figs. 30.8 and 30.9 provide little support for this nomenclature.

Although striated muscle differentiation is well recognized in Wilms' tumour, convincing myofilaments and Z-lines have not been found in *malignant rhabdoid tumour of the kidney*. By LM the neoplastic cells possess eosinophilic PAS-positive cytoplasmic bodies conferring a resemblance to rhabdomyoblasts. The ultrastructural appearances are characterized by non-specific filaments concentrated in the paranuclear cytoplasm; measuring 4–11 nm in diameter, they may form concentric filamentous whorls, curving parallel arrays, or sheaves resembling tonofilaments.[1004,1008]

'Rhabdoid' tumours of this type are not restricted to the kidney. Gonzalez-Crussi et al[2195] have studied four such malignancies they designated as 'infantile sarcoma with intracytoplasmic filamentous inclusions', two of renal origin, one developing in the liver, and the last situated in the chest wall (we have also examined an apparently identical intracerebral neoplasm). Once again, myosin filaments and Z-line-like material could not be demonstrated. Instead, the cells were characterized by phagocytic activity, cell-surface complement receptors and cytoplasmic muramidase, suggesting histiocytic differentiation. In contrast, immuno-cytochemical investigation of one of the two cases reported by Schmidt et al[1027] revealed negative reactions for muramidase, $\alpha_1$-antitrypsin, $\alpha_1$-antichymotrypsin, myoglobin and cyto-keratins.

## RETINOBLASTOMA

The neuroblastoma-like appearances of retinoblastoma by LM extend to the ultrastructural level, and therefore this tumour is not illustrated separately in this atlas (see Figs. 13.7 and 13.8).

One poorly differentiated retinoblastoma grown in tissue culture which we examined recently consisted predominantly of primitive embryonal cells with abundant nuclear euchromatin and numerous cytoplasmic ribosomes. Rarely, the cells formed rudimentary rosettes, but classical rosettes with apical cilia showing a 9 + 0 configuration[2149] were not evident. Distinct neuritic features were also observed, in the form of elongated cell processes containing clustered neurosecretory granules and numerous microtubules 22 nm in diameter; the granules averaged 110 nm in diameter, with a range of 85–130 nm, but in other cases they have ranged from 120–180 nm in size.[2143] Although concentrated in the cytoplasmic processes, granules were also present in the cell bodies and granulogenesis was seen in relation to Golgi complexes. Intercellular junctions were sparse and rudimentary.

Photoreceptor differentiation may occur in highly

**Table 30.1  Major ultrastructural features of gynaecological neoplasms I: Tumours of the cervix and uterus**

| Tumour | Characteristics and figure numbers |
| --- | --- |
| *UTERINE CERVIX* | |
| Clear cell adenocarcinoma | Vaginal and cervical tumours seen particularly in diethylstilboestrol progeny.[1153] Similar clear cell adenocarcinomas also occur in endometrium and ovary. Characterized by glandular epithelial differentiation, with copious glycogen, abundant RER and prominent Golgi complexes. See Fig. 5.27 |
| Squamous cell carcinoma | Squamous differentiation. See Figs. 4.1–4.11 |
| Cervical adenocarcinoma | Glandular differentiation, with mucin granules, prominent RER and well developed Golgi complexes. Membrane-bound microfibrillary bodies may also be seen; apparently restricted to the human endocervix, these structures probably represent a distinctive type of mucin granule formed by coalescence of other mucin granules. See Fig. 5.11 |
| Undifferentiated cervical carcinomas | Appear to represent a collection of extremely poorly differentiated squamous and adeno-carcinomas, analogous to large cell undifferentiated carcinomas of lung. In one series of 18 cases,[1152] 14 were found by EM to be squamous carcinomas, 2 showed glandular differentiation and the remaining 2 were devoid of differentiating features |
| Glassy cell carcinoma | Two separate reports claim evidence of adenosquamous differentiation[1205, 1207] |
| Carcinoid tumours | Wide histological spectrum by LM, poorly differentiated cases conforming to small cell anaplastic carcinomas. Stroma may contain amyloid. Neoplastic cells contain neurosecretory granules with diameters in the range 120–500 nm; highly differentiated tumours tend to have small to large rounded granules, while those in the poorly differentiated group tend to be pleomorphic. See Table 16.2, and Chapters 6 and 16 |
| *UTERINE CORPUS* | |
| Endometrial adenocarcinoma | Glandular differentiation with paranuclear aggregates of intermediate filaments approximately 8 nm in diameter. Cilia are frequent in highly differentiated carcinomas, but are fewer than in normal and hyperplastic endometria; they are further depleted in poorly differentiated tumours, as are microvilli. See Figs. 5.28 and 5.29 |
| | In epithelial cells the ultrastructural findings said to be suggestive of Müllerian differentiation include the combination of microvilli, whorled paranuclear intermediate filaments, prominent lysosomes, plasmalemmal interdigitations, squamous features and seemingly intracytoplasmic collagen[1171] |
| Small cell carcinoma of endometrium | One case.[1246] The component cells formed sporadic intermediate junctions and desmosomes. Cytoplasmic processes were also evident and the cells contained neurosecretory granules 100–160 nm in diameter |
| Endometrial stromal sarcomas | Component cells have fibroblastoid characteristics. Collagen synthesis present, but collagen fibres may be sparse in high grade tumours. In comparison to haemangiopericytoma (Figs. 23.8 and 23.9), external lamina, microfilaments and micropinocytotic vesicles are inconspicuous. Bimorphic epithelial-stromal differentiation with the development of acini is described[1248] |
| Malignant mixed Müllerian tumours | Rhabdomyoblastic differentiation may be present (see Table 22.1 and Figs. 22.6–22.8). Carcinomatous elements form cell clusters bordered by basal lamina; intercellular and/or subcellular acini may be present |
| Leiomyoma and leiomyosarcoma of myometrium | Smooth muscle differentiation. See Figs. 21.1-21.8 |
| Plexiform tumourlet of myometrium | Smooth muscle differentiation. See Fig. 21.1 |
| Adenomatoid tumour | Mesothelial differentiation, whereas angiomas simulating adenomatoid tumour by LM have endothelial characteristics by EM. See Figs. 9.7 and 9.8 |

References: 1152–1158; 1159–1171 (vulva and vagina); 1172–1207 (cervix); 1208–1260 (uterine corpus)

differentiated tumours and is indicated by so-called fleurettes.[2146,2149] The cells comprising these structures form lumina with subjacent intermediate junctions, in mimicry of the retinal external limiting membrane. Cytoplasmic projections with bulbous ends extend beyond the junctions, and contain parallel membranes or clustered mitochondria, simulating the outer and inner photoreceptor segments respectively.[2146,2149] Melanogenesis is also described.[2161]

## OTHER BLASTOMAS

Other blastomas are considered elsewhere in this atlas. Hepatoblastoma is discussed briefly in the caption to Fig. 5.32. Neuroblastoma and ganglioneuroblastoma are covered in Chapter 13, while medulloblastoma is illustrated in Chapter 17 (see Figs. 17.3 and 17.4).

**Table 30.2  Major ultrastructural features of gynaecological neoplasms II: Trophoblastic and ovarian tumours**

| Tumour | Characteristics and figure numbers |
| --- | --- |
| *TROPHOBLAST* | |
| Hydatidiform mole | The superficial syncytiotrophoblastic layer possesses numerous elaborate surface microvilli, with intervening micropinocytotic and coated vesicles. Cytoplasm contains lipid droplets, ribosomes, RER and well developed Golgi complexes. Cytofilaments may also be seen. Cytotrophoblast includes light and dark cells, and rests on a basal lamina; may show evidence of transformation to syncytiotrophoblast in the form of plasmalemmal discontinuities. Desmosomes link adjoining cyto- and syncytio-trophoblastic cells |
| Choriocarcinoma | Both cytotrophoblastic and syncytiotrophoblastic cells recognizable. Former are larger than normal, with irregular large mitochondria which contain few cristae. Golgi apparatus may be prominent. Intracytoplasmic crypts lined by microvilli are described |
| *OVARY* | |
| Mucinous cystadenocarcinoma | Tumours of borderline malignancy contain mixture of endocervical- and intestinal-type cells. In frankly carcinomatous cases the endocervical-type cells are depleted, leaving mucinous cells of intestinal-type only; these resemble neoplastic colonic epithelium with goblet cells (Fig. 5.8). Enterochromaffin (EC) cells are also seen (Fig. 7.1). Other gastroenteropancreatic endocrine-type cells are reported in mucinous ovarian tumours, including somatostatin (D) and gastrin (G) cells, as well as composite muco-endocrine cells (see Tables 14.1 and 14.2) |
| Serous cystadenocarcinoma | Ciliated and non-ciliated cells in highly differentiated tumours. Elliptical electron-dense suprabasal granules may be seen in poorly differentiated cases |
| Brenner tumour | Epithelial component displays urothelial differentiation (Figs. 4.12 and 4.13); stromal cells are fibroblastoid.[1338] Similar features in malignant Brenner tumour. Presence of serotonin-storing endocrine cells is also recorded in Brenner tumour.[1284,1310] See also Table 7.2 |
| Ovarian carcinoid tumours, including strumal carcinoid tumour | Numerous cytoplasmic neurosecretory granules present. In strumal carcinoid tumours, the cells lining the follicles contain neurosecretory granules with an average diameter of 185 nm; nevertheless, the presence of intrafollicular thyroglobulin has also been demonstrated by immunocytochemistry. In an analysis of 2 cases, Ulbright et al[1350] identified thyroxin in both follicles and lining cells resembling follicular epithelium by EM and showing a transition to calcitonin-containing granulated cells of parafollicular type |
| Sertoli cell tumour | Light and dark tumour cells with thin (5 nm) paranuclear filaments, and 'hyaline' bodies composed of filaments about 30 nm in diameter: Charcot-Böttcher 'crystalloids' formed by parallel elongated filaments may also be seen[1349] |
| Fibroma-thecoma | Morphological continuum of cells from fibroma to thecoma. See Fig. 2.20 |
| Granulosa-theca cell tumour | Cells show deep nuclear indentations. Foci of central cell degeneration conform to Call-Exner bodies. Cytoplasmic filaments become less numerous with loss of differentiation. Small mitochondria and lipid bodies also present.<br><br>In some cases, 2 cell types are seen, representing both granulosa cells and luteinized theca-type cells. The granulosa cells are characterized by dense cytoplasm, small mitochondria with lamellar cristae and a paucity of SER. In contrast, the luteinized cells contain abundant SER, large mitochondria with disarrayed tubulovesicular cristae, and myelinoid figures resembling poorly-formed spironolactone bodies |
| Hilar cell tumour | Abundant SER. Reinke crystals may be present, and spironolactone-like bodies (Fig. 13.1) are also reported. See Figs. 30.1 and 30.2 |
| Dysgerminoma | Cell population resembles primitive germ cells, with nucleolar spiremes, annulate lamellae, and a paucity of organelles. Glycogen may be abundant. Associated inflammatory cells. See Fig. 30.3 (testicular seminoma) and Table 26.1 (mediastinal germinoma) |
| Endodermal sinus tumour | Glandular differentiation, abundant glycogen, and apparently proteinaceous material within cisternae of RER and in extracellular spaces; the interstitial material appears to represent basal lamina. See Figs. 30.5–30.7 (testicular yolk sac carcinoma) |

References: 1152–1155; 1214, 1220, 1222, 1224, 1237, 1238, 1258, 1259; 1261–1357

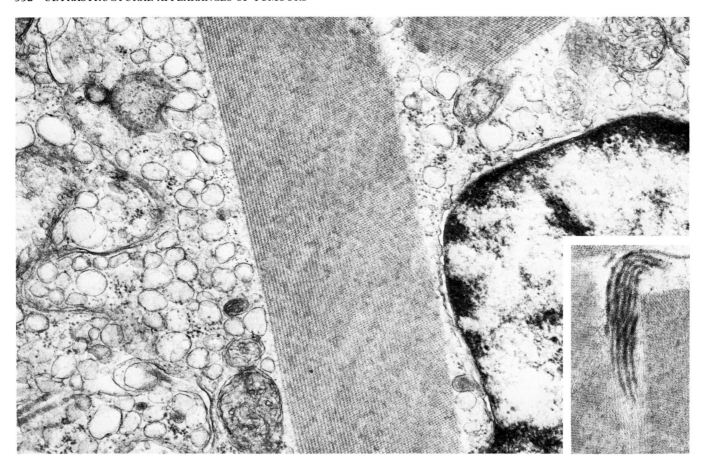

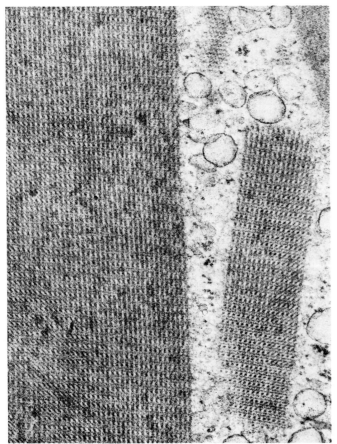

**Fig. 30.1** *(Above)* **Testicular Leydig cell tumour: Cell detail**

A Reinke crystal is present in the paranuclear region, while much of the abundant smooth endoplasmic reticulum consists of tubular profiles. (× 36 000)

**Inset:** 'Rice'-like bodies appear to blend with the lattice of the Reinke crystal. (× 29 300)

See Table 30.2.

References: 39, 1116, 1117, 1121, 1134, 1135, 1137, 1154, 1294, 1319, 1335

**Fig. 30.2** *(Left)* **Leydig cell tumour: Reinke crystal**

The lattice-like substructure of the crystal is seen in various planes. Same case as Fig. 30.1. (× 51 100)

**Fig. 30.3** *(Facing page)* **Testicular seminoma: Cell types and intercellular junctions**

The neoplastic cells (S) have complex fragmented nucleoli and evenly dispersed chromatin, but the characteristic ribbon-like nucleolonema is not shown (see Figs. 1.6 and 7.2). Cytoplasmic organelles are generally sparse, but particulate glycogen (G) is present and the middle cell contains a small stack of annulate lamellae (arrow). The cells are closely apposed, but there are few junctions, only infrequent intermediate junctions being apparent (arrowheads). Lymphocytes (L) and a mononuclear phagocyte (MP) lie next to the tumour cells. **Inset:** Intermediate junction and one of the few desmosomes found in the same tumour. (× 7000. Inset: × 38 000)

**Discussion:** The ultrastructural appearances of germinomas do not vary with the anatomical location of the tumour. The nuclei of the neoplastic cells are characteristically round to oval, with much euchromatin and fragmented filamentous nucleoli. Clumps of dense nuclear material and pseudoinclusions are occasionally seen. Nuclear pockets and reduplications are also described, as well as saccular and tubular invaginations of the nuclear envelope. The cells are usually polyhedral, but they sometimes possess processes which may have pseudopodial features; microvillous plasmalemmal projections are also recorded. Organelles are usually sparse, although glycogen, lipid, annulate lamellae, RER, microtubules, Golgi complexes and lysosomes are often present.[1123,1124]

See Table 26.1 (mediastinal germinoma).

References: 70, 1112, 1119, 1120, 1123, 1124, 1127, 1133, 1154, 1265, 1287, 1300, 1305, 1312, 1916–1918, 2669, 2683

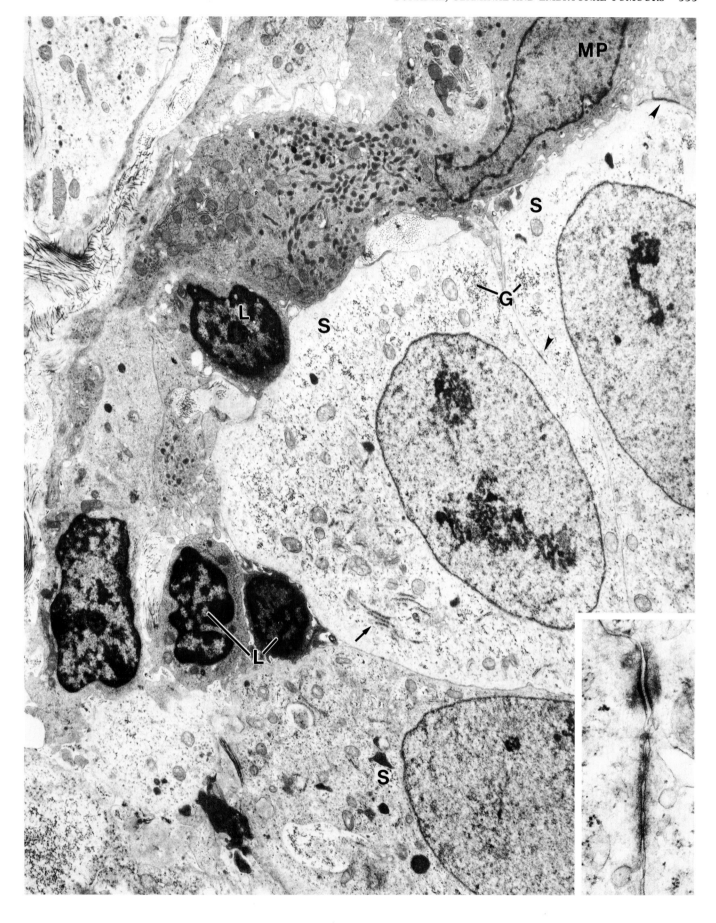

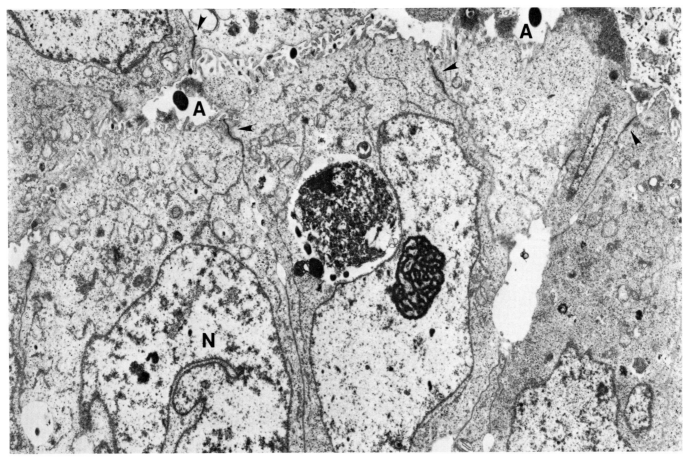

**Fig. 30.4   Malignant teratoma: Area of embryonal carcinoma**

Testicular tumour in a 31-year-old. The nuclei show little heterochromatin, while the nucleolonema is complex and filamentous; one nuclear profile (N) is quite irregular. An intercellular acinar space (A) is evident, with lining microvilli and subluminal junctional complexes (arrowheads). An autophagic vacuole is recognizable in the cell near the centre. Islands of cartilage ultrastructurally resembling the appearances illustrated in Fig. 25.3 were also present in this case. (× 5500)

**Discussion:** Albrechtsen et al[1112] have also reported dense-core vesicles and 'nuages' in neoplastic germ cells in testicular carcinoma in situ. The dense-core vesicles consist of homogeneous electron-dense material in an otherwise empty vacuole. The 'nuages' take the form of aggregated, moderately dense, finely granular material lying free in the cytoplasm.

References: 1112, 1127, 1939

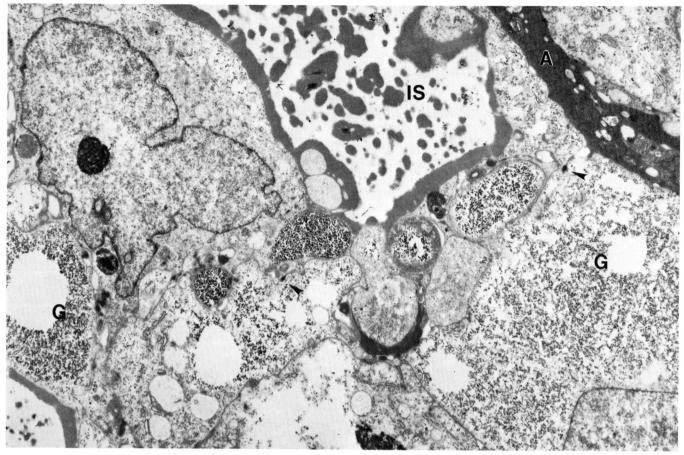

**Fig. 30.5   Endodermal sinus tumour: Survey**

Testicular yolk sac carcinoma, said to have been present since birth, in a 2-year-old infant; the tumour labelled strongly for α-fetoprotein (AFP) by the immunoperoxidase method. The neoplastic cells contain plentiful glycogen (G). They are closely apposed, and are joined by a few desmosomes (arrowheads). The intercellular space (IS) contains layered and clustered moderately electron-dense material, presumably including basal lamina. An apoptotic cell (A) is also present. (× 6900)

**Discussion:** A germinomatous component consisting of primitive cells with sparse organelles, annulate lamellae and occasional glycogen deposits has been described in a suprasellar yolk sac carcinoma, as have trophoblastic cells.[1151]

Areas of 'hepatoid' differentiation may also be seen.[1147] The cells comprising these areas often contain rounded hyaline bodies on LM. EM reveals polyhedral cells with intercellular acinar spaces resembling bile canaliculi, but without detectable bile.[1147] The nuclei contain plentiful euchromatin and prominent nucleoli. Moulding of RER around mitochondria may be evident. The cytoplasm also contains rounded membrane-bound dense structures resembling lysosomes, presumably correlating with the hyaline globules on LM; these appear to represent sites of immunoreactivity for α₁-antitrypsin.[1147]

In addition to AFP, these tumours produce albumin, prealbumin, α₁-antitrypsin, transferrin, carcinoembryonic antigen and human chorionic gonadotrophin.[1150] Synthesis of laminin by a yolk sac carcinoma in the rat has also been documented.[1142]

References: 1140–1151

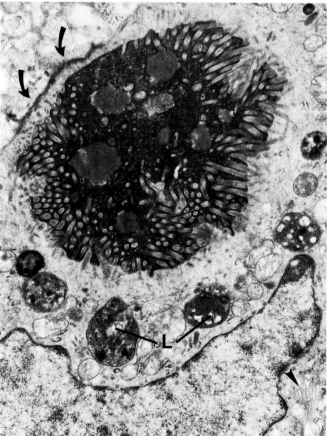

**Fig. 30.6   Endodermal sinus tumour: Intracytoplasmic crypt**

The crypt is filled with secretion, while pleomorphic lysosomes (L) are present in the surrounding cytoplasm. A Golgi complex (arrowhead) and an intercellular junction (curved arrows) are also evident. (× 13 000)

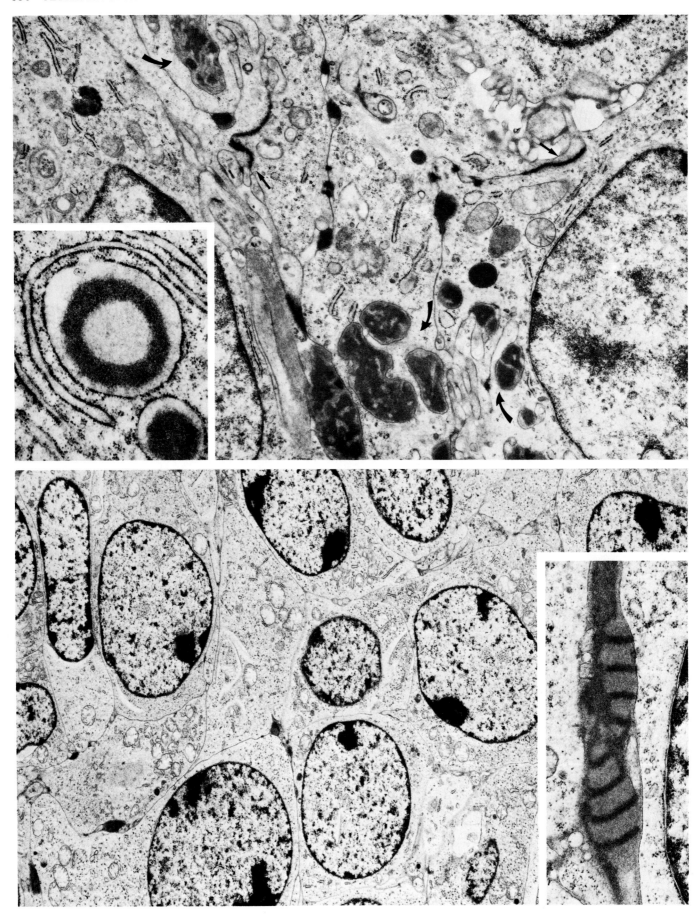

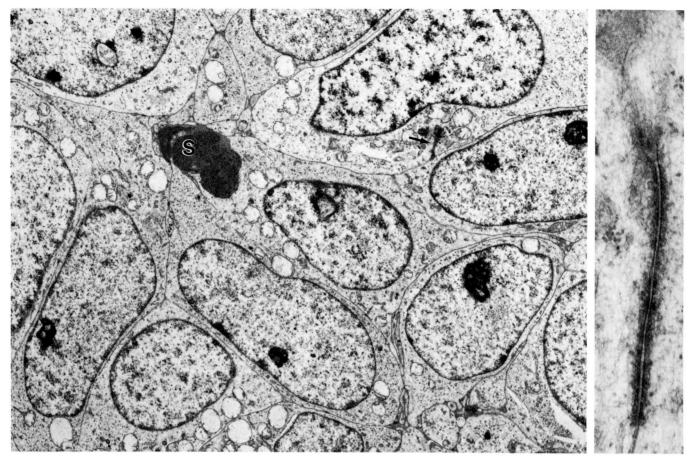

**Fig. 30.9  Monomorphic blastemal Wilms' tumour: Primitive tubule formation and intercellular junction**

Here there is a suggestion of radial orientation of the malignant cells around a central space (S) containing amorphous material of medium density. A budding cilium (arrow) can also be seen. **Inset:** Subluminal intercellular junction in the same tumour; this may represent a defective (leaky) tight junction or an intermediate-type junction. ($\times$ 5400. Inset: $\times$ 59 300)

'Oligocilogenesis' is often evident in Wilms' tumour. The cilia may be found in blastemal and epithelial cells, and in stromal fibroblasts; their presence lacks specificity (see Fig. 2.14).

**Fig. 30.7** *(Facing page — top)* **Endodermal sinus tumour: Proteinaceous material, endoplasmic reticulum, and intercellular junctions**

The cytoplasmic processes show complex interdigitations; there are many desmosomes, and junctional complexes (straight arrows) are evident. Mottled, apparently proteinaceous material is present in intercellular spaces (curved arrows), and also within the cisternae of the RER (inset). Annulate lamellae may also be present, sometimes in continuity with the RER.[1150] ($\times$ 12 700. Inset: $\times$ 27 000)

**Fig. 30.8** *(Facing page — bottom)* **Blastemal Wilms' tumour: Survey and intercellular banded structure**

Monomorphic blastemal tumour of kidney in a 13-year-old youth (nephrectomy specimen). The neoplastic cells in this field show close apposition, with scattered intercellular junctions. Groups of cell processes can be seen and electron-dense extracellular material is also evident. Mitochondria are moderately frequent. Note the prominent nucleolar margination. ($\times$ 5400)

**Inset:** Electron-dense extracellular material was found in this case, occasionally producing banded structures with a periodicity of approximately 475 nm, as shown here; this material lacks the filamentous substructure and 100 nm periodicity of fibrous long-spacing collagen, and may represent proteinaceous matter. ($\times$ 23 200)

**Discussion:** Small numbers of fine filaments can be found in the blastemal cells in most Wilms' tumours, but prominent filamentous aggregates are rare. Profuse autophagosomes resembling those of granular cell tumour (see Table 18.2) are exceptional. On the other hand, confronting cisternae of RER are commonly encountered.

References: 109, 991, 994, 1015, 1019, 1022, 1026, 1031, 1032

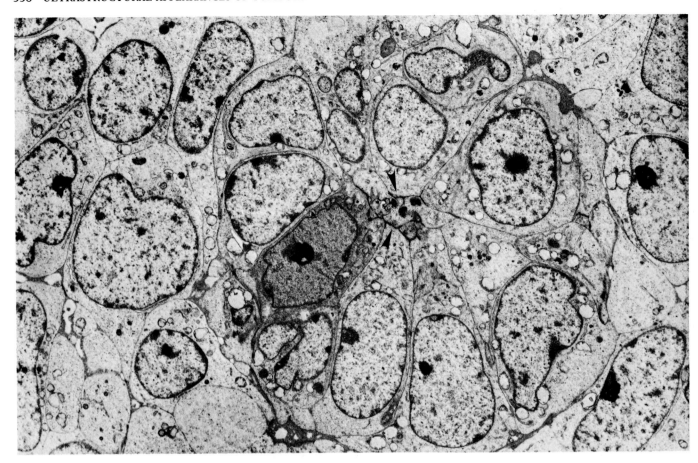

## Fig. 30.10  Wilms' tumour: Tubular differentiation I

Tumour from a 2-year-old boy. A fine needle aspiration biopsy of the abdominal mass was interpreted by LM as a small cell tumour consistent with neuroblastoma. However, ultrastructural examination of the aspirate revealed embryonic cells devoid of neuritic features, but possessing a well developed, if fragmentary, layer of fuzzy external laminal material. Accordingly, a diagnosis of Wilms' tumour was suggested and was verified on the subsequent nephrectomy specimen.

The cells comprising this rudimentary tubule are radially arranged around a central point, where there are intercellular junctions (arrowheads), but a tubular lumen is not evident. Blastemal cells occupy the peritubular area. (× 3700)

References: 109, 991, 994, 1000, 1015, 1026, 1031, 1032

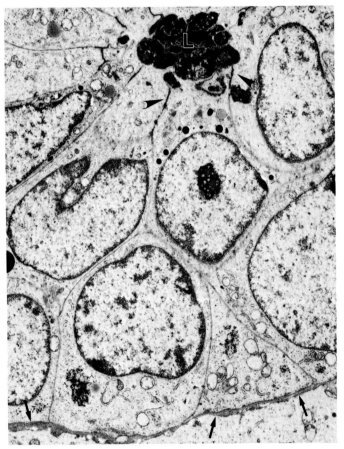

## Fig. 30.11  Wilms' tumour: Tubular differentiation II

A lumen (L) containing electron-dense material occupies the central area of this primitive tubule. Luminal microvilli are not present, but apical junctional complexes (arrowheads) can be discerned. Basal lamina (arrows) surrounds the tubule. (× 4500)

Luminal microvilli may be seen in the tubular structures in Wilms' tumour and infolding of the basal plasma membrane is described. Lipid and glycogen are sometimes present in the cytoplasm, as are tonofibrils on rare occasions.

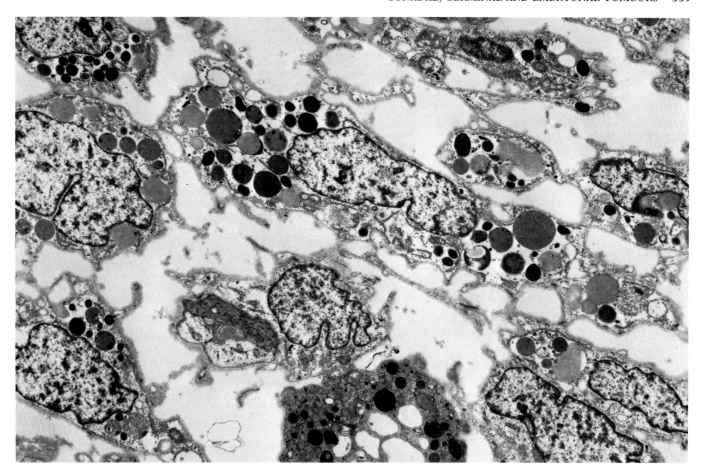

**Fig. 30.12 Wilms' tumour: Spindle cell area**

The cells are elongated, contain numerous rounded granules of varying density — possibly lysosomal in type — and are invested by a layer of external lamina-like matter. Intercellular spaces are wide and almost devoid of collagen and elastin fibres. (× 5400)

(Case contributed by Drs. R.F. Carter and G.F. Binns).

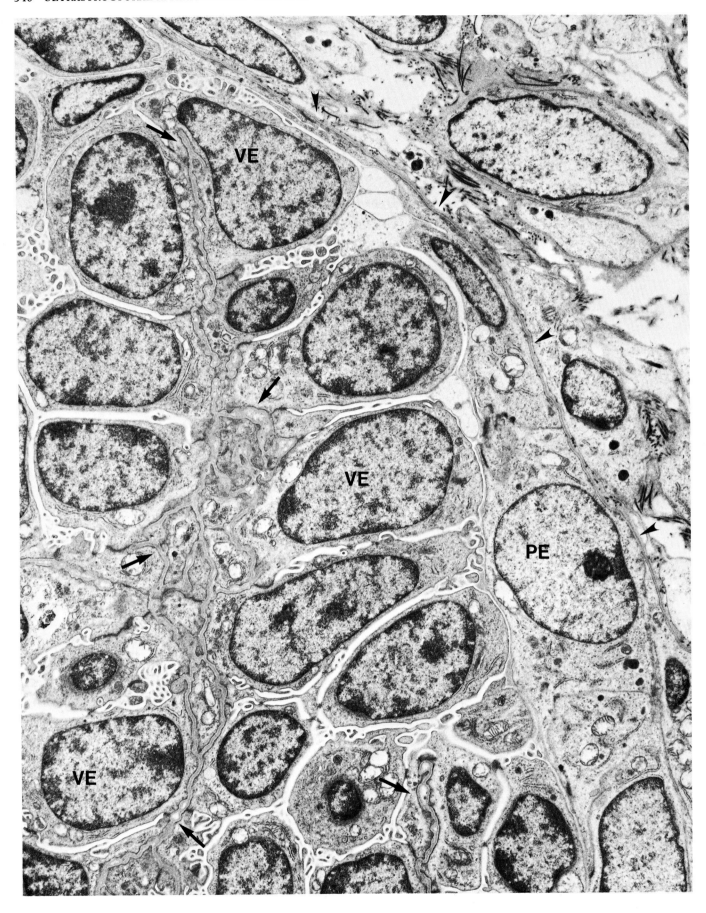

**Fig. 30.13** *(Facing page)*   **Wilms' tumour: Glomeruloid body**

This glomeruloid body consists of visceral epithelial cells (VE) in close contact with external lamina (arrows). Microvillous processes protrude from the apical and lateral surfaces of the cells, but there are no foot processes. Capillary formations and endothelial cells are not evident. A layer of parietal epithelial cells (PE) surrounds the tuft, being accompanied by basal lamina in mimicry of Bowman's capsule (arrowheads). (× 7000)

**Discussion:** Most glomeruloid bodies in Wilms' tumours appear to consist only of epithelial cells and basal lamina. To the best of our knowledge, unequivocal endothelial and mesangial cells have not been found in the tufts by EM, but capillarized glomeruloid bodies have been observed by LM.[1026] The absence of capillaries in these structures appears to reflect a process of abnormal epithelial differentiation rather than a direct recapitulation of glomerular development. Glomerular capillaries normally develop from the extraglomerular mesenchymal vasculature; at no stage do they arise in solid collections of epithelial cells.

References: 109, 991, 1026

# References

## 1 HISTORICAL ASPECTS

1. Majno G, Joris I 1973 The microscope in the history of pathology: with a note on the pathology of fat cells. Virchows Archiv A Pathologische Anatomie 360: 273–286
2. Ruge C 1890 The microscope in gynaecology and diagnosis. Zeitschrift für Geburtshilfe und Perinatologie 20: 178–205

## 2 GENERAL ASPECTS OF NEOPLASTIC FINE STRUCTURE, AND THE ROLE OF ELECTRON MICROSCOPY IN THE DIAGNOSIS OF TUMOURS

3. Abelev G I 1971 Alpha-fetoprotein in ontogenesis and its association with malignant tumors. Advances in Cancer Research 14: 295–358
4. Abercrombie M 1961 Behaviour of normal and malignant connective tissue cells in vitro. Proceedings of the Canadian Cancer Research Conference 4: 110–117
5. Adcock E W, Teasdale F, August C S, Meschia G, Battaglia F C, Naughton M A 1973 Human chorionic gonadotropin: its possible role in maternal lymphocyte suppression. Science 181: 845–847
6. Akhtar M, Ali M A, Owen E W 1981 Application of electron microscopy in the interpretation of fine-needle aspiration biopsies. Cancer 48: 2458–2463
7. Alexander P 1972 Foetal 'antigens' in cancer. Nature 235: 137–140
8. Avis P, Lewis M G 1973 Brief communication: tumour associated fetal antigens in human tumors. Journal of the National Cancer Institute 51: 1063–1065
9. Azar H A, Espinoza C G, Richman A V, Saba S R, Wang T-Y 1982 'Undifferentiated' large cell malignancies: an ultrastructural and immunocytochemical study. Human Pathology 13: 323–333
10. Balinsky D 1980 Enzymes and isozymes in cancer. In: Sell S (ed) Cancer markers: diagnostic and developmental significance. The Humana Press Inc., New Jersey, p 191–224
11. Becker S N, Wong J Y, Marchiondo A A, Davis C P 1981 Scanning electron microscopy of alcohol-fixed cytopathology specimens. Acta Cytologica 25: 578–584
12. Berliner J A, Janssen M, McLatchie C 1978 The use of scanning electron microscopy in the diagnosis of malignancy in human serous effusions. Scanning Electron Microscopy 2: 797–802
13. Birbeck M S C 1976 Ultrastructure of tumour cells. In: Symington T, Carter R L (eds) Scientific foundations of oncology, Heinemann, London, ch 2, p 8–15
14. Bonikos D S, Bensch K G, Kempson R L 1976 The contribution of electron microscopy to the differential diagnosis of tumors. Beiträge zur Pathologie 158: 417–444
15. Borek E, Kerr S J 1972 Atypical transfer RNAs and their origin in neoplastic cells. Advances in Cancer Research 15: 163–190
16. Brady R O, Fishman P H 1974 Biosynthesis of glycolipids in virus transformed cells. Biochimica et Biophysica Acta 355: 121–148
17. Busch H 1977 Some aspects of the molecular biology of cancer. In: Gallo R C (ed) Recent advances in cancer research: cell biology, molecular biology and tumor virology, vol 1. CRC Press Inc., Cleveland, p 1–15
18. Carr I, Toner P G 1977 Electron microscopy for the diagnosis of tumours; editorial. Canadian Medical Association Journal 116: 341–342
19. Carr K E, Chung P, McLay A L C, Toner P G, Wong A L 1981 The role of scanning electron microscopy in diagnostic pathology. Diagnostic Histopathology 4: 237–244
20. Carter H W, Carr K E, Toner P G, Buss H 1980 Clinical applications of the scanning electron microscope. Scanning Electron Microscopy, Inc. AMF O'Hare, Il, U.S.A.
21. Caspersson T, Gahrton G, Lindsten J, Zech L 1970 Identification of the Philadelphia chromosome as a number 22 by quinacrine mustard fluorescence analysis. Experimental Cell Research 63: 238–244
22. Chaudhry A P, Cutler L S, Montes M, Satchidanand S, Raj M S 1980 Electron microscopy, its application in diagnostic pathology. New York State Journal of Medicine 80: 1809–1814
23. Chism S E 1980 Oncofetal transplantation antigens. In: Sell S (ed) Cancer markers: diagnostic and developmental significance. The Humana Press Inc., New Jersey, 115–132
24. Chiu J-F, Chytil F, Hnilica L S 1976 Onco-fetal antigens in chromatin of malignant cells. In: Fishman W H, Sell S (eds) Onco-developmental gene expression. Academic Press, Inc., New York, p 271–280
25. Chiu J-F, Hnilica L S 1976 DNA polymerase in developing and neoplastic tissues. In: Fishman W H, Sell S (eds) Onco-developmental gene expression. Academic Press Inc., New York, p 65–74
26. Coggin J H, Anderson N G 1974 Cancer, differentiation and embryonic antigens: some central problems. Advances in Cancer Research 19: 105–165
27. Collins V P, Ivarsson B 1981 Tumor classification by electron microscopy of fine needle aspiration biopsy material. Acta Pathologica et Microbiologica Scandinavica. Section A, Pathology 89: 103–105
28. Cox W F Jr., Pierce G B 1982 The endodermal origin of the endocrine cells of an adenocarcinoma of the colon of the rat. Cancer 50: 1530–1538
29. Criss W E 1971 A review of isoenzymes in cancer. Cancer Research 31: 1523–1542
30. Damjanov I 1979 Ultrastructural pathology of human tumors, vol 1. Eden Press, Montreal
31. David H 1978 Cellular pathology. In: Johannessen J V (ed) Electron microscopy in human medicine, vol 2. Cellular pathology, metabolic and storage diseases. McGraw-Hill, New York, pt I, p 1–48
32. Davis F M, Gyorkey F, Busch R K, Busch H 1979 Nucleolar antigen found in several human tumors but not in the nontumor tissues studied. Proceedings of the National Academy of Science USA 76: 892–896
33. de Harven E 1966 Electron microscopy of cancer cells: a review. Medical Clinics of North America 50: 887–900
34. de Harven E 1977 Electron microscopy: remarks on 40 years of ultrastructural explorations. CA. Cancer Journal for Clinicians 27: 281–288
35. Domagala W, Koss L G 1980 Configuration of surfaces of human cancer cells obtained by fine needle aspiration biopsy: a comparative light microscopic and scanning electron miscoscopic study. Acta Cytologica 24: 427–434
36. Domagala W, Woyke S 1975 Transmission and scanning electron microscopic studies of cells in effusions. Acta Cytologica 19: 214–224
37. Dvorak A M, Monahan R A 1982 Metastatic adenocarcinoma of unknown primary site. Diagnostic electron microscopy to determine the site of tumor origin. Archives of Pathology and Laboratory Medicine 106: 21–24
38. Edidin M, Weiss A 1974 Restriction of antigen mobility in the plasma membranes of some cultured fibroblasts. In: Clarkson B, Baserga R (eds) Cold Spring Harbor conferences on cell proliferation, vol 1. Control of proliferation in animal cells. Cold Spring Harbor Laboratory, New York p 213–220

39. Erlandson R A 1981 Diagnostic transmission electron microscopy of human tumors. The interpretation of submicroscopic structures in human neoplastic cells. Masson Publishing USA, New York

40. Folkman J, Merler E, Abernathy C, Williams G 1971 Isolation of a tumor factor responsible for angiogenesis. Journal of Experimental Medicine 133: 275–288

41. Forman J 1980 Antigens and the major histocompatibility complex. In: Sell S (ed) Cancer markers: diagnostic and developmental significance. The Humana Press Inc., New Jersey p 133–168

42. Gabbiani G, Csank-Brassert T, Schneeberger J C, Kapanci Y, Trenchev P, Holborow J 1976 Contractile proteins in human cancer cells. Immunofluorescent and electron microscopic study. American Journal of Pathology 83: 457–474

43. Geisinger K R, Naylor B, Beals T F, Novak P M 1980 Cytopathology, including transmission and scanning electron microscopy, of pleomorphic liposarcomas in pleural fluids. Acta Cytologica 24: 435–441

44. Ghadially F N 1975 Ultrastructural pathology of the cell. A text and atlas of physiological and pathological alterations in cell fine structure. Butterworths, London

45. Ghadially F N 1980 Diagnostic electron microscopy of tumours. Butterworths, London

46. Ghadially F N 1981 The role of electron microscopy in the determination of tumour histogenesis. Diagnostic Histopathology 4: 245–262

47. Ghadially F N 1982 Ultrastructural pathology of the cell and matrix. A text and atlas of physiological and pathological alterations in the fine structure of cellular and extracellar components, 2nd edn. Butterworths, London

48. Gillespie T J 1982 Ultrastructural diagnosis of large cell 'undifferentiated' neoplasia. Diagnostic Histopathology 5: 33–51

49. Gold D V, Goldenberg D M 1980 Antigens associated with human solid tumors. In: Sell S (ed) Cancer markers: diagnostic and developmental significance. The Humana Press Inc., New Jersey p 329–369

50. Gondos B, McIntosh K M, Renston R H, King E B 1978 Application of electron microscopy in the definitive diagnosis of effusions. Acta Cytologica 22: 297–304

51. Gould V E, Benditt E P 1973 Ultrastructural and functional relationships of some human endocrine tumors. Pathology Annual 8: 205–230

52. Gould V E, Memoli V A, Dardi L E 1981 Multidirectional differentiation in human epithelial cancers. Journal of Submicroscopic Cytology 13: 97–115

53. Goussev A I, Engelhardt N V, Masseyeff R , Camain R, Basteris B 1971 Immunofluorescent study of alpha-foetoprotein (afp) in liver and liver tumours II. Localization of afp in the tissues of patients with primary liver cancer (PLC). International Journal of Cancer 7: 207–217

54. Griffing G, Vaitukaitis J L 1980 Hormone secreting tumors. In: Sell S (ed) Cancer markers: diagnostic and developmental significance. The Humana Press Inc., New Jersey, p 169–190

55. Gyorkey F, Min K-W, Krisko I, Gyorkey P 1975 The usefulness of electron microscopy in the diagnosis of human tumors. Human Pathology 6: 421–441

56. Hagelqvist E 1978 Light and electron microscopic studies on material obtained by fine needle biopsy. A methodological study on aspirates from tumours of the head and neck region with special emphasis on salivary gland tumours. Acta Otolaryngologica suppl 354: 1–75

57. Hagelqvist E, Engstrom B 1973 Electron microscopy studies on cytologic material acquired by fine needle biopsy. Upsala Journal of Medical Science 78: 153–159

58. Haguenau F 1969 Ultrastructure of the cancer cell. In: Bittar E E, Bittar N (eds) The biological basis of medicine, vol 5. Academic Press, New York, ch 12, p 433–486

59. Hakomori S-I 1973 Glycolipids of tumor cell membranes. Advances in Cancer Research 18: 265–315

60. Harnden D G, Taylor A M R 1979 Chromosomes and neoplasia. In: Harris H, Hirschhorn K (eds) Advances in human genetics, vol 9. Plenum Press, New York, p 1–70

61. Harris M 1981 Differential diagnosis of spindle cell tumours by electron microscopy — personal experience and a review. Histopathology 5: 81–105

62. Harris R, Viza D, Todd R, Phillips J, Sugar R, Jennison R F, Marriott G, Gleeson M H 1971 Detection of human leukaemia associated antigens in leukaemic serum and normal embryos. Nature 233: 556–557

63. Henderson D W, Papadimitriou J M 1980 Electron microscopy in the diagnosis of tumors. Micron 11: 441–442

64. Henderson D W, Papadimitriou J M 1982 Ultrastructural appearances of tumours. A diagnostic atlas. 1st edn. Churchill Livingstone, Edinburgh

65. Hirai H 1979 Model systems of AFP and CEA expression. In: Fishman W H, Busch H (eds) Methods in Cancer Research, vol 18, Oncodevelopmental antigens. Academic Press Inc., New York, p 39–97

66. Hirsch F W, Nall N N, Hayes L C, Raju K S, Spohn W H, Busch H 1977 Adsorption of messenger RNA of Novikoff hepatoma, normal liver and regenerating liver on complementary DNA-cellulose affinity matrices. Cancer Research 37: 3694–3700

67. Hnilica L S, Briggs R C 1980 Nonhistone protein antigens. In: Sell S (ed) Cancer Markers: diagnostic and developmental significance. The Humana Press Inc., New York, p 463–483

68. Horne C H W, Bremner R D 1980 Pregnancy proteins as tumor markers. In: Sell S (ed) Cancer Markers: diagnostic and developmental significance. The Humana Press Inc., New Jersey, p 225–247

69. Isselbacher K J 1972 Sugar and amino acid transport by cells in culture: differences between normal and malignant cells. New England Journal of Medicine 286: 929–933

70. Johannessen J V 1982 Diagnostic electron microscopy. Hemisphere Publishing Corporation, Washington

71. Kaiser-McCaw B, Epstein A L, Kaplan H L, Hecht F 1977 Chromosome 14 translocation in African and North American Burkitt's lymphomas. International Journal of Cancer 19: 482–486

72. Kaneshima S, Kiyasu Y, Kudo H, Koga S, Tanaka K 1978 An application of scanning electron microscopy to cytodiagnosis of pleural and peritoneal fluids. Comparative observation of the same cells by light microscopy and scanning electron microscopy. Acta Cytologica 22: 490–499

73. Karcioglu Z, Someren A, Mathes S J 1977 Ecto-mesenchymoma: a malignant tumor of migratory neural crest (ectomesenchyme) remnants showing ganglionic, Schwannian, melanocytic and rhabdomyoblastic differentiation. Cancer 39: 2486–2496

74. Ketoh Y, Stoner G D, McIntire K R, Hill T A, Anthony R, McDowell E M 1979 Immunologic markers of human bronchial epithelial cells in vivo and in vitro. Journal of the National Cancer Institute 62: 1177–1185

75. Kindblom L-G 1983 Light and electron microscopic examination of embedded fine-needle aspiration biopsy specimens in the preoperative diagnosis of soft tissue and bone tumors. Cancer 51: 2264–2277

76. Kirby D R S, Cowell T P 1968 Trophoblast host interactions. In: Fleishmajer R, Gillingham R E (eds) Epithelial-mesenchymal interactions. Williams and Wilkins, Baltimore, p 64–77

77. Koss L G, Domagala W 1980 Configuration of surfaces of human cancer cells in effusions. A review. Scanning Electron Microscopy 3: 89–100

78. Kuzela D C, True L D, Eiseman B 1982 The role of electron microscopy in the management of surgical patients. Annals of Surgery 195: 1–11

79. Lattes R 1973 The pathological diagnosis of soft tissue tumors. Proceedings of the National Cancer Conference 7: 869–872

80. Legrand M, Pariente R 1976 Electron microscopy in the cytological examination of metastatic pleural effusions. Thorax 31: 443–449

81. Luning B, Redelius P, Wiklund B, Bjorklund B 1976 Biochemistry of TPA. In: Fishman W H, Sell S (eds) Onco-developmental gene expression. Academic Press Inc., New York, p 773–778

82. Lyon M F 1961 Gene action in the mouse (mus musculus). Nature 190: 372–373

83. Macartney J C, Trevithick M A, Kricka L, Kurran R C 1979 Identification of myosin in human epithelial cancers with immunofluorescence. Laboratory Investigation 41: 437–445

84. Mackay B 1972 Electron microscopy and tumor diagnosis. Cancer Bulletin 24: 42–45

85. Mackay B 1981 Introduction to diagnostic electron microscopy. Appleton–Century–Crofts, New York

86. Mackay B, Osborne B M 1978 The contribution of electron microscopy to the diagnosis of tumors. Pathobiology Annual 8: 359–405

87. Mackay B, Silva E G 1980 Diagnostic electron microscopy in oncology. Pathology Annual 15, pt 2: 241–270

88. Mark J 1974 The human meningioma: a benign tumour with specific chromosome characteristics. In: German J (ed) Chromosomes and cancer. Wiley, New York, p 495–517

89. Mason D, Pedraza M A, Doshi F A, Marsh R A 1981 Ultrastructural and immunological methods in diagnostic pathology in a community hospital. Ultrastructural Pathology 2: 373–381

90. McDonagh J 1981 Fibronectin. Archives of Pathology and Laboratory Medicine 105: 393–396

91. McLay A L C, Toner P G 1981 Diagnostic electron microscopy. Recent Advances in Histopathology 11: 241–261

92. McLay A L C, Toner P G 1981 The classification of ultrastructural topography in the context of an ultrastructural pathology service. Diagnostic Histopathology 4: 219–222

93. McManus L M, Naughton M A, Martinez-Hernandez A 1976 Human chorionic gonadotropin in human neoplastic cells. Cancer Research 36: 3476–3481

94. Metcalf D 1983 How many cancers are reversible or suppressible? Pathology 15: 1–3

95. Mierau G, Favara B 1976 Ultrastructure of tumors in infancy and childhood. The Children's Hospital, Denver

96. Montandon D Kocher O, Gabbiani G 1982 Cancer invasiveness: immunofluorescent and ultrastructural methods of assessment. Plastic and Reconstructive Surgery 69: 365–371

97. Morales A R 1980 Electron microscopy of human tumors. Progress in Surgical Pathology 1: 51–70

98. Mukherjee T M 1982 The role of electron microscopy in the diagnosis of neoplastic cells in effusion fluids. Journal of Submicroscopic Cytology 14: 717–743

99. Neustein H B 1973 Electron microscopy in diagnostic pathology. Perspectives in Pediatric Pathology 1: 369–392

100. Neville A M, Laurence D J R 1974 Report of the workshop on the carcinoembryonic antigen (CEA): the present position and proposals for future investigation. International Journal of Cancer 14: 1–18

101. Nicolson G L 1974 Interaction of lectins with animal cell surfaces: In: Bourne G H, Danielli J F (eds). International Review of Cytology, Academic Press Inc., New York, p 89–190

102. Nicolson G L 1976 Transmembrane control of the receptors on normal and tumour cells. II. Surface changes associated with transformation and malignancy. Biochimica et Biophysica Acta 459: 1–71

103. Nicolson G L 1980 Lectin interactions with normal and tumor cells and the affinity purification of tumor cell glycoproteins. In: Sell S (ed) Cancer Markers: diagnostic and developmental significance. The Humana Press Inc., New Jersey, p 403–443

104. Nicolson G L, Poste G 1976 The cancer cell: dynamic aspects and modifications in cell surface organisation (first of two parts). New England Journal of Medicine 295: 197–203

105. Nicolson G L, Poste G 1976 The cancer cell: dynamic aspects and modifications in cell surface organisation (second of two parts). New England Journal of Medicine 295: 253–258

106. Nordgren H, Åkerman M 1982 Electron microscopy of fine needle aspiration biopsy from soft tissue tumors. Acta Cytologica 26: 179–187

107. O'Riordan M L, Robinson J A, Buckton K E, Evans H J 1971 Distinguishing between the chromosomes involved in Down's syndrome (trisomy 21) and chronic myeloid leukaemia (Ph') by fluorescence. Nature, London 230: 167–168

108. Olsen E G J 1982 Electron microscopy: an essential tool for morphological diagnosis? British Medical Journal 284: 1897–1898

109. Raikhlin N T, David H, Lapish K (eds) 1981 Ultrastructure of tumours in man. (Guidebook on diagnosis). Meditsina, Moscow

110. Regezi J A, Batsakis J G 1978 Diagnostic electron microscopy of head and neck tumors. Archives of Pathology and Laboratory Medicine 102: 8–14

111. Rowley J D 1973 A new consistent chromosomal abnormality in chronic myelogenous leukaemia identified by quinacrine fluorescence and Giemsa staining. Nature, London 243: 290–293

112. Rowley J D, Testa J R 1982 Chromosome abonormalities in malignant hematologic diseases. In: Klein G, Weinhouse S (eds) Advances in Cancer Research, vol 36, Academic Press Inc., New York, p 103–148

113. Ruoslahti E, Hayman E G, Engvall E 1980 Fibronectin. In: Sell S (ed) Cancer markers: diagnostic and developmental significance. The Humana Press Inc., New Jersey, p 485–505

114. Sakaguchi H 1973 Scanning electron microscopy in a field of pathology. Journal of Electron Microscopy 22: 1–3

115. Sandberg A A, Hossfeld D K 1982 Chromosomes in the pathogenesis of cancer and leukaemia. In: Holland J F, Frei E (eds) Cancer Medicine, Lea and Febiger, Philadelphia, p 190–239

116. Schapira F 1973 Isozymes and cancer. Advances in Cancer Research 18: 77–153

117. Seifert W, Rudland P S 1974 Cyclic nucleotides and growth control in cultured mouse cells: correlation of changes in intracellular 3':5' cGMP concentration with a specific phase of the cycle. Proceedings of the National Academy of Science USA 71: 4920–4924

118. Sell S 1980 Alphafetoprotein. In: Sell S (ed) Cancer markers: diagnostic and developmental significance. The Humana Press Inc., New Jersey, p 249–293

119. Seymour A E, Henderson D W 1981 Electron microscopy in surgical pathology: a selective review. Pathology 13: 111–135

120. Sherman M I, Strickland S, Reich E 1976 Differentiation of early mouse embryonic and teratocarcinoma cells in vitro: plasminogen activator production. Cancer Research 36: 4208–4216

121. Shin S-I, Freedman V H, Risser R, Pollack R 1975 Tumorigenicity of virus-transformed cells in nude mice is correlated specifically with anchorage independent growth in vitro. Proceedings of the National Academy of Science USA 72: 4435–4439

122. Shin W Y, Ilardi C, Desner M 1982 Electron microscopy and biopsy: diagnostic clue provided on routine formalin-fixed material. New York State Journal of Medicine 82: 1060–1062

123. Shinitzky M, Inbar M 1974 Difference in microviscosity induced by different cholesterol levels in the surface membrane lipid layer of normal lymphocytes and malignant lymphoma cells. Journal of Molecular Biology 85: 603–615

124. Shires T K, Pilot H C, Kauffman F A 1974 The membron: a functional hypothesis for the translational regulation of genetic expression. Biomembranes 5: 81–145

125. Shively J E, Todd C W 1980 Carcinoembryonic antigen A: chemistry and biology. In: Sell S (ed) Cancer Markers: diagnostic and developmental significance. The Humana Press Inc., New Jersey, p 295–314

126. Sobel H J, Marquet E 1980 Usefulness of electron microscopy in the diagnosis of tumors. Pathology Research and Practice 167: 22–44

127. Sobrinho-Simoes M, Nesland J M, Johannessen J V 1981 Diagnostic ultrastructural pathology — sub-speciality or special stain? Diagnostic Histopathology 4: 223–236

128. Stark P, Hildebrandt-Stark H E 1982 Electron microscopy of cells obtained by fine needle aspiration biopsy of lung lesions. Radiologe 22: 327–328

129. Stein G, Stein J L, Thomson J A 1978 Chromosomal proteins in transformed and neoplastic cells: a review. Cancer Research 38: 1181–1201

130. Stoker M 1967 Contact and short range interactions affecting growth of animal cells in culture. Current Topics in Developmental Biology 2: 107–128

131. Strong J E 1980 Comparison of malignant cells and non malignant cells. In: Crooke S T, Bestayko A W (eds) Cancer and Chemotherapy, vol 1. Introduction to neoplasia and anti-neoplastic therapy. Academic Press Inc., New York, p 77–94

132. Teplitz R L, Barr K J, Laure H J 1972 Karyological and biochemical evidence for chromosomal dedifferentiation in neoplasia. In Vitro 7: 197–200

133. Tseng C H (ed) 1980 Atlas of ultrastructure. Ultrastructural features in pathology. Appleton-Century-Crofts, New York

134. Uriel J, Bouillon D, Aussel C, Dupiers M 1976 Alpha-fetoprotein: the major high-affinity estrogen binder in rat uterine cytosols. Proceedings of the National Academy of Science USA 73: 1452–1456

135. Wang K, Heggeness M H, Singer J S 1978 Mechanochemical proteins and cell-cell interactions. Birth Defects 14: 29–40

136. Weber G 1977 Enzymology of cancer cells (first of two parts). The New England Journal of Medicine 296: 486–493

137. Weber G 1977 Enzymology of cancer cells (second of two parts). The New England Journal of Medicine 296: 541–551

138. Weiss L, Poste G 1976 The tumour cell periphery. In: Symington T, Carter R L (eds) Scientific foundations of oncology. Heinemann, London, p 25–35

139. Williams M J 1981 Diagnostic electron microscopy in the U.S. Veterans Administration. Diagnostic Histopathology 4: 279–283

140. Wills E J 1983 Ultrathin section electron microscopy in the diagnosis of viral infections. Pathology Annual 18, pt 1: 139–180

141. Wolf B A, Goldberg A R 1976 Rous sarcoma virus tranformed fibroblasts having low levels of plasminogen activator. Proceedings of the National Academy of Science USA 73: 3613–3617

142. Woodruff M F A 1983 Cellular heterogeneity in tumours. British Journal of Cancer 47: 589–594

143. Yogeeswaran G 1980 Surface glycolipid and glycoprotein antigens. In: Sell S (ed) Cancer Markers: diagnostic and developmental significance. The Humana Press Inc., New Jersey, p 371–401

144. Zech L, Hoglund U, Nilsson K, Klein G 1976 Characteristic chromosomal abnormalities in biopsies and lymphoid-cell lines from patients with Burkitt and non Burkitt lymphomas. International Journal of Cancer 17: 47–56

145. Zimmermann L E, Font R L, Ts'o M O M, Fine B S 1972 Application of electron microscopy to histopathologic diagnosis. Transactions: American Academy of Ophthalmology and Otolaryngology 76: 101–107

## 3 TECHNIQUES IN DIAGNOSTIC ELECTRON MICROSCOPY

146. Aoki M, Tavassoli M 1981 OTO method for preservation of actin filaments in electron microscopy. Journal of Histochemistry and Cytochemistry 29: 682–683

147. Burns W A 1978 Thick sections: techniques and applications. In: Trump B F, Jones R T (eds) Diagnostic electron microscopy, vol 1. John Wiley & Sons, New York, ch 4, p 141–166

148. Burns W A, Bretschneider A M, Morrison A B 1979 Embedding in large plastic blocks. Diagnostic light and potential electron microscopy on the same block. Archives of Pathology and Laboratory Medicine 103: 177–179

149. Carr I, Toner P G 1977 Rapid electron microscopy in oncology. Journal of Clinical Pathology 30: 13–15

150. Carr K E, Toner P G, Saleh K M 1982 Scanning electron microscopy. Histopathology 6: 3–24

151. Carson F L, Martin J H, Lynn J A 1973 Formalin fixation for electron microscopy: a re-evaluation. American Journal of Clinical Pathology 59: 365–373

152. Chandler J A 1977 X-ray microanalysis in the electron microscope. In: Glauert A M (ed) Practical methods in electron microscopy, vol 5, pt II. North-Holland Publishing Company Amsterdam

153. Coppola A 1979 A rapid method for electron microscopic examination of blood cells. Journal of Clinical Pathology 32: 162–167

154. Ferguson D J P, Anderson T J 1981 A technique for identifying areas of interest in human breast tissue before embedding for electron microscopy. Journal of Clinical Pathology 34: 1187–1189

155. Gilchrist W, Kutchera A R, Albrecht R M, Benson R C Jr 1978 Scanning electron microscopy and light microscopy of the same area within surgical specimens. Scanning Electron Microscopy 2: 291–296

156. Glauert A M 1975 Fixation, dehydration and embedding of biological specimens. In: Glauert A M (ed) Practical methods in electron microscopy, vol 3, pt I. North-Holland Publishing Company, Amsterdam

157. Johannessen J V (ed) 1978 Electron microscopy in human medicine, vol 1. Instrumentation and techniques. McGraw-Hill, New York

158. Johannessen J V 1977 Use of paraffin material for electron microscopy. Pathology Annual 12: 189–224

159. Lazzaro A V 1983 Technical note: Improved preparation of fine needle aspiration biopsies for transmission electron microscopy. Pathology 15: 399–402

160. Lynne J A 1975 'Adjacent' sections — a bridge in the gap between light and electron microscopy. Human Pathology 6: 400–402

161. Martin J H, Marcus P B 1983 Simple technique to facilitate tissue processing for electron microscopy. Ultrastructural Pathology 4: 261–264

162. McDowell E M 1978 Fixation and processing. In: Trump B F, Jones R T (eds) Diagnostic electron microscopy, vol 1. John Wiley & Sons, New York, ch 3, p 113–139

163. McDowell E M, Trump B F 1976 Histologic fixatives suitable for diagnostic light and electron microscopy. Archives of Pathology and Laboratory Medicine 100: 405–414

164. Nesland J M, Millonig G, Wilson A, Johannessen J V 1982 Rapid techniques in diagnostic electron microscopy. Ultrastructural Pathology 3: 295–300

165. Orci L, Perrelet A 1975 Freeze-etch histology. A comparison between thin sections and freeze-etch replicas. Springer-Verlag, Berlin

166. Todd W J, Burgdorfer W 1982 Rapid processing of biopsy specimens for examination by electron microscopy. American Journal of Clinical Pathology 77: 95–99

## 4 IMMUNOCYTOCHEMISTRY IN TUMOUR DIAGNOSIS – GENERAL REFERENCES

167. DeLellis R A 1981 Diagnostic immunohistochemistry. Masson Publishing USA, New York

168. Dhillon A P, Rode J, Leathem A 1982 Neurone specific enolase: an aid to the diagnosis of melanoma and neuroblastoma. Histopathology 6: 81–92

169. Falini B, Taylor C R 1983 New developments in immunoperoxidase techniques and their application. Archives of Pathology and Laboratoy Medicine 107: 105–117

170. Harris J P, South M A 1981 Secretory component. A glandular epithelial cell marker. American Journal of Pathology 105: 47–53

171. Kahn H J, Marks A, Thom H, Baumal R 1983 Role of antibody to S100 protein in diagnostic pathology. American Journal of Clinical Pathology 79: 341–347

172. Larsson L-I 1981 Peptide immunocytochemistry. Progress in Histochemistry and Cytochemistry 13: 1–85

173. Polak J M, Van Noorden S 1983 Immunocytochemistry. Practical applications in pathology and biology. Wright P S G, Bristol

174. Ramaekers F, Puts J, Moesker O, Kant A, Jap P, Vooijs P 1983 Demonstration of keratin in human adenocarcinomas. American Journal of Pathology 111: 213–223

175. Taylor C R, Kledzik G 1981 Immunohistologic techniques in surgical pathology – a spectrum of 'new' special stains. Human Pathology 12: 590–596

## 5 GENERAL ACCOUNTS OF THE ULTRASTRUCTURAL APPEARANCES OF NORMAL CELLS AND TISSUES

176. Björkman N 1970 An atlas of placental fine structure. Baillière Tindall & Cassell, London

177. Bloom W, Fawcett D W 1975 A textbook of histology, 10th edn. W B Saunders Company, Philadelphia

178. Breathnach A S 1971 An atlas of the ultrastructure of human skin. Development, differentiation, and post-natal features. Churchill, London

179. Carr K E, Toner P G 1982 Cell structure. An introduction to biomedical electron microscopy, 3rd edn. Churchill Livingstone, Edinburgh

180. Fawcett D W 1981 The cell. 2nd edn. W B Saunders Company, Philadelphia

181. Kessel R G, Kardon R H 1979 Tissues and organs. A text-atlas of scanning electron microscopy. W H Freeman & Company, San Francisco

182. Krstić R V 1979 Ultrastructure of the mammalian cell. An atlas. Springer-Verlag, Berlin

183. Kurosumi K, Fujita H 1974 An atlas of electron micrographs: Functional morphology of endocrine glands. Igaku Shoin, Tokyo

184. Lagnens R P Gómez Dumm C L A 1969 Atlas of human electron microscopy. CV Mosby Company, St Louis

185. Lentz T L 1971 Cell fine structure. An atlas of drawings of whole-cell structure. W B Saunders Company, Philadelphia

186. Matthews J L, Martin J H 1973 Atlas of human histology and ultrastructure. Lea & Febiger, Philadelphia

187. Motta P, Andrews P M, Porter K R 1977 Microanatomy of cell and tissue surfaces. An atlas of scanning electron microscopy. Lea & Febiger, Philadelphia

188. Pfeiffer C J, Rowden G, Weibel J 1974 Gastrointestinal ultrastructure. An atlas of scanning and transmission electron micrographs. Igaku Shoin, Tokyo

189. Rhodin J A G 1974 Histology. A text and atlas. Oxford University Press, New York

190. Tanaka Y, Goodman J R 1972 Electron microscopy of human blood cells. Harper & Row, New York

191. Toner P G, Carr K E, Wyburn G M 1971 The digestive system – an ultrastructural atlas and review. Butterworths, London

## 6 GENERAL NUCLEAR FINE-STRUCTURAL ABNORMALITIES IN TUMOURS

192. Beltran G, Stuckey W J 1972 Nuclear lobulation and cytoplasmic fibrils in leukemic plasma cells. American Journal of Clinical Pathology 58: 159–164

193. Benjamin I, Rana M W, Xynos F P, Urhahn J 1980 Intranuclear filaments in xenografts of human squamous cell carcinoma in nude mice. Human Pathology 11: 87–89

194. Blackburn W R 1971 Pathobiology of nucleocytoplasmic exchange. Pathobiology Annual 1: 1–31

195. Blaustein A, Shenker L 1974 Ultrastructural demonstration of nuclear bodies in primary ovarian cancer. Gynecologic Oncology 2: 101–108

196. Christ M L, Haja J 1979 Intranuclear cytoplasmic inclusions (invaginations) in thyroid aspirations: frequency and specificity. Acta Cytologica 23: 327–331

197. Elias H, Fong B B 1978 Nuclear fragmentation in colon carcinoma cells. Human Pathology 9: 679–684

198. Elias H, Hyde D M 1982 Separation and spread of nuclear fragments ('nucleotesimals') in colonic neoplasms. Human Pathology 13: 635–639

199. Ferenczy A, Braun L, Shah K V 1981 Human papillomavirus (HPV) in condylomatous lesions of cervix. A comparative ultrastructural and immunohistochemical study. American Journal of Surgical Pathology 5: 661–670

200. Ferguson D J P, Anderson T J 1981 Ultrastructural observations on cell death by apoptosis in the 'resting' human breast. Virchows Archiv A Pathological Anatomy and Histology 393: 193–203

201. Franke W W, Scheer U, Krohne G, Jarasch E-D 1981 The nuclear envelope and the architecture of the nuclear periphery. Journal of Cell Biology 91: 39s–50s

202. Inoué S 1981 Cell division and the mitotic spindle. Journal of Cell Biology 91: 131s–147s

203. Itabashi M, Hruban Z, Wong T W, Chou S F 1976 Concentric nuclear inclusions. Virchows Archiv B Cell Pathology 20: 103–111

204. Kay S 1977 Morphologic aspects of nuclear bodies in a case of bronchiolar-alveolar carcinoma of the lung. Human Pathology 8: 224–230

205. Kerr J F R, Searle J, Bishop C J 1979 Apoptosis: a distinctive mode of cell death that plays an opposite role to mitosis in cell population kinetics. Australasian Radiology 23: 192–201

206. Lampert F, Lampert P 1975 Multiple sclerosis. Morphologic evidence of intranuclear paramyxovirus or altered chromatin fibers? Archives of Neurology 32: 425–427

207. Mazur M T, Hendrickson M R, Kempson R L 1983 Optically clear nuclei. An alteration of endometrial epithelium in the presence of trophoblast. American Journal of Surgical Pathology 7: 415–423

208. Min K W, Song J 1982 Virus-like intranuclear particles in bronchiolar-alveolar cell carcinoma. Journal of the Iowa Medical Society 72: 319–321

209. Mori M, Onoe T 1967 An electron microscope study on the formation of intranuclear inclusions. Journal of Electron Microscopy 16: 137–142

210. Padykula H A, Fitzgerald M, Clark J H, Hardin J W 1981 Nuclear bodies as structural indicators of estrogenic stimulation in uterine luminal epithelial cells. Anatomical Record 201: 679–696

211. Rivas C, Oliva H 1974 Nuclear bodies in Hodgkin's disease. Pathologia Europaea 9: 297–301

212. Searle J, Kerr J F R, Bishop C J 1982 Necrosis and apoptosis: distinct modes of cell death with fundamentally different significance. Pathology Annual 17, pt 2: 229–259

213. Smith H S, Springer E L, Hackett A J 1979 Nuclear ultrastructure of epithelial cell lines derived from human carcinomas and nonmalignant tissues. Cancer Research 39: 332–344

214. Sobrinho-Simoes M A, Gonçalves V 1974 Nuclear bodies in papillary carcinomas of the human thyroid gland. Archives of Pathology 98: 94–99

215. Sobrinho-Simoes M A, Gonçalves V 1978 Nucleolar abnormalities in human papillary thyroid carcinomas. Archives of Pathology and Laboratory Medicine 102: 635–638

216. Tani E, Ametani T 1975 Nuclear characteristics of malignant lymphoma in the brain. Acta Neuropathologica suppl 6: 167–171

217. Tani E, Ametani T, Kawamura Y, Handa H 1969 Nuclear structures of primary malignant lymphoma in the brain. Cancer 24: 617–624

218. Valenzuela R, McMahon J T, Deodhar S D, Braun W E 1981 Ultrastructural study of tissue and peripheral blood neutrophils in human renal allograft recipients. A clinicopathological description of an unusual abnormality discovered in three cases. Human Pathology 12: 355–359

219. Wyllie A H, Kerr J F R, Currie A R 1980 Cell death: the significance of apoptosis. International Review of Cytology 68: 251–306

## 7 INTRANUCLEAR FIBRILLARY AND TUBULAR INCLUSIONS

220. Boquist L 1969 Intranuclear rods in pancreatic islet β-cells. Journal of Cell Biology 43: 377–381

221. Gonzalez-Crussi F, Hull M T, Mirkin D L 1978 Intranuclear filaments in a soft tissue sarcoma. Human Pathology 9: 189–198

222. Gunning W T, Harris J H 1983 Intranuclear tubular inclusions and cytoplasmic bodies in a patient with chronic interstitial fibrosis. Micron 14: 81–82

223. Györkey F, Györkey P A, Sinkovics J G 1980 Origin and significance of intranuclear tubular inclusions in type II pulmonary alveolar epithelial cells of patients with bleomycin and busulfan toxicity. Ultrastructural Pathology 1: 211–221

224. Hou-Jensen K, Rawlinson D G, Hendrickson M 1973 Proliferating histiocytic lesion (histiocytosis X?). Association of an extensive mediastinal and retroperitoneal sclerosing lesion with Gagel's granuloma of the posterior lobe of the pituitary. Cancer 32: 809–821

225. Kawanami O, Ferrans V J, Fulmer J D, Crystal R G 1979 Nuclear inclusions in alveolar epithelium of patients with fibrotic lung disorders. American Journal of Pathology 94: 301–322

226. Schochet S S, McCormick W F 1973 Polymyositis with intranuclear inclusions. A light and electron microscopic study. Archives of Neurology 28: 280–283

227. Seïte R, Zerbib R, Vuillet-Luciani J, Vio M 1977 Nuclear inclusions in sympathetic neurons: a quantitative and ultrastructural study in the superior cervical and celiac ganglia of the cat. Journal of Ultrastructure Research 61: 254–259

228. Shaw C-M, Sumi S M 1975 Non-viral intranuclear filamentous inclusions. Archives of Neurology 32: 428–432

229. Sheibani K, Tubbs R D, Savage R A, Sebek B A 1978 Intranuclear filaments in aleukemic histiomonocytic leukemia. Human Pathology 9: 608–609

230. Sherwin R P, Kaufman C, Dermer G R, Monroe S A 1977 Intranuclear rodlets in an intrathyroid tumor associated with hyperparathyroidism. Cancer 39: 178–185

231. Tamura H, Aronson B E 1978 Intranuclear fibrillary inclusions in influenza pneumonia. Archives of Pathology and Laboratory Medicine 102: 252–257

232. Tanaka R, Santoli D, Koprowski H 1976 Unusual intranuclear filaments in the circulating lymphocytes of patients with multiple sclerosis and optic neuritis. American Journal of Pathology 83: 245–254

233. Torikata C, Ishiwata K 1977 Intranuclear tubular structures observed in the cells of an alveolar cell carcinoma of the lung. Cancer 40: 1194–1201

234. Yunis E J, Samaha F J 1971 Inclusion body myositis. Laboratory Investigation 25: 240–245

## 8 GENERAL CYTOPLASMIC ABNORMALITIES IN TUMOURS

235. Allison A C 1974 Lysosomes in cancer cells. Journal of Clinical Pathology 27, suppl 7: 43–50

236. Altmannsberger M, Osborn M, Weber K, Schauer A 1982 Expression of intermediate filaments in different human epithelial and mesenchymal tumors. Pathology Research and Practice 175: 227–237

237. Bainton D F 1981 The discovery of lysosomes. Journal of Cell Biology 91: 66s–76s

238. Bannasch P, Zerban H, Mayer D 1982 The cytoskeleton in tumor cells. Pathology Research and Practice 175: 196–211

239. Brawn P N, Mackay B 1980 Intracristal crystalline inclusions in mitochondria of a neuroblastoma. Ultrastructural Pathology 1: 495–497

240. Cain H 1982 Introduction to the pathobiology of the cytoskeleton. Pathology Research and Practice 175: 119–127

241. Caselitz J, Osborn M, Wustrow J, Seifert G, Weber K 1982 The expression of different intermediate-sized filaments in human salivary glands and their tumours. Pathology Research and Practice 175: 266–278

242. Cheung W Y 1982 Calmodulin. Scientific American 246: 48–56

243. Chu H, Foucar K, Barlogie B, Middleman E 1982 Tubular complexes of endoplasmic reticulum in lymphoblastic lymphoma: case report. Cancer 49: 1629–1635

244. Cohen M L, Dawkins R L, Henderson D W, Sterrett G F, Papadimitriou J M 1979 Pulmonary lymphomatoid granulomatosis with immunodeficiency terminating as malignant lymphoma. Pathology 11: 537–550

245. Coudrier E, Reggio H, Louvard D 1981 Immunolocalization of the 110,000 molecular weight cytoskeletal protein of intestinal microvilli. Journal of Molecular Biology 152: 49–66

246. Djaldetti M, Mandel E M, Fishman P, Bessler H, Lewinski U 1974 Intramitochondrial crystalline inclusions in metastatic hypernephroma of the liver. Biomedicine Express 21: 158–163

247. Dustin P, Tondeur M, Libert J 1978 Metabolic and storage diseases. In: Johannessen J V (ed) Electron microscopy in human medicine, vol 2. Cellular pathology, metabolic and storage diseases. McGraw-Hill, New York, pt 2, p 151–245

248. Espinoza C G, Azar H A 1982 Immunohistochemical localization of keratin-type proteins in epithelial neoplasms. Correlation with electron microscopic findings. American Journal of Clinical Pathology 78: 500–507

249. Farquhar M G, Palade G E 1963 Junctional complexes in various epithelia. Journal of Cell Biology 17: 375–412

250. Farquhar M G, Palade G E 1981 The Golgi apparatus (complex) — (1954–1981) — from artifact to center stage. Journal of Cell Biology 91: 77s–103s

251. Felix H, Sträuli P 1978 Intermediate-sized filaments in leukemia cells. Virchows Archiv B Cell Pathology 28: 59–75

252. Foa C, Foa J, Carcassonne Y 1976 Morphologic study of virus-like particles in a case of acute leukemia. Cancer 37: 1718–1724

253. Franke W W, Zerban H, Grund C, Schmid E 1981 Electron microscopy of vimentin filaments and associated whisker structures in thin sections and freeze-fractures. Biology of the Cell 41: 173–178

254. Gabbiani G, Csank-Brassert J, Schneeberger J-C, Kapanci Y, Trenchev P, Holborow E J 1976 Contractile proteins in human cancer cells. Immunofluorescent and electron microscopic study. American Journal of Pathology 83: 457–474

255. Geiger B, Dutton A H, Tokuyasu K T, Singer S J 1981 Immunoelectron microscope studies of membrane-microfilament interactions: distributions of $\alpha$-actinin, tropomyosin, and vinculin in intestinal epithelial brush border and chicken gizzard smooth muscle cells. Journal of Cell Biology 91: 614–628

256. Hammar S P, Bockus D, Remington F 1983 Zipper-like structures in hepatocytes (letter). Ultrastructural Pathology 4: 283–284

257. Inoue S, Dionne G P 1977 Tonofilaments in normal human bronchial epithelium and in squamous cell carcinoma. American Journal of Pathology 88: 345–354

258. Jesudason M L, Iseri O A 1980 Host-tumor cellular junctions: an ultrastructural study of hepatic metastases of bronchogenic oat cell carcinoma. Human Pathology 11: 67–70

259. Kocher O, Amaudruz M, Schindler A M, Gabbiani G 1981 Desmosomes and gap junctions in precarcinomatous and carcinomatous conditions of squamous epithelia. An electron microscopic and morphometrical study. Journal of Submicroscopic Cytology 13: 267–281

260. Krepler R, Denk H, Artlieb U, Fichtinger E, Davidovits A 1982 Antibodies to intermediate filament proteins as molecular markers in clinical tumor pathology. Differentiation of carcinomas by their reaction with different cytokeratin antibodies. Pathology Research and Practice 175: 212–226

261. Lake J A 1981 The ribosome. Scientific American 245: 56–69

262. Lazarides E, Revel J P 1979 The molecular basis of cell movement. Scientific American 240: 88–100

263. Leblond C P, Sarkar K, Kallenbach E, Clermont Y 1966 Fibrillar structures (cell web) in the cells of human adenocarcinomas. Cancer Research 26: 2259–2266

264. Löning Th, Viac J, Caselitz J, Thivolet J, Otto H F, Seifert G 1982 Comparative investigation of keratin-filaments in normal tissues and tumours of skin, oral mucosa, salivary glands and thymus. Pathology Research and Practice 175: 256–265

265. Maciejewski W, Dabrowski J, Jakubowicz K 1973 Studies on cytoplasmic tubular inclusions in papilloma and other epithelial tumours. Folia Histochemica et Cytochemica 11: 339–340

266. Martinez-Palomo A 1971 Intercellular junctions in normal and malignant cells. Pathobiology Annual 1: 261–270

267. Maupin-Szamier P, Pollard T D 1978 Actin filament destruction by osmium tetroxide. Journal of Cell Biology 77: 837–852

268. Metz S A, Levine R J 1977 Neuroendocrine tumours that secrete biologically active peptides and amines. Clinics in Endocrinology and Metabolism 6: 719–744

269. Moll R, Franke W W 1982 Intermediate filaments and their interaction with membranes. The desmosome-cytokeratin filament complex and epithelial differentiation. Pathology Research and Practice 175: 146–161

270. Mukai K, Schollmeyer J V, Rosai J 1981 Immunohistochemical localization of actin. Applications in surgical pathology. American Journal of Surgical Pathology 5: 91–97

271. Osborn M, Altmannsberger M, Shaw G, Schauer A, Weber K 1982 Various sympathetic derived human tumors differ in neuro-filament expression. Use in diagnosis of neuroblastoma, ganglioneuroblastoma and pheochromocytoma. Virchows Archiv B Cell Pathology 40: 141–156

272. Osborn M, Weber K 1983 Tumor diagnosis by intermediate filament typing: a novel tool for surgical pathology. Laboratory Investigation 48: 372–394

273. Panel discussion 1982 Zipper-like structures in hepatocytes. Ultrastructural Pathology 3: 91–94

274. Perez-Atayde A R, Kozakewich H P W, Seiler M W 1981 Ribosome-lamellae complexes in non-leukemic tumor cells: an ultrastructural study. Laboratory Investigation 44: 52A

275. Pollard T D 1981 Cytoplasmic contractile proteins. Journal of Cell Biology 91: 156s–165s

276. Ramaekers F, Huysmans A, Moesker O, Kant A, Jap P, Herman C, Vooijs P 1983 Monoclonal antibody to keratin filaments, specific for glandular epithelia and their tumors. Use in surgical pathology. Laboratory Investigation 49: 353–361

277. Robertson J D 1981 Membrane structure. Journal of Cell Biology 91: 189s–204s

278. Rungger-Brändle E, Gabbiani G 1983 The role of cytoskeletal and cytocontractile elements in pathologic processes. American Journal of Pathology 110: 359–392

279. Scott R E, Furcht L T 1976 Membrane pathology of normal and malignant cells — a review. Human Pathology 7: 519–532

280. Seman G, Gallager H S 1979 Intramitochondrial rod-like inclusions in human breast tumors. Anatomical Record 194: 267–272

281. Sieinski W, Dorsett B, Ioachim H L 1981 Identification of prekeratin by immunofluorescence staining in the differential diagnosis of tumors. Human Pathology 12: 452–458

282. Sinha A A, Bentley M D, Blackard C E 1977 Freeze-fracture observations on the membranes and junctions in human prostatic carcinoma and benign prostatic hypertrophy. Cancer 40: 1128–1188

283. Sobrinho-Simoes M, Johannessen J V, Gould V E 1981 The diagnostic significance of intracytoplasmic lumina in metastatic neoplasms. Ultrastructural Pathology 2: 327–335

284. Staehelin L A 1974 Structure and function of intercellular junctions. International Review of Cytology 39: 191–283

285. Stoebner P, Renversez J C, Groulade J, Vialtel P, Cordonnier D 1979 Ultrastructural study of human IgG and IgG-IgM crystalcryoglobulins. American Journal of Clinical Pathology 71: 404–410

286. Sun C N 1976 Abnormal mitochondria in retinoblastoma. Experientia 32: 630–632

287. Szekely I E, Fischer D R, Schumacher H R 1976 Leukemic mitochondria. II. Acute monoblastic leukemia. Cancer 37: 805–811

288. Tandler B, Erlandson R A 1983 Giant mitochondria in a pleomorphic adenoma of the submandibular gland. Ultrastructural Pathology 4: 85–96

289. Tani E, Ametani T, Higashi N, Fujihara E 1971 Atypical cristae in mitochondria of human glioblastoma multiforme cells. Journal of Ultrastructure Research 36: 211–221

290. Thornell L-E, Bjelle A 1981 Eosinophilic fasciitis: an ultrastructural and immunohistochemical study of the intermediate filament protein skeletin in regenerating muscle fibres. Neuropathology and Applied Neurobiology 7: 435–449

291. Trump B F, Jesudason M L, Jones R T 1978 Ultrastructural features of diseased cells. In: Trump B F, Jones R T (eds) Diagnostic electron microscopy, vol 1. John Wiley & Sons, New York, ch 1, p 1–88

292. Trump B F, Mergner W J 1974 Cell injury. In: Zweifach B W, Grant L, McCluskey R T (eds) The inflammatory process, 2nd edn, vol 1. Academic Press, New York, ch 3 p 115–257

293. von Bassewitz D B, Roessner A, Grundmann E 1982 Intermediate-sized filaments in cells of normal human colonic mucosa, adenomas and carcinomas. Pathology Research and Practice 175: 238–255

294. Warner T F C S, Seo I S 1980 Aggregates of cytofilaments as the cause of the appearance of hyaline tumor cells. Ultrastructural Pathology 1: 395–401

295. Watanabe H, Burnstock G, Jarrott B, Louis W J 1976 Mitochondrial abnormalities in human pheochromocytoma. Cell and Tissue Research 172: 281–288

296. Weber K, Osborn M 1981 Aspects of the cytoskeleton of mammalian cells. In: Lloyd C W, Rees D A (eds) Cellular controls in differentiation. Academic Press, London, p 11–28

297. Weber K, Osborn M 1982 Cytoskeleton: definition, structure and gene regulation. Pathology Research and Practice 175: 128–145

298. Weinstein R S, Merk F B, Alroy J 1976 The structure and function of intercellular junctions in cancer. Advances in Cancer Research 23: 23–89

299. Wills E J 1983 Zipper-like structures in hepatocytes (letter). Ultrastructural Pathology 4: 277–278

300. Wilson P D, Nathrath W B J, Trejdosiewicz L K 1982 Immunoelectron microscopic localisation of keratin and luminal epithelial antigens in normal and neoplastic urothelium. Pathology Research and Practice 175: 289–298

301. Witaliński W, Goniakowska-Witalińska L 1981 Atypical mitochondria in the lung of newts Triturus alpestris, Laur. Journal of Ultrastructure Research 77: 223–231

302. Woods G L, Espinoza C G, Azar H A 1982 Carcinomas with spindle cell (sarcomatoid) component: an immunocytochemical and electron microscopic study. Laboratory Investigation 46: 91A

## 9 TUBULORETICULAR ARRAYS

303. Grimley P M, Schaff Z 1976 Significance of tubuloreticular inclusions in the pathobiology of human diseases. Pathobiology Annual 6: 221–257

304. Györkey F, Sinkovics J G, Györkey P 1971 Electron microscopic observations on structures resembling myxovirus in human sarcomas. Cancer 27: 1449–1454

305. Jenson A B, Spjut H J, Smith M N, Rapp F 1971 Intracellular branched tubular structures in osteosarcoma. An ultrastructural and serological study. Cancer 27: 1440–1448

306. Landolt A M, Ryffel U, Hosbach H U, Wyler R 1976 Ultrastructure of tubular inclusions in endothelial cells of pituitary tumors associated with acromegaly. Virchows Archiv A Pathological Anatomy and Histology 370: 129–140

307. Popoff N A, Malinin T I 1975 Myxovirus-like particles in cells of American Burkitt's-type lymphoma. Acta Neuropathologica suppl 6: 47–52

308. Popoff N A, Malinin T I 1976 Cytoplasmic tubular arrays in cells of American Burkitt's type lymphoma. Cancer 37: 275–284

309. Schaff Z, Barry D W, Grimley P M 1973 Cytochemistry of tubuloreticular structures in lymphocytes from patients with systemic lupus erythematosus and in cultured human lymphoid cells. Comparison to a paramyxovirus. Laboratory Investigation 29: 577–586

310. Uzman B G, Saito H, Kasac M 1971 Tubular arrays in the endoplasmic reticulum in human tumor cells. Laboratory Investigation 24: 492–498

311. Vernick S H, Kay S, Escobar M, Sperber E, Rosato F 1977 Intracisternal tubules in myxoid chondrosarcoma. Archives of Pathology and Laboratory Medicine 101: 556

## 10 ANNULATE LAMELLAE

312. Ancla M, De Brux J 1965 Occurrence of intranuclear tubular structures in the human endometrium during the secretory phase, and of annulate lamellae in hyperestrogenic states. Obstetrics and Gynecology 26: 23–33

313. Bhawan J, Ceccacci L, Cranford J 1978 Annulate lamellae in a malignant mesenchymal tumor. Virchows Archiv B Cell Pathology 26: 261–265

314. Freedman R S, Pihl E, Kusyk C, Gallager H S, Rutledge F 1978 Characterization of an ovarian carcinoma cell line. Cancer 42: 2352–2359

315. Gang D L, Long J C, Zamecnik P C, Chi S-Y, Dvorak A M 1979 Electron microscopy of Hodgkin's disease tissue cultures. Cancer 44: 543–557

316. Kadin M E, Bensch K G 1971 Comparison of pheochromocytes with ganglion cells and neuroblasts grown in vitro. An electron microscopic and histochemical study. Cancer 27: 1148–1160

317. Nakayama I, Moriuchi A, Taira Y, Takahara O, Itoga T 1977 Fine structural study of annulate lamellae complexes in human tumours. Acta Pathologica Japonica 27: 25–39

318. Seshadri R, Matthews C, Gardiakos C, Moore H, Zola H, Henderson D W, Jackey P, Morley A A 1984 FMC-HV-1-B cell line: a lymphoma B cell line with unusual characteristics. Leukaemia Research (in press)

319. Sun C N, White H J 1979 Annulate lamellae in human tumor cells. Tissue & Cell 11: 139–146

320. Tschang T-P, Kasin J V, Parnell D, Kraus F T 1978 Annulate lamellae in human malignant tumors. Report of three cases. Archives of Pathology and Laboratory Medicine 102: 426–430

321. Uzman B G, Foley G E, Farber S, Lazarus H 1966 Morphologic variations in human leukemic lymphoblasts (CCRF-CEM cells) after long-term culture and exposure to chemotherapeutic agents. A study with the electron microscope. Cancer 19: 1725–1742

322. Wielinski S T, Seiler M W 1980 Annulate lamellae in human tumors. Laboratory Investigation 42: 167A

## 11 STROMAL FINE STRUCTURE

323. Balázs M, Kovács A 1982 The 'transitional' mucosa adjacent to large bowel carcinoma — electron microscopic features and myofibroblast reaction. Histopathology 6: 617–629

324. Banfield W G, Lee C K, Lee C W 1973 Myocardial collagen of the fibrous long-spacing type. Archives of Pathology 95: 262–266

325. Bender B L, Jaffe R, Carlin B, Chung A E 1981 Immunolocalization of entactin, a sulfated basement membrane component, in rodent tissues, and comparison with GP-2 (laminin). American Journal of Pathology 103: 419–426

326. Bitterman P B, Rennard S I, Crystal R G 1981 Environmental lung disease and the interstitium. Clinics in Chest Medicine 2: 393–412

327. Blom J, Wiik A 1983 Russell bodies — immunoglobulins? American Journal of Clinical Pathology 79: 262–263

328. Bloom G D 1974 Structural and biochemical characteristics of mast cells. In: Zweifach B W, Grant L, McCluskey R T (eds) The inflammatory process, 2nd edn, vol 1. Academic Press, New York, ch 10, p 545–599

329. Catchpole H R 1982 Connective tissue, basement membrane, extracellular matrix. Pathobiology Annual 12: 1–33

330. Chambers T J 1978 Multinucleate giant cells. Journal of Pathology 126: 125–148

331. Connolly C E 1981 'Crystalline' collagen production by an unusual benign soft tissue tumour ('amianthioma'). Histopathology 5: 11–20

332. Cooper P H, Goodman M D 1974 Multilayering of the capillary basal lamina in the granular cell tumor. A marker of cellular injury. Human Pathology 5: 327–338

333. Dictor M, Hasserius R 1981 Systemic amyloidosis and non-hematologic malignancy in a large autopsy series. Acta Pathologica et Microbiologica Scandinavica. Section A. Pathology 89: 411–416

334. Erickson H P, Carrell N, McDonagh J 1981 Fibronectin molecule visualized in electron microscopy: a long, thin, flexible strand. Journal of Cell Biology 91: 673–678

335. Factor S M, Biempica L, Ratner I, Ahuja K K, Biempica S 1977 Carcinoma of the breast with multinucleated reactive stromal giant cells. A light and electron microscopic study of two cases. Virchows Archiv A Pathological Anatomy and Histology 374: 1–12

336. Fromme H G, Voss B, Pfautsch M, Grote M, von Figura K, Beeck H 1982 Immunoelectron-microscopic study on the location of fibronectin in human fibroblast cultures. Journal of Ultrastructure Research 80: 264–269

337. Gould V E, Battifora H 1976 Origin and significance of the basal lamina and some interstitial fibrillar components in epithelial neoplasms. Pathology Annual 11: 353–386

338. Hay E D 1981 Collagen and embryonic development. In: Hay E D (ed) Cell biology of extracellular matrix. Plenum Press, New York, ch 12, p 379–409

339. Hay E D 1981 Extracellular matrix. Journal of Cell Biology 91: 205s–223s

340. Hirano A, Matsui T 1975 Vascular structures in brain tumors. Human Pathology 6: 611–621

341. Hsu S-M, Hsu P-L, McMillan P N, Fanger H 1982 Russell bodies. A light and electron microscopic immunoperoxidase study. American Journal of Clinical Pathology 77: 26–31

342. Hynes R O 1981 Fibronectin and its relation to cellular structure and behaviour. In: Hay E D (ed) Cell biology of extracellular matrix. Plenum Press, New York, ch 10, p 295–334

343. Ingber D E, Madri J A, Jamieson J D 1981 Role of the basal lamina in neoplastic disorganization of tissue architecture. Proceedings of the National Academy of Science USA 78: 3901–3905

344. Kamiyama R 1982 Fibrous long spacing-like fibers in the bone marrow of myeloproliferative disorder. Virchows Archiv B Cell Pathology 39: 285–291

345. Kawamura J, Kamijyo Y, Sunaga T, Nelson E 1974 Tubular bodies in vascular endothelium of a cerebellar neoplasm. Laboratory Investigation 30: 358–365

346. Kleinman H K, Klebe R J, Martin G R 1981 Role of collagenous matrices in adhesion and growth of cells. Journal of Cell Biology 88: 473–485

347. Lagacé R, Schürch W, Seemayer T A 1980 Myofibroblasts in soft tissue sarcomas. Virchows Archiv A Pathological Anatomy and Histology 389: 1–11

348. Liotta L A 1982 Tumor extracellular matrix. Laboratory Investigation 47: 112–113

349. Lipper S, Kahn L B, Reddick R L 1980 The myofibroblast. Pathology Annual 15, pt. 1: 409–441

350. Ludatscher R M, Gellei B, Barzilai D 1979 Ultrastructural observations on the capillaries of human thyroid tumours. Journal of Pathology 128: 57–62

351. Majno G 1979 The story of the myofibroblasts. American Journal of Surgical Pathology 3: 535–542

352. Martin G R, Kleinman H K 1981 Extracellular matrix proteins give new life to cell culture. Hepatology 1: 264–266

353. Martinez-Hernandez A, Catalano E 1980 Stromal reaction to neoplasia: colonic carcinomas. Ultrastructural Pathology 1: 403–410

354. Martinez-Hernandez A, Francis D J, Silverberg S G 1977 Elastosis and other stromal reactions in benign and malignant breast tissue. An ultrastructural study. Cancer 40: 700–706

355. McDonagh J 1981 Fibronectin. A molecular glue. Archives of Pathology and Laboratory Medicine 105: 393–396

356. McGee J O'D, Al-Adnani M S 1976 Stroma in tumours. In: Symington T, Carter R L (eds) Scientific foundations of oncology. Heinemann, London, ch 2, p 45–52

357. Min K-W, Song J 1981 Long-spaced collagen in Hodgkin's disease: an ultrastructural observation. Laboratory Investigation 44: 44A

358. Mollo F, Monga G 1971 Banded structures in connective tissues of lymphomas, lymphadenitis and thymomas. Virchows Archiv B Zellpathologie 7: 356–366

359. Nakanishi I, Kajikawa K, Okada Y, Eguchi K 1981 Myofibroblasts in fibrous tumours and fibrosis in various organs. Acta Pathologica Japonica 31: 423–437

360. Nakanishi I, Masuda S, Kitamura T, Moriizumi I, Kajikawa K 1981 Distribution of fibrous long-spacing fibers in normal and pathological lymph nodes. Acta Pathologica Japonica 31: 733–745

361. Neyazaki T, Ikeda M, Mitsui K, Kimura S, Suzuki M, Suzuki C 1970 Angioarchitecture of pulmonary malignancies in humans. Cancer 26: 1246–1255

362. Orenstein J M 1983 Amianthoid fibers in a synovial sarcoma and a malignant Schwannoma. Ultrastructural Pathology 4: 163–176

363. Pasyk K A, Grabb W C, Cherry G W 1983 Ultrastructure of mast cells in growing and involuting stages of hemangiomas. Human Pathology 14: 174–181

364. Povýsil C, Matejovsky Z 1979 Ultrastructural evidence of myofibroblasts in pseudomalignant myositis ossificans. Virchows Archiv A Pathological Anatomy and Histology 381: 189–203

365. Ryan G B, Cliff W J, Gabbiani G, Irlé C, Montandon D, Statkov P R, Majno G 1974 Myofibroblasts in human granulation tissue. Human Pathology 5: 55–67

366. Säve-Söderbergh J 1975 Basal lamina in granular cell tumors. Human Pathology 6: 637–638

367. Scholtz C L 1975 Banded structures in cauda equina. Pathology 7: 129–132

368. Schürch W, Seemayer T A, Lagacé R 1981 Stromal myofibroblasts in primary invasive and metastatic carcinomas. A combined immunological, light and electron microscopic study. Virchows Archiv A Pathological Anatomy and Histology 391: 125–139

369. Scully R E 1981 Smooth-muscle differentiation in genital tract disorders. Archives of Pathology and Laboratory Medicine 105: 505–507

370. Seemayer T A, Lagacé R, Schürch W, Thelmo W L 1980 The myofibroblast: biologic, pathologic and theoretical considerations. Pathology Annual 15, pt 1: 443–470

371. Seemayer T A, Schürch W, Lagacé R 1981 Myofibroblasts in human pathology. Human Pathology 12: 491–492

372. Seemayer T A, Schürch W, Lagacé R, Tremblay G 1979 Myofibroblasts in the stroma of invasive and metastatic carcinoma. A possible host response to neoplasia. American Journal of Surgical Pathology 3: 525–533

373. Slavkin H C 1983 Extracellular matrix influences on gene expression (editorial). Journal of Craniofacial Genetics and Developmental Biology 2: 97–98

374. Toole B P 1981 Glycosaminoglycans in morphogenesis. In: Hay E D (ed) Cell biology of extracellular matrix. Plenum Press, New York, ch 9, p 259–294

375. Tremblay G 1976 Ultrastructure of elastosis in scirrhous carcinoma of the breast. Cancer 37: 307–316

376. Vaheri A, Alitalo K 1981 Pericellular matrix glycoproteins in cell differentiation and in malignant transformation. In: Lloyd C W, Rees D A (eds) Cellular controls in differentiation. Academic Press, London, p 29–56

377. Wang W, Campiche M 1982 Microvasculature of human colorectal epithelial tumors. An electron microscopic study. Virchows Archiv A Pathological Anatomy and Histology 397: 131–147

378. Ward J D, Hadfield M G, Becker D P, Lovings E T 1974 Endothelial fenestrations and other vascular alterations in primary melanoma of the central nervous system. Cancer 34: 1982–1991

379. Wilander E, Westermark P, Grimelius L 1980 Intracellular and extracellular fibrillar structures in gastroduodenal endocrine tumors. Ultrastructural Pathology 1: 49–54

380. Wirman J A 1976 Nodular fasciitis, a lesion of myofibroblasts. An ultrastructural study. Cancer 33: 2378–2389

381. Yamada K M 1981 Fibronectin and other structural proteins. In: Hay E D (ed) Cell biology of extracellular matrix. Plenum Press, New York, ch 4, p 95–114

## 12 TUMOURS OF THE UPPER RESPIRATORY TRACT, INCLUDING NASAL CAVITY, NASOPHARYNX AND LARYNX

382. Ahmed M M 1981 Studies on human laryngeal papilloma. Degeneration of lymphocytes within the neoplastic cells. Acta Otolaryngologica 92: 563–567

383. Albert R W 1981 Esthesioneuroblastoma. Ear, Nose and Throat Journal 60: 522–526

384. Arnold W, Huth F 1978 Electron microscopic findings in four cases of nasopharyngeal fibroma. Virchows Archiv A Pathological Anatomy and Histology 379: 285–298

385. Benisch B M, Tawfik B, Breitenbach E E 1975 Primary oat cell carcinoma of the larynx: an ultrastructural study. Cancer 36: 145–148

386. Boysen M, Reith A 1980 Surface structures in normal, metaplastic and dysplastic nasal mucosa of nickel workers. A SEM and post SEM histopathological study. Scanning Electron Microscopy 3: 35–41

387. Boysen M, Reith A 1982 The surface structure of the human nasal mucosa II. Metaplasia, dysplasia and carcinoma in nickel workers. A correlated study by scanning/transmission electron and light microscopy. Virchows Archiv B Cell Pathology 40: 295–309

388. Chaudhry A P, Haar J G, Koul A, Nickerson P A 1979 Olfactory neuroblastoma (esthesioneuroblastoma). A light and ultrastructural study of two cases. Cancer 44: 564–579

389. Cook T A, Brunschwig J P, Butel J S, Cohn A M, Gozepfert H, Rawls W E 1973 Laryngeal papilloma: etiologic and therapeutic considerations. Annals of Otology, Rhinology and Laryngology 82: 649–655

390. Curtis J L, Rubinstein L J 1982 Pigmented olfactory neuroblastoma. A new example of melanotic neuroepithelial neoplasm. Cancer 49: 2136–2143

391. Dahm L J, Schaefer S D, Carder H M, Vellios F 1978 Osteosarcoma of the soft tissue of the larynx: report of a case with light and electron microscopic studies. Cancer 42: 2343–2351

392. De Thé G, Geser A 1974 Nasopharyngeal carcinoma: recent studies and outlook for a viral etiology. Cancer Research 34: 1196–1206

393. DiMaio S J, DiMaio V J, DiMaio T M, Nicastri A D, Chen C K 1980 Oncocytic carcinoma of the nasal cavity. Southern Medical Journal 73: 803–806

394. Ferlito A, Gale N, Hvala H 1981 Laryngeal salivary duct carcinoma: a light and electron microscopic study. Journal of Laryngology and Otology 95: 731–738

395. Gallivan M V E, Chun B, Rowden G, Lack EE 1979 Laryngeal paraganglioma. Case report with ultrastructural analysis and literature review. American Journal of Surgical Pathology 3: 85–92

396. Gebhart W, Hohlbrugger H, Lassmann H, Ramadan W 1982 Nasal glioma. International Journal of Dermatology 21: 212–215

397. Giffer R F, Gillespie J J, Ayala A G, Newland J R 1977 Lymphoepithelioma in cervical lymph nodes of children and young adults. American Journal of Surgical Pathology 1: 293–302

398. Gnepp D R, Ferlito A, Hyams V 1983 Primary anaplastic small cell (oat cell) carcinoma of the larynx. Review of the literature and report of 18 cases. Cancer 51: 1731–1745

399. Hassoun J, Gambarelli D, Grisoli F, Henric A, Toga M 1981 Esthesioneuroepithelioma, a true neurosensorial tumor. Light- and electron-microscopic study of a case with endocranial extension. Acta Neuropathologica 55: 77–80

400. Incze J S, Lue P S, Strong M S, Vaughan C W, Clemente M P 1977 The morphology of human papillomas of the upper respiratory tract. Cancer 39: 1634–1646

401. Jin G, Gang Y, Ke-Xue X, Bao-Gui L, Yi-Lin S 1982 Characteristics of invasiveness of human nasopharyngeal carcinoma cells in organ culture, as observed by scanning electron microscopy. Pathology Research and Practice 174: 325–341

402. Kahn L B 1974 Esthesioneuroblastoma: a light and electron microscopic study. Human Pathology 5: 364–371

403. Kameya T, Shimosato Y, Adachi I, Abe K, Ebihara S, Ono I 1980 Neuroendocrine carcinoma of the paranasal sinus. A morphological and endocrinological study. Cancer 45: 330–339

404. Katenkamp D, Stiller D, Küttner K 1982 Inverted papillomas of nasal cavity and paranasal sinuses. Ultrastructural investigations on epithelial-stromal interface. Virchows Archiv A Pathological Anatomy and Histology 397: 215–226

405. Lasser K H, Naeim F, Higgins J, Cove H, Waisman J 1979 'Pseudosarcoma' of the larynx. American Journal of Surgical Pathology 3: 397–404

406. Lin H-S, Lin C-S, Yeh S, Tu S-M 1969 Fine structure of nasopharyngeal carcinoma with special reference to the anaplastic type. Cancer 23: 390–405

407. Martinez M A, Navas J J, Blanco M, Alvarez J J 1982 Esthesioneuroblastoma: a light and electron microscopic study. Morfología Normal y Patológica 6: 259–269

408. Mills S E, Cooper P H, Garland T A, Johns M E 1983 Small cell undifferentiated carcinoma of the larynx. Report of two patients and review of 13 additional cases. Cancer 51: 116–120

409. Mullins J D, Newman R K, Coltman C A Jr 1979 Primary oat cell carcinoma of the larynx: a case report and review of the literature. Cancer 43: 711–717

410. Osamura R Y, Fine G 1976 Ultrastructure of the esthesioneuroblastoma. Cancer 38: 173–179

411. Paladugu R R, Nathwani B N, Goodstein J, Dardi L E, Memoli V E, Gould V E 1982 Carcinoma of the larynx with mucosubstance production and neuroendocrine differentiation. An ultrastructural and immunohistochemical study. Cancer 49: 343–349

412. Papavasiliou A, Michaels L 1981 Unusual leiomyoma of the nose (leiomyoblastoma): report of a case. Journal of Laryngology and Otology 95: 1281–1286

413. Patterson S D, Ballard R W 1980 Nasal blastoma: a light and electron microscopic study. Ultrastructural Pathology 1: 487–494

414. Perzin K H, Cantor J O, Johannessen J V 1981 Acinic cell carcinoma arising in nasal cavity: report of a case with ultrastructural observations. Cancer 47: 1818–1822

415. Prasad U, Gogusev J 1978 Intracisternal tubular inclusions in nasopharyngeal carcinoma. Journal of Laryngology and Otology 92: 979–989

416. Quick C A, Faras A, Krzysek R 1978 The etiology of laryngeal papillomatosis. Laryngoscope 88: 1789–1795

417. Rosai J 1981 Letter to the editor. Ultrastructural Pathology 2: 193

418. Sanchez-Casis G, Devine K D, Weiland L H 1971 Nasal adenocarcinomas that closely simulate colonic carcinomas. Cancer 28: 714–720

419. Schenk P 1980 Gap junctions in laryngeal carcinoma. Archives of Otorhinolaryngology 228: 51–56

420. Schmid K O, Auböck L, Albegger K 1979 Endocrine-amphicrine enteric carcinoma of the nasal mucosa. Virchows Archiv A Pathological Anatomy and Histology 383: 329–343

421. Schwarz R, Marquet E, Sobel H J 1982 Another look at the 'anemone cell' (letter). Ultrastructural Pathology 3: 209–211

422. Sciubba J J 1981 Letter to the editor. Ultrastructural Pathology 2: 193

423. Sibley R, Rosai J, Froehlich W 1980 A case for the panel: anemone cell tumor. Ultrastructural Pathology 1: 449–453

424. Sidhu G S 1982 Another look at the 'anemone cell' (letter). Ultrastructural Pathology 3: 211–212

425. Silva E G, Butler J J, Mackay B, Goepfert H 1982 Neuroblastomas and neuroendocrine carcinomas of the nasal cavity. A proposed new classification. Cancer 50: 2388–2405

426. Stiller D, Katenkamp D, Kuttner K 1976 Cellular differentiations and structural characteristics in naso-pharyngeal angiofibromas. An electron microscopic study. Virchows Archiv A Pathological Anatomy and Histology 371: 273–282

427. Svoboda D J, Kirchner F 1966 Ultrastructure of nasopharyngeal angiofibromas. Cancer 19: 1949–1962

428. Tamai S, Iri H, Maruyama T, Kasahara M, Akatsuka S, Sakurai S, Murakami Y 1981 Laryngeal carcinoid tumor: light and electron microscopic studies. Cancer 48: 2256–2259

429. Taxy J B 1977 Juvenile nasopharyngeal angiofibroma. An ultrastructural study. Cancer 39: 1044–1054

430. Taxy J B, Hidvegi D F 1977 Olfactory neuroblastoma. An ultrastructural study. Cancer 39: 131–138

431. Tomita T, Lotuaco L, Talbott L, Watanabe I 1977 Mucoepidermoid carcinoma of the subglottis. An ultrastructural study. Archives of Pathology and Laboratory Medicine 101: 145–148

432. Trojanowski J Q, Lee V, Pillsbury N, Lee S 1982 Neuronal origin of human esthesioneuroblastoma demonstrated with anti-neurofilament monoclonal antibodies. New England Journal of Medicine 307: 159–161

433. Wetmore R F, Tronzo R D, Lane R J, Lowry L D 1981 Nonfunctional paraganglioma of the larynx: clinical and pathological considerations. Cancer 48: 2717–2723

434. Wilander E, Nordlinder H, Grimelius L, Larsson L-I, Angelborg C 1977 Esthesioneuroblastoma. Histological, histochemical and electron microscopic studies of a case. Virchows Archiv A Pathological Anatomy and Histology 375: 123–128

## 13 BRONCHOPULMONARY TUMOURS

435. Ahmed A 1974 Some ultrastructural observations of haematoxyphil vascular change in oat-cell carcinoma. Journal of Pathology 112: 1–3

436. Alvarez-Fernandez E 1980 Intracytoplasmic fibrillary inclusions in bronchial carcinoid. Cancer 46: 144–151

437. Alvarez-Fernandez E, Folque-Gomez E 1981 Atypical bronchial carcinoid with oncocytoid features. Its ultrastructure, with special reference to its granular content. Archives of Pathology and Laboratory Medicine 105: 428–431

438. Alves de Matos A P 1974 Tubuloreticular structures in a case of bronchial adenoma (carcinoid type). Experientia 30: 1465–1466

439. An T 1978 Cytoplasmic inclusions in bronchial carcinoid. Human Pathology 9: 241–242

440. Auerbach O, Frasca J M, Parks V R, Carter H W 1982 A comparison of World Health Organization (WHO) classification of lung tumors by light and electron microscopy. Cancer 50: 2079–2088

441. Azumi N, Churg A 1981 Intravascular and sclerosing bronchioloalveolar tumor. A pulmonary sarcoma of probable vascular origin. American Journal of Surgical Pathology 5: 587–596

442. Basset F, Soler P, Wyllie L, Abelanet R, Le Charpentier M, Kreis B, Breathnach A S 1974 Langerhans cell in a bronchiolar-alveolar tumour of lung. Virchows Archiv A Pathological Anatomy and Histology 362: 315–330

443. Becker N H, Soifer I 1971 Benign clear cell tumor ('sugar tumor') of the lung. Cancer 27: 712–719

444. Bedrossian C W M, Verani R, Unger K M, Salman J 1979 Pulmonary malignant fibrous histiocytoma. Light and electron microscopic studies of one case. Chest 75: 186–189

445. Bedrossian C W M, Weilbaecher D G, Bentinck D C, Greenberg S D 1975 Ultrastructure of human bronchiolo-alveolar cell carcinoma. Cancer 36: 1399–1413

446. Bell R M, Bullock J D, Albert D M 1975 Solitary choroidal metastasis from bronchial carcinoid. British Journal of Ophthalmology 59: 155–163

447. Bensch K G, Corrin B, Pariente R, Spencer H 1968 Oat-cell carcinoma of the lung. Its origin and relationship to bronchial carcinoid. Cancer 22: 1163–1172

448. Bensch K G, Gordon G B, Miller L R 1965 Electron microscopic and biochemical studies on the bronchial carcinoid tumor. Cancer 18: 592–602

449. Bensch K, Kuhn C (discussants) 1981 A case for the panel. Vacuolated epithelial lesion in lung. Ultrastructural Pathology 2: 303–307

450. Bhagavan B S, Dorfman H D, Murthy M S N, Eggleston J C 1982 Intravascular bronchiolo-alveolar tumor (IVBAT). A low-grade sclerosing epithelioid angiosarcoma of lung. American Journal of Surgical Pathology 6: 41–52

451. Black W C III 1969 Pulmonary oncocytoma. Cancer 23: 1347–1357

452. Block P, Wuketich S, Gorgas K 1977 Fine structure of a bronchial oncocytoma. Oesterreichische Zeitschrift für Onkologie 4: 14–20

453. Bolen J W, Thorning D 1982 Histogenetic classification of lung carcinomas. Small cell carcinomas studied by light and electron microscopy. Journal of Submicroscopic Cytology 14: 499–514

454. Bolen J W, Thorning D 1982 Histogenetic classification of pulmonary carcinomas. Peripheral adenocarcinomas studied by light microscopy, histochemistry and electron microscopy. Pathology Annual 17: 77–100

455. Bonikos D S, Archibald R, Bensch K G 1976 On the origin of the so-called tumorlets of the lung. Human Pathology 7: 461–469

456. Bonikos D S, Bensch K G, Jamplis R W 1976 Peripheral pulmonary carcinoid tumors. Cancer 37: 1977–1998

457. Bonikos D S, Hendrickson M, Bensch K G 1977 Pulmonary alveolar cell carcinoma. Fine structural and in vitro study of a case and critical review of the literature. American Journal of Surgical Pathology 1: 93–108

458. Brown B L, Scharifker D A, Gordon R, Deppe G G, Cohen C J 1980 Bronchial carcinoid tumor with ovarian metastasis. A light microscopic and ultrastructural study. Cancer 46: 543–546

459. Burkhardt A, Otto H F, Kaukel E 1981 Multiple pulmonary (hamartomatous?) leiomyomas. Light and electron microscopic study. Virchows Archiv A Pathological Anatomy and Histology 394: 133–141

460. Capella C, Gabrielli M, Polak J M, Buffa R, Solcia E, Bordi C 1979 Ultrastructural and histological study of 11 bronchial carcinoids. Evidence for different types. Virchows Archiv A Pathological Anatomy and Histology 381: 313–329

461. Carstens P H B 1983 Electron microscopy of small cell carcinoma of the lung with special reference to the crush phenomenon. Ultrastructural Pathology 4: 253–260

462. Cebelin M S 1980 Melanocytic bronchial carcinoid tumor. Cancer 46: 1843–1848

463. Cebelin M S 1981 Melanotic bronchial carcinoid tumor. Laboratory Investigation 44: 9A

464. Chaffin J C Jr, Herrera G A, Roberts C 1983 Oat cell carcinoma of the trachea: a case report with electron microscopy. Ultrastructural Pathology 4: 61–65

465. Chan K W, Gibbs A R, Lo W S, Newman G R 1982 Benign sclerosing pneumocytoma of lung (sclerosing haemangioma). Thorax 37: 404–412

466. Chumas J C, Lorelle C A 1982 Pulmonary meningioma. A light- and electron-microscopic study. American Journal of Surgical Pathology 6: 795–801

467. Churg A 1977 Large spindle cell variant of peripheral bronchial carcinoid tumor. Archives of Pathology and Laboratory Medicine 101: 216–218

468. Churg A 1978 The fine structure of large cell undifferentiated carcinoma of the lung. Evidence for its relation to squamous cell carcinomas and adenocarcinomas. Human Pathology 9: 143–156

469. Churg A M, Warnock M L 1976 So-called 'minute pulmonary chemodectoma'. A tumor not related to paragangliomas. Cancer 37: 1759–1769

470. Churg A, Johnston W H, Stulbarg M 1980 Small cell squamous and mixed small cell squamous-small cell anaplastic carcinomas of the lung. American Journal of Surgical Pathology 4: 255–263

471. Churg A, Warnock M L 1976 Pulmonary tumorlet. A form of peripheral carcinoid. Cancer 37: 1469–1477

472. Coalson J J, Mohr J A, Pirtle J K, Dee A L, Rhoades E R 1970 Electron microscopy of neoplasms in the lung with special emphasis on the alveolar cell carcinoma. American Review of Respiratory Disease 101: 181–197

473. Corrin B 1980 Lung endocrine tumours. Investigative & Cell Pathology 3: 195–206

474. Corrin B, Manners B, Millard M, Weaver L 1979 Histogenesis of the so-called 'intravascular bronchioloalveolar tumour.' Journal of Pathology 128: 163–167

475. Dail D H, Liebow A A, Gmelich J T, Friedman P J, Miyai K, Myer W, Patterson S D, Hammar S P 1983 Intravascular, bronchiolar, and alveolar tumor of the lung (IVBAT). An analysis of twenty cases of a peculiar sclerosing endothelial tumor. Cancer 51: 452–464

476. Dairaku M, Sueishi K, Tanaka K, Horie A 1983 Immunohistological analysis of surfactant-apoprotein in the bronchiolo-alveolar carcinoma. Virchows Archiv A Pathological Anatomy and Histopathology 400: 223–234

477. Fabich D R, Hafez G R 1980 Glomangioma of the trachea. Cancer 45: 2337–2341

478. Falini B, Bucciarelli E, Grignani F, Martelli M F 1980 Erythrophagocytosis by undifferentiated lung carcinoma cells. Cancer 46: 1140–1145

479. Fantone J C, Geisinger K R, Appelman H D 1982 Papillary adenoma of the lung with lamellar and electron dense granules. An ultrastructural study. Cancer 50: 2839–2844

480. Fechner R E, Bentinck B R 1973 Ultrastructure of bronchial oncocytoma. Cancer 31: 1451—1457

481. Fechner R E, Bentinck B R, Askew J B Jr 1972 Acinic cell tumor of the lung. A histologic and ultrastructural study. Cancer 29: 501–508

482. Feldman P S, Innes D J Jr 1980 Pulmonary alveolar cell carcinoma: a new variant. Laboratory Investigation 42: 116A

483. Fisher E R, Palekar A, Paulson J D 1978 Comparative histopathologic, histochemical, electron microscopic and tissue culture studies of bronchial carcinoids and oat cell carcinomas of lung. American Journal of Clinical Pathology 69: 165–172

484. Fu Y-S, McWilliams N B, Stratford T P, Kay S 1974 Bronchial carcinoid with choroidal metastasis in an adolescent. Case report and ultrastructural study. Cancer 33: 707–715

485. Fung C H, Lo J W, Yonan T N, Milloy F J, Hakami M M, Changus G W 1977 Pulmonary blastoma. An ultrastructural study with a brief review of literature and a discussion of pathogenesis. Cancer 39: 153–163

486. Gillespie J J, Luger A M, Callaway L A 1979 Peripheral spindled carcinoid tumor: a review of its ultrastructure, differential diagnosis and biologic behavior. Human Pathology 10: 601–606

487. Gordon H W, Miller R Jr, Mittman C 1973 Medullary carcinoma of the lung with amyloid stroma: a counterpart of medullary carcinoma of the thyroid. Human Pathology 4: 431–436

488. Gould V E, Chejfec G 1978 Ultrastructural and biochemical analysis of 'undifferentiated' pulmonary carcinomas. Human Pathology 9: 377–384

489. Gould V E, Linnoila R I, Memoli V A, Warren W H 1983 Neuroendocrine cells and neuroendocrine neoplasms of the lung. Pathology Annual 18, pt 1: 287–330

490. Grazer R, Cohen S M, Jacobs J B, Lucas P 1982 Melanin-containing peripheral carcinoid of lung. American Journal of Surgical Pathology 6: 73–78

491. Greenberg S D, Harness M K, Levy M L, Fechner R E 1975 Diagnosing bronchial carcinoid tumors by electron microscopy. Texas Medicine 71: 50–54

492. Greenberg S D, Smith M N, Spjut H J 1975 Bronchiolo-alveolar carcinoma — cell of origin. American Journal of Clinical Pathology 63: 153–167

493. Greene J G, Divertie M B, Brown A L, Lambert E H 1968 Small cell carcinoma of lung. Observations on four patients including one with a myasthenic syndrome. Archives of Internal Medicine 122: 333–339

494. Haas J E, Yunis E J, Totten R S 1972 Ultrastructure of a sclerosing hemangioma of the lung. Cancer 30: 512–518

495. Hage E 1973 Histochemistry and fine structure of bronchial carcinoid tumours. Virchows Archiv A Pathological Anatomy and Histology 361: 121–128

496. Hammar S P, Bockus D, Remington F, Hallman K O, Winterbauer R H, Hill L D, Bauermeister D E, Jones H W, Mennemeyer R P, Wheelis R F 1980 Langerhans cells and serum precipitating antibodies against fungal antigens in bronchioloalveolar cell carcinoma: possible association with pulmonary eosinophilic granuloma. Ultrastructural Pathology 1: 19–37

497. Hashimoto K, Fukuoka M, Nagasawa S, Tamai S, Kusunoki Y, Kawahara M, Furuse K, Sawamura K, Fujimoto T 1979 Small cell carcinoma of the lung and its histological origin. Report of a case. American Journal of Surgical Pathology 3: 343–351

498. Hattori S, Matsuda M, Tateishi R, Nishimara H, Horai T 1972 Oat-cell carcinoma of the lung. Clinical and morphological studies in relation to its histogenesis. Cancer 30: 1014–1024

499. Hattori S, Matsuda M, Tateishi R, Terazawa T 1967 Electron microscopic studies on human lung cancer cells. Gann 58: 283–290

500. Hayakawa K, Takahashi M, Sasaki K, Kawaoi A, Okano T 1977 Primary choriocarcinoma of the lung: case report of two male subjects. Acta Pathologica Japonica 27: 123–135

501. Heard B E, Dewar A 1982 Squamous cell carcinoma of bronchus: polypoid granules and mitochondrial densities found by electron microscopy. Diagnostic Histopathology 5: 189–195

502. Heard B E, Dewar A, Firmkin R K, Lennox S C 1982 One very rare and one new tracheal tumour found by electron microscopy: glomus tumour and acinic cell tumour resembling carcinoid tumours by light microscopy. Thorax 37: 97–103

503. Heilman E, Feiner H 1978 The role of electron microscopy in the diagnosis of unusual peripheral lung tumors. Human Pathology 9: 589–593

504. Hill G S, Eggleston J C 1972 Electron microscopic study of so-called 'pulmonary sclerosing hemangioma'. Report of a case suggesting epithelial origin. Cancer 30: 1092–1106

505. Hoch W S, Patchefsky A S, Takeda M, Gordon G 1974 Benign clear cell tumor of the lung. An ultrastructural study. Cancer 33: 1328–1336

506. Hollmann K H, Verley J M 1982 Ultrastructural study of small cell carcinoma. Bulletin du Cancer (Paris) 69: 66–68

507. Horie A, Ohta M 1981 Ultrastructural features of large cell carcinoma of the lung with reference to the prognosis of patients. Human Pathology 12: 423–432

508. Incze J S 1977 Morphology of the epithelial component of human lung hamartomas. Human Pathology 8: 411–419

509. Jacques J, Currie W 1977 Bronchiolo-alveolar carcinoma: a Clara cell tumor? Cancer 40: 2171–2180

510. Kameya T, Shimosato Y, Kodama T, Tsumuraya M, Koide T, Yamaguchi K, Abe K 1983 Peptide hormone production by adenocarcinomas of the lung: its morphologic basis and histogenetic considerations. Virchows Archiv A Pathological Anatomy and Histopathology 400: 245–257

511. Kandawalla N, Kasnic G Jr, Azar H A 1977 An ultrastructural study of lung tumors. Laboratory Investigation 36: 342A

512. Katz D R, Bubis J J 1976 Acinic cell tumor of the bronchus. Cancer 38: 830–832

513. Katzenstein A-L A, Maurer J J 1979 Benign histiocytic tumor of lung. A light- and electron-microscopic study. American Journal of Surgical Pathology 2: 61–68

514. Katzenstein A-L A, Weise D L, Fulling K, Battifora H 1983 So-called sclerosing hemangioma of the lung. Evidence for mesothelial origin. American Journal of Surgical Pathology 7: 3–14

515. Kay S, Still W J, Borochovitz D 1977 Sclerosing hemangioma of the lung: an endothelial or epithelial neoplasm? Human Pathology 8: 468–474

516. Keane J, Fretzin D F, Jao W, Shapiro C M 1980 Bronchial carcinoid metastatic to skin. Light and electron microscopic findings. Journal of Cutaneous Pathology 7: 43–49

517. Kemnitz P, Spormann H, Heinrich P 1982 Meningioma of the lung: first report with light and electron microscopic findings. Ultrastructural Pathology 3: 359–365

518. Kennedy A 1973 Sclerosing haemangioma of the lung: an alternative view of its development. Journal of Clinical Pathology 26: 792–799

519. Kennedy A 1979 The diagnosis of pulmonary carcinoid tumours. British Journal of Diseases of the Chest 73: 71–80

520. Kern W H, Hughes R K, Meyer B W, Harley D P 1979 Malignant fibrous histiocytoma of the lung. Cancer 44: 1793–1801

521. Kimula Y 1978 A histochemical and ultrastructural study of adenocarcinoma of the lung. American Journal of Surgical Pathology 2: 253–264

522. Klacson P G, Olsen J L, Eggleston J C 1979 Mucoepidermoid carcinoma of the bronchus. An electron microscopic study of the low grade and the high grade variants. Cancer 43: 1720–1733

523. Kodama T, Kameya T, Shimosato Y, Koketsu H, Yoneyama T, Tamai S 1980 Cell incohesiveness and pattern of extension in a rare case of bronchioloalveolar carcinoma. Ultrastructural Pathology 1: 177–188

524. Kradin R L, Young R H, Dickersin G R, Kirkham S E, Mark E J 1982 Pulmonary blastoma with argyrophil cells and lacking sarcomatous features (pulmonary endodermal tumor resembling fetal lung). American Journal of Surgical Pathology 6: 165–172

525. Kuhn C 1972 Fine structure of bronchiolo-alveolar cell carcinoma. Cancer 30: 1107–1118

526. Kuhn C III 1979 The lung. In: Johannessen J V (ed) Electron microscopy in human medicine, vol 6. Nervous system, sensory organs and respiratory tract. McGraw-Hill, New York, ch 11, p 387–446

527. Kuhn C III, Askin F B 1975 The fine structure of so-called minute pulmonary chemodectomas. Human Pathology 6: 681–691

528. Kuhn C III, Askin F B, Katzenstein A-L A 1980 Diagnostic light and electron microscopy. In: Diagnostic Techniques in Pulmonary Disease, pt I. Sackner M A (ed) Lung Biology in Health and Disease, vol 16. Marcel Dekker, New York, p 89–202

529. Leong A S-Y 1982 The relevance of ultrastructural examination in the classification of primary lung tumours. Pathology 14: 37–46

530. Li W-i, Hammar S P, Jolly P C, Hill L D, Anderson R P 1981 Unpredictable course of small cell undifferentiated lung carcinoma. Journal of Thoracic and Cardiovascular Surgery 81: 34–43

531. Lupulescu A, Boyd C B 1972 Lung cancer: a transmission and scanning electron microscopic study. Cancer 29: 1530–1538

532. Marcus P B, Dieb T M, Martin J H 1982 Pulmonary blastoma: an ultrastructural study emphasizing intestinal differentiation in lung tumors. Cancer 49: 1829–1833

533. Marks C, Lamberty J 1977 The cellular structure of bronchial carcinoids. Postgraduate Medical Journal 53: 360–363

534. Matthews M J, Mackay B, Lukeman J 1983 The pathology of non-small cell carcinoma of the lung. Seminars in Oncology 10: 34–55

535. McCann M P, Fu Y-S, Kay S 1976 Pulmonary blastoma. A light and electron microscopic study. Cancer 38: 789–797

536. McDowell E M, Barrett L A, Trump B F 1976 Observations on small granule cells in adult human bronchial epithelium and in carcinoid and oat cell tumors. Laboratory Investigation 34: 202–206

537. McDowell E M, Becci P J, Barrett L A, Trump B F 1978 Morphogenesis and classification of lung cancer. In: Harris C C (ed) Pathogenesis and therapy of lung cancer. Lung biology in health and disease, vol 10. Marcel Dekker, New York, ch 9, p 445–519

538. McDowell E M, Hess F G Jr, Trump B F 1980 Epidermoid metaplasia, carcinoma in situ, and carcinomas of the lung. In: Trump B F, Jones R T (eds) Diagnostic Electron Microscopy, vol 3. John Wiley & Sons, New York, ch 2, p 37–96

539. McDowell E M, McLaughlin J S, Merrenyl D K, Kieffer R F, Harris C C 1978 The respiratory epithelium. V. Histogenesis of lung carcinomas in the human. Journal of the National Cancer Institute 61: 587–606

540. McDowell E M, Sorokin S P, Hoyt R F Jr, Trump B F 1981 An unusual bronchial carcinoid tumor: light and electron microscopy. Human Pathology 12: 338–348

541. McDowell E M, Trump B F 1980 Pulmonary endocrine tumors with mixed phenotypes — a hypothesis to explain their existence. Laboratory Investigation 42: 134A

542. McDowell E M, Trump B F 1981 Pulmonary small cell carcinoma showing tripartite differentiation in inividual cells. Human Pathology 12: 286–294

543. McDowell E M, Wilson T S, Trump B F 1981 Atypical endocrine tumors of the lung. Archives of Pathology and Laboratory Medicine 105: 20–28

544. Michel R P, Limacher J J, Kimoff R J 1982 Mallory bodies in scar adenocarcinoma of the lung. Human Pathology 13: 81–85

545. Mikuz G, Szinicz G, Fischer H 1979 Sclerosing angioma of the lung. Case report and electron microscope investigation. Virchows Archiv A Pathological Anatomy and Histology 385: 93–101

546. Mills S A, Breyer R H, Johnston F R, Hudspeth A S, Marshall R B, Choplin R H, Cordell A R, Myers R T 1982 Malignant fibrous histiocytoma of the mediastinum and lung: a report of three cases. Journal of Thoracic and Cardiovascular Surgery 84: 367–372

547. Mills S E, Cooper P H, Walker A N, Kron I L 1982 Atypical carcinoid tumor of the lung. A clinicopathologic study of 17 cases. American Journal of Surgical Pathology 6: 643–654

548. Mollo F, Canese M G, Campobasso O 1973 Human peripheral lung tumors: light and electron microscopic correlation. British Journal of Cancer 27: 173–182

549. Montes M, Binette J P, Chaudhry A P, Adler R H, Guarino R 1977 Clara cell adenocarcinoma. Light and electron microscopic studies. American Journal of Surgical Pathology 1: 245–253

550. Morningstar W A, Hassan M O 1979 Bronchiolo-alveolar carcinoma with nodal metastases. An ultrastructural study. American Journal of Surgical Pathology 3: 273–278

551. Morohoshi T, Nakamura N, Hayashi K, Kanda M 1980 Amylase producing lung cancer. Electronmicroscopical and biochemical studies. Virchows Archiv A Pathological Anatomy and Histology 387: 125–132

552. Mukherjee T M, Swift J G, Smith K, Smith L A 1983 Exocytosis of neurosecretory granules in small cell undifferentiated carcinoma. Ultrastructural Pathology 4: 187–195

553. Mullins J D, Barnes R P 1979 Childhood bronchial mucoepidermoid tumors. A case report and review of the literature. Cancer 44: 315–322

554. Nagaishi C, Okada Y, Daido S, Genka K, Ikeda S, Kitano M 1965 Electron microscopic observations of the human lung cancer. Experimental Medicine and Surgery 25: 177–202

555. Nair S, Nair K, Weisbrot I M 1974 Fibrous histiocytoma of the lung: sclerosing hemangioma variant? Chest 65: 465–468

556. Nakamura M, Itoh K, Honda Y, Koba H, Asakawa M, Suzuki A, Yoshida Y, Satoh M, Akino T 1983 A case of bronchioloalveolar carcinoma. Ultrastructural and lipid-biochemical studies. Cancer 52: 861–867

557. Nash G, Langlinais P C, Greenawald K A 1972 Alveolar cell carcinoma: does it exist? Cancer 29: 322–326

558. Ng W-L, Ma L 1983 Is sclerosing hemangioma of lung an alveolar mixed tumour? Pathology 15: 205–211

559. Obiditsch-Mayer I, Breitfellner G 1968 Electron microscopy in cancer of the lung. Cancer 21: 945–951

560. Oyasu R, Battifora H A, Buckingham W B, Hidvegi D 1977 Metaplastic squamous cell carcinoma of bronchus simulating giant cell tumor of bone. Cancer 39: 1119–1128

561. Palacios J J N, Escribano P M, Toledo J, Garzon A, Larrú E, Palomera J 1979 Sclerosing hemangioma of the lung. An ultrastructural study. Cancer 44: 949–955

562. Paulsen S M, Egebald K, Christensen J 1981 Malignant fibrous histiocytoma of the lung. Virchows Archiv A Pathological Anatomy and Histology 391: 167–176

563. Rainio P 1983 Ultrastructure of neoplastic cells in different histologic subtypes of pulmonary adenocarcinoma. Pathology Research and Practice 176: 216–235

564. Rainio P, Sutinen S, Väänänen R 1982 A scanning and transmission electron microscopic study of pulmonary adenocarcinoma with histological correlation. Acta Pathologica, Microbiologica et Immunologica Scandinavica. Section A. Pathology 90: 463–470

565. Ranchod M 1977 The histogenesis and development of pulmonary tumorlets. Cancer 39: 1135–1145

566. Ranchod M, Levine G D 1980 Spindle cell carcinoid tumors of the lung: a clinicopathologic study of 35 cases. American Journal of Surgical Pathology 4: 315–331

567. Saba S R, Azar H A, Richman A V, Solomon D A, Spurlock R G, Mardelli I G, Kasnic G Jr 1981 Dual differentiation in small cell carcinoma (oat cell carcinoma) of the lung. Ultrastructural Pathology 2: 131–138

568. Said J W, Nash G, Tepper G, Banks-Shlegel S 1983 Keratin proteins and carcinoembryonic antigen in lung carcinoma: an immunoperoxidase study of fifty-four cases, with ultrastructural correlations. Human Pathology 14: 70–76

569. Sajjad S M, Mackay B, Lukeman J M 1980 Oncocytic carcinoid tumor of the lung. Ultrastructural Pathology 1: 171–176

570. Sale G E, Kulander B G 1976 Benign clear cell tumor of lung with necrosis. Cancer 37: 2355–2358

571. Santos-Briz A, Terrón J, Sastre R, Romero L, Valle A 1977 Oncocytoma of the lung. Cancer 40: 1330–1336

572. Scharifker D, Marchevsky A 1981 Oncocytic carcinoid of lung: an ultrastructural analysis. Cancer 47: 530–532

573. Sherwin R P 1982 When are electron microscopy, histoculture, and other procedures useful in the clinical evaluation of lung cancer? American Journal of Surgery 143: 680–684

574. Sidhu G S 1982 The ultrastructure of malignant epithelial neoplasms of the lung. Pathology Annual 17: 235–266

575. Sidhu G S, Forrester E M 1977 Glycogen-rich Clara cell-type bronchiolo-alveolar carcinoma. Light and electron microscopic study. Cancer 40: 2209–2215

576. Silverman J F, Leffers B R, Kay S 1976 Primary pulmonary neurilemoma. Report of a case with ultrastructural examination. Archives of Pathology and Laboratory Medicine 100: 644–648

577. Singh G, Katyal S L, Torikata C 1981 Carcinoma of type II pneumocytes. Immunodiagnosis of a subtype of 'bronchioloalveolar carcinomas'. American Journal of Pathology 102: 195–208

578. Singh G, Lee R E, Brooks D H 1977 Primary pulmonary paraganglioma. Report of a case and review of the literature. Cancer 40: 2286–2289

579. Sklar J L, Churg A, Bensch K G 1980 Oncocytic carcinoid tumor of the lung. American Journal of Surgical Pathology 4: 287–292

580. Smith M N, Greenberg S D, Spjut H J 1979 The Clara cell: a comparative ultrastructural study in mammals. American Journal of Anatomy 155: 15–30

581. Smith P S, McClure J 1982 A papillary endobronchial tumor with a transitional cell pattern. Archives of Pathology and Laboratory Medicine 106: 503–506

582. Stoebner P, Cussac Y, Porte A, Le Gal Y 1967 Ultrastructure of anaplastic bronchial carcinomas. Cancer 20: 286–294

583. Stone F J, Churg A M 1977 The ultrastructure of pulmonary hamartoma. Cancer 39: 1064–1070

584. Takenaga A, Matsuda M, Horai T, Ikegami H, Hattori S 1977 Scanning electron microscopy in the study of lung cancer. New technique of comparative studies on the same lung cancer cells by light microscopy and scanning electron microscopy. Acta Cytologica 21: 90–95

585. Takenaga A, Matsuda M, Horai T, Ikegami H, Hattori S 1980 Giant cell carcinoma of the lung: comparative studies of the same cancer cells by light microscopy and scanning electron microscopy. Acta Cytologica 24: 190–196

586. Tamai S, Kameya T, Shimosato Y, Tsumuraya M, Wada T 1980 Pulmonary blastoma. An ultrastructural study of a case and its transplanted tumor in athymic nude mice. Cancer 46: 1389–1396

587. Tamai S, Kameya T, Yamaguchi K, Yanai N, Abe K, Yanaihara N, Yamazaki H, Kageyama K 1983 Peripheral lung carcinoid tumor producing predominantly gastrin-releasing peptide (GRP). Morphologic and hormonal studies. Cancer 52: 273–281

588. Tateishi R, Horai T, Hattori S 1978 Demonstration of argyrophil granules in small cell carcinoma of the lung. Virchows Archiv A Pathological Anatomy and Histology 377: 203–210

589. Toker C 1966 Observations on the ultrastructure of a bronchial adenoma, carcinoid type. Cancer 19: 1943–1948

590. Tosi P, Luzi P, Leoncini L, Sforza V, Gotti G, Grossi A 1983 Scanning electron microscopy in the diagnosis of bronchogenic squamous cell and small cell anaplastic carcinoma. Applied Pathology 1: 82–88

591. Tsumuraya M, Kodama T, Kameya T, Shimosato Y, Koketsu H, Uei Y 1981 Light and electron microscopic analysis of intranuclear inclusions in papillary adenocarcinoma of the lung. Acta Cytologica 25: 523–532

592. Vera-Román J M, Sobonya R E, Gomez-Garcia J L, Sanz-Bondia J R, Paris-Romeu F 1983 Leiomyoma of the lung. Literature review and case report. Cancer 52: 936–941

593. Walter P, Warter A, Morand G 1978 Bronchial oncocytic carcinoid. Histological, histochemical and ultrastructural study. Virchows Archiv A Pathological Anatomy and Histology 379: 85–97

594. Wang N S, Seemayer T A, Ahmed M N, Knaack J 1976 Giant cell carcinoma of lung. A light and electron microscopic study. Human Pathology 7: 3–16

595. Warter A, Walter P, Sabountchi M, Jory A 1981 Oncocytic bronchial adenoma. Histological, histochemical and ultrastructural study. Virchows Archiv A Pathological Anatomy and Histology 392: 231–239

596. Weldon-Linne C M, Victor T A, Christ M L, Fry W A 1981 Angiogenic nature of the 'intravascular bronchioloalveolar tumor' of the lung. Archives of Pathology and Laboratory Medicine 105: 174–179

597. Wick M R, Scheithauer B W, Piehler J M, Pairolero P C 1982 Primary pulmonary leiomyosarcomas. A light and electron microscopic study. Archives of Pathology and Laboratory Medicine 106: 510–514

598. Williams L J Jr, Greenberg S D, Mace M L Jr 1982 Pulmonary sclerosing hemangioma: sometimes a form of pulmonary hamartoma. Southern Medical Journal 75: 665–670

599. Wilson B O, Battifora H A 1974 The histological classification of malignant lung tumours. Annals of Clinical and Laboratory Science 4: 4—12

600. Yokayama M, Natsuizaka T, Ishii Y, Ohshima S, Kasagi A, Tateno S 1977 Amylase-producing lung cancer. Ultrastructural and biochemical studies. Cancer 40: 766–772

601. Zimmerman K G, Sobonya R E, Payne C M 1981 Histochemical and ultrastructural features of an unusual pulmonary carcinosarcoma. Human Pathology 12: 1046–1051

602. Zolliker A S, Jacques J 1981 Clara cell carcinoma of the lung. Human Pathology 12: 748–750

603. Zolliker A, Jacques J, Goldstein A S 1979 Benign clear cell tumor of the lung. Archives of Pathology and Laboratory Medicine 103: 526–530

## 14 MESOTHELIAL NEOPLASMS, INCLUDING ADENOMATOID TUMOUR

604. Akhtar M, Reyes F, Young I 1976 Elastogenesis in adenomatoid tumor. Histochemical and ultrastructural observations. Cancer 37: 338–345

605. Alvarez-Fernandez E, Escalona-Zapata J 1982 Intrapulmonary mesotheliomas: their identification by tissue culture. Virchows Archiv A Pathological Anatomy and Histology 395: 331–343

606. Bell D A, Flotte T J 1982 Factor VIII related antigen in adenomatoid tumors. Implications for histogenesis. Cancer 50: 932–938

607. Benisch B, Peison B, Sobel H J, Marquet E 1981 Fibrous mesotheliomas (pseudofibroma) of the scrotal sac: a light and ultrastructural study. Cancer 47: 731–735

608. Bolen J W, Thorning D 1980 Mesotheliomas. A light- and electron-microscopic study concerning histogenetic relationships between the epithelial and the mesenchymal variants. American Journal of Surgical Pathology 4: 451–464

609. Boon M E, Posthuma H S, Ruiter D J, von Andel J G 1981 Secreting peritoneal mesothelioma. Report of a case with cytological, ultrastructural, morphometric and histological studies. Virchows Archiv A Pathological Anatomy and Histology 392: 33–44

610. Briselli M, Mark E J, Dickersin G R 1981 Solitary fibrous tumors of the pleura: eight new cases and review of 360 cases in the literature. Cancer 47: 2678–2689

611. Corson J M, Pinkus G S 1982 Mesothelioma: profile of keratin proteins and carcinoembryonic antigen. An immunoperoxidase study of 20 cases and comparison with pulmonary adenocarcinomas. American Journal of Pathology 108: 80–87

612. Craig J R, Hart W R 1979 Extragenital adenomatoid tumor. Evidence for the mesothelial theory of origin. Cancer 43: 1678–1681

613. Davis J M 1974 Ultrastructure of human mesotheliomas. Journal of the National Cancer Institute 52: 1715–1725

614. Davy C L, Tang C-K 1980 Are all adenomatoid tumors mesothelial in origin? Laboratory Investigation 42: 110A

615. Davy C L, Tang C-K 1981 Are all adenomatoid tumors adenomatoid mesotheliomas? Human Pathology 12: 360–369

616. Dionne G P, Wang N S 1977 A scanning electron microscopic study of diffuse mesothelioma and some lung carcinomas. Cancer 40: 707–715

617. Dumke K, Schnoy N, Specht G, Buse H 1983 Comparative light and electron microscopic studies of cystic and papillary tumors of the peritoneum. Virchows Archiv A Pathological Anatomy and Histopathology 399: 25–39

618. Echevarria R A, Arean V M 1968 Ultrastructural evidence of secretory differentiation in a malignant pleural mesothelioma. Cancer 22: 323–332

619. Eimoto T, Inoue I 1977 Malignant fibrous mesothelioma of the tunica vaginalis. A histologic and ultrastructural study. Cancer 39: 2059–2066

620. Fenoglio J J Jr, Jacobs D W, McAllister H A Jr 1977 Ultrastructure of the mesothelioma of the atrioventricular node. Cancer 40: 721–727

621. Ferenczy A, Fenoglio J, Richart R M 1972 Observations on benign mesothelioma of the genital tract (adenomatoid tumor). A comparative ultrastructural study. Cancer 30: 244–260

622. Goepel J R 1981 Benign papillary mesothelioma of peritoneum: a histological, histochemical and ultrastructural study of six cases. Histopathology 5: 21–30

623. Henderson D W 1982 Asbestos-related pleuropulmonary diseases: asbestosis, mesothelioma and lung cancer. Pathology 14: 239–243

624. Hernandez F J, Fernandez B B 1974 Localized fibrous tumors of pleura: a light and electron microscopic study. Cancer 34: 1667–1674

625. Japko L, Horta A A, Schreiber K, Mitsudo S, Karwa G L, Singh G, Koss L G 1982 Malignant mesothelioma of the tunica vaginalis testis: Report of first case with preoperative diagnosis. Cancer 49: 119–127

626. Kannerstein M, Churg J, McCaughey W T E 1978 Asbestos and mesothelioma: a review. Pathology Annual 13, pt 1: 81–129

627. Katsube Y, Mukai K, Silverberg S G 1982 Cystic mesothelioma of the peritoneum. A report of five cases and review of the literature. Cancer 50: 1615–1622

628. Kawai T, Mikata A, Torikata C, Yakumaru K, Kageyama K, Shimosato Y 1978 Solitary (localized) pleural mesothelioma. A light- and electron-microscopic study. American Journal of Surgical Pathology 2: 365–375

629. Klima M, Spjut H J, Bossart M I, Frazier O H, Cooley D H 1982 Malignant pleural mesothelioma with a 14-year survival: a case report and electronmicroscopic study. Journal of Surgical Oncology 20: 253–259

630. Legrand M, Pariente R 1974 Ultrastructural study of pleural fluid in mesothelioma. Thorax 29: 164–171

631. Lehto V P, Virtanen I 1978 Intermediate 10 nm filaments in human malignant mesothelioma. Virchows Archiv B Cell Pathology 28: 229–234

632. Lehto V-P, Miettinen M, Virtanen I 1983 Adenomatoid tumor: immunohistological features suggesting a mesothelial origin. Virchows Archiv B Cell Pathology 42: 153–159

633. Mackay B, Bennington J L, Skoglund R W 1971 The adenomatoid tumor: fine structural evidence for a mesothelial origin. Cancer 27: 109–115

634. Marcus J B, Lynn J A 1970 Ultrastructural comparison of an adenomatoid tumor, lymphangioma, hemangioma, and mesothelioma. Cancer 25: 171–175

635. Mennemayer R, Smith M 1979 Multicystic peritoneal mesothelioma. A report with electron microscopy of a case mimicking intra-abdominal cystic hygroma (lymphangioma). Cancer 44: 692–698

636. Mikuz G, Höpfel-Kreiner I 1982 Papillary mesothelioma of the tunica vaginalis propria testis. Case report and ultrastructural study. Virchows Archiv A Pathological Anatomy and Histology 396: 231–238

637. Moore J H Jr, Crum C P, Chandler J G, Feldman P S 1980 Benign cystic mesothelioma. Cancer 45: 2395–2399

638. Mucientes F 1983 Adenomatoid tumor of the epididymis. Ultrastructural study of three cases. Pathology Research and Practice 176: 258–268

639. Osamura R Y 1977 Ultrastructure of localized fibrous mesothelioma of the pleura. Report of a case with histogenetic considerations. Cancer 39: 139–142

640. Osculati F, Parravicini C, Cinti S, Mosca L 1982 Human malignant diffuse mesothelioma: submicroscopic study on the epithelial component. Journal of Submicroscopic Cytology 14: 203–213

641. Paulsen S M, Kristensen I B 1981 So-called mesothelioma of the atrioventricular node. Journal of Submicroscopic Cytology 13: 667–674

642. Rich S, Presant C A, Meyer J, Stevens S C, Carr D 1979 Human chorionic gonadotrophin and malignant mesothelioma. Cancer 43: 1457–1462

643. Salazar H, Kanbour A, Burgess F 1972 Ultrastructure and observations on the histogenesis of mesotheliomas 'adenomatoid tumors' of the female genital tract. Cancer 29: 141–152

644. Sidhu G S, Fresko O 1980 Adenomatoid tumor of the epididymis: ultrastructural evidence of its biphasic nature. Ultrastructural Pathology 1: 39–47

645. Söderström K-O 1982 Origin of adenomatoid tumor. A comparison between the structure of adenomatoid tumor and epididymal duct cells. Cancer 49: 2349–2357

646. Stoebner P, Brambilla E 1982 Ultrastructural diagnosis of pleural tumors. Pathology Research and Practice 173: 402–416

647. Suzuki Y, Churg J, Kannerstein M 1976 Ultrastructure of human malignant diffuse mesothelioma. American Journal of Pathology 85: 241–262

648. Tang C K, Gray G F, Keuhnelian J G 1976 Malignant peritoneal mesothelioma in an inguinal hernial sac. Cancer 37: 1887–1890

649. Taxy J B, Battifora H, Oyasu R 1974 Adenomatoid tumors: a light microscopic, histochemical and ultrastructural study. Cancer 34: 306–316

650. Uys C J 1979 Observations on the pathology and ultrastructure of mesothelioma. In: Muggia F M, Rozencweig M (eds) Lung cancer: progress in therapeutic research. Progress in cancer research and therapy, vol 11. Raven Press, New York, p 117–127

651. Wang N-S 1973 Electron microscopy in the diagnosis of pleural mesotheliomas. Cancer 31: 1046–1054

652. Warhol M J, Hickey W F, Corson J M 1982 Malignant mesothelioma. Ultrastructural distinction from adeno-carcinoma. American Journal of Surgical Pathology 6: 307–314

653. Whitaker D, Sterrett G F, Shilkin K B 1982 Detection of tissue CEA-like substance as an aid in the differential diagnosis of malignant mesothelioma. Pathology 14: 255–258

## 15 OTHER THORACIC AND PLEUROPULMONARY TUMOURS

654. Askin F B, Rosai J, Sibley R K, Dehner L P, McAlister W H 1979 Malignant small cell tumor of the thoracopulmonary region in childhood. A distinctive clinicopathologic entity of uncertain histogenesis. Cancer 43: 2438–2451

655. Barson A J, Ahmed A, Gibson A A, Macdonald A M 1978 Chest wall sarcoma of childhood with a good prognosis. Archives of Disease in Childhood 53: 882–889

656. Linnoila R I, Tsokos M, Triche T J, Chandra R 1983 Evidence for neural origin and periodic acid-Schiff-positive variants of the malignant small cell tumor of thoracopulmonary region. Laboratory Investigation 48: 51A

657. Meijer S, Hoitsma H F W 1982 Malignant intrathoracic oncocytoma. Cancer 49: 97–100

658. Ursell P C, Albala A, Fenoglio J J Jr 1982 Malignant neurogenic tumor of the heart. Human Pathology 13: 640–645

## 16 GENERAL ASPECTS OF GASTROINTESTINAL TRACT TUMOURS

659. Buchan A M J, Polak J M 1980 The classification of the human gastroenteropancreatic endocrine cells. Investigative & Cell Pathology 3: 51–71

660. Marcus P B 1981 Glycocalyceal bodies and their role in tumor typing. Journal of Submicroscopic cytology 13: 483–500

661. Marcus P B, Martin J H, Green R H, Krouse M A 1979 Glycocalyceal bodies and microvillous core rootlets. Archives of Pathology and Laboratory Medicine 103: 89–92

662. Solcia E, Capella C, Buffa R, Fiocca R, Frigerio B, Usellini L 1980 Identification, ultrastructure and classification of gut endocrine cells and related growths. Investigative & Cell Pathology 3: 37–49

663. Toner P G, Carr K E, Al Yassin T M 1980 The gastrointestinal tract. In: Johannessen J V (ed) Electron microscopy in human medicine, vol 7. Digestive system. McGraw-Hill, New York, pt 2, p 87–207

664. Yang K, Ulich T, Cheng L, Lewin K J 1983 The neuroendocrine products of intestinal carcinoids. An immunoperoxidase study of 35 carcinoid tumors stained for serotonin and eight polypeptide hormones. Cancer 51: 1918–1926

## 17 TUMOURS OF THE ORAL CAVITY

665. Chen S-Y, Miller A S 1980 Canalicular adenoma of the upper lip. An electron microscopic study. Cancer 46: 522–556

666. Fejerskov O, Andersen L, Philipsen H P 1980 Oral mucous membrane. In: Johannessen J V (ed) Electron microscopy in human medicine, vol 7. McGraw-Hill, New York, ch 5, p 25–58

667. Leifer C, Miller A S, Putong P B, Min B H 1974 Spindle cell carcinoma of the oral mucosa. A light and electron microscopic study of apparent sarcomatous metastasis to cervical lymph nodes. Cancer 34: 597–605

668. Nesland J M, Olafsson J, Sobrinho-Simoes M 1981 Plasmacytoid myoepithelioma of the palate. Journal of Oral Pathology 10: 14–21

669. Prioleau P G, Santa Cruz D J, Meyer J S, Bauer W C 1980 Verrucous carcinoma: a light and electron microscopic, autoradiographic, and immunofluorescence study. Cancer 45: 2849–2857

670. Reichart P A, Althoff J 1981 The surface cell structure of oral carcinoma: a scanning electron microscope study of 32 cases. International Journal of Oral Surgery 10 suppl 1: 11–15

## 18 ODONTOGENIC TUMOURS

671. Anderson H C, Kim B, Minkowitz S 1969 Calcifying epithelial odontogenic tumor of Pindborg. Cancer 24: 585–596

672. Chaudhry A P, Hanks C T, Leifer C, Gargiulo E A 1972 Calcifying epithelial odontogenic tumor. A histochemical and ultrastructural study. Cancer 30: 519–529

673. Chen S Y, Miller A S 1975 Ultrastructure of the keratinizing and calcifying odontogenic cyst. Oral Surgery, Oral Medicine, Oral Pathology 39: 769–780

674. Chomette G, Auriol M, Guilbert F, Delcourt A 1983 Ameloblastic fibrosarcoma of the jaws — report of three cases. Clinico-pathologic, histoenzymological and ultrastructural study. Pathology Research and Practice 178: 40–47

675. Fejerskov O, Andersen L, Philipsen H P 1980 Odontogenic cysts and tumors. In: Johannessen J V (ed) Electron microscopy in human medicine, vol 7. Digestive system. McGraw-Hill, New York, ch 4, p 14–24

676. Gould A R, Farman A G, DeJean E K, van Arsdall L R 1982 Peripheral ameloblastoma: an ultrastructural analysis. Journal of Oral Pathology 11: 90–101

677. Hanna R J, Regezi J A, Hayward J R 1976 Ameloblastic fibro-odontoma: report of case with light and electron microscopic observations. Journal of Oral Surgery 34: 820–825

678. Hatakeyama S, Suzuki A 1978 Ultrastructural study of adenomatoid odontogenic tumor. Journal of Oral Pathology 7: 295–300

679. Honma T 1982 Multilobulated nuclear cells in squamous metaplasia of the ameloblastoma. Journal of Submicroscopic cytology 14: 691–695

680. Khan M Y, Kwee H, Schneider L C, Saber I 1977 Adenomatoid odontogenic tumor resembling a globulomaxillary cyst. Light and electron microscopic studies. Journal of Oral Surgery 35: 739–742

681. Lee K W, El-Labban N G, Kramer I R H 1972 Ultrastructure of a simple ameloblastoma. Journal of Pathology 108: 173–176

682. Mincer H H, McGinnis J P 1972 Ultrastructure of three histologic variants of the ameloblastoma. Cancer 30: 1036–1045

683. Nasu M, Ishikawa G 1983 Ameloblastoma. Light and electron microscopic study. Virchows Archiv A Pathological Anatomy and Histopathology 399: 163–175

684. Navarrete A R, Smith M 1971 Ultrastructure of granular cell ameloblastoma. Cancer 27: 948–955

685. Page D L, Weiss S W, Eggleston J C 1975 Ultrastructural study of amyloid material in the calcifying epithelial odontogenic tumor. Cancer 36: 1426–1435

686. Rothouse L S, Majack R A, Fay J T 1980 An ameloblastoma with myofibroblasts and intracellular septate junctions. Cancer 45: 2858–2863

687. Schlosnagle D C, Someren A 1981 The ultrastructure of the adenomatoid odontogenic tumour. Oral Surgery 52: 154–161

688. Slootweg P J 1980 Epithelio-mesenchymal morphology in ameloblastic fibro-odontoma: a light and electron microscopic study. Journal of Oral Pathology 9: 29–40

689. Smith R R, Olson J L, Hutchins G M, Crawley W A, Levin L S 1979 Adenomatoid odonotogenic tumor: ultrastructural demonstration of two cell types and amyloid. Cancer 43: 505–511

690. Soames J V 1982 A pigmented calcifying odontogenic cyst. Oral Surgery 53: 395–400

691. Solomon M P, Vuletin J C, Pertschuk L P, Gormley M B, Rosen Y 1975 Calcifying epithelial odontogenic tumor. A histologic, histochemical, fluorescent and ultrastructural study. Oral Surgery, Oral Medicine, Oral Pathology 40: 522–530

692. Takagi M 1967 Adenomatoid ameloblastoma. An analysis of nine cases by histopathological and electron microscopic study. Bulletin of Tokyo Medical and Dental University 14: 487–506

693. Westwood R M, Alexander R W, Bennett D E 1974 Giant odontogenic myxofibroma. Report of a case with histochemical and ultrastructural studies and a review of the literature. Oral Surgery, Oral Medicine, Oral Pathology 37: 83–92

694. Yamamoto H, Kozawa Y, Hirai G, Hagiwara T, Nakamura T 1981 Adenomatoid odontogenic tumour: light and electron microscopic study. International Journal of Oral Surgery 10: 272–278

## 19 TUMOURS OF SALIVARY GLANDS

695. Allegra S R 1971 Warthin's tumor: a hypersensitivity disease? Ultrastructural, light and immunofluorescent study. Human Pathology 2: 403–420

696. Benjamin E, Wells S, Fox H, Reeve N L, Knox F 1982 Malignant fibrous histiocytomas of salivary glands. Journal of Clinical Pathology 35: 946–953

697. Bloom G D, Carlsoo B, Diamant H, Thyberg J 1982 Fine structure of – and some histochemical observations on – chondroid regions of benign mixed parotid tumours. Acta Otolaryngologica 93: 131–138

698. Caselitz J, Löning T 1981 Specific demonstration of actin and keratin filaments in pleomorphic adenomas by means of immunoelectron microscopy. Virchows Archiv A Pathological Anatomy and Histology 393: 153–158

699. Caselitz J, Osborn M, Seifert G, Weber K 1981 Intermediate-sized filament proteins (prekeratin, vimentin, desmin) in the normal parotid gland and parotid gland tumours. Immunofluorescence study. Virchows Archiv A Pathological Anatomy and Histology 393: 273–286

700. Chaudhry A P, Cutler L S, Satchidanand S, Labay G, Raj M S, Lin C-C 1983 Monomorphic adenomas of the parotid glands. Their ultrastructure and histogenesis. Cancer 52: 112–120

701. Chaudhry A P, Cutler L S, Satchidanand S, Labay G, Raj M S, Lin C-C 1983 Glycogen-rich tumor of the oral minor salivary glands. A histochemical and ultrastructural study. Cancer 52: 105–111

702. Chaudry A P, Satchidanand S, Peer R, Cutler L S 1982 Myoepithelial cell adenoma of the parotid gland: a light and ultrastructural study. Cancer 49: 288–293

703. Chen S Y, Brannon R B, Miller A S, White D K, Hooker S P 1978 Acinic cell adenocarcinoma of minor salivary glands. Cancer 42: 678–685

704. Chisholm D M, Waterhouse J P, Kraucunas E, Sciubba J J 1974 A quantitative ultrastructural study of the pleomorphic adenoma (mixed tumor) of human minor salivary glands. Cancer 34: 1631–1641

705. Chomette G, Auriol M, Tranbaloc P, Vaillant J M 1982 Adenoid cystic carcinoma of minor salivary glands. Analysis of 86 cases. Clinico-pathological, histoenzymological and ultrastructural studies. Virchows Archiv A Pathological Anatomy and Histology 395: 289–301

706. Crissman J D, Wirman J A, Harris A 1977 Malignant myoepithelioma of the parotid gland. Cancer 40: 3042–3049

707. Dardick I, van Nostrand A W P, Jeans M T D, Rippstein P, Edwards V 1983 Pleomorphic adenoma I: ultrastructural organization of 'epithelial' regions. Human Pathology 14: 780–797

708. Dardick I, van Nostrand A W P, Jeans M T D, Rippstein P, Edwards V 1983 Pleomorphic adenoma II: ultrastructural organization of 'stromal' regions. Human Pathology 14: 798–809

709. Dardick I, van Nostrand A W P, Phillips M J 1982 Histogenesis of salivary gland pleomorphic adenoma (mixed tumor) with an evaluation of the role of the myoepithelial cell. Human Pathology 13: 62–75

710. David R, Buchner A 1978 Amyloid stroma in a tubular carcinoma of palatal salivary gland: histochemical and ultrastructural study. Cancer 41: 1836–1844

711. David R, Buchner A 1980 Elastosis in benign and malignant salivary gland tumors. A histochemical and ultrastructural study. Cancer 45: 2301–2310

712. David R, Buchner A 1980 Langerhans' cells in a pleomorphic adenoma of submandibular salivary gland. Journal of Pathology 131: 127–135

713. David R, Kim K M 1982 β-fibrillary bodies in low-grade adenocarcinoma of parotid gland: a histochemical and ultrastructural study. Human Pathology 13: 1028–1038

714. Deppisch L M, Toker C 1969 Mixed tumors of the parotid gland. An ultrastructural study. Cancer 24: 174–184

715. Donath K, Seifert G, Sunder-Plassmann E 1982 Ultrastructural subclassification of undifferentiated carcinoma of the parotid gland. Analysis of 11 cases. Journal of Cancer Research and Clinical Oncology 103: 75–92

716. Doyle L E, Lynn J A, Panopio I T, Grass G 1968 Ultrastructure of the chondroid regions of benign mixed tumor of salivary gland. Cancer 22: 225–233

717. Echevarria R A 1967 Ultrastructure of the acinic cell carcinoma and clear cell carcinoma of the parotid gland. Cancer 20: 563–571

718. Eneroth C M, Wersall J 1966 Fine structure of the epithelial cells in mixed tumors of the parotid gland. Annals of Otology, Rhinology and Laryngology 75: 95–102

719. Erlandson R A, Tandler B 1972 Ultrastructure of acinic cell carcinoma of the parotid gland. Archives of Pathology 93: 130–140

720. Fejerskov O, Andersen L, Philipsen H P 1980 Salivary glands. In: Johannessen J V (ed) Electron microscopy in human medicine, vol 7. Digestive System. McGraw-Hill, New York, ch 6, p 59–84

721. Freedman S I, Van de Velde R L, Kagan A R, Perzik S L 1972 Primary malignant mixed tumor of the mandible. Cancer 30: 167–173

722. Hagelqvist E 1978 Light and electron microscopic studies on material obtained by fine needle biopsy. A methodological study on aspirates from tumours of the head and neck region with special emphasis on salivary gland tumours. Acta Otolaryngologica suppl: 1–75

723. Hayashi Y, Aoki N 1983 Undifferentiated carcinoma of the parotid gland with bizarre giant cells. Clinicopathologic report with ultrastructural study. Acta Pathologica Japonica 33: 169–176

724. Headington J T, Batsakis J G, Beals T F, Campbell T E, Simmons J L, Stone W D 1977 Membranous basal cell adenoma of parotid gland, dermal cylindromas, and trichoepitheliomas. Comparative histochemistry and ultrastructure. Cancer 39: 2460–2469

725. Hoshino M, Yamamoto I 1970 Ultrastructure of adenoid cystic carcinoma. Cancer 25: 186–198

726. Hübner G, Klein H J, Kleinsasser O, Schiefer H G 1971 Role of myoepithelial cells in the development of salivary gland tumors. Cancer 27: 1255–1261

727. Hübner G, Kleinsasser O, Klein H J 1969 Fine structure and genesis of cylindroma (adenoidcystic carcinoma) of salivary glands: further investigations on the role of myoepithelial differentiated cells in salivary gland tumors. Virchows Archiv A Pathologische Anatomie 347: 296–315

728. Hübner G, Kleinsasser O, Klein H J 1971 Fine structure of basal cell adenoma of the salivary gland: cellular differentiation in tumors of salivary glands. Virchows Archiv A Pathologische Anatomie 353: 333–346

729. Jao W, Keh P C, Swerdlow M A 1976 Ultrastructural studies of the basal cell adenoma of parotid gland. Cancer 37: 1322–1333

730. Kahn L B, Schoub L 1973 Myoepithelioma of the palate. Histochemical and ultrastructural observations. Archives of Pathology 95: 209–212

731. Kay S, Schatzki P F 1972 Ultrastructure of acinic cell carcinoma of the parotid salivary gland. Cancer 29: 235–244

732. Kay S, Still W J S 1973 Electron microscopic observations on a parotid oncocytoma. Archives of Pathology 96: 186–188

733. Kierszenbaum A L 1968 The ultrastructure of human mixed salivary tumors. Laboratory Investigation 18: 391–396

734. Kim S-K, Weatherbee L, Nasjleti C E 1973 Lysosomes in the epithelial component of Warthin's tumor. Archives of Pathology 95: 56–62

735. Koss L G, Spiro R H, Hajdu S 1972 Small cell (oat cell) carcinoma of minor salivary gland origin. Cancer 30: 737–741

736. Kraemer B B, Mackay B, Batsakis J G 1983 Small cell carcinomas of the parotid gland: a clinicopathologic study of three cases. Laboratory Investigation 48: 46A

737. Lawrence J B, Mazur M T 1982 Adenoid cystic carcinoma: a comparative pathologic study of tumors in salivary gland, breast, lung, and cervix. Human Pathology 13: 916–924

738. Lee S C, Roth L M 1976 Malignant oncocytoma of the parotid gland. A light and electron microscopic study. Cancer 37: 1606–1614

739. Leifer C, Miller A S, Putong P B, Harwick R D 1974 Myoepithelioma of the parotid gland. Archives of Pathology 98: 312–319

740. Levin J M, Robinson D W, Lin F 1975 Acinic cell carcinoma: collective review, including bilateral cases. Archives of Surgery 110: 64–68

741. Luna M A, Mackay B 1976 Basal cell adenoma of the parotid gland: case report with ultrastructural observations. Cancer 37: 1615–1621

742. Luna M A, Mackay B, Gamez-Araujo J 1973 Myoepithelioma of the palate. Report of a case with histochemical and electron microscopic observations. Cancer 32: 1429–1435

743. Mills S E, Cooper P H 1981 An ultrastructural study of cartilaginous zones and surrounding epithelium in mixed tumors of salivary glands and skin. Laboratory Investigation 44: 6–12

744. Min B H, Miller A S, Leifer C, Putong P B 1974 Basal cell adenoma of the parotid gland. Archives of Otolaryngology 99: 88–93

745. Mohamed A H, Cherrick H M 1975 Glycogen-rich adenocarcinoma of minor salivary glands. A light and electron microscopic study. Cancer 36: 1057–1066

746. Moosavi H, Ryan C, Schwartz S, Donnelly J A 1980 Malignant adenolymphoma. Human Pathology 11: 80–83

747. Nagao K, Matsuzaki O, Saiga H, Sugano I, Shigematsu H, Kaneko T, Katoh T, Kitamura T 1981 Histopathologic studies on carcinoma in pleomorphic adenoma of the parotid gland. Cancer 48: 113–121

748. Nagao K, Matsuzaki O, Saiga H, Sugano I, Shigematsu H, Kaneko T, Katoh T, Kitamura T 1982 Histopathologic studies of basal cell adenoma of the parotid gland. Cancer 50: 736–745

749. Nakashima N, Goto K, Takeuchi J 1983 Malignant papillary cystadenoma lymphomatosum. Light and electron microscopic study. Virchows Archiv A Pathological Anatomy and Histopathology 399: 207–219

750. Osborn D A 1977 Morphology and the natural history of cribriform adenocarcinoma-adenoid cystic carcinoma. Journal of Clinical Pathology 30: 195–205

751. Regezi J A, Batsakis J G 1977 Histogenesis of salivary gland neoplasms. Otolaryngologic Clinics of North America 10: 297–307

752. Sciubba J J, Brannon R B 1982 Myoepithelioma of salivary glands: report of 23 cases. Cancer 49: 562–572

753. Shulman J, Waisman J, Morledge D 1973 Sebaceous carcinoma of the parotid gland. Archives of Otolaryngology 98: 417–421

754. Sidhu G S, Forrester E M 1977 Acinic cell carcinoma: long-term survival after pulmonary metastases. Light and electron microscopic study. Cancer 40: 756–765

755. Sidhu G S, Waldo E D 1975 Oncocytic change in mucoepidermoid carcinoma of the parotid gland. Archives of Pathology 99: 663–666

756. Stromayer F W, Haggitt R C, Nelson J F, Hardman J M 1975 Myoepithelioma of minor salivary gland origin. Light and electron microscopical study. Archives of Pathology 99: 242–245

757. Sun C N, White H J, Thompson B W 1975 Oncocytoma: mitochondrioma of the parotid gland. An electron microscopic study. Archives of Pathology 99: 208–214

758. Suzuki K 1982 Basal cell adenoma with acinic differentiation. Acta Pathologica Japonica 32: 1085–1092

759. Takeuchi J, Sobue M, Yoshida M, Esaki T, Kato Y 1975 Pleomorphic adenoma of the salivary gland. With special reference to histochemical and electron microscopic studies and biochemical analysis of glycosaminoglycans in vivo and in vitro. Cancer 36: 1771–1789

760. Tandler B 1966 Fine structure of oncocytes in human salivary glands. Virchows Archiv A Pathologische Anatomie 341: 317–326

761. Tandler B 1966 Warthin's tumor. Electron microscopic studies. Archives of Otolaryngology 84: 68–76

762. Tandler B 1971 Ultrastructure of adenoid cystic carcinoma of salivary gland origin. Laboratory Investigation 24: 504–512

763. Tandler B 1981 Amyloid in a pleomorphic adenoma of the parotid gland. Electron microscopic observations. Journal of Oral Pathology 10: 158–163

764. Thackray A C, Lucas R B 1974 Tumors of the major salivary glands. Atlas of tumor pathology, 2nd series, fascicle 10. Armed Forces Institute of Pathology, Washington D C, p 81–90

765. Tomec R, Ahmad I, Fu Y S, Jaffe S 1979 Malignant hemangioendothelioma (angiosarcoma) of the salivary gland. An ultrastructural study. Cancer 43: 1664–1671

766. Wassef M, Le Charpentier Y, Monteil J-P, Le Tien K, Galian A 1982 Undifferentiated carcinoma with lymphoid stroma of the parotid (undifferentiated carcinoma nasopharyngeal type?). Optical, electron microscopical and immunofluorescence study. Bulletin du Cancer (Paris) 69: 11–21

767. Wirman J A, Battifora H 1976 Small cell undifferentiated carcinoma of salivary gland origin. An ultrastructural study. Cancer 37: 1840–1848

768. Yaku Y, Kanda T, Yoshihara T, Kaneko T, Nagao K 1983 Undifferentiated carcinoma of the parotid gland. Case report with electron microscopic findings. Virchows Archiv A Pathological Anatomy and Histopathology 401: 89–97

773. Cook M G, Eusebi V, Betts C M 1976 Oat cell carcinoma of the esophagus. A recently recognized entity. Journal of Clinical Pathology 29: 1068–1073

774. Du Boulay C E H, Isaacson P 1981 Carcinoma of the oesophagus with spindle cell features. Histopathology 5: 403–414

775. Go A T, Zirkin R M 1982 Primary malignant melanoma of the esophagus: a case report with endoscopic and electron microscopic studies. American Journal of Gastroenterology 77: 840–843

776. Imai T, Sannohe Y, Okano H 1978 Oat cell carcinoma (apudoma) of the esophagus. A case report. Cancer 41: 358–364

777. Kishida H, Sodemoto Y, Ushigome S, Kubota S, Kataba Y 1983 Non-oat cell small cell carcinoma of the esophagus. Report of a case with ultrastructural observation. Acta Pathologica Japonica 33: 403–413

778. Martin M R, Kahn L B 1977 So-called pseudosarcoma of the esophagus. Nodal metastases of the spindle cell element. Archives of Pathology and Laboratory Medicine 101: 604–609

779. Osamura R Y, Shimamura K, Hata J, Tamaoki N, Watanabe K, Kubota M, Yamazaki S, Mitomi T 1978 Polypoid carcinoma of the esophagus. A unifying term for 'carcinosarcoma' and 'pseudosarcoma'. American Journal of Surgical Pathology 2: 201–208

780. Reid H A, Richardson W W, Corrin B 1980 Oat cell carcinoma of the esophagus. Cancer 45: 2342–2347

781. Reyes C V, Chejfec G, Jao W, Gould V E 1980 Neuroendocrine carcinomas of the esophagus. Ultrastructural Pathology 1: 367–376

782. Rivera F, Matilla A, Fernandez-Sanz J, Galera II 1981 Oat cell carcinoma of the oesophagus. Case description and review of the literature. Virchows Archiv A Pathological Anatomy and Histology 391: 337–344

783. Robinson K M, Gregory M A 1981 Transmission electron microscopy of human oesophageal carcinomas. Journal of Pathology 135: 97–109

784. Rosen Y, Moon S, Kim B 1975 Small cell epidermoid carcinoma of the esophagus. An oat-cell-like carcinoma. Cancer 36: 1042–1049

785. Sasaki K, Tani S, Nagamine Y, Takahashi M 1978 Pseudosarcomatous carcinoma of the esophagus – reference to its histogenesis. Acta Pathologica Japonica 28: 779–785

786. Sweeney E C, Cooney T 1980 Adenoid cystic carcinoma of the esophagus: a light and electron microscopic study. Cancer 45: 1516–1525

787. Tateishi R, Taniguchi K, Horai T, Iwanaga T, Taniguchi H 1976 Argyrophil cell carcinoma: apudoma of the oesophagus. A histopathologic entity. Virchows Archiv A Pathological Anatomy and Histology 371: 283–294

## 20 OESOPHAGEAL TUMOURS

769. Banner B F, Memoli V A, Warren W H, Gould V E 1983 Carcinoma with multidirectional differentiation arising in Barrett's esophagus. Ultrastructural Pathology 4: 205–217

770. Banner B F, Memoli V A, Warren W H, Gould V E 1983 Multidifferentiated carcinoma arising in Barrett's esophagus. Laboratory Investigation 48: 6A

771. Briggs J C, Ibrahim N B N 1983 Oat cell carcinoma of the oesophagus: a clinico-pathological study of 23 cases. Histopathology 7: 261–277

772. Burke J S, Ranchod M 1981 Hemangiopericytoma of the oesophagus. Human Pathology 12: 96–100

## 21 TUMOURS OF THE STOMACH

788. Bansal M, Kaneko M, Gordon R E 1982 Carcinosarcoma and separate carcinoid tumor of the stomach. A case report with light and electron microscopic studies. Cancer 50: 1876–1881

789. Black W C, Haffner H E 1968 Diffuse hyperplasia of gastric argyrophil cells and multiple carcinoid tumors. An historical and ultrastructural study. Cancer 21: 1080–1099

790. Burns D K, Silva F G, Forde K A, Mount P M, Clark H B 1983 Primary melanocytic Schwannoma of the stomach. Evidence of dual melanocytic and Schwannian differentiation in an extra-axial site in a patient with neurofibromatosis. Cancer 52: 1432–1441

791. Capella C, Polak J M, Timson C M, Frigerio B, Solcia E 1980 Gastric carcinoids of argyrophil ECL cells. Ultrastructural Pathology 1: 411–418

792. Chejfec G, Gould V E 1977 Malignant gastric neuroendocrinomas. Ultrastructural and biochemical characterization of their secretory activity. Human Pathology 8: 433–440

793. Dajee A, Dajee H, Hinrichs S, Lilington G 1982 Pulmonary chondroma, extra-adrenal paraganglioma, and gastric leiomyosarcoma: Carney's triad. Journal of Thoracic and Cardiovascular Surgery 84: 377–381

794. Eimoto T, Hayakawa H 1980 Oat cell carcinoma of the stomach. Pathology Research and Practice 168: 229–236

795. Goldman H, French S, Burbidge E 1981 Kulchitsky cell hyperplasia and multiple metastasising carcinoids of the stomach. Cancer 47: 2620–2626

796. Hajdu S I, Erlandson R A, Paglia M A 1972 Light and electron microscopic studies of a gastric leiomyoblastoma. Archives of Pathology 93: 36–41

797. Heitz P U, Wegmann W 1980 Identification of neoplastic Paneth cells in an adenocarcinoma of the stomach, using lysozyme as a marker, and electron microscopy. Virchows Archiv A Pathological Anatomy and Histology 386: 107–116

798. Hinrichs S, Goodnight J, Tesluk H, Ruebner B H 1982 Extraadrenal paraganglioma, pulmonary chondromas, and gastric leiomyosarcoma: a triad of tumors in young adults. Laboratory Investigation 46: 7P

799. Hull M T, Jesseph J E 1982 Ultrastructure of gastric myxofibroma with intracytoplasmic collagen. Ultrastructural Pathology 3: 25–30

800. Kanwar Y S, Manaligod J R 1975 Glomus tumor of the stomach. An ultrastructural study. Archives of Pathology 99: 392–397

801. Kim B-H, Rosen Y, Suen K C 1975 Endocrine-type granules in cells of glomus tumor of the stomach. Archives of Pathology 99: 544–547

802. Kondo K, Nagatomo T 1974 Ultrastructure of serosal surface in gastric carcinoma. Journal of Electron Microscopy 23: 147–159

803. Kubo T, Watanabe H 1971 Neoplastic argentaffin cells in gastric and intestinal carcinomas. Cancer 27: 447–454

804. Marcus F S, Friedman M A, Callen P W, Churg A, Harbour J 1980 Successful therapy of an ACTH-producing gastric carcinoid APUD tumor. Report of a case and review of the literature. Cancer 46: 1263–1269

805. Mazur M T, Clark H B 1983 Gastric stromal tumors. Reappraisal of histogenesis. American Journal of Surgical Pathology 7: 507–519

806. Mingazzini P L, Barsotti P, Malchiodi Albedi F 1983 Adenosquamous carcinoma of the stomach: histological, histochemical and ultrastructural observations. Histopathology 7: 433–443

807. Murayama H, Imai T, Kikuchi M 1983 Solid carcinomas of the stomach. A combined histochemical, light and electron microscopic study. Cancer 51: 1673–1681

808. Murayama H, Kamio A, Imai T, Kikuchi M 1982 Gastric carcinoma with psammomatous calcification: report of a case, with reference to calculogenesis. Cancer 49: 788–796

809. Nevalainen T J, Jarvi O H 1977 Ultrastructure of intestinal and diffuse type gastric carcinoma. Journal of Pathology 122: 129–136

810. Saigo P E, Rosen P P, Brigati D J, Turnbull A D, Sternberg S S 1981 Primary gastric choriocarcinoma. An immunohistological study. American Journal of Surgical Pathology 5: 333–342

811. Salazar H, Totten R S 1970 Leiomyoblastoma of the stomach. An ultrastructural study. Cancer 25: 176–185

812. Sato A, Maie O, Kato T 1973 Ultrastructure of signet ring cells in cutaneous metastases of gastric carcinoma. Archiv für Dermatologische Forschung 247: 99–109

813. Tahara E, Ito H, Shimamoto F, Taniyama K, Iwamoto T 1982 Argyrophil cells in early gastric carcinoma: an immunohistochemical and ultrastructural study. Journal of Cancer Research and Clinical Oncology 103: 187–202

814. Wick M R, Carney J A 1980 An electron microscopic study of gastric epithelioid leiomyosarcoma. Laboratory Investigation 42: 160A

815. Wick M R, Ruebner B H, Carney J A 1981 Gastric tumors in patients with pulmonary chondroma or extra-adrenal paraganglioma. An ultrastructural study. Archives of Pathology and Laboratory Medicine 165: 527–531

816. Yamashiro K, Suzuki H, Nagayo T 1977 Electron microscopic study of signet ring cells in diffuse carcinoma of the human stomach. Virchows Archiv A Pathological Anatomy and Histology 374: 275–284

## 22 TUMOURS OF THE SMALL INTESTINE

817. Bjerregaard E 1974 Adenoacanthoma of the small bowel. Report of a case. Acta Pathologica et Microbiologica Scandinavica. Section A. Pathology 82: 113–115

818. Carstens P H B, Broghamer W L, Hire D 1976 Malignant fibrillo-caveolated cell carcinoma of the human intestinal tract. Human Pathology 7: 505–517

819. Carstens P H, Broghamer W L Jr 1978 Duodenal carcinoid with cytoplasmic whorls of microfilaments. Journal of Pathology 124: 235–238

820. Cooney T, Sweeney E C 1978 Paraganglioneuroma of the duodenum: an evolutionary hybrid? Journal of Clinical Pathology 31: 233–244

821. Dayal Y, Doos W G, O'Brien M J, Nunnemacher G, DeLellis R A, Wolfe H J 1983 Psammomatous somatostatinomas of the duodenum. American Journal of Surgical Pathology 7: 653–665

822. Elliott R L, Williams R D, Bayles D, Griffin J 1966 Lymphangioma of the duodenum: case report with light and electron microscopic observation. Annals of Surgery 163: 86–92

823. Gould V E, Valaitis J, Trujillo Y, Chejfec G, Gruhn J G 1980 Neuroendocrinoma of the jejunum: electron microscopic and biochemical analysis. Cancer 46: 713–717

824. Hamilton C W, Shelburne J D, Bossen E H 1982 A glomus tumor of the jejunum masquerading as a carcinoid tumor. Human Pathology 13: 859–861

825. Kaneko H, Yanaihara N, Ito S, Kusumoto Y, Fujita T, Ishikawa S, Sumida T, Sekiya M 1979 Somatostatinoma of the duodenum. Cancer 44: 2273–2279

826. Murayama H, Imai T, Kikuchi M, Kamio A 1979 Duodenal carcinoid (apudoma) with psammoma bodies. A light and electron microscopic study. Cancer 43: 1411–1417

827. Qizilbash A H 1973 Benign paraganglioma of the duodenum. Case report with light and electron microscopic examination and brief review of literature. Archives of Pathology 96: 276–280

828. Toker C 1974 Oat cell tumor of the small bowel. American Journal of Gastroenterology 61: 481–483

829. Weichert R F III, Roth L M, Harkin J C 1971 Carcinoid-islet cell tumor of the duodenum and associated multiple carcinoid tumors of the ileum. An electron microscopic study. Cancer 27: 910–918

## 23 TUMOURS OF THE VERMIFORM APPENDIX

830. Abt A B, Carter S L 1976 Goblet cell carcinoid of the appendix. An ultrastructural and histochemical study. Archives of Pathology and Laboratory Medicine 100: 301–306
831. Cooper P H, Warkel R L 1978 Ultrastructure of the goblet cell type of adenocarcinoid of the appendix. Cancer 42: 2687–2695
832. Johnston W H, Waisman J 1971 Carcinoid tumor of the vermiform appendix with Cushing's syndrome. Ultrastructural study of a case. Cancer 27: 681–686
833. Rodriguez F H, Sarma D P, Lunseth J H 1982 Goblet cell carcinoid of the appendix. Human Pathology 13: 286–288
834. Warner T F C S, Seo I S 1979 Goblet cell carcinoid of the appendix. Ultrastructural features and histogenetic aspects. Cancer 44: 1700–1706

## 24 TUMOURS OF THE COLON, RECTUM AND ANUS

835. Ahnen D J, Nakane P K, Brown W R 1982 Ultrastructural localization of carcinoembryonic antigen in normal intestine and colon cancer. Abnormal distribution of CEA on the surfaces of colon cancer cells. Cancer 49: 2077–2090
836. Allen M S Jr, Mills S E 1983 Small cell undifferentiated carcinomas of the colon arising in adenomas. Laboratory Investigation 48: 2A
837. Balázs M 1981 Electron microscopy of polyps of the colon. I. Comparative study of the epithelial cells of adenomatous and adenopapillary polyps. Experimental Pathology 19: 112–121
838. Balázs M 1981 Electron microscopy of polyps of the colon. II. Inclusion bodies of Leuchtenberger. Experimental Pathology 19: 164–171
839. Balázs M, Kovács A 1981 Electron microscopic study of carcinoma of the colon. Experimental Pathology 20: 203–214
840. Balázs M, Kovács A 1982 The 'transitional' mucosa adjacent to large bowel carcinoma – electron microscopic features and myofibroblast reaction. Histopathology 6: 617–629
841. Chumas J C, Lorelle C A 1981 Melanotic adenocarcinoma of the anorectum. American Journal of Surgical Pathology 5: 711–717
842. Damjanov I, Amenta P S, Bosman F T 1983 Undifferentiated carcinoma of the colon containing exocrine, neuroendocrine and squamous cells. Virchows Archiv A Pathological Anatomy and Histopathology 401: 57–66
843. Fenoglio C M, Richart R M, Kaye G I 1975 Comparative electron microscopic features of normal, hyperplastic and adenomatous human colonic epithelium. II. Variations in surface architecture found by scanning electron microscopy. Gastroenterology 69: 100–109
844. Fisher E R 1969 The basal cell nature of the so-called transitional cloacogenic carcinoma of anus as revealed by electron microscopy. Cancer 24: 312–322
845. Gabbert H, Höhn P 1980 Grades of atypia in tubular and villous adenomas of the human colon. An electron microscopic study. Virchows Archiv B Cell Pathology 33: 1–15
846. Gillespie J J, Mackay B 1978 Histogenesis of cloacogenic carcinoma. Fine structure of anal transitional epithelium and cloacogenic carcinoma. Human Pathology 9: 579–587
847. Goldenburg D M, Fisher E R 1970 Histogenetic relationship between carcinoids and mucin-secreting carcinomas of colon as revealed by heterotransplantation. British Journal of Cancer 24: 610–614
848. Gould V E, Chejfec G 1978 Neuroendocrine carcinomas of the colon. Ultrastructural and biochemical evidence of their secretory function. American Journal of Surgical Pathology 2: 31–38

849. Hall-Craggs M, Toker C 1982 Basaloid tumor of the sigmoid colon. Human Pathology 13: 497–500
850. Hernandez F J, Fernandez B B 1974 Mucus-secreting colonic carcinoid tumors: light and electron microscopic study of three cases. Diseases of the Colon and Rectum 17: 387–396
851. Hickey W F, Seiler M W 1981 Ultrastructural markers of colonic adenocarcinoma. Cancer 47: 140–145
852. Ioachim N-J, Delaney W E, Madrazo A 1974 Villous adenoma of the colon and rectum: an ultrastructural study. Cancer 34: 586–596
853. Kleir S, Hickey R C, Martin R G, Mackay B, Gallagher H S 1972 Cloacogenic carcinoma of the anal canal. Archives of Surgery 104: 407–415
854. Lewin K 1968 Neoplastic Paneth cells. Journal of Clinical Pathology 21: 476–479
855. Mughal S, Filipe M I, Jass J R 1981 A comparative ultrastructural study of hyperplastic and adenomatous polyps, incidental and in association with colorectal cancer. Cancer 48: 2746–2755
856. Nakamura K, Nakaya T, Sato E, Sasano N 1974 Ultramorphometry of the nucleus of human rectal cancer compared with normal mucosal gland. Tohoku Journal of Experimental Medicine 112: 177–188
857. Orloff M J 1971 Carcinoid tumors of the rectum. Cancer 28: 175–180
858. Polack-Charcon S, Shoham J, Ben-Shaul Y 1980 Tight junctions in epithelial cells of human fetal hindgut, normal colon, and colon adenocarcinoma. Journal of the National Cancer Institute 65: 53–62
859. Riddell R H, Eisenstat L, Levin B, Golomb H 1976 Surface ultrastructure of human adenomatous and hyperplastic polyps. Scanning Electron Microscopy 2: 19–24
860. Riddell R H, Levin B 1977 Ultrastructure of the transitional mucosa adjacent to large bowel carcinoma. Cancer 40: 2509–2522
861. Sato E, Goto M, Nakamura T 1981 Nuclear ultrastructure in carcinoma, adenoma, Peutz-Jeghers polyp and dysplasia of the large bowel: a morphometric analysis. Gann 72: 245–253
862. Shousha S 1979 Paneth cell-rich papillary adenocarcinoma and a mucoid adenocarcinoma occurring synchronously in colon: a light and electron microscopic study. Histopathology 3: 489–501
863. Shousha S 1982 Signet-ring cell adenocarcinoma of rectum: a histological, histochemical and electron microscopic study. Histopathology 6: 341–350
864. Siew S 1976 Scanning electron microscopy of neoplastic lesions of the human colon. Scanning Electron Microscopy 2: 11–18
865. Ulich T R, Cheng L, Glover H, Yang K, Lewin K J 1983 A colonic adenocarcinoma with argentaffin cells. An immunoperoxidase study demonstrating the presence of numerous endocrine products. Cancer 51: 1483–1489

## 25 HEPATO-BILIARY TUMOURS

866. Alpert L I, Zak F G, Werthamer S, Bochetto J F 1974 Cholangiocarcinoma. A clinicopathologic study of five cases with ultrastructural observations. Human Pathology 5: 709–728
867. An T, Ghatak N, Kastner R, Kay S, Lee H M 1983 Hyaline globules and intracellular lumina in a hepatocellular carcinoma. American Journal of Clinical Pathology 79: 392–396
868. Baithun S I, Pollock D J 1983 Oncocytic hepatocellular tumour. Histopathology 7: 107–112

869. Balázs M 1976 Electron microscopic study of benign hepatoma in a patient on oral contraceptives. Beiträge zur Pathologie 159: 299–306

870. Balázs M 1978 Comparative electron microscopic studies of benign hepatoma and icterus in patients on oral contraceptives. Virchows Archiv A Pathological Anatomy and Histology 381: 97–109

871. Barsky S H, Linnoila R I, Triche T J, Costa J 1981 Hepatocellular carcinomas with carcinoid components. Laboratory Investigation 44: 3A

872. Becker F F 1974 Hepatoma: nature's model tumor. A review. American Journal of Pathology 74: 179–210

873. Chang W W L, Agha F P, Morgan W S 1983 Primary sarcoma of the liver in the adult. Cancer 51: 1510–1517

874. Cozzutto C, De Bernardi B, Comelli A, Soave F 1981 Malignant mesenchymoma of the liver in children: a clinicopathologic and ultrastructural study. Human Pathology 12: 481–485

875. Craig J R, Peters R L, Edmonson H A, Omata M 1980 Fibrolamellar carcinoma of the liver: a tumor of adolescents and young adults with distinctive clinico-pathologic features. Cancer 46: 372–379

876. Dehner L P, Ewing S L, Sumner H W 1975 Infantile mesenchymal hamartoma of the liver. Histologic and ultrastructural observations. Archives of Pathology 99: 379–382

877. Denk H, Krepler R, Lackinger E, Artlieb U, Franke W W 1982 Biochemical and immunocytochemical analysis of the intermediate filament cytoskeleton in human hepatocellular carcinomas and in hepatic neoplastic nodules in mice. Laboratory Investigation 46: 584–596

878. Enat R, Buschmann R J, Chomet B 1973 Ultrastructure of cytoplasmic hyaline inclusions in a case of human hepatocarcinoma. Gastroenterology 65: 802–810

879. Farhi D C, Shikes R H, Silverberg S G 1982 Ultrastructure of fibrolamellar oncocytic hepatoma. Cancer 50: 702–709

880. Fechner R E 1977 Hepatic tumors and oral contraceptives. Pathology Annual 12, pt 1: 293–310

881. Garancis J C, Tang T, Panares R, Jurevics I 1969 Hepatic adenoma. Biochemical and electron microscopic study. Cancer 24: 560–568

882. Ghadially F N, Parry E W 1966 Ultrastructure of a human hepatocellular carcinoma and surrounding non-neoplastic liver. Cancer 19: 1989–2004

883. Gonzalez-Crussi F, Manz H J 1972 Structure of a hepatoblastoma of pure epithelial type. Cancer 29: 1272–1280

884. Grimelius L, Stenram U, Westman J, Westman-Naeser S 1977 Hyaline cytoplasmic inclusions in human hepatoma. A case report. Acta Cytologica 21: 469–476

885. Horie A, Kotoo Y, Hayashi I 1979 Ultrastructural comparison of hepatoblastoma and hepatocellular carcinoma. Cancer 44: 2184–2193

886. Horvath E, Kovacs K, Ross R C 1972 Ultrastructural findings in a well differentiated hepatoma. Digestion 7: 74–82

887. Kay S, Schatzki P F 1971 Ultrastructure of a benign liver cell adenoma. Cancer 28: 755–762

888. Keeley A F, Iseri O A, Gottlieb L S 1972 Ultrastructure of hyaline cytoplasmic inclusions in a human hepatoma: relationship to Mallory's alcoholic hyalin. Gastroenterology 62: 280–293

889. Kihara I, Suzuki T, Takamiya H, Hirono S 1973 Cholangiocarcinoma with hypercalcemia: a case report studied by electron microscope and radioimmunoassay. Acta Pathologica Japonica 23: 791–804

890. Lapis K 1979 The liver. In: Johannessen J V (ed) Electron microscopy in human medicine, vol. 2. The liver. McGraw-Hill, New York, pt 1, ch 9, p 188–197

891. Misugi K, Okojima H, Misugi N, Newton W A Jr 1967 Classification of primary malignant tumors of liver in infancy and childhood. Cancer 20: 1760–1771

892. Munoz P A, Rao M S, Reddy J K 1980 Osteoclastoma-like giant cell tumor of the liver. Cancer 46: 771–779

893. Nakanuma Y, Kono N, Ohta G, Shirasaki S, Takeshita H, Watanabe K, Tsuda S, Yoshizawa H 1982 Pale eosinophilic inclusions simulating ground-glass appearance of cells of hepatocellular carcinoma. Acta Pathologica Japonica 32: 71–81

894. Phillips M J, Langer B, Stone R, Fisher M M, Ritchie S 1973 Benign liver cell tumors. Classification and ultrastructural pathology. Cancer 32: 463–470

895. Platt M S, Agamanolis D P, Krill C E Jr, Boeckman C, Potter J L, Robinson H, Lloyd J 1983 Occult hepatic sinusoid tumor of infancy simulating neuroblastoma. Cancer 52: 1183–1189

896. Pollice L 1981 Primary pediatric tumors of the liver. Progress in Surgical Pathology 3: 195–219

897. Primack A, Wilson J, O'Connor G T, Engelman K, Hull E, Canellos G P 1971 Hepatocellular carcinoma with the carcinoid syndrome. Cancer 27: 1182–1189

898. Raju U B, Fine G 1980 Ultrastructure of the gallbladder paraganglia. Archives of Pathology and Laboratory Medicine 104: 379–383

899. Rhodes R H, Marchildon M B, Luebke D C, Edmondson H A, Mikity V G 1978 A mixed hamartoma of the liver: light and electron microscopy. Human Pathology 9: 211–221

900. Rosa F, Grases P J 1980 Ultrastructural studies in a case of hepatoblastoma. Human Pathology 11: 70–72

901. Roth J A, Berman E, Befeler D, Johnson F B 1982 A black hepatocellular carcinoma with Dubin-Johnson-like pigment and Mallory bodies. A histochemical and ultrastructural study. American Journal of Surgical Pathology 6: 375–382

902. Ruebner B H, Gonzalez-Licea A, Slusser R J 1967 Electron microscopy of some human hepatomas. Gastroenterology 53: 18–30

903. Schaffner F 1972 Electron microscopy in the study of human liver disease. Human Pathology 3: 293–294

904. Scotto J, Homberg J C, Stralin H, Caroli J 1974 Ultrastructural study of cytoplasmic inclusions in cases of viral hepatitis and hepatomas. Pathologia Europaea 9: 211–216

905. Silverman J F, Fu Y-S, McWilliams N B, Kay S 1975 An ultrastructural study of mixed hepatoblastoma with osteoid elements. Cancer 36: 1436–1443

906. Swift J G, Mukherjee T M, Rowland R 1983 Intercellular junctions in hepatocellular carcinoma. Journal of Submicroscopic Cytology 15: 799–810

907. Tanikawa K 1979 Ultrastructural aspects of the liver and its disorders, 2nd edn. Igaku-Shoin, Tokyo, p 338–348

908. Toker C, Trevino N 1966 Ultrastructure of human primary hepatic carcinoma. Cancer 19: 1594–1606

909. Toner P G, Carr K E, McLay A L C 1979 The gallbladder and biliary ducts. In: Johannessen J V (ed) Electron microscopy in human medicine, vol 3. The liver. McGraw-Hill, New York, pt 2, ch 10, p 201–210

910. Wada A, Ishiguro S, Tateishi R, Ishikawa O, Matsui Y 1983 Carcinoid tumor of the gallbladder associated with adenocarcinoma. Cancer 51: 1911–1917

911. Warner T F C S, Soo I S, Madura J A, Polak J M, Pearse A G E 1980 Pancreatic-polypeptide-producing apudoma of the liver. Cancer 46: 1146–1151

912. Willén R, Willén H 1982 Primary sarcoma of the gallbladder. A light and electron microscopic study. Virchows Archiv A Pathological Anatomy and Histology 396: 91–102

913. Wills E J 1968 Fine structure and surface adenosinetriphosphatase activity of a human hepatoma. Cancer 22: 1046–1052

914. Woyke S, Domagala W, Olszewski W 1974 Ultrastructure of hepatoma cells detected in peritoneal fluid. Acta Cytologica 18: 130–136

915. Wu P C, Lai C L, Lam K C, Lok A S F, Lin H J 1983 Clear cell carcinoma of liver. An ultrastructural study. Cancer 52: 504–507

## 26 TUMOURS OF THE EXOCRINE AND ENDOCRINE PANCREAS

916. Akagi T, Fujii Y 1981 Histology, ultrastructure, and tissue culture of human insulinomas. Cancer 47: 417–424

917. Alguacil-Garcia A, Weiland L H 1977 The histologic spectrum, prognosis, and histogenesis of the sarcomatoid carcinoma of the pancreas. Cancer 39: 1181–1189

918. An T, Kaye G I 1978 Amyloid formation in insulinoma. Archives of Pathology and Laboratory Medicine 102: 227–232

919. Berger M, Teuscher A, Halban P, Trimble E, Studer P P, Wollheim C B, Zimmerman-Telschow H, Muller W A 1980 In vitro and in vivo studies on glucagonoma tissue. Hormone and Metabolic Research 12: 144–150

920. Bordi C, Bussolati G 1974 Immunofluorescence, histochemical and ultrastructural studies for the detection of multiple endocrine polypeptide tumours of the pancreas. Virchows Archiv B Zellpathologie 17: 13–27

921. Bordi C, Bussolati G, Ballerio G, Togni R 1975 Endocrine tumor of the pancreas composed of argyrophil and B cells. A correlated light, immunofluorescent and ultrastructural study. Cancer 35: 436–444

922. Bordi C, Tardini A 1980 Electron microscopy of islet cell tumors. Progress in Surgical Pathology 1: 135–155

923. Burns W A, Matthews M J, Hamosh M, Weide G V, Blum R, Johnson F B 1974 Lipase-secreting acinar cell carcinoma of the pancreas with polyarthropathy. A light and electron microscopic, histochemical and biochemical study. Cancer 33: 1002–1009

924. Cantrell B B, Cubilla A L, Erlandson R A, Fortner J, Fitzgerald P J 1981 Acinar cell cystadenocarcinoma of human pancreas. Cancer 47: 410–416

925. Capella C, Solcia E, Frigerio B, Buffa R, Usellini L, Fontana P 1977 The endocrine cells of the pancreas and related tumours. Ultrastructural study and classification. Virchows Archiv A Pathological Anatomy and Histology 373: 327–352

926. Carney C N 1976 Congenital insulinoma (nesidioblastoma). Ultrastructural evidence for histogenesis from pancreatic duct epithelium. Archives of Pathology and Laboratory Medicine 100: 352–356

927. Creutzfeldt W 1980 Endocrine tumors of the pancreas: clinical, chemical and morphological findings. In: Fitzgerald P J, Morrison A B (eds) The pancreas. International Academy of Pathology Monograph No 21. Williams & Wilkins, Baltimore, ch 13, p 208–230

928. Creutzfeldt W, Arnold R, Creutzfeldt C, Deuticke U, Frerichs H, Track N S 1973 Biochemical and morphological investigations of 30 human insulinomas. Correlation between the tumour content of insulin and proinsulin-like components and the histological and ultrastructural appearance. Diabetologia 9: 217–231

929. Creutzfeldt W, Arnold R, Creutzfeldt C, Track N S 1975 Pathomorphologic, biochemical and diagnostic aspects of gastrinomas (Zollinger-Ellison syndrome). Human Pathology 6: 47–76

930. Feiner H 1978 Electron microscopy of neoplasms of pancreatic islet cells. Journal of Dermatologic Surgery and Oncology 4: 751–757

931. Frable W J, Still W J S, Kay S 1971 Carcinoma of the pancreas, infantile type. A light and electron microscopic study. Cancer 27: 667–673

932. Frerichs H, Creutzfeldt W 1976 Hypoglycaemia. I. Insulin secreting tumours. Clinics in Endocrinology and Metabolism 5: 747–767

933. Friesen S R 1982 Tumors of the endocrine pancreas. New England Journal of Medicine 306: 580–590

934. Gammil S L, Weichert R, Smith S L, Font R, Ingraffia R 1973 Carcinoid islet cell tumours. Acta Radiologica 12: 229–240

935. Goldenberg V E, Goldenberg N S, Benditt E P 1969 Ultrastructural features of functioning alpha- and beta-cell tumors. Cancer 24: 236–247

936. Gould V E, Memoli V A, Dardi L E, Gould N S 1981 Nesidiodysplasia and nesidioblastosis of infancy: ultrastructural and immunohistochemical analysis of islet cell alterations with and without associated hyper-insulinaemic hypoglycaemia. Scandinavian Journal of Gastroenterology suppl 70: 129–142

937. Greider M H, Elliott D W 1964 Electron microscopy of human pancreatic tumors of islet cell origin. American Journal of Pathology 44: 663–678

938. Greider M H, Rosai J, McGuigan J E 1974 The human pancreatic islet cells and their tumors. II. Ulcerogenic and diarrheogenic tumors. Cancer 33: 1423–1443

939. Guillan R A, McMahon J 1973 Pleomorphic adenocarcinoma of the pancreas. American Journal of Gastroenterology 60: 379–386

940. Håkanson R, Alumets J, Rehfeld J F, Ekelund M, Sundler F 1982 The life cycle of the gastrin granule. Cell and Tissue Research 222: 479–491

941. Hammar S, Sale G 1975 Multiple hormone producing islet cell carcinomas of the pancreas. A morphological and biochemical investigation. Human Pathology 6: 349–362

942. Heitz P U, Kasper M, Polak J M, Klöppel G 1982 Pancreatic endocrine tumors. Immunocytochemical analysis of 125 tumors. Human Pathology 13: 263–271

943. Heitz P U, Kloppel G, Hacki W H, Polak J M, Pearse A G 1977 Nesidioblastosis: the pathologic basis of persistent hyperinsulinemic hypoglycemia in infants. Morphologic and quantitative analysis of seven cases based on specific immuno-staining and electron microscopy. Diabetes 26: 632–642

944. Hernandez Sanchez L, Navas Palacios J, De Agustin de Agustin P 1981 Acinar cell carcinoma of the pancreas: light and electron microscopic study. Morfología Normal y Patológica 5: 273–284

945. Horie A, Yano Y, Kotoo Y, Miwa A 1977 Morphogenesis of pancreatoblastoma, infantile carcinoma of the pancreas. Report of two cases. Cancer 39: 247–254

946. Huntrakoon M 1983 Oncocytic carcinoma of the pancreas. Cancer 51: 332–336

947. Jacob E T, Golan M, Griffel B, Deutsch V 1973 Giant islet cell tumor of the pancreas with alpha-like granules. An ultrastructural study. Israel Journal of Medical Sciences 9: 1028–1035

948. Kahan R S, Perez-Figaredo R A, Neimanis A 1977 Necrolytic migratory erythema: distinctive dermatosis of the glucagonoma syndrome. Archives of Dermatology 113: 792–797

949. Katz R, Fischmann A B, Galotto J, Guccio J G, Higgins G A, Ortega L G, West W H, Recant L 1979 Necrolytic migratory erythema, presenting as candidiasis, due to a pancreatic glucagonoma. Cancer 44: 558–563

950. Kostianovsky M 1980 Endocrine pancreatic tumors: ultrastructure. Annals of Clinical and Laboratory Science 10: 65–76

951. Kovi J 1982 Adenosquamous carcinoma of the pancreas: a light and electron microscopic study. Ultrastructural Pathology 3: 17–23

952. Larsson L-I 1978 Endocrine pancreatic tumors. Human Pathology 9: 401–416

953. Larsson L-I 1978 PP-producing and mixed endocrine pancreatic tumours. In: Bloom S R (ed) Gut hormones. Churchill Livingstone, Edinburgh, ch 98, p 605–610

954. Larsson L-I, Grimelius L, Håkanson R, Rehfeld J F, Stadil F, Holst J, Angervall L, Sundler F 1975 Mixed endocrine pancreatic tumors producing several peptide hormones. American Journal of Pathology 79: 271–284

955. Larsson L-I, Hirsch M A, Holst J J, Ingmansson S, Kuhl C, Jensen S L, Lundqvist G, Rehfeld J F, Schwartz T W 1977 Pancreatic somatostatinoma. Clinical features and physiological implications. Lancet i: 666–668

956. Lechago J, Weinstein W M 1978 Morphological aspects of the G-cells. In: Bloom S R (ed) Gut hormones. Churchill Livingstone, Edinburgh, p 140–144

957. Leong A S, Slavotinek A H, Higgins B A 1980 Nesidioblastosis, islet cell hyperplasia, and adenomatosis in a case of metastasizing insulinoma: contribution to the genesis of the islets of Langerhans. Diabetes Care 3: 537– 542

958. Liu T H, Zeng X J, Zhu Y, Wu W R 1981 Insulinoma. Light and electron microscopic study of 65 cases. Chinese Medical Journal 94: 21–30

959. Lo J W, Fung C H K, Yonan T N, Martinez N 1977 Cystadenoma of the pancreas. An ultrastructural study. Cancer 39: 2470–2474

960. McGavran M H, Unger R H, Recant L, Polk H C, Kilo C, Levin M E 1966 A glucagon-secreting alpha cell carcinoma of the pancreas. New England Journal of Medicine 274: 1408–1413

961. Navas Palacios J J, Garzon Martin A 1979 Functioning islet cell tumors of the pancreas: light and electron microscopic study of seven cases. Morfología Normal y Patológica 3: 595–618

962. Osborne B M, Culbert S J, Cangir A, Mackay B 1977 Acinar cell carcinoma of the pancreas in a 9-year-old child: case report with electron microscopic observations. Southern Medical Journal 70: 370–372

963. Patchefsky A S, Gordon G S 1974 Endocrine tumors of the pancreas associated with elevated urinary serotonin excretion. Annals of Clinical and Laboratory Science 4: 383–393

964. Patchefsky A S, Gordon G, Harrer W V, Hoch W S 1974 Carcinoid tumor of the pancreas. Ultrastructural observations of a lymph node metastasis and comparison with bronchial carcinoid. Cancer 33: 1349–1354

965. Perez-Atayde A R, Hartman A S, Seiler M W 1982 Ribosome-lamellae complexes in a symptomatic insulinoma. An ultrastructural study. Archives of Pathology and Laboratory Medicine 106: 221–223

966. Posen J A 1981 Giant cell tumor of the pancreas of the osteoclastic type associated with a mucous secreting cystadenocarcinoma. Human Pathology 12: 944–947

967. Rawlinson D G 1973 Electron microscopy of an ACTH-secreting islet cell carcinoma. Cancer 31: 1015–1018

968. Rawlinson D G, Christiansen R O 1973 Light and electron microscopic observations on a congenital insulinoma. Cancer 32: 1470–1476

969. Reid J D, Yuh S-L, Petrelli M, Jaffe R 1982 Ductuloinsular tumors of the pancreas: a light, electron microscopic and immunohistochemical study. Cancer 49: 908–915

970. Robinson L, Damjanov I, Brezina P 1977 Multinucleated giant cell neoplasm of the pancreas. Light and electron microscopy features. Archives of Pathology and Laboratory Medicine 101: 590–593

971. Rosai J 1968 Carcinoma of pancreas simulating giant cell tumor of bone. Electron microscopic evidence of its acinar cell origin. Cancer 22: 333–344

972. Ruttman E, Klöppel G, Bommer G, Kiehn M, Heitz Ph U 1980 Pancreatic glucagonoma with and without syndrome: immunocytochemical study of 5 tumor cases and review of the literature. Virchows Archiv A Pathological Anatomy and Histology 388: 51–67

973. Schlosnagle D C, Campbell W G Jr 1981 The papillary and solid neoplasm of the pancreas: a report of two cases with elecron microscopy, one containing neurosecretory granules. Cancer 47: 2603–2610

974. Solcia E, Capella C, Buffa R, Frigerio B, Fiocca R 1980 Pathology of the Zollinger-Ellison syndrome. Progress in Surgical Pathology 1: 119–133

975. Solcia E, Capella C, Buffa R, Frigerio B, Usellini L, Fontana P 1981 The endocrine pancreas. In: Johannessen J V (ed) Electron microscopy in human medicine, vol 10. Endocrine organs. McGraw-Hill, New York, pt 5, p 189–212

976. Suzuki H, Matsuyama M 1971 Ultrastructure of functioning beta cell tumors of the pancreatic islets. Cancer 28: 1302–1313

977. Takemiya M, Miyayama H, Takeya M, Takeuchi T, Konno T, Kitoh M, Fukushima H 1981 A post mortem study of malignant glucagonoma with heart muscle hypertrophy, including chemical, histochemical, immunohistological, and ultrastructural observations. Human Pathology 12: 988–999

978. Taxy J B 1976 Adenocarcinoma of the pancreas in childhood: report of a case and a review of the English language literature. Cancer 37: 1508–1518

979. Thomson O F 1979 Pancreatic beta-cell tumours studied by immunofluorescence and electron microscopy. A report of four cases and a review of the literature. Acta Pathologica et Microbiologica Scandinavica. Section A. Pathology 87: 463–478

980. Toker C 1967 Some observations on the ultrastructure of a malignant islet cell tumor associated with duodenal ulceration and severe diarrhea. Journal of Ultrastructure Research 19: 522–531

981. Tomita T 1974 Pathology of ulcerogenic and diarrheogenic tumors of the pancreas. Acta Pathologica Japonica 24: 189–205

982. Toner P G, Carr K E, McKay A L C 1980 The exocrine pancreas. In: Johannessen J V (ed) Electron microscopy in human medicine, vol 7. Digestive system. McGraw-Hill, New York, pt 3, p 211–245

983. Trepeta R W, Mathur B, Lagin S, Li Volsi V A 1981 Giant cell tumor ('osteoclastoma') of the pancreas. A tumor of epithelial origin. Cancer 48: 2022–2028

984. Ulich T, Cheng L, Lewin K J 1982 Acinar-endocrine cell tumor of the pancreas. Report of a pancreatic tumor containing both zymogen and neuroendocrine granules. Cancer 50: 2099–2105

985. Urbanski S J, Medline A 1982 Giant cell carcinoma of pancreas with clear cell pattern in metastases. Human Pathology 13: 1047–1049

986. Van Obberghen E, Somers G, Devis G, Ravazzola M, Malaisse-Lagae F, Orci L, Malaisse W J 1975 Dynamics of insulin release and the microtubular-microfilamentous system. VII. Do microfilaments provide motive force for translocation and extrusion of beta granules? Diabetes 24: 892–901

987. Verner J V, Morrison A B 1974 Endocrine pancreatic islet disease with diarrhea. Report of a case due to diffuse hyperplasia of nonbeta islet tissue with a review of 54 additional cases. Archives of Internal Medicine 133: 492–499

988. Warner T F C S, Block M, Hafez G R, Mack E, Lloyd R V, Bloom S R 1983 Glucagonomas. Ultrastructure and immunocytochemistry. Cancer 51: 1091–1096

989. Wilander E, El-Salhy M, Willén R, Grimelius L 1981 Immunocytochemistry and electron microscopy of an argentaffin endocrine tumour of the pancreas. Virchows Archiv A Pathological Anatomy and Histology 392: 263–269

990. Woodtli W, Hedinger C 1976 Histologic characteristics of insulinomas and gastrinomas. Value of argyrophilia, metachromasia, immunohistology and elecron microscopy for the identification of gastrointestinal and pancreatic endocrine cells and their tumors. Virchows Archiv A Pathological Anatomy and Histology 371: 331–350

## 27 TUMOURS OF THE KIDNEY, INCLUDING JUXTAGLOMERULAR CELL TUMOUR

991. Balsaver A N, Gibley C W Jr, Tessmer C F 1968 Ultrastructural studies in Wilms's tumor. Cancer 22: 417–427

992. Bannayan G A, Lamm D L 1980 Renal cell tumors. Pathology Annual 15, pt 2: 271–308

993. Barajas L, Bennett C M, Connor G, Lindstrom R R 1977 Structure of a juxtaglomerular cell tumor: the presence of a neural component. A light and electron microscopic study. Laboratory Investigation 37: 357–368

994. Bennington J L, Beckwith J B 1975 Tumors of the kidney, renal pelvis, and ureter. Atlas of tumor pathology, 2nd series, fascicle 12. Armed Forces Institute of Pathology, Washington, D C, p 156–159

995. Bossart M I, Spjut H J, Wright J E, Pranke D W 1982 Multilocular cystic leiomyoma of the kidney. Ultrastructural Pathology 3: 367–374

996. Brown J J, Fraser R, Lever A F, Morton J J, Robertson J I, Tree M, Bell P R, Davidson J K, Ruthven I S 1973 Hypertension and secondary hyperaldosteronism associated with a renin-secreting renal juxtaglomerular cell tumor. Lancet ii: 1228–1232

997. Busuttil A, More I A 1974 Two malignant soft tissue tumors of the kidney: an ultrastructural appraisal. Journal of Urology 112: 24–29

998. Chalvardjian A, Kovacs K, Horvath E 1978 Renal angiomyolipoma: ultrastructural study. Urology 12: 717–720

999. Chatelanat F 1981 Sarcomatous tumors of the kidney. Progress in Surgical Pathology 3: 181–194

1000. Coleman M 1980 Multilocular renal cyst. Case report, ultrastructure and review of the literature. Virchows Archiv A Pathological Anatomy and Histology 387: 207–219

1001. Deitchman B, Sidhu G S 1980 Ultrastructural study of a sarcomatoid variant of renal cell carcinoma. Cancer 46: 1152–1157

1002. Ericsson J L, Seljelid R, Orrenius S 1966 Comparative light and electron microscopic observations of the cytoplasmic matrix in renal carcinomas. Virchows Archiv A Pathologische Anatomie 341: 204–223

1003. Fu Y-S, Kay S 1973 Congenital mesoblastic nephroma and its recurrence. An ultrastructural observation. Archives of Pathology 96: 66–70

1004. Fung C H K, Gonzalez-Crussi F, Yonan T N, Martinez N 1981 'Rhabdoid' Wilms' tumor. An ultrastructural study. Archives of Pathology and Laboratory Medicine 105: 521–523

1005. Glick A D, Tham K T, Leung N K, Wong S W 1981 Unusual clear cell tumor of the kidney in infancy. American Journal of Surgical Pathology 5: 581–585

1006. Gondos B 1981 Diagnosis of tumors of the kidney: ultrastructural classification. Annals of Clinical and Laboratory Science 11: 308–315

1007. Gonzalez-Crussi F, Baum E S 1983 Renal sarcomas of childhood. A clinicopathologic and ultrastructural study. Cancer 51: 898–912

1008. Haas J E, Palmer N F, Weinberg A G, Beckwith J B 1981 Ultrastructure of malignant rhabdoid tumor of the kidney. A distinctive renal tumor of children. Human Pathology 12: 646–657

1009. Herman C J, Moesker O, Kant A, Huysmans A, Vooijs G P, Ramaekers F C S 1983 Is renal cell (Grawitz) tumor a carcinosarcoma? Evidence from analysis of intermediate filament types. Virchows Archiv B Cell Pathology 44: 73–83

1010. Hollifield J W, Page D L, Smith C, Michelakis A M, Staab E, Rhamy R 1975 Renin-secreting clear cell carcinoma of the kidney. Archives of Internal Medicine 135: 859–864

1011. Holthöfer H, Miettinen A, Paasivuo R, Lehto V-P, Linder E, Alfthan O, Virtanen I 1983 Cellular origin and differentiation of renal carcinomas. A fluorescence microscopic study with kidney-specific antibodies, antiintermediate filament antibodies, and lectins. Laboratory Investigation 49: 317–326

1012. Kay S, Armstrong K S 1980 Oncocytic tubular adenoma of the kidney – report of three cases with 28-year follow-up on one. Progress in Surgical Pathology 2: 259–268

1013. Kimura K, Ohnishi Y, Morishita H, Amezaki M, Irikura K 1983 Giant cell tumor of the kidney. Virchows Archiv A Pathological Anatomy and Histopathology 398: 357–365

1014. Klein M J, Valensi Q J 1976 Proximal tubular adenomas of kidney with so-called oncocytic features. A clinico-pathologic study of 13 cases of a rarely reported neoplasm. Cancer 38: 906–914

1015. Kurtz S M 1979 A unique ultrastructural variant of Wilms' tumor. American Journal of Surgical Pathology 3: 257–264

1016. Lam A S, Bedard Y C, Buckspan M B, Logan A G, Steinhardt M I 1982 Surgically curable hypertension associated with reninoma. Journal of Urology 128: 572–575

1017. Levin N P, Damjanov I, Depillis V J 1982 Mesoblastic nephroma in an adult patient. Recurrence 21 years after removal of the primary lesion. Cancer 49: 573–577

1018. Lindop G B M, Stewart J A, Downie T T 1983 The immunocytochemical demonstration of renin in a juxtaglomerular cell tumour by light and electron microscopy. Histopathology 7: 421–431

1019. Mahoney J P, Saffos R O 1981 Fetal rhabdomyomatous nephroblastoma with a renal pelvic mass simulting sarcoma botryoides. American Journal of Surgical Pathology 5: 297–306

1020. Mitchell K M, Shilkin K B 1982 Renal oncocytoma. Pathology 14: 75–80

1021. More I A R, Jackson A M, MacSween R N M 1974 Renin-secreting tumor associated with hypertension. Cancer 34: 2093–2102

1022. Novak R W, Caces J N, Johnson W W 1980 Sarcomatous renal tumor of childhood. An electron microscopic study. American Journal of Clinical Pathology 73: 622–625

1023. Phillips G, Mukherjee T M 1972 A juxtaglomerular cell tumour: light and electron microscopic studies of a renin-secreting kidney tumour containing both juxtaglomerular cells and mast cells. Pathology 4: 193–204

1024. Pratt-Thomas H R, Spicer S S, Upshur J K, Greene W B 1973 Carcinoma of the kidney in a 15-year-old boy. Unusual histologic features with formation of microvilli. Cancer 31: 719–725

1025. Sanfilippo F, Pizzo S V, Croker B P 1982 Immunohistochemical studies of cell differentiation in a juxtaglomerular tumor. Archives of Pathology and Laboratory Medicine 106: 604–607

1026. Schmidt D, Dickersin G R, Vawter G F, Mackay B, Harms D 1982 Wilms' tumor: review of ultrastructure and histogenesis. Pathobiology Annual 12: 281–300

1027. Schmidt D, Harms D, Zieger G 1982 Malignant rhabdoid tumor of the kidney. Histopathology, ultrastructure and comments on differential diagnosis. Virchows Archiv A Pathological Anatomy and Histology 398: 101–108

1028. Shen S C, Yunis E J 1980 A study of the cellularity and ultrastructure of congenital mesoblastic nephroma. Cancer 45: 306–314

1029. Stahl R E, Sidhu G S 1979 Primary carcinoid of the kidney. Light and electron microscopic study. Cancer 44: 1345–1349

1030. Sun C N, Bissada N K, White H J, Redman J F 1977 Spectrum of ultrastructural patterns of renal cell adenocarcinoma. Urology 9: 195–200

1031. Tannenbaum M 1971 Ultrastructural pathology of human renal cell tumors. Pathology Annual 6: 249–277

1032. Tannenbaum M 1979 Renal tumors. In: Johannessen J V (ed) Electron microscopy in human medicine, vol 9. Urogenital system and breast. McGraw-Hill, New York, ch 14, p 166–190

1033. Taxy J B 1981 Renal adenocarcinoma presenting as a solitary metastasis: contribution of electron microscopy to diagnosis. Cancer 48: 2056–2062

1034. van der Walt J D, Reid H A S, Risdon R A, Shaw J H F 1983 Renal oncocytoma. A review of the literature and report of an unusual multicentric case. Virchows Archiv A Pathological Anatomy and Histopathology 398: 294–304

1035. Vanatta P R, Silva F G, Taylor W E, Costa J C 1983 Renal cell carcinoma and systemic amyloidosis: demonstration of AA protein and review of the literature. Human Pathology 14: 195–201

1036. Ward S P, Dehner L P 1974 Sacrococcygeal teratoma with nephroblastoma (Wilms tumor): a variant of extragonadal teratoma in childhood. A histologic and ultrastructural study. Cancer 33: 1355–1363

1037. Wigger H J 1975 Fetal mesenchymal hamartoma of kidney. A tumor of secondary mesenchyme. Cancer 36: 1002–1008

1038. Yu G S M, Rendler S, Herskowitz A, Molnar J J 1980 Renal oncocytoma. Report of five cases and review of literature. Cancer 45: 1010–1018

1039. Zak F G, Jindrak K, Capozzi F 1983 Carcinoidal tumor of the kidney. Ultrastructural Pathology 4: 51–59

1040. Zanetti G, Giangaspero F 1982 Rhabdomyoblastic nature of cytoplasmic inclusions in malignant rhabdoid tumour. Human Pathology 13: 410

1041. Zollinger H U, Mihatsch M J 1978 Renal pathology in biopsy. Light, electron and immunofluorescence microscopy and clinical aspects. Springer-Verlag, Berlin, ch 29, p 553–563

## 28 TUMOURS OF THE URINARY TRACT

1042. Alroy J, Gould V E 1980 Epithelial-stromal interface in normal and neoplastic human bladder epithelium. Ultrastructural Pathology 1: 201–210

1043. Alroy J, Miller A W III, Coon J S IV, James K K, Gould V E 1980 Inverted papilloma of the urinary bladder. Ultrastructural and immunologic studies. Cancer 46: 64–70

1044. Alroy J, Pauli B U, Hayden J E, Gould V E 1979 Intracytoplasmic lumina in bladder carcinomas. Human Pathology 10: 549–555

1045. Alroy J, Pauli B U, Weinstein R S 1981 Association of therapeutic radiation with Golgi complex hypertrophy in human urinary bladder carcinomas: quantitative electron microscopy studies. Ultrastructural Pathology 2: 43–52

1046. Alroy J, Pauli B U, Weinstein R S 1981 Correlation between numbers of desmosomes and the aggressiveness of transitional cell carcinoma in human urinary bladder. Cancer 47: 104–112

1047. Alroy J, Roganovic D, Banner B F, Jacobs J B, Merk F B, Ucci A A, Kwan P W L, Coon J S IV, Miller A W III 1981 Primary adenocarcinomas of the human urinary bladder: histochemical, immunological and ultrastructural studies. Virchows Archiv A Pathological Anatomy and Histology 393: 165–181

1048. Alroy J, Ucci A A, Roganovic D, Jacobs J B, Merk F B 1982 Ultrastructural changes in surface topography, glycocalyx and plasma membrane interior of tumor cells during exocytosis of mucus. Journal of Submicroscopic Cytology 14: 171–177

1049. Aronson P, Ronan S G, Briele H A, Bardawil W A, Manaligod J R 1982 Adenoid cystic carcinoma of the female periurethral area. Light and electron microscopic study. Urology 20: 312–315

1050. Bhagavan B S, Tiamson E M, Wenk R E, Berger B W, Hamamoto G, Eggleston J C 1981 Nephrogenic adenoma of the urinary bladder and urethra. Human Pathology 12: 907–916

1051. Chasko S B, Keuhnelian J G, Gutowski W T III, Gray G F 1980 Spindle cell cancer of the bladder during cyclophosphamide therapy for Wegener's granulomatosis. American Journal of Surgical Pathology 4: 191–196

1052. Colby T V 1980 Carcinoid tumor of the bladder. A case report. Archives of Pathology and Laboratory Medicine 104: 199–200

1053. Cramer S F, Aikawa M, Cebelin M 1981 Neurosecretory granules in small cell invasive carcinoma of the urinary bladder. Cancer 47: 724–730

1054. Croft W A, Nelson C E, Nilsson T 1979 Scanning electron microscopy of exfoliated malignant and non malignant human urothelial cells. Scandinavian Journal of Urology and Nephrology 13: 49–57

1055. Davis B H, Ludwig M E, Cole S R, Pastuszak W T 1983 Small cell neuroendocrine carcinoma of the urinary bladder: report of three cases with ultrastructural analysis. Ultrastructural Pathology 4: 197–204

1056. Duong H D, Jackson A G, Kovi J, Ransome J R, Jones G W 1981 Mixed mesodermal tumor of urinary bladder: a light and electron microscopic study. Urology 17: 377–380

1057. Fulker M J, Cooper E H, Tanaka T 1971 Proliferation and ultrastructure of papillary transitional cell carcinoma of the human bladder. Cancer 27: 71–82

1058. Gilchrist K W, Benson R C Jr, Albrecht R M, Kutchera A R, Inhorn S L 1982 Scanning electron microscopy after cytologic examination of urinary cells: lack of diagnostic advantage using combined microscopy. Acta Cytologica 26: 92–95

1059. Gilchrist K W, Benson R C Jr, Kutchera A R 1980 Pleomorphic microvilli and low-grade human urothelial cancer: need to correlate diagnostic modalities. Urology 15: 69–73

1060. Gonzalez E, Fowler M R, Venable D D 1982 Primary signet ring cell adenocarcinoma of the bladder (linitis plastica of the bladder): report of a case and review of the literature. Journal of Urology 128: 1027–1030

1061. Hodges G M 1978 Normal and neoplastic urothelium of human bladder in vivo and in vitro: an assessment of SEM studies. Scanning Electron Microscopy 2: 983–990

1062. Imahori S 1980 Nephrogenic adenoma of the urinary bladder: a light and electron microscopic study. Laboratory Investigation 42: 124–125A

1063. Imahori S C, Magoss I V 1980 Nephrogenic adenoma of bladder. Clinical and ultrastructural study. Urology 16: 310–312

1064. Iwata H, Yokoyama M, Morita M, Bekku T, Ochi K, Takeuchi M 1982 Inverted papilloma of urinary bladder. Scanning and transmission electron microscopic observation. Urology 19: 322–324

1065. Jacobs J B, Cohen S M, Farrow G M, Friedell G H 1981 Scanning electron microscopic features of human urinary bladder cancer. Cancer 48: 1399–1409

1066. Jao W, Soto J M, Gould V E 1975 Squamous carcinoma of bladder with pseudosarcomatous stroma. Archives of Pathology 99: 461–466

1067. Kjaer T B, Carlson S D, Nilsson T, Madsen P O 1976 Scanning electron microscopy of normal and malignant human urothelium. Urology 8: 59–62

1068. Koss L G 1977 Some ultrastructural aspects of experimental and human carcinoma of the bladder. Cancer Research 37: 2824–2835

1069. Kunze E, Schauer A, Schmitt M 1983 Histology and histogenesis of two different types of inverted urothelial papillomas. Cancer 51: 348–358

1070. Molland E A, Trott P A, Paris A M, Blandy J P 1976 Nephrogenic adenoma: a form of adenomatous metaplasia of the bladder. A clinical and electron microscopical study. British Journal of Urology 48: 453–462

1071. Nelson C E, Croft W A, Nilsson T 1979 Surface characteristics of malignant human urinary bladder epithelium studied with scanning electron microscopy. Scandinavian Journal of Urology and Nephrology 13: 31–42

1072. Newman J, Hicks R M 1978 Detection of neoplastic and preneoplastic urothelia by combined scanning and transmission electron microscopy of urinary surface of human and rat bladders. Histopathology 1: 125–135

1073. Newman J, Hicks R M 1981 Diffuse neoplastic change in urothelium from tumour-bearing human lower urinary tract. Scanning Electron Microscopy 3: 1–10

1074. Price D A, Morley A R, Hall R R 1980 Scanning electron microscopy in the study of normal, inflamed and neoplastic human urothelium. British Journal of Urology 52: 370–376

1075. Schnoy N, Leistenschneider W 1982 Tumor of mesonephric origin in a diverticulum of the urethra. An ultrastructural study. Virchows Archiv A Pathological Anatomy and Histology 397: 335–345

1076. Smith A F 1981 An ultrastructural and morphometric study of bladder tumours (I). Virchows Archiv A Pathological Anatomy and Histology 390: 11–21

1077. Smith A F 1982 An ultrastructural and morphometric study of bladder tumours (II). Virchows Archiv A Pathological Anatomy and Histology 396: 291–301

1078. Tanabe E T, Mazur M T, Schaeffer A J 1982 Clear cell adenocarcinoma of the female urethra: clinical and ultrastructural study suggesting a unique neoplasm. Cancer 49: 372–378

1079. Tannenbaum M 1976 Light and electron microscopy of urothelial cancer, carcinoma in situ. Urology 8: 498–501

1080. Tannenbaum M 1979 Lower urinary tract. In: Johannessen J V (ed) Electron microscopy in human medicine, vol 9. Urogenital system and breast. McGraw-Hill, New York, ch 15, p 193–224

1081. Tannenbaum M 1979 Ultrastructural pathology of the human urinary bladder. In: Trump B F, Jones R T (eds) Diagnostic electron microscopy, vol 2. John Wiley & Sons, New York, ch 5, p 163–219

1082. Tannenbaum M, Tannenbaum S, Carter H W 1978 SEM, BEI and TEM ultrastructural characteristics of normal, preneoplastic, and neoplastic human transitional epithelia. Scanning Electron Microscopy 2: 949–958

1083. Weinstein R S 1976 Changes in plasma membrane structure associated with malignant transformation in human urinary bladder epithelium. Cancer Research 36: 2518–2524

## 29 PROSTATIC TUMOURS

1084. Azzopardi J G, Evans D J 1971 Argentaffin cells in prostatic carcinoma: differentiation from lipofuscin and melanin in prostatic epithelium. Journal of Pathology 104: 247–251

1085. Brandes D, Kirchheim D 1977 Histochemistry of the prostate. In: Tannenbaum M (ed) Urologic pathology: the prostate. Lea & Febiger, Philadelphia, p 99–128

1086. Capella C, Usellini L, Buffa R, Frigerio B, Solcia E 1981 The endocrine component of prostatic carcinomas, mixed adenocarcinoma-carcinoid tumours and non-tumour prostate. Histochemical and ultrastructural identification of the endocrine cells. Histopathology 5: 175–192

1087. Epstein N A 1977 Primary papillary carcinoma of the prostate: report of a histologic, cytologic and electron microscopic study on one case. Acta Cytologica 21: 543–546

1088. Fisher E R, Sieracki J C 1970 Ultrastructure of human normal and neoplastic prostate. Pathology Annual 5: 1–26

1089. Gaeta J F, Berger J E, Gamarra M C 1977 Scanning electron microscopic study of prostatic cancer. Cancer Treatment Reports 61: 227–253

1090. Hassan M O, Maksem J 1980 The prostatic perineural space and its relation to tumor spread: an ultrastructural study. American Journal of Surgical Pathology 4: 143–148

1091. Heidger P M Jr, Feuchter F A, Hawtrey C E 1977 Scanning and transmission electron microscopy of human prostatic adenocarcinoma. In: Yates R D, Gordon M (eds) Male reproductive system. Fine structure analysis by scanning and transmission electron microscopy. Masson Publishing, U.S.A., New York, ch 11, p 185–205

1092. Kastendieck H, Altenähr E 1976 Cyto- and histomorphogenesis of the prostate carcinoma. A comparative light- and electron microscopic study. Virchows Archiv A Pathological Anatomy and Histology 370: 207–224

1093. Kern W H 1978 Well differentiated adenocarcinoma of the prostate. Cancer 41: 2046–2054

1094. Kirchheim D 1976 A critical review of histochemical and electronmicroscopical studies of total prostatectomy specimens. In: Marberger H et al (eds) Prostatic disease. New York, Liss, p 357–361

1095. Kudo S 1967 Electron microscopical studies on the prostatic epithelium. II. Fine structures of the human prostatic cancer. Kumamoto Medical Journal 20: 86–101

1096. Mao P, Nakao K, Angrist A 1966 Human prostatic carcinoma: an electron microscope study. Cancer Research 26: 955–973

1097. Melicow M M, Pachter M R 1967 Endometrial carcinoma of prostatic utricle — uterus masculinus. Cancer 20: 1715–1722

1098. Mickey D D, Stone K R, Stone M P, Paulson D F 1977 Morphologic and immunologic studies of human prostatic carcinoma. Cancer Treatment Reports 61: 133–138

1099. Mostofi F K, Price E B Jr 1973 Tumors of the male genital system. Atlas of tumor pathology, 2nd series, fascicle 8. Armed Forces Institute of Pathology, Washington DC, p 208–213

1100. Ohtsuki Y, Seman G, Maruyama K, Bowen J M, Johnson D E, Dmochowski L 1976 Ultrastructural studies of human prostatic neoplasia. Cancer 37: 2295–2305

1101. Sinha A A, Blackard C E 1973 Ultrastructure of prostatic benign hyperplasia and carcinoma. Urology 2: 114–120

1102. Stone M P, Stone K R, Paulson D F 1976 Scanning electron microscopy of hyperplastic and neoplastic human prostate. Urological Research 4: 71–75

1103. Tannenbaum M 1975 Carcinoma with sarcomatoid changes or carcinosarcoma of prostate. Urology 6: 91–93

1104. Tannenbaum M 1979 Male accessory organs: seminal vesicle, prostate, and testis. In: Johannessen J V (ed) Electron microscopy in human medicine, vol 9. Urogenital system and breast. McGraw-Hill, New York, ch 16, p 227–278

1105. Tannenbaum M, Tannenbaum S 1980 Ultrastructural pathology of human prostatic carcinoma. In: Trump B F, Jones R T (eds) Diagnostic electron microscopy, vol 3. John Wiley & Sons, New York, ch 4, p 175–201

1106. Tannenbaum M, Tannenbaum S, de Sanctis P N, Olsson C A 1982 Prognostic significance of nucleolar surface area in prostatic cancer. Urology 19: 546–551

1107. Trump B F, Heatfield B M, Phelps P C 1981 The role of the cytoskeleton and related components in normal and neoplastic prostatic epithelium. Progress in Clinical and Biological Research 75A: 25–53

1108. Wasserstein P W, Goldman R L 1981 Diffuse carcinoid of prostate. Urology 18: 407–409

1109. Zaloudek C, Williams J W, Kempson R L 1976 'Endometrial' adenocarcinoma of the prostate. A distinctive tumor of probable prostatic duct origin. Cancer 37: 2255–2262

## 30 TESTICULAR TUMOURS

1110. Able M E, Lee J C 1969 Ultrastructure of a Sertoli-cell adenoma of the testis. Cancer 23: 481–486

1111. Akhtar M, Sidiki Y 1979 Undifferentiated intratubular germ cell tumor of the testis. Light and electron microscopic study of a unique case. Cancer 43: 2332–2339

1112. Albrechtsen R, Nielsen M H, Skakkebaeck N E, Wewer U 1982 Carcinoma in situ of the testis. Some ultrastructural characteristics of germ cells. Acta Pathologica Microbiologica et Immunologica Scandinavica. Section A. Pathology 90: 301–303

1113. Altaffer L F III, Dufour D R, Castleberry G M, Steele S M Jr 1982 Coexisting rete testis adenoma and gonadoblastoma. Journal of Urology 127: 332–335

1114. Chakraborty J, Franco-Saenz R, Kropp K 1983 Electron microscopic study of testicular tumor of congenital adrenal hyperplasia. Human Pathology 14: 151–157

1115. Damjanov I, Klauber G 1980 Microscopic gonadoblastoma in dysgenetic gonad of an infant: an ultrastructural study. Urology 15: 605–609

1116. Dhom G, Hohbach Ch 1980 Case 10: benign interstitial cell tumor of the testes. Ultrastructural Pathology 1: 127–132

1117. Feldman P S, Kovacs K, Horvath E, Adelson G L 1982 Malignant Leydig cell tumor: clinical, histologic and electron microscopic features. Cancer 49: 714–721

1118. Fukunaga M, Aizawa S, Furusato M, Akasaka Y, Machida T 1982 Papillary adenocarcinoma of the rete testis. A case report. Cancer 50: 134–138

1119. Holstein A F, Körner F 1974 Light and electron microscopical analysis of cell types in human seminoma. Virchows Archiv A Pathological Anatomy and Histology 363: 97–112

1120. Janssen M, Johnston W H 1978 Anaplastic seminoma of the testis: ultrastructural analysis of three cases. Cancer 41: 538–544

1121. Kay S, Fu Y, Koontz W W, Chen A T 1975 Interstitial cell tumor of the testis: tissue culture and ultrastructural studies. American Journal of Clinical Pathology 63: 366–376

1122. Kirkland R T, Kirkland J L, Kennan B S, Bongiovanni A M, Rosenberg H S, Clayton G W 1977 Bilateral testicular tumors in congenital adrenal hyperplasia. Journal of Clinical Endocrinology and Metabolism 44: 369–378

1123. Koide O 1981 The fine structure of the seminoma cell nucleus. Journal of Clinical Electron Microscopy 14: 25–34

1124. Koide O, Iwai S 1981 An ultrastructural study on germinoma cells. Acta Pathologica Japonica 31: 755–766

1125. Nogales F F Jr, Matilla A, Ortega I, Alvarez T 1979 Mixed Brenner and adenomatoid tumor of the testis: an ultrastructural study and histogenetic considerations. Cancer 43: 539–543

1126. Perez-Atayde A R, Nunez A E, Carroll W L, Murthy A S K, Vaitukaitis J L, Watson D J, Bauer S B, Kozakewich H P W 1983 Large-cell calcifying Sertoli cell tumor of the testis. An ultrastructural, immunocytochemical, and biochemical study. Cancer 51: 2287–2292

1127. Pierce G B Jr 1966 Ultrastructure of human testicular tumors. Cancer 19: 1963–1983

1128. Pierce G B, Abell M R 1970 Embryonal carcinoma of the testis. Pathology Annual 5: 27–60

1129. Proppe K H, Dickersin G R 1982 Large-cell calcifying Sertoli cell tumor of the testis: light microscopic and ultrastructural study. Human Pathology 13: 1109–1114

1130. Raghavan D, Heyderman E, Monaghan P, Gibbs J, Rouslahti E, Peckham M J, Neville A M 1981 Hypothesis: when is a seminoma not a seminoma? Journal of Clinical Pathology 34: 123–128

1131. Rosai J, Khodadoust K, Silber I 1969 Spermatocytic seminoma. II. Ultrastructural study. Cancer 24: 103–116

1132. Saliba N S, Sawyer K C, Hall W W, Sawyer R B, Proctor H M, Shand J A 1966 Choriocarcinoma in the male patient presenting as gastrointestinal hemorrhage. American Journal of Surgery 112: 764–769

1133. Schulze C, Holstein A F 1977 On the histology of human seminoma: development of the solid tumor from intra-tubular seminoma cells. Cancer 39: 1090–1100

1134. Sohval A R, Churg J, Gabrilove J L, Freiberg E K, Katz N 1982 Ultrastructure of feminizing testicular Leydig cell tumors. Ultrastructural Pathology 3: 335–345

1135. Sohval A R, Churg J, Suzuki Y, Katz N, Gabrilove J L 1977 Electron microscopy of a feminizing Leydig cell tumor of the testis. Human Pathology 8: 621–634

1136. Sullivan J L, Packer J T, Bryant M 1981 Primary malignant carcinoid of the testis. Archives of Pathology and Laboratory Medicine 105: 515–517

1137. Sworn M J, Buchanan R 1981 Malignant interstitial cell tumor of the testis. Human Pathology 12: 72–77

1138. Talerman A, Gratama S, Miranda S, Okagaki T 1978 Primary carcinoid tumor of the testis: case report, ultrastructure and review of the literature. Cancer 42: 2696–2706

1139. Ueda G, Yamasaki M, Sato Y, Hiramatsu K, Matsumoto K 1976 Light and electron microscopic study of an intermediate Sertoli-Leydig cell tumor with a review of literatures in Japan. Acta Obstetrica et Gynaecologica Japonica 23: 14–22

## 31 ENDODERMAL SINUS TUMOUR

1140. Gonzalez-Crussi F 1979 The human yolk sac and yolk sac (endodermal sinus) tumors. A review. Perspectives in Pediatric Pathology 5: 179–215

1141. Gonzalez-Crussi F, Roth L M 1976 The human yolk sac and yolk sac carcinoma. An ultrastructural study. Human Pathology 7: 675–691

1142. Martinez-Hernandez A, Miller E J, Damjanov I, Gay S 1982 Laminin-secreting yolk sac carcinoma of the rat. Biochemical and electron immunohistochemical studies. Laboratory Investigation 47: 247–257

1143. Mukai K, Adams W R 1979 Yolk sac tumor of the anterior mediastinum. Case report with light- and electron microscopic examination and immunohistochemical study of alpha-fetoprotein. American Journal of Surgical Pathology 3: 77–83

1144. Nakanishi I, Kawahara E, Kajikawa K, Miwa A, Terahata S 1982 Hyaline globules in yolk sac tumor. Histochemical, immunohistochemical and electron microscopic studies. Acta Pathologica Japonica 32: 733–739

1145. Nogales F F Jr, Matilla A, Nogales-Ortiz F, Galera-Davidson H L 1978 Yolk sac tumors with pure and mixed polyvesicular vitelline patterns. Human Pathology 9: 553–566

1146. Nogales-Fernandez F, Silverberg S G, Bloustein P A, Martinez-Hernandez A, Pierce G B 1977 Yolk sac carcinoma (endodermal sinus tumor). Ultrastructure and histogenesis of gonadal and extragonadal tumors in comparison with normal human yolk sac. Cancer 39: 1462–1474

1147. Prat J, Bhan A K, Dickersin G R, Robboy S J, Scully R E 1982 Hepatoid yolk sac tumor of the ovary (endodermal sinus tumor with hepatoid differentiation). A light microscopic, ultrastructural and immunohistochemical study of seven cases. Cancer 50: 2355–2368

1148. Sass M, Jao W, Horn T, Keh P C 1983 Mediastinal yolk sac tumor: ultrastructural and immunofluorescent studies. Ultrastructural Pathology 4: 67–73

1149. Stachura I, Mendelow H 1980 Endodermal sinus tumor originating in the region of the pineal gland. Ultrastructural and immunohistochemical study. Cancer 45: 2131–2137

1150. Suganuma T, Takao S, Suzuki S, Tsuyama S, Nishi M, Murata F 1981 Ultrastructure and immunohistochemical staining of a transplanted endodermal sinus tumor. Virchows Archiv B Cell Pathology 38: 177–187

1151. Takei Y, Pearl G S 1981 Ultrastructural study of intracranial yolk sac tumor: with special reference to the oncologic phylogeny of germ cell tumors. Cancer 48: 2038–2046

## 32 GENERAL ASPECTS OF GYNAECOLOGICAL TUMOURS

1152. Ferenczy A 1976 The ultrastructural morphology of gynecologic neoplasms. Cancer 38: 463–486

1153. Ferenczy A 1979 Diagnostic electron microscopy in gynecologic pathology. Pathology Annual 14, pt 1: 353–381

1154. Ferenczy A, Fenoglio C M 1979 Female genital tract. In: Johannessen J V (ed) Electron microscopy in human medicine, vol 9. Urogenital system and breast. McGraw-Hill, New York, ch 18, p 297–384

1155. Ferenczy A, Richart R M 1979 Gynecology. In: Trump B F, Jones R T (eds) Diagnostic electron microscopy, vol 2. John Wiley & Sons, New York, ch 6, p 269–308

1156. Roth L M 1974 Clear-cell adenocarcinoma of the female genital tract. A light and electron microscopic study. Cancer 33: 990–1001

1157. Steeper T A, Piscioli F, Rosai J 1983 Squamous cell carcinoma with sarcoma-like stroma of the female genital tract. Clinicopathologic study of four cases. Cancer 52: 890–898

1158. Tang C K, Toker C, Wybel R E, Desai R G 1981 An unusual pelvic tumor with benign glandular, sarcomatous, and Wilms' tumor-like components. Human Pathology 12: 940–944

## 33 TUMOURS OF THE VAGINA AND VULVA

1159. Dickersin G R, Welch W R, Erlandson R, Robboy S J 1980 Ultrastructure of 16 cases of clear cell adenocarcinoma of the vagina and cervix in young women. Cancer 45: 1615–1624

1160. Fenoglio C M, Ferenczy A, Richart R M, Townsend D 1976 Scanning and transmission electron microscopic studies of vaginal adenosis and the cervical transformation zone in progeny exposed in utero to diethylstilbestrol. American Journal of Obstetrics and Gynecology 126: 170–180

1161. Genton C Y, Kunz J, Schreiner W E 1981 Primary malignant melanoma of the vagina and cervix uteri. Report of a case with ultrastructural study. Virchows Archiv A Pathological Anatomy and Histology 393: 245–250

1162. Hasumi K, Sakamoto G, Sugano H, Kasuga T, Masubuchi K 1978 Primary malignant melanoma of the vagina: study of four autopsy cases with ultrastructural findings. Cancer 42: 2675–2686

1163. Hinchey W W, Silva E G, Guarda L A, Ordonez N G, Wharton J T 1983 Paravaginal Wolffian duct (mesonephros) adenocarcinoma: a light and electron microscopic study. American Journal of Clinical Pathology 80: 539–544

1164. Kuzuya K, Matsuyama M, Nishi Y, Chihara T, Suchi T 1981 Ultrastructure of adenocarcinoma of Bartholin's gland. Cancer 48: 1392–1398

1165. Okagaki T, Ishida T, Hilgers R D 1976 A malignant tumor of the vagina resembling synovial sarcoma. A light and electron microscopic study. Cancer 37: 2306–2320

1166. Rastkar G, Okagaki T, Twiggs L B, Clark B A 1982 Early invasive and in situ warty carcinoma of the vulva: clinical, histologic, and electron microscopic study with particular reference to viral association. American Journal of Obstetrics and Gynecology 143: 814–820

1167. Rich P M, Okagaki T, Clark B, Prem K A 1981 Adenocarcinoma of the sweat gland of the vulva: light and electron microscopic study. Cancer 47: 1352–1357

1168. Sherman A I, Steger R W, Hafez E S, Brown S 1975 Human vaginal adenosis and adenocarcinoma. Journal of Reproductive Medicine 14: 221–227

1169. Shevchuk M M, Fenoglio C M, Lattes R, Frick H C II, Richart R M 1978 Malignant mixed tumor of the vagina probably arising in mesonephric rests. Cancer 42: 214–223

1170. Silverberg S G, DeGiorgi L S 1972 Clear cell carcinoma of the vagina. A clinical, pathologic, and electron microscopic study. Cancer 29: 1680–1690

1171. Ulbright T M, Alexander R W, Kraus F T 1981 Intramural papilloma of the vagina: evidence of Müllerian histogenesis. Cancer 48: 2260–2266

## 34 TUMOURS OF THE UTERINE CERVIX

1172. Albores-Saavedra J, Larraza O, Poucell S, Martinez H A R 1976 Carcinoid tumor of the uterine cervix. Additional observations on a new tumor entity. Cancer 38: 2328–2342

1173. Albores-Saavedra J, Rodrígues-Martínez H A, Larraza-Hernández O 1979 Carcinoid tumors of the cervix. Pathology Annual 14, pt 1: 273–291

1174. Bhowmick K D, Mitra A 1968 Ultrastructural morphology of squamous carcinoma of human exocervix. Indian Journal of Medical Research 56: 282–287

1175. Ferenczy A 1977 Carcinoma and other malignant tumors of the cervix. In: Blaustein A (ed) Pathology of the female genital tract. Springer-Verlag, New York, ch 9, p 171–205

1176. Habib A, Kaneko M, Cohen C J, Walker G 1979 Carcinoid of the uterine cervix. A case report with light and electron microscopic studies. Cancer 43: 535–538

1177. Hall-Craggs M, Toker C, Nedwich A 1981 Carcinosarcoma of the uterine cervix: a light and electron microscopic study. Cancer 48: 161–169

1178. Ito E, Kudo R 1982 Scanning electron microscopy of normal cells, dyskaryotic cells and malignant cells exfoliated from the uterine cervix. Acta Cytologica 26: 457–465

1179. Kaufman R H 1967 Dysplasia and carcinoma in situ of the cervix. Clinical Obstetrics and Gynecology 10: 748–784

1180. Kott M M, Silva E G, Ordonez N G 1983 Neuroendocrine carcinoma, carcinoid type, of the cervix. Laboratory Investigation 48: 46A

1181. Lawrence W D, Shingleton H M, Gore H, Soong S J 1980 Ultrastructural and morphometric study of diethylstilbestrol-associated lesions diagnosed as cervical intraepithelial neoplasia III. Cancer Research 40: 1558–1567

1182. Mackay B, Osborne B M, Wharton J T 1979 Small cell tumor of cervix with neuroepithelial features. Ultrastructural observations in two cases. Cancer 43: 1138–1145

1183. Matsuyama M, Inoue T, Ariyoshi Y, Doi M, Suchi T, Sato T, Tashiro K, Chihara T 1979 Argyrophil cell carcinoma of the uterine cervix with ectopic production of ACTH, β-MSH, serotonin, histamine, and amylase. Cancer 44: 1813–1823

1184. Mazur M T, Battifora H A 1982 Adenoid cystic carcinoma of the uterine cervix: ultrastructure, immunofluorescence, and criteria for diagnosis. American Journal of Clinical Pathology 77: 494–500

1185. Mullins J D, Hilliard G D 1981 Cervical carcinoid ('argyrophil cell' carcinoma) associated with an endocervical adenocarcinoma: a light and ultrastructural study. Cancer 47: 785–790

1186. Murphy J F, Allen J M, Jordan J A, Williams A E 1975 Scanning electron microscopy of normal and abnormal exfoliated cervical squamous cells. British Journal of Obstetrics and Gynaecology 82: 44–51

1187. Murphy J F, Jordan J A, Allen J M, Williams A E 1974 Correlation of scanning electron microscopy, colposcopy and histology in 50 patients presenting with abnormal cervical cytology. Journal of Obstetrics and Gynaecology of the British Commonwealth 81: 236–241

1188. Paulsen S M, Hansen K C, Nielsen V T 1980 Glassy-cell carcinoma of the cervix: case report with a light and electron microscopy study. Ultrastructural Pathology 1: 377–384

1189. Pilotti S, Rilke F, DePalo G, Della Torre G, Alasio L 1981 Condylomata of the uterine cervix and koilocytosis of cervical intraepithelial neoplasia. Journal of Clinical Pathology 34: 532–541

1190. Praphat H, Ruffolo E H, Copeland W J, Richman A V, Cavanagh D 1980 Carcinoma of the cervix: a diagnostic problem. American Journal of Obstetrics and Gynecology 137: 514–516

1191. Puri S, Fenoglio C M, Richart R M, Townsend D 1977 Clear cell carcinoma of cervix and vagina in progeny of women who received diethylstilbestrol. Three cases with scanning and transmission electron microscopy. American Journal of Obstetrics and Gynecology 128: 550–555

1192. Richart R M 1973 Cervical intraepithelial neoplasia. Pathology Annual 8: 301–328

1193. Roth L M, Pride G L, Sharma H M 1976 Müllerian adenosarcoma of the uterine cervix with heterologous elements. A light and electron microscopic study. Cancer 37: 1725–1736

1194. Rubio C A, Einhorn N 1977 The exfoliating epithelial surface of the uterine cervix. IV. Scanning electron microscopical study in invasive squamous carcinoma of human subjects. Beiträge zur Pathologie 161: 72–81

1195. Rubio C A, Kranz I 1976 The exfoliating cervical epithelial surface in dysplasia, carcinoma in situ and invasive squamous carcinoma. I. Scanning electron microscopic study. Acta Cytologica 20: 144–150

1196. Ruiter D J, Boon M E 1982 Atypical indifferent (reserve) cells in the cervical epithelium and their exfoliative pattern. Acta Cytologica 26: 292–298

1197. Searle J, Collins D J, Harmon B, Kerr J F R 1973 The spontaneous occurrence of apoptosis in squamous carcinomas of the uterine cervix. Pathology 5: 163–169

1198. Shingleton H M, Lawrence W D, Gore H 1977 Cervical carcinoma with adenoid cystic pattern. A light and electron microscopic study. Cancer 40: 1112–1121

1199. Shingleton H M, Richart R M, Wiener J, Spiro D 1968 Human cervical intraepithelial neoplasia: fine structure of dysplasia and carcinoma in situ. Cancer Research 28: 695–706

1200. Shingleton H M, Wilbanks G D 1974 Fine structure of human cervical intraepithelial neoplasia in vivo and in vitro. Cancer 33: 981–989

1201. Stanbridge D M, Butler E B, Langley F A 1980 Problems in cervicovaginal cytology: fine structure as an aid to diagnosis. Acta Cytologica 24: 335–343

1202. Stegner H E 1981 Precursors of cervical cancer: ultrastructural morphology. Current Topics in Pathology 70: 171–193

1203. Tang C K, Toker C, Harriman B 1981 Müllerian adenosarcoma of the uterine cervix. Human Pathology 12: 579–581

1204. Tateishi R, Wada A, Hayakawa K, Hongo J, Ishii S, Terakawa N 1975 Argyrophil cell carcinomas (apudomas) of the uterine cervix: light and electron microscopic observations of five cases. Virchows Archiv A Pathological Anatomy and Histology 366: 257–274

1205. Ulbright T M, Gersell D J 1983 Glassy cell carcinoma of the uterine cervix. A light and electron microscopic study of five cases. Cancer 51: 2255–2263

1206. Wiernick G, Bradbury S, Plant M, Cowdell R H, Williams E A 1973 A quantitative comparison between normal and carcinomatous squamous epithelia of the uterine cervix. British Journal of Cancer 28: 488–499

1207. Zaino R J, Nahhas W A, Mortel R 1982 Glassy cell carcinoma of the uterine cervix. An ultrastructural study and review. Archives of Pathology and Laboratory Medicine 106: 250–254

## 35 TUMOURS OF THE UTERINE CORPUS AND FALLOPIAN TUBES

1208. Aikawa M, Ng A B P 1973 Mixed (adenosquamous) carcinoma of the endometrium: electron microscopic observations. Cancer 31: 385–397

1209. Akhtar M, Kim P Y, Young I 1975 Ultrastructure of endometrial stromal sarcoma. Cancer 35: 406–412

1210. Bibro M C, Livolsi V A, Schwartz P E 1979 Adenosarcoma of the uterus: ultrastructural observations. American Journal of Clinical Pathology 71: 112–117

1211. Böcker W, Stegner H-E 1975 A light and electron microscopic study of endometrial sarcomas of the uterus. Virchows Archiv A Pathological Anatomy and Histology 368: 141–156

1212. Böcker W, Stegner H-E 1975 Mixed Müllerian tumors of the uterus. Ultrastructural studies on the differentiation of rhabdomyoblasts. Virchows Archiv A Pathological Anatomy and Histology 365: 337–349

1213. Boram L H, Erlandson R A, Hajdu S I 1972 Mesodermal mixed tumor of the uterus. A cytologic, histologic, and electron microscopic correlation. Cancer 30: 1295–1306

1214. Cash J B, Powell D E 1980 Placental chorioangioma: presentation of a case with electron microscopic and immunochemical studies. American Journal of Surgical Pathology 4: 87–92

1215. Cozzutto C 1981 Uterus-like mass replacing ovary. Archives of Pathology and Laboratory Medicine 105: 508–511

1216. Crum C P, Rogers B H, Andersen W 1980 Osteosarcoma of the uterus: case report and review of the literature. Gynecologic Oncology 9: 256–268

1217. Demopoulos R I, Sitelman A, Flotte T, Bigelow B 1980 Ultrastructural study of a female adnexal tumor of probable Wolffian origin. Cancer 46: 2273–2280

1218. Fenoglio C M, Crum C P, Ferenczy A 1982 Endometrial hyperplasia and carcinoma. Are ultrastructural, biochemical and immunocytochemical studies useful in distinguishing between them? Pathology Research and Practice 174: 257–284

1219. Ferenczy A 1982 Cytodynamics of endometrial hyperplasia and carcinoma. I. Histology and ultrastructure. Progress in Surgical Pathology 4: 95–113

1220. Ferenczy A, Richart R M 1972 Scanning electron microscopic study of normal and molar trophoblast. Gynecologic Oncology 1: 95–110

1221. Fisher E R, Paulson J D, Gregorio R M 1978 The myofibroblastic nature of the uterine plexiform tumor. Archives of Pathology and Laboratory Medicine 102: 477–480

1222. Gloor E, Hürlimann J 1981 Trophoblastic pseudotumor of the uterus. Clinicopathologic report with immuno-histochemical and ultrastructural studies. American Journal of Surgical Pathology 5: 5–13

1223. Gompel C 1971 Ultrastructure of endometrial carcinoma. Review of fourteen cases. Cancer 28: 745–754

1224. Gonzalez-Angulo A, Marquez-Monter H, Zavala B J, Yabur E, Salazar H 1966 Electron microscopic observations in hydatidiform mole. Obstetrics and Gynecology 27: 455–467

1225. Goodhue W W, Susin M, Kramer E E 1974 Smooth muscle origin of uterine plexiform tumors. Archives of Pathology 97: 263–268

1226. Grimalt M, Arguelles M, Ferenczy A 1975 Papillary cystadenofibroma of endometrium: a histochemical and ultrastructural study. Cancer 36: 137–144

1227. Hameed K, Morgan D A 1972 Papillary adenocarcinoma of endometrium with psammoma bodies. Histology and fine structure. Cancer 29: 1326–1335

1228. Hendrickson M R, Kempson R L 1980 Surgical pathology of the uterine corpus. W B Saunders, Philadelphia

1229. Joelsson I, Ingelman-Sundberg A, Granberg I, Nilsson L 1975 Scanning electron microscopy of carcinoma of the uterine corpus. Journal of Reproductive Medicine 14: 219–220

1230. Johnson L, Diamond I, Jolly G 1978 Ultrastructure of fallopian tube carcinoma. Cancer 42: 1291–1297

1231. Kanbour A I, Burgess F, Salazar H 1973 Intramural adenofibroma of the fallopian tube. Light and electron microscopy. Cancer 31: 1433–1439

1232. Katzenstein A-L, Askin F B, Feldman P S 1977 Müllerian adenosarcoma of the uterus. An ultrastructural study of four cases. Cancer 40: 2233–2242

1233. Kindblom L-G, Seidal T 1981 Malignant giant cell tumor of the uterus. A clinico-pathologic, light- and electron-microscopic study of a case. Acta Pathologica et Microbiologica Scandinavica. Section A. Pathology 89: 179–184

1234. Klemi P J, Grönroos M, Rauramo L, Punnonen R 1980 Ultrastructural features of endometrial atypical adenomatous hyperplasia and adenocarcinoma and the plasma level of oestrogens. Gynecologic Oncology 9: 162–169

1235. Komorowski R A, Garancis J C, Clowry L J Jr 1970 Fine structure of endometrial stromal sarcoma. Cancer 26: 1042–1047

1236. Kudo R, Komori A, Hashimoto M 1973 Ultrastructural study of endometrial stromal sarcoma or stromal endometriosis. Acta Obstetrica et Gynaecologica Japonica 20: 72–78

1237. Larsen J F 1973 Ultrastructure of the abnormal human trophoblast. Acta Anatomica 86, suppl 61: 47–74

1238. Larsen J F, Ehrmann R L, Bierring F 1967 Electron microscopy of human choriocarcinoma transplanted into hamster liver. American Journal of Obstetrics and Gynecology 99: 1109–1124

1239. Mazur M T, Askin F B 1978 Endolymphatic stromal myosis. Unique presentation and ultrastructural study. Cancer 42: 2661–2667

1240. Mazur M T, Kraus F T 1980 Histogenesis of morphologic variations in tumors of the uterine wall. American Journal of Surgical Pathology 4: 59–74

1241. McCarty K S Jr, Barton T K, Peete C H Jr, Creasman W T 1978 Gonadal dysgenesis with adenocarcinoma of the endometrium: an electron microscopic and steroid receptor analysis with a review of the literature. Cancer 42: 512–520

1242. Miles P A, Herrera G A, Greenberg H, Trujillo I 1982 Müllerian adenofibroma of the endometrium. A report of a case with ultrastructural study. Diagnostic Gynecology and Obstetrics 4: 215–221

1243. Mukai K, Varela-Duran J, Nochomovitz L E 1980 The rhabdomyoblast in mixed Müllerian tumors of the uterus and ovary. Laboratory Investigation 42: 138A

1244. Nunez-Alonso C, Battifora H 1979 Plexiform tumors of the uterus. Ultrastructural study. Cancer 44: 1707–1714

1245. Ober S B, Labay G R 1972 The histopathology of the endometrium: selected topics. Obstetrics and Gynecology Annual 1: 373–420

1246. Olson N, Twiggs L, Sibley R 1982 Small-cell carcinoma of the endometrium: light microscopic and ultrastructural study of a case. Cancer 50: 760–765

1247. Orenstein H H, Richart R M, Fenoglio C M 1980 Müllerian adenosarcoma of the uterus: literature review, case report, and ultrastructural observations. Ultrastructural Pathology 1: 189–200

1248. Paulsen S M, Nielsen V T, Hansen P, Ferenczy A 1982 Endolymphatic stromal myosis with focal tubular-glandular differentiation (biphasic endometrial stromal sarcoma). Ultrastructural Pathology 3: 31–42

1249. Perkins D G, Kopp C M, Haust M D 1980 Placental infiltration in congenital neuroblastoma: a case study with ultrastructure. Histopathology 4: 383–389

1250. Rorat E, Ferenczy A, Richart R M 1974 The ultrastructure of clear cell adenocarcinoma of endometrium. Cancer 33: 880–887

1251. Silverberg S G, DeGiorgi L S 1973 Clear cell carcinoma of the endometrium. Clinical, pathologic, and ultrastructural findings. Cancer 31: 1127–1140

1252. Silverberg S G, Wilson M A, Board J A 1971 Hemangiopericytoma of the uterus: an ultrastructural study. American Journal of Obstetrics and Gynecology 110: 397–404

1253. Talamo T S, Bender B L, Ellis L D, Scioscia E A 1982 Adenocarcinoma of the fallopian tube. An ultrastructural study. Virchows Archiv A Pathological Anatomy and Histology 397: 363–368

1254. Tang C K, Toker C, Ances I G 1979 Stromomyoma of the uterus. Cancer 43: 308–316

1255. Thrasher T V, Richart R M 1972 An ultrastructural comparison of endometrial adenocarcinoma and normal endometrium. Cancer 29: 1713–1723

1256. Ulbright T M, Kraus F T 1981 Endometrial stromal tumors of extra-uterine tissue. American Journal of Clinical Pathology 76: 371–377

1257. White A J, Buchsbaum H J 1974 Scanning electron microscopy of the human endometrium. II. Hyperplasia and adenocarcinoma. Gynecologic Oncology 2: 1–8

1258. Wynn R M, Ferenczy A 1979 Placenta. In: Johannessen J V (ed) Electron microscopy in human medicine, vol 9. Urogenital system and breast. McGraw-Hill, New York, ch 19, p 387–405

1259. Wynn R M, Harris J A 1967 Ultrastructure of trophoblast and endometrium in invasive hydatidiform mole (chorioadenoma destruens). American Journal of Obstetrics and Gynecology 99: 1125–1135

1260. Zaharopoulos P, Wong J Y, Lamke C R 1982 Endometrial stromal sarcoma. Cytology of pulmonary metastasis including ultrastructural study. Acta Cytologica 26: 49–54


## 36 OVARIAN TUMOURS

1261. Addis B J, Fox H 1983 Papillary mesothelioma of ovary. Histopathology 7: 287–298

1262. Amin H K, Okagaki T, Richart R M 1971 Classification of fibroma and thecoma of the ovary. An ultrastructural study. Cancer 27: 438–446

1263. Arhelger R B, Kelly B 1974 Strumal carcinoid: report of a case with electron microscopical observations. Archives of Pathology 97: 323–325

1264. Bigelow B, Blaustein A 1978 Paneth cells in a mucinous cystadenoma of the ovary: light and electron microscopic study. Gynecologic Oncology 6: 391–394

1265. Bjersing L, Cajander S 1977 Ultrastructure of gonadoblastoma and dysgerminoma (seminoma) in a patient with XY gonadal dysgenesis. Cancer 40: 1127–1137

1266. Bjersing L, Frankendal B, Angstrom T 1973 Studies on a feminizing ovarian mesenchymoma (granulosa cell tumor). I. Aspiration biopsy cytology, histology and ultrastructure. Cancer 32: 1360–1369

1267. Blaustein A 1979 Calcitonin secreting struma-carcinoid tumor of the ovary. Human Pathology 10: 223–228

1268. Bransilver B R, Ferenczy A, Richart R M 1974 Brenner tumors and Walthard cell nests. Archives of Pathology 98: 76–86

1269. Chalvardjian A, Derzko C 1982 Gynandroblastoma. Its ultrastructure. Cancer 50: 710–721

1270. Cramer S F, Bruns D E 1979 Amylase-producing ovarian neoplasm with pseudo-Meigs' syndrome and elevated pleural fluid amylase. Case report and ultrastructure. Cancer 44: 1715–1721

1271. Cummins P A, Fox H, Langley F A 1973 An electron microscope study of a dysgenetic gonad containing a focus of apparent gonadoblastoma. Journal of Pathology 110: P iv

1272. Cummins P A, Fox H, Langley F A 1973 An ultrastructural study of the nature and origin of the Brenner tumour of the ovary. Journal of Pathology 110: 167–176

1273. Cummins P A, Fox H, Langley F A 1974 Electron microscopic study of endometrioid adenocarcinoma of the ovary and comparison of its fine structure with that of normal endometrium and that of adenocarcinoma of the endometrium. Journal of Pathology 113: 165–173

1274. Czernobilsky B 1977 Primary epithelial tumors of the ovary. In: Blaustein A (ed) Pathology of the female genital tract. Springer-Verlag, New York, ch 24, p 453–504

1275. Czernobilsky B, Dgani R, Roth L M 1983 Ovarian mucinous cystadenocarcinoma with mural nodule of carcinomatous derivation. A light and electron microscopic study. Cancer 51: 141–148

1276. Damjanov I, Drobnjak P, Grizelj V 1975 Ultrastructure of gonadoblastoma. Archives of Pathology 99: 25–31

1277. Dickersin G R, Kline I W, Scully R E 1982 Small cell carcinoma of the ovary with hypercalcemia: a report of eleven cases. Cancer 49: 188–197

1278. Fenoglio C M 1980 Overview article: ultrastructural features of the common epithelial tumors of the ovary. Ultrastructural Pathology 1: 419–444

1279. Fenoglio C M, Castadot M J, Ferenczy A, Cottral G A, Richart R M 1977 Serous tumors of the ovary. I. Ultrastructural and histochemical studies of the epithelium of the benign serous neoplasms, serous cystadenoma and serous cystadenofibroma. Gynecologic Oncology 5: 203–218

1280. Fenoglio C M, Ferenczy A, Richart R M 1975 Mucinous tumors of the ovary. Ultrastructural studies of mucinous cystadenomas with histogenetic considerations. Cancer 36: 1709–1722

1281. Fenoglio C M, Ferenczy A, Richart R M 1976 Mucinous tumors of the ovary. II. Ultrastructural features of mucinous cystadenocarcinomas. American Journal of Obstetrics and Gynecology 125: 990–999

1282. Fenoglio C M, Puri S, Richart R M 1978 The ultrastructure of endometrioid carcinomas of the ovary. Gynecologic Oncology 6: 152–164

1283. Ferenczy A, Talens M, Zoghby M, Hussain S S 1977 Ultrastructural studies on the morphogenesis of psammoma bodies in ovarian serous neoplasia. Cancer 39: 2451–2459

1284. Fetissof F, Dubois M P, Arbeille-Brassart B, Lanson Y, Boivin F, Jobard P 1983 Endocrine cells in the prostate gland, urothelium and Brenner tumors. Immunohistological and ultrastructural studies. Virchows Archiv B Cell Pathology 42: 53–64

1285. Flotte T J, Bell D A 1980 Langerhans cells in ovarian benign cystic teratomas. Laboratory Investigation 42: 117A

1286. Garcia-Bunuel R, Brandes D 1976 Luteoma of pregnancy: ultrastructural features. Human Pathology 7: 205–214

1287. Garrido F S, Herrera I, Alonso F S 1976 Ovarian dysgerminoma: an ultrastructural study. Journal of Reproductive Medicine 16: 310–314

1288. Genton C Y 1979 Ultrastructure of clear cell carcinoma of the ovary. Case report and review of the literature. Virchows Archiv A Pathological Anatomy and Histology 385: 77–91

1289. Genton C Y 1980 Ovarian Sertoli-Leydig cell tumors. A clinical, pathological and ultrastructural study with particular reference to the histogenesis of these tumors. Archives of Gynecology 230: 49–75

1290. Genton C Y 1980 Some observations on the fine structure of human granulosa cell tumors. Virchows Archiv A Pathological Anatomy and Histology 387: 353–369

1291. Gondos B 1969 Ultrastructure of a metastatic granulosa-theca cell tumor. Cancer 24: 954–959

1292. Gondos B 1971 Electron microscope study of papillary serous tumors of the ovary. Cancer 27: 1455–1464

1293. Greco M A, Li Volsi V A, Pertschuk L P, Bigelow B 1979 Strumal carcinoid of the ovary. An analysis of its components. Cancer 43: 1380–1388

1294. Green J A, Maqueo M 1966 Histopathology and ultrastructure of an ovarian hilar cell tumor. American Journal of Obstetrics and Gynecology 96: 478–485

1295. Guérard M J, Ferenczy A, Arguelles M A 1982 Ovarian Sertoli-Leydig cell tumor with rhabdomyosarcoma: an ultrastructural study. Ultrastructural Pathology 3: 347–358

1296. Haid M, Victor T A, Weldon-Linne M, Danforth D N 1983 Malignant Brenner tumor of the ovary. Electron microscopic study of a case responsive to radiation and chemotherapy. Cancer 51: 498–508

1297. Harris M, Balgobin B 1978 Pure Sertoli cell tumor of the ovary: report of a case with ultrastructural observations. Histopathology 2: 449–459

1298. Hayden M T 1981 Bilateral malignant Brenner tumor: report of a case with ultrastructural study. Human Pathology 12: 89–92

1299. Hertel B F, Kempson R L 1977 Ovarian sex cord tumors with annular tubules. An ultrastructural study. American Journal of Surgical Pathology 1: 145–153

1300. Hou-Jensen K, Kempson R L 1974 The ultrastructure of gonadoblastoma and dysgerminoma. Human Pathology 5: 79–91

1301. Ioachim H L, Dorsett B H, Sabbath M, Barber H R 1975 Electron microscopy, tissue culture and immunology of ovarian carcinoma. National Cancer Institute Monograph 42: 45–62

1302. Ishida T, Okagaki T, Tagatz G E, Jacobsen M E, Doe R P 1977 Lipid cell tumor of the ovary: an ultrastructural study. Cancer 40: 234–243

1303. Ishida T, Tagatz G E, Okagaki T 1976 Gonadoblastoma. Ultrastructural evidence for testicular origin. Cancer 37: 1770–1781

1304. Kao G F, Norris H J 1978 Benign and low grade variants of mixed mesodermal tumor (adenosarcoma) of the ovary and adnexal region. Cancer 42: 1314–1324

1305. Kay S, Silverberg S G, Schatzki P F 1972 Ultrastructure of an ovarian dysgerminoma. Report of a case featuring neurosecretory-type granules in stromal cells. American Journal of Clinical Pathology 58: 458–468

1306. Klemi P J, Nevalainen T J 1978 Pathology of mucinous ovarian cystadenomas. 2. Ultrastructural findings. Acta Pathologica et Microbiologica Scandinavica. Section A. Pathology 86: 471–481

1307. Koss L G, Rothschild E O, Fleisher M, Francis J E Jr 1969 Masculinizing tumor of the ovary, apparently with adrenocortical activity. A histologic, ultrastructural and biochemical study. Cancer 23: 1245–1258

1308. Lack E E, Perez-Atayde A R, Murthy A S K, Goldstein D P, Crigler J F Jr, Vawter G F 1981 Granulosa theca cell tumors in premenarchal girls: a clinical and pathologic study of ten cases. Cancer 48: 1846–1854

1309. Livnat E J, Scommegna A, Racant W, Jao W 1977 Ultrastructural observations of the so-called strumal carcinoid of the ovary. Archives of Pathology and Laboratory Medicine 101: 585–589

1310. Ludena M D, Bullon A, Merchan M A 1982 Brenner tumor with argentaffin cells. An ultrastructural study. Morfología Normal y Patológica 6: 331–335

1311. Luse S A, Vietti T 1968 Ovarian teratoma. Ultrastructure and neural component. Cancer 21: 38–52

1312. Lynn J A, Varon H H, Kingsley W P, Martin J H 1967 Ultrastructural and biochemical analysis of estrogen secretory capacity of a nonfunctional ovarian neoplasm (dysgerminoma). American Journal of Pathology 51: 639–661

1313. Macaulay M A, Weliky I, Schulz R A 1967 Ultrastructure of a biosynthetically active granulosa cell tumor. Laboratory Investigation 17: 562–570

1314. Mackay A M, Pettigrew N, Symington T, Neville A M 1974 Tumors of dysgenetic gonads (gonadoblastoma): ultrastructural and steroidogenic aspects. Cancer 34: 1108–1125

1315. Murad T M, Mancini R, George J 1973 Ultrastructure of a virilizing ovarian Sertoli-Leydig cell tumor with familial incidence. Cancer 31: 1440–1450

1316. Ohkawa K, Amasaki H, Terashima Y, Aizawa S, Ishikawa E 1977 Clear cell carcinoma of the ovary: light and electron microscopic studies. Cancer 40: 3019–3029

1317. Okagaki T, Richart R M 1970 'Mesonephroma ovarii (hypernephroid carcinoma)'. Light microscopy and ultrastructural study of a case. Cancer 26: 453–461

1318. Papadaki L, Beilby J O 1975 Ovarian cystadenofibroma: a consideration of the role of estrogen in its pathogenesis. American Journal of Obstetrics and Gynecology 121 501–512

1319. Paradisi R, Venturoli S, Martinelli G, Serra L, Govoni E, Fabbri R, Flamigni C 1982 In vivo endocrine studies and morphological features in a case of hilus cell tumor in mesovarium. Gynecologic and Obstetric Investigation 14: 184–194

1320. Pardo-Mindan F J, Vazquez J J 1983 Malignant struma ovarii. Light and electron microscopic study. Cancer 51: 337–343

1321. Pratt-Thomas H R, Kreutner A Jr, Underwood P B, Dowdeswell R H 1976 Proliferative and malignant Brenner tumors of ovary. Report of two cases, one with Meigs' syndrome: review of literature and ultrastructural comparisons. Gynecologic Oncology 4: 176–193

1322. Ramzy I 1976 Signet-ring stromal tumor of ovary. Histochemical, light, and electron microscopic study. Cancer 38: 166–172

1323. Ramzy I, Bos C 1976 Sertoli cell tumors of ovary. Light microscopic and ultrastructural study with histogenetic considerations. Cancer 38: 2447–2456

1324. Ranchod M, Kempson R L, Dorgeloh J R 1976 Strumal carcinoid of the ovary. Cancer 37: 1913–1922

1325. Reddick R L, Walton L A 1982 Sertoli-Leydig cell tumor of the ovary with teratomatous differentiation. Clinico-pathologic considerations. Cancer 50: 1171–1176

1326. Robboy S J, Norris H F, Scully R E 1975 Insular carcinoid primary in the ovary. A clinicopathologic analysis of 48 cases. Cancer 36: 404–418

1327. Roberts D K, Marshall R B, Wharton J T 1970 Ultrastructure of ovarian tumors. I. Papillary serous cystadenocarcinoma. Cancer 25: 947–958

1328. Roberts D K, Wharton J T, Marshall R B, Horbelt D V 1975 Ovarian tumors: the ultrastructure of benign serous cystadenomas. Journal of the Kansas Medical Society 76: 132–134

1329. Roth L M 1971 Fine structure of the Brenner tumor. Cancer 27: 1482–1488

1330. Roth L M 1974 The Brenner tumor and the Walthard cell nest. An electron microscopic study. Laboratory Investigation 31: 15–23

1331. Roth L M, Liban E, Czernobilsky B 1982 Ovarian endometrioid tumors mimicking Sertoli and Sertoli-Leydig cell tumors. Sertoliform variant of endometrioid carcinoma. Cancer 50: 1322–1331

1332. Roth L M, Nicholas T R, Ehrlich C E 1979 Juvenile granulosa cell tumor. A clinicopathological study of three cases with ultrastructural observations. Cancer 44: 2194–2205

1333. Russell P, Bannatyne P 1983 Test and teach, number thirty-seven. Mucinous ovarian tumor with giant cell mural nodule. Pathology 15: 13–14, 99–100

1334. Russell P, Wills E J, Schweitzer P, Bannatyne P M 1981 Mucinous ovarian tumours with giant cell nodules: A report of two cases. Diagnostic Gynecology and Obstetrics 3: 233–249

1335. Schnoy N 1982 Ultrastructure of a virilizing ovarian Leydig-cell-tumor. Hilar cell tumor. Virchows Archiv A Pathological Anatomy and Histology 397: 17–27

1336. Sens M A, Levenson T B, Metcalf J S 1982 A case of metastatic carcinoid arising in an ovarian teratoma. Cancer 49: 2541–2546

1337. Serratoni F T, Robboy S J 1975 Ultrastructure of primary and metastatic ovarian carcinoids: analysis of 11 cases. Cancer 36: 157–160

1338. Shevchuk M M, Fenoglio C M, Richart R M 1980 Histogenesis of Brenner tumors, I: histology and ultrastructure. Cancer 46: 2607–2616

1339. Shikary A, Petrelli M, Hamilton P, Reid J D 1981 The Brenner tumor. A report of multiple tumors. Archives of Pathology and Laboratory Medicine 105: 207–213

1340. Stapleton J J, Haber M H, Lindner L E 1981 Paramesonephric papillary serous cystadenocarcinoma: a case report with scanning electron microscopy. Acta Cytologica 25: 310–316

1341. Stenbäck F 1980 Morphology of ovarian mucinous cystadenoma: surface ultrastructure, development and biologic behaviour. International Journal of Gynaecology and Obstetrics 18: 157–167

1342. Stenbäck F 1981 Benign, borderline and malignant serous cystadenomas of the ovary. A transmission and scanning electron microscopical study. Pathology Research and Practice 172: 58–72

1343. Stenbäck F 1982 Morphological characteristics of different types of cystic teratoma of the ovary. A study of surface ultrastructure in relation to tumor classification and development. Gynecologic and Obstetric Investigation 14: 161–175

1344. Stenbäck F, Kauppila A 1981 Endometrioid ovarian tumors: morphology and relation to other endometrial conditions. Gynecologic and Obstetric Investigation 12: 57–70

1345. Takeda A, Ishizuka T, Goto T, Goto S, Ohta M, Tomoda Y, Hoshino M 1982 Polyembryoma of ovary producing alpha-fetoprotein and HCG: Immunoperoxidase and electron microscopic study. Cancer 49: 1878–1889

1346. Takeda A, Matsuyama M, Chihara T, Suchi T, Sato T, Tomoda Y 1982 Ultrastructure and immunohistochemistry of gastro-entero-pancreatic (GEP) endocrine cells in mucinous tumors of the ovary. Acta Pathologica Japonica 32: 1003–1015

1347. Takeda A, Matsuyama M, Sugimoto Y, Suzumori K, Ishiwata T, Ishida S, Nakanishi Y, 1983 Oncocytic adenocarcinoma of the ovary. Virchows Archiv A Pathological Anatomy and Histopathology 399: 345–353

1348. Tavassoli F A 1983 A combined germ cell-gonadal stromal-epithelial tumor of the ovary. American Journal of Surgical Pathology 7: 73–84

1349. Tavassoli F A, Norris H J 1980 Sertoli tumors of the ovary. A clinicopathologic study of 28 cases with ultrastructural observations. Cancer 46: 2281–2297

1350. Ulbright T M, Roth L M, Ehrlich C E 1982 Ovarian strumal carcinoid. An immunocytochemical and ultra-structural study of two cases. American Journal of Clinical Pathology 77: 622–631

1351. Waxman M 1979 Pure and mixed Brenner tumors of the ovary. Clinicopathologic and histogenetic observations. Cancer 43: 1830–1839

1352. Waxman M, Damjanov I, Alpert L, Sardinsky T 1981 Composite mucinous ovarian neoplasms associated with Sertoli-Leydig and carcinoid tumors. Cancer 47: 2044–2052

1353. Waxman M, Vuletin J C, Pertschuk L P 1979 Lysosomes in Brenner's tumor simulating secretory argentaffin granules. Archives of Pathology and Laboratory Medicine 103: 183–186

1354. Williams R M 1979 A light and electron microscopic study of an ovarian and rectal carcinoid. Histopathology 3: 19–30

1355. Young R H, Dickersin G R, Scully R E 1983 A distinctive ovarian sex cord-stromal tumor causing sexual precocity in the Peutz-Jeghers syndrome. American Journal of Surgical Pathology 7: 233–243

1356. Young R H, Welch W R, Dickersin G R, Scully R E 1982 Ovarian sex cord tumor with annular tubules. Review of 74 cases including 27 with Peutz-Jeghers syndrome and four with adenoma malignum of the cervix. Cancer 50: 1384–1402

1357. Yutani C, Maeda H, Nakajima N, Takeuchi N, Kimura M, Kitamura H 1982 Primary ovarian lymphoma associated with Meigs' syndrome: a case report. Acta Cytologica 26: 44–48

## 37 TUMOURS OF THE BREAST

1358. Agnantis N T, Rosen P P 1979 Mammary carcinoma with osteoclast-like giant cells. A study of eight cases with follow up data. American Journal of Clinical Pathology 72: 383–389

1359. Ahmed A 1974 Electron-microscopic observations of scirrhous and mucin-producing carcinomas of the breast. Journal of Pathology 112: 177–181

1360. Ahmed A 1974 The myoepithelium in human breast fibroadenoma. Journal of Pathology 114: 135–138

1361. Ahmed A 1978 Atlas of the ultrastructure of human breast diseases. Churchill Livingstone, Edinburgh

1362. Ahmed A 1979 Ultrastructural aspects of human breast disease. In: Azzopardi J G Problems in breast pathology. Bennington J L (ed) Major problems in pathology, vol. 11. W. B. Saunders Company, Philadelphia, ch 17, p 407–436

1363. Ahmed A 1980 The ultrastructure of medullary carcinoma of the breast. Virchows Archiv A Pathological Anatomy and Histology 388: 175–186

1364. Ahmed A 1980 Ultrastructural aspects of human breast lesions. Pathology Annual 15, pt 2: 411–443

1365. Akhtar M, Robinson C, Ali M A, Godwin J T 1983 Secretory carcinoma of the breast in adults. Light and electron microscopic study of three cases with review of the literature. Cancer 51: 2245–2254

1366. Al-Hariri J A 1980 Primary signet ring cell carcinoma of the breast. Virchows Archiv A Pathological Anatomy and Histology 388: 105–111

1367. Allegra S R 1980 Virus-like particles in lactating adenoma of human breast. Journal of Submicroscopic Cytology 12: 283–291

1368. Azzopardi J G, Muretto P, Goddeeris P, Eusebi V, Lauweryns J M 1982 'Carcinoid' tumours of the breast: the morphological spectrum of argyrophil carcinomas. Histopathology 6: 549–569

1369. Battifora H 1975 Intracytoplasmic lumina in breast carcinoma. A helpful histopathologic feature. Archives of Pathology 99: 614–617

1370. Benisch B, Peison B, Newman R, Sobel H J, Marquet E 1983 Solid glycogen-rich clear cell carcinoma of the breast (a light and ultrastructural study). American Journal of Clinical Pathology 79: 243–245

1371. Bussolati G 1980 Actin-rich (myoepithelial) cells in lobular carcinoma in situ of the breast. Virchows Archiv B Cell Pathology 32: 165–176

1372. Bussolati G, Botto Micca F, Eusebi V, Betts C M 1981 Myoepithelial cells in lobular carcinoma in situ of the breast: a parallel immunocytochemical and ultrastructural study. Ultrastructural Patholgy 2: 219–230

1373. Carstens P H 1974 Ultrastructure of human fibroadenoma. Archives of Pathology 98: 23–32

1374. Clayton F, Sibley R K, Ordonez N G, Hanssen G 1982 Argyrophilic breast carcinomas. Evidence of lactational differentiation. American Journal of Surgical Pathology 6: 323–333

1375. Cubilla A L, Woodruff J M 1977 Primary carcinoid tumor of the breast. A report of eight patients. American Journal of Surgical Pathology 1: 283–292

1376. Douglas J G, Shivas A A 1974 The origins of elastica in breast carcinoma. Journal of the Royal College of Surgeons of Edinburgh 19: 89–93

1377. Dvorak H F, Dickersin G R, Dvorak A M, Manseau E J, Pyne K 1981 Human breast carcinoma: fibrin deposits and desmoplasia. Inflammatory cell type and distribution. Microvasculature and infarction. Journal of the National Cancer Institute 67: 335–345

1378. Erlandson R A, Carstens P H B 1972 Ultrastructure of tubular carcinoma of the breast. Cancer 29: 987–995

1379. Erlandson R A, Rosen P P 1982 Infiltrating myoepithelioma of the breast. American Journal of Surgical Pathology 6: 785–793

1380. Eusebi V, Azzopardi J G 1980 Lobular endocrine neoplasia in fibroadenoma of the breast. Histopathology 4: 413–428

1381. Factor S M, Biempica L, Ratner I, Ahuja K K, Biempica S 1977 Carcinoma of the breast with multinucleated reactive stromal giant cells. A light and electron microscopic study of two cases. Virchows Archiv A Pathological Anatomy and Histology 374: 1–12

1382. Feller W F, Chopra H C 1968 A small virus-like particle observed in human breast cancer by means of electron microscopy. Journal of the National Cancer Institute 40: 1359–1373

1383. Fernandez B B, Hernandez F J, Spindler W 1976 Metastatic cystosarcoma phyllodes. A light and electron microscopic study. Cancer 37: 1737–1746

1384. Fetissof F, Dubois M P, Arbeille-Brassart B, Lansac J, Jobard P 1983 Argyrophilic cells in mammary carcinoma. Human Pathology 14: 127–134

1385. Fisher E R 1976 Ultrastructure of the human breast and its disorders. American Journal of Clinical Pathology 66: 291–375

1386. Fisher E R, Palekar A S, Gregorio R M, Paulson J D 1983 Mucoepidermoid and squamous cell carcinomas of breast with reference to squamous metaplasia and giant cell tumors. American Journal of Surgical Pathology 7: 15–27

1387. Gersell D J, Katzenstein A-L A 1981 Spindle cell carcinoma of the breast. A clinicopathologic and ultrastructural study. Human Pathology 12: 550–561

1388. Ghosh L 1980 Ultrastructural study of myoepithelial cells in breast carcinoma. Journal of Surgical Oncology 15: 19–28

1389. Ghosh L, Nassauer J, Faiferman I, Ghosh B C 1980 Ultrastructure study of membrane glycocalyx in primary and metastatic human breast carcinoma. Clinical Oncology 6: 21–24

1390. Ghosh L, Nassauer J, Faiferman I, Ghosh B C 1981 Ultrastructural study of membrane glycocalyx in primary and metastatic human and rat mammary carcinoma. Journal of Surgical Oncology 17: 395–401

1391. Goldenberg V E, Goldenberg N S, Sommers S C 1969 Comparative ultrastructure of atypical ductal hyperplasia, intraductal carcinoma, and infiltrating ductal carcinoma of the breast. Cancer 24: 1152–1169

1392. Gould V E, Chejfec G 1980 Case 13: lobular carcinoma of the breast with secretory features. Ultrastructural Pathology 1: 151–156

1393. Gould V E, Jao W, Battifora H 1980 Ultrastructural analysis in the differential diagnosis of breast tumors. The significance of myoepithelial cells, basal lamina, intra-cytoplasmic lumina and secretory granules. Pathology Research and Practice 167: 45–70

1394. Gould V E, Snyder R W 1974 Ultrastructural features of papillomatosis and carcinoma of nipple ducts. The significance of myoepithelial cells and basal lamina in benign, 'questionable', and malignant lesions. Pathology Annual 9: 441–469

1395. Govoni E, Bazzocchi F, Pileri S, Martinelli G 1981 Lobular endocrine neoplasia in a fibroadenoma of the breast. An ultrastructural study. Virchows Archiv A Pathological Anatomy and Histology 393: 299–306

1396. Hamazaki M, Tanaka T 1978 Hemangiosarcoma of the breast. Case report with scanning electron microscopic study. Acta Pathologica Japonica 28: 605–613

1397. Harris M 1977 Pseudoadenoid cystic carcinoma of the breast. Archives of Pathology and Laboratory Medicine 101: 307–309

1398. Harris M, Vasudev K S, Amfield C, Wells S 1978 Mucin-producing carcinomas of the breast: ultrastructural observations. Histopathology 2: 177–188

1399. Hassan M O, Olaizola M Y 1979 Male breast carcinoma. An ultrastructural study. Archives of Pathology and Laboratory Medicine 103: 191–195

1400. Horie A 1981 Fine structure of cystosarcoma phyllodes with reference to smooth muscle tumors. Acta Pathologica Japonica 31: 1015–1028

1401. Hull M T, Priest J B, Broadie T A, Ransburgh R C, McCarthy L J 1981 Glycogen-rich clear cell carcinoma of the breast: a light and electron microscopic study. Cancer 48: 2003–2009

1402. Jao W, Recant W, Swerdlow M A 1976 Comparative ultrastructure of tubular carcinoma and sclerosing adenosis of the breast. Cancer 38: 180–186

1403. Jao W, Vazquez L T, Keh P C, Gould V E 1978 Myoepithelial differentiation and basal lamina deposition in fibroadenoma and adenosis of the breast. Journal of Pathology 126: 107–112

1404. Kaneko H, Sumida T, Sekiya M, Toshima M, Kobayashi H, Naito K 1982 A breast carcinoid tumor with special reference to ultrastructural study. Acta Pathologica Japonica 32: 327–332

1405. Koss L G, Brannan C D, Ashikari R 1970 Histologic and ultrastructural features of adenoid cystic carcinoma of the breast. Cancer 26: 1271–1279

1406. Lim-Co R, Gisser S D 1978 Unusual variant of lipid-rich mammary carcinoma. Archives of Pathology and Laboratory Medicine 102: 193–195

1407. Llombart-Bosch A, Peydro A 1974 Malignant mixed osteogenic tumours of the breast. Virchows Archiv A Pathological Anatomy and Histology 366: 1–14

1408. Lucas J G, Sharma H M, O'Toole R V 1981 Unusual giant cell tumor arising in a male breast. Human Pathology 12: 840–844

1409. McClure J, Smith P S, Jamieson G G 1982 'Mixed' salivary type adenoma of the human female breast. Archives of Pathology and Laboratory Medicine 106: 615–619

1410. Merino M J, Livolsi V A 1981 Signet ring cell carcinoma of the female breast: a clinicopathologic analysis of 24 cases. Cancer 48: 1830–1837

1411. Min K-W 1983 Argyrophilia in breast carcinomas: histochemical, ultrastructural, and immunocytochemical study. Laboratory Investigation 48: 58A

1412. Morris J A, Kelly J F 1982 Multiple breast adenomata in identical adolescent Negro twins. Histopathology 6: 539–547

1413. Mossler J A, Barton T K, Brinkhous A D, McCarty K S, Moylan J A, McCarty K S Jr 1980 Apocrine differentiation in human mammary carcinoma. Cancer 46: 2463–2471

1414. Murad T M 1971 A proposed histochemical and electron microscopic classification of human breast cancer according to cell of origin. Cancer 27: 288–299

1415. Murad T M 1971 Ultrastructure of ductular carcinoma of the breast (in situ and infiltrating lobular carcinoma). Cancer 27: 18–28

1416. Murad T M, Greider M H, Scarpelli D G 1967 The ultrastructure of human mammary fibroadenoma. American Journal of Pathology 51: 663–679

1417. Murad T M, Scarpelli D G 1967 The ultrastructure of medullary and scirrhous mammary duct carcinoma. American Journal of Pathology 50: 335–360

1418. Navas J J, Battifora H 1977 Primary lymphoma of the breast. Ultrastructural study of two cases. Cancer 39: 2025–2032

1419. Nesland J M, Johannessen J V 1982 Malignant breast lesions. Journal of Submicroscopic Cytology 4: 553–575

1420. Nielsen B B 1981 Oncocytic breast papilloma. Virchows Archiv A Pathological Anatomy and Histology 393: 345–351

1421. Ohtani H, Sasano N 1980 Myofibroblasts and myoepithelial cells in human breast carcinoma. An ultrastructural study. Virchows Archiv A Pathological Anatomy and Histology 385: 247–261

1422. Ozzello L 1971 Ultrastructure of intra-epithelial carcinomas of the breast. Cancer 28: 1508–1515

1423. Ozzello L 1971 Ultrastructure of the human mammary gland. Pathology Annual 6: 1–59

1424. Ozzello L 1979 Breast. In: Johannessen J V (ed) Electron microscopy in human medicine, vol 9. Urogenital system and breast. McGraw-Hill, New York, ch 20, p 409–450

1425. Ozzello L, Sanpitak P 1970 Epithelial-stromal junction of intraductal carcinoma of the breast. Cancer 26: 1186–1198

1426. Partanen S, Syrjänen K 1981 Argyrophilic cells in carcinoma of the female breast. Virchows Archiv A Pathological Anatomy and Histology 391: 45–51

1427. Qizilbash A H 1976 Cystosarcoma phyllodes with liposarcomatous stroma. American Journal of Clinical Pathology 65: 321–327

1428. Qizilbash A H, Patterson M C, Oliveira K F 1977 Adenoid cystic carcinoma of the breast. Light and electron microscopy and a brief review of the literature. Archives of Pathology and Laboratory Medicine 101: 302–306

1429. Raju U, Fine G 1983 The controversial mammary carcinoid tumor. Laboratory Investigation 48: 69A

1430. Ramos C V, Taylor H B 1974 Lipid-rich carcinoma of the breast. A clinicopathologic analysis of 13 examples. Cancer 33: 812–819

1431. Richters A, Sherwin R P 1974 Human breast cancer and the autochthonous lymph node cell responses: a tissue culture and ultrastructural study. Cancer 34: 328–337

1432. Roddy H J, Silverberg S G 1980 Ultrastructural analysis of apocrine carcinoma of the human breast. Ultrastructural Pathology 1: 385–393

1433. Rosen P P 1979 Multinucleated mammary stromal giant cells. A benign lesion that simulates invasive carcinoma. Cancer 44: 1305–1308

1434. Seman G, Dmochowski L 1973 Electron microscope observations of viruslike particles in comedo-carcinoma of the human breast. Cancer 32: 822–829

1435. Shivas A A, MacKenzie A 1974 The origins of stromal reaction in breast carcinoma. Journal of the Royal College of Surgeons of Edinburgh 19: 345–350

1436. Spring-Mills E, Elias J J 1975 Cell surface differences in ducts from cancerous and non-cancerous human breasts. Science 188: 947–949

1437. Stegner H-E, Bahnsen J, Fischer E 1981 Tumor grading in breast cancer by light microscopic and electron microscopic criteria. Part I: Relation between light microscopic grading and electron microscopic criteria. Pathology Research and Practice 173: 159–171

1438. Steinbrecher J S, Silverberg S G 1976 Signet-ring cell carcinoma of the breast. The mucinous variant of infiltrating lobular carcinoma? Cancer 37: 828–840

1439. Sugano I, Nagao K, Kondo Y, Nabeshima S, Murakami S 1983 Cytologic and ultrastructural studies of a rare breast carcinoma with osteoclast-like giant cells. Cancer 52: 74–78

1440. Sykes J A, Recher L, Jernstrom P H, Whitescarver J 1968 Morphological investigation of human breast cancer. Journal of the National Cancer Institute 40: 195–223

1441. Tang P H, Petrelli M, Robechek P J 1979 Stromal sarcoma of breast: a light and electron microscopic study. Cancer 43: 209–217

1442. Tateno M, Yoshiki T, Itoh T, Takamuro M, Saito C 1983 A case of primary B-cell lymphoma of the breast. Light and electron microscopy, and immunologic cell markers. Cancer 52: 671–674

1443. Taxy J B, Tischler A S, Insalaco S J, Battifora H 1981 'Carcinoid' tumor of the breast. A variant of conventional breast cancer? Human Pathology 12: 170–179

1444. Tobon H, Price H M 1972 Lobular carcinoma in situ. Some ultrastructural observations. Cancer 30: 1082–1091

1445. Tobon H, Salazar H 1977 Tubular carcinoma of the breast. Clinical, histological and ultrastructural observations. Archives of Pathology and Laboratory Medicine 101: 310–316

1446. Toker C, Tang C-K, Whitely J F, Berkheiser S W, Rachman R 1981 Benign spindle cell breast tumor. Cancer 48: 1615–1622

1447. Toth J 1977 Benign human mammary myoepithelioma. Virchows Archiv A Pathological Anatomy and Histology 374: 263–269

1448. Tsuchiya S 1981 Intracytoplasmic lumina of human breast cancer — a microscopic study and practical implication in cytological diagnosis. Acta Pathologica Japonica 31: 45–54

1449. Tsuchiya S, Takayama S, Higashi Y 1983 Electron microscopy of intraductal papilloma of the breast. Ultrastructural comparison of papillary carcinoma with normal mammary large duct. Acta Pathologica Japonica 33: 97–112

1450. Tulusan A H, Grünsteidel W, Ramming I, Egger H 1982 A contribution to the natural history of breast cancer. III. Changes in the basement membranes in breast cancers with stromal invasion. Archives of Gynecology 231: 209–218

1451. Tulusan A H, Hamann M, Prestele H, Ramming I, von Maillot K, Egger H 1982 Correlations of the receptor content and ultrastructure of breast cancer cells. Archives of Gynecology 231: 177–184

1452. Wade P M Jr, Mills S E, Read M, Cloud W, Lambert M J III, Smith R E 1983 Small cell neuroendocrine (oat cell) carcinoma of the breast. Cancer 52: 121–125

1453. Yogore M G III, Sahgal S 1977 Small cell carcinoma of the male breast. Report of a case. Cancer 39: 1748–1751

*38 NON-MELANOCYTIC TUMOURS OF THE SKIN*

1454. Alguacil-Garcia A, Unni K K, Goellner J R, Winkelmann R K 1977 Atypical fibroxanthoma of the skin. An ultrastructural study of two cases. Cancer 40: 1471–1480

1455. Asai Y, Ishii M, Hamada T 1982 Acral syringoma: electron microscopic studies on its origin. Acta Dermato-Venereologica 62: 64–68

1456. Barr R J, Wuerker R B, Graham J H 1977 Ultrastructure of atypical fibroxanthoma. Cancer 40: 736–743

1457. Battifora H 1976 Spindle cell carcinoma. Ultrastructural evidence of squamous origin and collagen production by the tumor cells. Cancer 37: 2275–2282

1458. Belcher R W 1972 Extramammary Paget's disease. Enzyme histochemical and electron microscopic study. Archives of Pathology 94: 59–64

1459. Brownstein M H, Shapiro L 1975 The sweat gland adenomas. International Journal of Dermatology 14: 397–411

1460. Candiani P, Rainoldi R, Sideri M, Le Grazie C, De Virgiliis G, Donati L 1981 Ultrastructural aspects of the dermatofibroma. Tumori 67: 249–252

1461. Castro C, Winkelmann R K 1974 Spiradenoma: histochemical and electron microscopic study. Archives of Dermatology 109: 40–48

1462. Challa V R, Jona J 1977 Eccrine angiomatous hamartoma: a rare skin lesion with diverse histological features. Dermatologica 155: 206–209

1463. Daróczy J 1980 The significance of electron microscopy in dermatology. Pathology Research and Practice 168: 36–64

1464. Demopoulos R I 1971 Fine structure of the extramammary Paget's cell. Cancer 27: 1202–1210

1465. Faber M, Hagedorn M 1981 A light and electron microscopic study of Bowenoid papulosis. Acta Dermato-Venereologica 61: 397–403

1466. Ferenczy A, Richart R M 1972 Ultrastructure of perianal Paget's disease. Cancer 29: 1141–1149

1467. Ferguson-Smith M A, Wallace D C, James Z H, Renwick J H 1971 Multiple self-healing squamous epitheliomas. Birth Defects 7: 157–163

1468. Fisher E R, McCoy M M, Wechsler H L 1972 Analysis of histopathologic and electron microscopic determinants of keratoacanthoma and squamous cell carcinoma. Cancer 29: 1387–1397

1469. Frigerio B, Capella C, Eusebi V, Tenti P, Azzopardi J G 1983 Merkel cell carcinoma of the skin: the structure and origin of normal Merkel cells. Histopathology 7: 229–249

1470. Gallager H S, Creasman W T, Mackay B 1976 Paget's disease of the vulva. In: Neoplasms of the skin and malignant melanoma. Year Book Medical Publishers, Chicago, p 231–242

1471. Gomez L G, DiMaio S, Silva E G, Mackay B 1983 Association betweeen neuroendocrine (Merkel cell) carcinoma and squamous carcinoma of the skin. American Journal of Surgical Pathology 7: 171–177

1472. Gould V E, Dardi L E, Memoli V A, Johannessen J V 1980 Neuroendocrine carcinomas of the skin: light microscopic, ultrastructural and immunohistochemical analysis. Ultrastructural Pathology 1: 499–509

1473. Gross B G 1965 The fine structure of apocrine hidrocystoma. Archives of Dermatology 92: 706–712

1474. Harris M 1982 Spindle cell squamous carcinoma: ultrastructural observations. Histopathology 6: 197–220

1475. Hashimoto K, Brownstein M H 1973 Localized amyloidosis in basal cell epitheliomas. Acta Dermato-Venereologica 53: 331–339

1476. Hashimoto K, Dibella R J, Borsuk G M, Lever W F 1967 Eruptive hiradenoma and syringoma. Histological, histochemical and electron microscopic studies. Archives of Dermatology 96: 500–519

1477. Hashimoto K, Dibella R J, Lever W F 1967 Clear cell hidradenoma. Histological, histochemical and electron microscopic studies. Archives of Dermatology 96: 18–38

1478. Hashimoto K, Gross B G, Lever W F 1966 Syringoma: histochemical and electron microscopic studies. Journal of Investigative Dermatology 46: 150–166

1479. Hashimoto K, Gross B G, Nelson R G, Lever W F 1966 Eccrine spiradenoma: histochemical and electron microscopic studies. Journal of Investigative Dermatology 46: 347–365

1480. Hashimoto K, Lever W F 1969 Histogenesis of skin appendage tumors. Archives of Dermatology 100: 356–369

1481. Hashimoto K, Nelson R G, Lever W F 1966 Calcifying epithelioma of Malherbe: histochemical and electron microscopic studies. Journal of Investigative Dermatology 46: 391–408

1482. Hashimoto K, Yamanishi Y, Maeyens E, Dabbous M K, Kanzaki T 1973 Collagenolytic activities of squamous cell carcinoma of the skin. Cancer Research 33: 2790–2801

1483. Headington J T 1977 Primary mucinous carcinoma of skin: histochemistry and electron microscopy. Cancer 39: 1055–1063

1484. Headington J T, Nederhuber J E, Beals T F 1978 Malignant clear cell acrospiroma. Cancer 41: 641–647

1485. Hull M T, Eble J N, Priest J B, Mulcahy J J 1981 Ultrastructure of Buschke-Loewenstein tumor. Journal of Urology 126: 485–489

1486. Iwasaki H, Mitsui T, Kikuchi M, Imai T, Fukushima K 1981 Neuroendocrine carcinoma (trabecular carcinoma) of the skin with ectopic ACTH production. Cancer 48: 753–756

1487. Johannessen J V, Gould V E 1980 Neuroendocrine skin carcinoma associated with calcitonin production: a Merkel cell carcinoma? Human Pathology 11: 586–588

1488. Kao G F, Graham J H, Helwig E B 1982 Carcinoma cuniculatum (verrucous carcinoma of the skin): a clinicopathologic study of 46 cases with ultrastructural observations. Cancer 49: 2395–2403

1489. Kimura S, Yamasaki Y, Nishikawa T, Kurihara S, Hatano H 1980 A comparative study of seborrhoeic keratoses and basal cell epitheliomas by complement immunofluorescence and electron microscopy. Acta Dermato-Venereologica 60: 203–207

1490. Kirkam N, Isaacson P 1983 Merkel cell carcinoma: a report of three cases with neurone-specific enolase activity. Histopathology 7: 251–259

1491. Kitajima Y, Mori S 1980 Ultrastructural characterisation of the extramammary Paget cell plasma membrane: a freeze fracture study. Journal of Cutaneous Pathology 7: 364–372

1492. Koss L G, Brockunier A Jr 1969 Ultrastructural aspects of Paget's disease of the vulva. Archives of Pathology 87: 592–600

1493. Kwittken J 1974 Muciparous epidermal tumor. Archives of Dermatology 109: 554–555

1494. Lichtiger B, Mackay B, Tessmer C F 1970 Spindle-cell variant of squamous carcinoma. A light and electron microscopic study of 13 cases. Cancer 26: 1311–1320

1495. Lipper S, Peiper S C 1979 Sweat gland carcinoma with syringomatous features. A light microscopic and ultrastructural study. Cancer 44: 157–163

1496. Lopez D A, Silvers D N, Helwig E B 1974 Cutaneous meningiomas: a clinicopathologic study. Cancer 34: 728–744

1497. Macadam R F 1978 An electron microscopic study of basal cell carcinoma. Journal of Pathology 126: 149–156

1498. Manglani K S, Manaligod J R, Ray B 1980 Spindle cell carcinoma of the glans penis: a light and electron microscopic study. Cancer 46: 2266–2272

1499. Massarelli G, Tanda F, Bosincu L, Denti S 1983 Myofibroblasts in the epithelial-stromal junction of basal cell carcinoma. Applied Patholgy 1: 25–30

1500. McGavran M H 1965 Ultrastructure of pilomatrixoma (calcifying epithelioma). Cancer 18: 1445–1456

1501. McNutt N S 1976 Ultrastructural comparison of the interface between epithelium and stroma in basal cell carcinoma and control human skin. Laboratory Investigation 35: 132–142

1502. Medenica M, Sahili T 1972 Ultrastructural study of a case of extramammary Paget's disease of the vulva. Archives of Dermatology 105: 236–243

1503. Miettinen M, Lehto V-P, Virtanen I, Asko-Seljavaara S, Pitkänen J, Dahl D 1983 Neuroendocrine carcinoma of the skin (Merkel cell carcinoma): ultrastructural and immunohistochemical demonstration of neurofilaments. Ultrastructural Patholgy 4: 219–225

1504. Mihara M, Kanbe N, Shimao S, Nakakuki S 1981 Atypical fibroxanthoma of the skin. A histological and electron microscopic study. Journal of Dermatology 8: 411–417

1505. Mitchell R E 1974 Mammary and extramammary Paget's disease. Australasian Journal of Dermatology 15: 51–63

1506. Morley S M, Rennison A, Macadam R F 1983 Membrane-bound structures at the interface between tumour and dermis in basal cell carcinoma. An ultrastructural study. Journal of Pathology 140: 267–274

1507. Nadji M, Morales A R, Girtanner R E, Ziegels-Weissman J, Penneys N S 1982 Paget's disease of the skin. A unifying concept of histogenesis. Cancer 50: 2203–2206

1508. Niizuma K 1977 An electron microscopic study of sebaceous epithelioma. A case report with two new observations on lipid droplet formation. Dermatologica 154: 98–106

1509. Niizuma K 1977 Lipid droplet of sebaceous carcinoma. Electron microscopic study utilizing glycol methacrylate glutaraldehyde urea procedure. Archives of Dermatological Research 260: 111–119

1510. Ono T, Sakazaki Y, Jono M, Muto K 1982 Banded structure in solitary trichoepithelioma. Acta Dermato-Venereologica 62: 68–72

1511. Ose D, Vollmer R, Shelburne J, McComb R, Harrelson J 1983 Histiocytoid hemangioma of the skin and scapula: a case report with electron microscopy and immunohistochemistry. Cancer 51: 1656–1662

1512. Penneys N S, Nadji M, Ziegels-Weissman J, Morales A R 1983 Prekeratin in spindle cell tumors of the skin. Archives of Dermatology 119: 476–479

1513. Pilotti S, Rilke F, Lombardi L 1982 Neuroendocrine (Merkel cell) carcinoma of the skin. American Journal of Surgical Pathology 6: 243–254

1514. Posalaky Z, McGinley D, Cutler B, Katz H I 1979 Intercellular junctional specializations in human basal cell carcinoma. A freeze fracture study. Virchows Archiv A Pathological Anatomy and Histology 384: 53–63

1515. Redono C, Rocamora A, Villoria F, Garcia M 1982 Malignant mixed tumor of the skin: malignant chondroid syringoma. Cancer 49: 1690–1696

1516. Rosen Y, Kim B, Yermakov V A 1975 Eccrine sweat gland tumor of clear cell origin involving the eyelids. Cancer 36: 1034–1041

1517. Roth L M, Lee S C, Ehrlich C E 1977 Paget's disease of the vulva. A histogenetic study of five cases including ultrastructural observations and review of the literature. American Journal of Surgical Pathology 1: 193–206

1518. Santa Cruz D J, Bauer E A 1982 Merkel cells in the outer follicular sheath. Ultrastructural Pathology 3: 59–63

1519. Sarma D P 1980 Metastatic basal cell carcinoma: electron microscopic study of the primary and metastatic lesion. Southern Medical Journal 73: 799–801

1520. Sato A, Seiji M 1973 Electron microscopic observations of malignant dyskeratosis in leukoplakia and Bowen's disease. Acta Dermato-Venereologica, suppl 73: 101–110

1521. Sibley R K, Rosai J, Foucar E, Dehner L P, Bosl G 1980 Neuroendocrine (Merkel cell) carcinoma of the skin. A histologic and ultrastructural study of two cases. American Journal of Surgical Pathology 4: 211–221

1522. Silva E G, Mackay B 1980 Small cell neuroepithelial tumor of the skin. Laboratory Investigation 42: 151A

1523. Silva E, Mackay B 1981 Neuroendocrine (Merkel cell) carcinomas of the skin: an ultrastructural study of nine cases. Ultrastructural Pathology 2: 1–9

1524. Sperling L C, Sakas E L 1982 Eccrine hidrocystomas. Journal of the American Academy of Dermatology 7: 763–770

1525. Starink T H Hausman R, Van Delden L, Neering H 1977 Atypical fibroxanthoma of the skin. Presentation of 5 cases and a review of the literature. British Journal of Dermatology 97: 167–177

1526. Sugar F 1968 An electron microscopic study of early invasive growth in human skin tumors and laryngeal carcinoma. European Journal of Cancer 4: 33–38

1527. Szpak C A, Woodard B H, Bossen E H 1981 Neuroendocrine carcinoma of the skin: ultrastructural contrast with oat cell carcinoma. Laboratory Investigation 44: 65A

1528. Tang C K, Toker C 1978 Trabecular carcinoma of the skin: an ultrastructural study. Cancer 42: 2311–2321

1529. Taxy J B, Ettinger D S, Wharam M D 1980 Primary small cell carcinoma of the skin. Cancer 46: 2308–2311

1530. Tulman L S, Jack M K 1965 Porosyringoma: report of a case. American Journal of Ophthalmology 60: 1116–1121

1531. Turner J J, Maxwell L, Bursle G A 1982 Eccrine porocarcinoma: a case report with light microscopy and ultrastructure. Pathology 14: 469–475

1532. Underwood J W, Adcock L L, Okagaki T 1978 Adenosquamous carcinoma of skin appendages (adenoid squamous cell carcinoma, pseudoglandular squamous cell carcinoma, adenoacanthoma of sweat gland of Lever) of the vulva. A clinical and ultrastructural study. Cancer 42: 1851–1858

1533. Varela-Duran J, Diaz-Flores L, Varela-Nunez R 1979 Ultrastructure of chondroid syringoma. Role of the myoepithelial cell in the development of the mixed tumor of the skin and soft tissues. Cancer 44: 148–156

1534. Veda K, Komori Y, Maruo M, Kusaba K 1981 Ultrastructure of trichoepithelioma papulosum multiplex. Journal of Cutaneous Pathology 8: 188–198

1535. Warner T F C S, Uno H, Hafez R, Burgess J, Bolles C, Lloyd R V, Oka M 1983 Merkel cells and Merkel cell tumors. Ultrastructure, immunocytochemistry and review of the literature. Cancer 52: 238–245

1536. Webb J N, Stott W G 1975 Malignant chondroid syringoma of the thigh. Report of a case with electron microscopy of the tumour. Journal of Pathology 116: 43–46

1537. Weedon D, Kerr J F 1975 Atypical fibroxanthoma of skin: an electron microscope study. Pathology 7: 173–177

1538. Wick M R, Goellner J R, Scheithauer B W, Thomas J R III, Sanchez N P, Schroeter A L 1983 Primary neuroendocrine carcinomas of the skin (Merkel cell tumors). A clinical, histologic, and ultrastructural study of thirteen cases. American Journal of Surgical Pathology 7: 6–13

1539. Wilborn W H, Pitts W J, Montes L F 1981 Sebaceous adenocarcinoma. Journal of Cutaneous Pathology 8: 266–270

1540. Willemze R, Ruiter D J, Scheffer E, van Vloten W A 1980 Diffuse cutaneous mastocytosis with multiple cutaneous mastocytomas. Report of a case with clinical, histopathological and ultrastructural aspects. British Journal of Dermatology 102: 601–607

1541. Wong S W, Dao A H, Glick A D 1981 Trabecular carcinoma of the skin: a case report. Human Pathology 12: 838–840

1542. Wood C, Hu C-H 1980 Diagnostic electron microscopy of the skin. In: Trump B F, Jones R T (eds) Diagnostic electron microscopy, vol 3. John Wiley & Sons, New York, ch 6, p 315–357

1543. Woyke S, Domagala W, Olszewski W, Korabiec M 1974 Pseudosarcoma of the skin. An electron miscroscopic study and comparison with the fine structure of spindle cell variant of squamous carcinoma. Cancer 33: 970–980

1544. Wright J D, Font R L 1979 Mucinous sweat gland adenocarcinoma of eyelid. A clinicopathologic study of 21 cases with histochemical and electron microscopic observations. Cancer 44: 1757–1768

1545. Yeh S, Chen H C, How S W, Deng C S 1974 Fine structure of Bowen's disease in chronic arsenicalism. Journal of the National Cancer Institute 53: 31–44

1546. Yeung K-Y, Stinson J C 1977 Mucinous (adenocystic) carcinoma of sweat glands with widespread metastasis. Case report with ultrastructural study. Cancer 39: 2556–2562

1547. Zelickson A S 1967 The pigmented basal cell epithelioma. Archives of Dermatology 96: 524–527

1548. Zina A M, Bundino S 1980 Multiple cutaneous fibromyxomas: a light and electron microscopic study. Journal of Cutaneous Pathology 7: 335–341

## 39 MELANOCYTIC TUMOURS

1549. Abrahams C, Skudowitz R B 1979 An ultrastructural study of a juvenile melanoma. South African Medical Journal 55: 47–49

1550. Aichner F, Schuler G 1982 Primary leptomeningeal melanoma. Diagnosis by ultrastructural cytology and cerebrospinal fluid and cranial computed tomography. Cancer 50: 1751–1756

1551. Ainsworth A M, Clark W H Jr, Mastrangelo M, Conger K B 1976 Primary malignant melanoma of the urinary bladder. Cancer 37: 1928–1936

1552. Anderson C W, Stevens M H, Moatamed F 1981 Electron microscopy and L-dopa reaction in the evaluation of an unusual amelanotic malignant melanoma of the neck. Otolaryngology and Head and Neck Surgery 89: 594–598

1553. Arbuckle S, Weedon D 1982 Eosinophilic globules in the Spitz nevus. Journal of the American Academy of Dermatology 7: 324–327

1554. Berman M L, Tobon H, Surti U 1981 Primary malignant melanoma of the vagina: clinical, light and electron microscopic observations. American Journal of Obstetrics and Gynecology 139: 963–965

1555. Bigotti A, De Martino C, Natali P, Sciarretta F, Colizza S 1981 Malignant lentigo–melanoma – a comparative histological and electron microscopy study. Journal of Surgical Oncology 18: 31–37

1556. Bleehen S S, Hartley L, Senior J 1976 Lentigo maligna melanoma. An ultrastructural study. British Journal of Dermatology 95, suppl 14: 14–15

1557. Bryant E, Ronan S G, Felix E L, Manaligod J R 1982 Desmoplastic malignant melanoma: a study by conventional and electron microscopy. American Journal of Dermatopathology 4: 467–474

1558. Burgess J H, Warner T F C S, Mohs F E, Lantis S 1982 Giant melanosomes in the B-K mole syndrome. Journal of Cutaneous Pathology 9: 241–248

1559. Carstens P H B, Kuhns J G 1981 Ultrastructural confirmation of malignant melanoma. Ultrastructural Pathology 2: 147–149

1560. Caselitz J, Jänner M, Breitbart E, Weber K, Osborn M 1983 Malignant melanomas contain only the vimentin type of intermediate filaments. Virchows Archiv A Pathological Anatomy and Histopathology 400: 43–51

1561. Conley J, Lattes R, Orr W 1971 Desmoplastic malignant melanoma (a rare variant of spindle cell melanoma). Cancer 28: 914–936

1562. Coppeto J R, Jaffe R, Gillies C G 1978 Primary orbital melanoma. Archives of Ophthalmology 96: 2255–2258

1563. Dehner L P, Sibley R K, Sauk J J Jr, Vickers R A, Nesbit M E, Leonard A S, Waite D E, Neeley J E, Ophoven J 1979 Malignant melanotic neuroectodermal tumor of infancy. A clinical, pathologic, ultrastructural and tissue culture study. Cancer 43: 1389–1410

1564. DiMaio S M, Mackay B, Smith J L Jr, Dickersin G R 1982 Neurosarcomatous transformation in malignant melanoma. An ultrastructural study. Cancer 50: 2345–2354

1565. Drzewiecki K T 1977 The surface morphology of the melanoma cell. A scanning electron microscope study on the primary cutaneous melanoma. Scandinavian Journal of Plastic and Reconstructive Surgery 11: 9–16

1566. Elomaa M, Sainio P, Calonius P E, Hietanen J 1973 Melanotic neuroectodermal tumor of infancy. A case report and review. Proceedings of the Finnish Dental Society 69: 227–243

1567. Erlandson R A, Rosen P P 1982 Electron microscopy of a nevus cell aggregate associated with an axillary lymph node. Cancer 49: 269–272

1568. Foa C, Aubert C 1977 Ultrastructural comparison between cultured and tumor cells of human malignant melanoma. Cancer Research 37: 3957–3963

1569. Font R L, Zimmerman L E, Armaly M F 1974 The nature of the orange pigment over a choroidal melanoma. Histochemical and electron microscopical observations. Archives of Ophthalmology 91: 359–362

1570. Fresko O, Sidhu G S 1980 Clefts in intradermal nevi: an ultrastructural study. Ultrastructural Pathology 1: 361–366

1571. Fu Y-S, Kaye G I, Lattes R 1975 Primary malignant melanocytic tumors of the sympathetic ganglia with an ultrastructural study of one. Cancer 36: 2029–2041

1572. Hashimoto K 1974 Ultrastructural studies of halo nevus. Cancer 34: 1653–1666

1573. Hashimoto K, Bale G F 1972 An electron microscopic study of balloon cell nevus. Cancer 30: 530–540

1574. Hatae Y, Kikuchi M, Segawa M, Yonemitsu K 1978 Malignant melanoma of the gallbladder. Pathology Research and Practice 163: 281–287

1575. Hendrickson M R, Ross J C 1981 Neoplasms arising in congenital giant nevi. Morphologic study of seven cases and a review of the literature. American Journal of Surgical Pathology 5: 109–135

1576. Hu F 1982 Melanocyte morphology in normal skin, melanocytic nevi, and malignant melanomas. A review. In: Ackerman A B (ed) Pathology of malignant melanoma. Masson Publishing USA, New York, p 1–21

1577. Hull M T, Epinette W W 1982 Ultrastructure of giant melanosomes in the B-K mole syndrome. Laboratory Investigation 46: 37A

1578. Hunter J A 1976 Cutaneous malignant melanoma. International Journal of Dermatology 15: 633–649

1579. Hunter J A, Paterson W D, Fairley D J 1978 Human malignant melanoma. Melanosomal polymorphism and the ultrastructural dopa reaction. British Journal of Dermatology 98: 381–390

1580. Hunter J A, Zaynoun S, Paterson W D, Bleehen S S, Mackie R, Cochran A J 1978 Cellular fine structure of the invasive nodules of different histogenetic types of malignant melanoma. British Journal of Dermatology 98: 255–272
1581. Hunter J A, Zaynoun S, Paterson W D, Mackie R M, Cochran A J, Bleehen S S 1976 Malignant melanoma. A comparison of cellular fine structure in invasive nodules of different histogenetic type. British Journal of Dermatology 95, suppl 14: 13–14
1582. Jakobiec F A, Ellsworth R, Tannenbaum M 1974 Primary orbital melanoma. American Journal of Ophthalmology 78: 24–39
1583. Jensen O A, Povlsen A 1979 Melanomas of the choroid. In: Johannessen J V (ed) Electron microscopy in human medicine, vol 6. Nervous system, sensory organs and respiratory tract. McGraw-Hill, New York, ch 9, p 346-368
1584. Johnson R E, Scheithauer B W, Dahlin D C 1982 Melanotic neuroectodermal tumor of infancy: a malignant tumor of the femur. Mayo Clinic Proceedings 57: 719–722
1585. Juarez C P, Tso M O 1980 An ultrastructural study of melanocytomas (magnocellular nevi) of the optic disc and uvea. American Journal of Ophthalmology 90: 48–62
1586. Koaresen R 1974 The immune reaction against malignant melanoma studied in a biopsy material. Acta Pathologica et Microbiologica Scandinavica. Section A. Pathology 82: 116–126
1587. Kudo M, Nagayama T, Miura M, Fukunaga N 1983 Blue nevus of the uterine cervix. An ultrastructural study of two cases. Archives of Pathology and Laboratory Medicine 107: 87–90
1588. Labrecque P G, Hu C-H, Winkelmann R K 1976 On the nature of desmoplastic melanoma. Cancer 38: 1205–1213
1589. Lee W R 1973 The fine structure of three malignant melanomas of the iris. Albrecht von Graefes Archiv für Klinische und Experimentelle Ophthalmologie 188: 91–108
1590. Mackay B, Ayala A G 1980 Intracisternal tubules in human melanoma cells. Ultrastructural Pathology 1: 1–6
1591. Mazur M T, Katzenstein A-L A 1980 Metastatic melanoma: the spectrum of ultrastructural morphology. Ultrastructural Pathology 1: 337–356
1592. Merkow L P, Burt R C, Hayeslip D W, Newton F J, Slifkin M, Pardo M 1969 A cellular and malignant blue nevus: a light and electron microscopic study. Cancer 24: 888–896
1593. Milton C W, Lane-Brown M M, Gilder M 1967 Malignant melanoma with an occult primary lesion. British Journal of Surgery 54: 651–658
1594. Mintzis M M, Silvers D N 1978 Ultrastructural study of superficial spreading melanoma and benign simulants. Cancer 42: 502–511
1595. Mishima Y 1967 Melanocytic and nevocytic malignant melanomas. Cellular and subcellular differentiation. Cancer 20: 632–649
1596. Misugi K, Okajima H, Newton W A Jr, Kmetz D R, deLorimier A A 1965 Mediastinal origin of a melanotic progonoma or retinal anlage tumor. Ultrastructural evidence for neural crest origin. Cancer 18: 477–484
1597. Navas Palacios J J 1980 Malignant melanotic neuro-ectodermal tumor. Light and electron microscopic study. Cancer 46: 529–536
1598. Neustein H B 1967 Fine structure of a melanotic progonoma or retinal anlage tumor of the anterior fontanel. Experimental and Molecular Pathology 6: 131–142
1599. Nikai H, Ijuhin N, Yamasaki A, Niitani K, Imai K 1977 Ultrastructural evidence of neural crest origin of the melanotic neuroectodermal tumor of infancy. Journal of Oral Pathology 6: 221–232
1600. Nozicka Z, Spacek J 1978 Melanotic neuroectodermal tumor of infancy with highly differentiated neural component. Light and electron microscopic study. Acta Neuropathologica 44: 229–233
1601. Okun M R, Donnellan B, Edelstein L 1974 An ultrastructural study of balloon cell nevus. Relationship of mast cells to nevus cells. Cancer 34: 615–625
1602. Persky B, Meyskens F L Jr, Hendrix M J C 1983 Diagnostic electron microscopy for amelanotic melanoma: correlation of patient biopsy, soft agar assay, and xenograft. Journal of Pathology 141: 17–27
1603. Pomeranz G A, Bunt A H, Kalina R E 1981 Multifocal choroidal melanoma in ocular melanocytosis. Archives of Ophthalmology 99: 857–863
1604. Radnot M 1976 Scanning electron microscopy of melanoblastomas of the choroid. Ophthalmologica 173: 352–363
1605. Ranchod M 1972 Metastatic melanoma with balloon cell changes. Cancer 30: 1006–1013
1606. Roth A M 1978 Malignant change in melanocytomas of the uveal tract. Survey of Ophthalmology 22: 404–412
1607. Schlappner O L, Rowden G, Philips T M, Rahim Z 1978 Melanoacanthoma. Ultrastructural and immunological studies. Journal of Cutaneous Pathology 5: 127–141
1608. Schuler G, Hönigsmann H, Wolff K 1980 Diffuse melanosis in metastatic melanoma. Further evidence for disseminated single cell metastases in the skin. Journal of the American Academy of Dermatology 3: 363–369
1609. Shields M B, Klintworth G K 1980 Anterior uveal melanomas and intraocular pressure. Opthalmology 87: 503–517
1610. Silbert S W, Smith K R Jr, Horenstein S 1978 Primary leptomeningeal melanoma. An ultrastructural study. Cancer 41: 519–527
1611. Silverberg G D, Kadin M E, Dorfman R F, Hanbery J W, Prolo D J 1971 Invasion of the brain by a cellular blue nevus of the scalp. A case report with light and electron microscopic studies. Cancer 27: 349–355
1612. Silverberg I, Kopf A W, Gumport S L 1968 Diffuse melanosis in malignant melanoma. Report of a case and of studies by light and electron microscopy. Archives of Dermatology 97: 671–677
1613. Søndergaard K, Henschel A, Hou-Jensen K 1980 Metastatic melanoma with balloon cell changes: an electron microscopic study. Ultrastructural Pathology 1: 357–360
1614. Szaniawski W 1974 Ultrastructure of four cases of choroidal malignant melanoma. Annals of the Medical Section of the Polish Academy of Sciences 19: 149–150
1615. Szekeres L, Daróczy J 1981 Electron microscopic investigation on the local cellular reaction to primary malignant melanoma. Dermatologica 163: 137–144
1616. Szpack C A, Shelburne J D, Lindner J, Klintworth G K 1983 The significance of premelanosomes (stage II melanosomes) in non-melanocytic neoplasms. Laboratory Investigation 48: 83A
1617. Valensi Q J 1979 Desmoplastic malignant melanoma. A light and electron microscopic study of two cases. Cancer 43: 1148–1155
1618. Verdaguer J, Valenzuela H, Strozzi L 1974 Melanocytoma of the conjunctiva. Archives of Ophthalmology 91: 363–366
1619. Warner T F C S, Hafez G R, Buchler D A 1982 Neurotropic melanoma of the vulva. Cancer 49: 999–1004
1620. Warner T F C S, Hafez G R, Finch R E, Brandenberg J H 1981 Schwann cell features in neurotropic melanoma. Journal of Cutaneous Pathology 8: 177–187
1621. Yannopoulos K 1980 Desmoplastic malignant melanoma. Progress in Surgical Pathology 2: 269–289

*40 GENERAL ENDOCRINE REFERENCES AND APUD
TUMOURS*

1622. Black W C III 1968 Enterochromaffin cell types and corresponding carcinoid tumors. Laboratory Investigation 19: 473–486

1623. Bloodworth J M B Jr, Horvath E, Kovacs K 1980 Fine structural pathology of the endocrine system. In: Trump B F, Jones R T (eds) Diagnostic electron microscopy, vol 3. John Wiley & Sons, New York, ch 7, p 359–527

1624. Chow C W, Sane S, Campbell P E, Carter R F 1982 Malignant carcinoid tumors in children. Cancer 49: 802–811

1625. Gould R P 1978 The APUD cell system. In: Anthony P P, Woolf N (eds) Recent advances in histopathology, no 10. Churchill Livingstone, Edinburgh, ch1, p 1–22

1626. Gould V E 1977 Neuroendocrinomas and neuroendocrine carinomas. APUD cell system neoplasms and their aberrant secretory activities. Pathology Annual 12: 33–62

1627. Gould V E 1982 Neuroendocrine tumors in 'miscellaneous' primary sites: clinical, pathologic and histogenetic implications. Progress in Surgical Pathology 4: 181–198

1628. Gould V E, Banner B F, Baerwaldt M 1981 Neuroendocrine neoplasms in unusual primary sites. Diagnostic Histopathology 4: 263–277

1629. Gould V E, Memoli V A, Dardi L E, Sobel H J, Somers S C, Johannessen J V 1981 Neuroendocrine carcinomas with multiple immunoreactive peptides and melanin production. Ultrastructural Pathology 2: 199–217

1630. Heitz P U, Klöppel G, Polak J M, Staub J-J 1981 Ectopic hormone production by endocrine tumors: localization of hormones at the cellular level by immunocytochemistry. Cancer 48: 2029–2037

1631. Kameya T, Shimosato Y, Abe K, Takeuchi T 1980 Morphologic and functional aspects of hormone-producing tumors. Pathology Annual 15, pt 1: 351–386

1632. Lechago J 1978 Endocrine cells of the gastrointestinal tract and their pathology. Pathology Annual 13, pt 2: 329–350

1633. Min K-W, Song J 1980 Ultrastructural observation of neural elements in carcinoid tumors. Laboratory Investigation 42: 136A

1634. Pearse A G E 1974 The APUD cell concept and its implications in pathology. Pathology Annual 9: 27–41

1635. Pearse A G E, Polak J M 1978 The diffuse neuroendocrine system and the APUD concept. In: Bloom S R (ed) Gut hormones. Churchill Livingstone, Edinburgh, ch 4, p 33–39

1636. Solcia E, Capella C, Buffa R, Frigerio B, Usellini L, Fontana P 1978 Endocrine cells of the gut and related growths: recent developments and classification. In: Bloom S R (ed) Gut hormones. Churchill Livingstone, Edinburgh, ch 10, p 77–81

1637. Solcia E, Capella C, Buffa R, Usellini L, Fontana P, Frigerio B 1978 Endocrine cells of the gastrointestinal tract: general aspects, ultrastructure and tumour pathology. Advances in Experimental Medicine and Biology 106: 11–22

1638. Solcia E, Polak J M, Pearse A G E, Forssmann W G, Larsson L-I, Sundler F, Lechago J, Grimelius L, Fuyita T, Creutzfeldt W, Gepts W, Falkmer S, Lefranc G, Heitz Ph, Hage E, Buchan A M J, Bloom S R, Grossman M I 1978 Lausanne 1977 classification of gastroenteropancreatic endocrine cells. In: Bloom S R (ed) Gut hormones. Churchill Livingstone, Edinburgh, ch 5, p 40–48

1639. Tapia F J, Barbosa A J A, Marangos P J, Polak J M, Bloom S R, Dermody C, Pearse A G E 1981 Neuron-specific enolase is produced by neuroendocrine tumours. Lancet i: 808–811

1640. Westermark P, Grimelius L, Polak J M, Larsson L-I, Van Noorden S, Wilander E, Pearse A G E 1977 Amyloid in polypeptide hormone-producing tumors. Laboratory Investigation 37: 212–215

1641. Wick M R, Carney J A, Bernatz P E, Brown L R 1982 Primary mediastinal carcinoid tumors. American Journal of Surgical Pathology 6: 195–205

*41 PITUITARY TUMOURS*

1642. Anniko M, Wersäll J 1982 Morphological effects in pituitary tumours following radiotherapy. Virchows Archiv A Pathological Anatomy and Histology 395: 45–58

1643. Bauserman S C, Hardman J M, Schochet S S Jr, Earle K M 1978 Pituitary oncocytoma: indispensable role of electron microscopy in its identification. Archives of Pathology and Laboratory Medicine 102: 456–459

1644. Bilbao J M, Horvath E, Hudson A R, Kovacs K 1975 Pituitary adenoma producing amyloid-like substance. Archives of Pathology 99: 411–415

1645. Bilbao J M, Horvath E, Kovacs K, Singer W, Hudson A R 1978 Intrasellar paraganglioma associated with hypopituitarism. Archives of Pathology and Laboratory Medicine 102: 95–98

1646. Bilbao J M, Kovacs K, Horvath E, Higgins H P, Horsey W J 1975 Pituitary melanocorticotrophinoma with amyloid deposition. Canadian Journal of Neurological Sciences 2: 199–202

1647. Capella C, Buffa R, Usellini L, Frigerio B, Johenson P, Sessa F, Solcia E 1983 Alpha and beta subunits of glycoprotein hormones in argyrophil pituitary tumors with small granule cells. Ultrastructural Pathology 4: 35–50

1648. Cardell R R Jr, Knighton R S 1966 The cytology of a human pituitary tumor: an electron microscopic study. Transactions of the American Microscopical Society 85: 58–78

1649. Charpin C, Hassoun J, Oliver C, Jaquet P, Argemi B, Grisoli F, Toga M 1982 Immunohistochemical and immuno-electron-microscopic study of pituitary adenomas associated with Cushing's disease. A report of 13 cases. American Journal of Pathology 109: 1–7

1650. Corenblum B, Sirek A M, Horvath E, Kovacs K, Ezrin C 1976 Human mixed somatotrophic and lactotrophic pituitary adenomas. Journal of Clinical Endocrinology and Metabolism 42: 857–863

1651. Cravioto H, Fukaya T, Zimmerman E A, Kleinberg D L, Flamm E S 1981 Immunohistochemical and electron-microscopic studies of functional and non-functional pituitary adenomas including one TSH secreting tumor in a thyrotoxic patient. Acta Neuropathologica 53: 281–292

1652. De Cicco F A, Dekker A, Yunis E J 1972 Fine structure of Crooke's hyaline change in the human pituitary gland. Archives of Pathology 94: 65–70

1653. Dingemans K P, Assies J, Jansen N, Diegenbach P C 1982 Sparsely granulated prolactin cell adenomas of the pituitary gland. Correlation of ultrastructure with plasma hormone level. Virchows Archiv A Pathological Anatomy and Histology 396: 167–186

1654. Doniach I 1977 Histopathology of the anterior pituitary. Clinics in Endocrinology and Metabolism 6: 21–52

1655. El-Etreby M F, Gunzel P 1973 Prolactin cell tumors in animal experiments and in man. Arzneimittel-Forschung 23: 1768–1790

1656. Farmer P M 1979 Electron microscopy in the diagnosis of pituitary tumors. Annals of Clinical and Laboratory Science 9: 275–288

1657. Felix I A, Horvath E, Kovacs K 1981 Massive Crooke's hyalinization in corticotroph cell adenomas of the human pituitary. A histological, immunocytological, and electron microscopic study of three cases. Acta Neurochirurgica 58: 235–243

1658. Furth J, Nakane P, Pasteels J L 1977 Tumours of the pituitary gland. IARC Science Publication 1: 201–237

1659. Ghatak N R, Hirano A, Zimmerman H M 1971 Ultrastructure of a craniopharyngioma. Cancer 27: 1465–1475

1660. Gjerris A, Lindholm J, Riishede J 1978 Pituitary oncocytic tumor with Cushing's disease. Cancer 42: 1818–1822

1661. Gray A B 1977 Analysis of diameters of human pituitary hormone secretory granules. Acta Endocrinologica 85: 249–255

1662. Halmi N S 1982 Occurrence of both growth hormone- and prolactin-immunoreactive material in the cells of human somatotropic pituitary adenomas containing mammotropic elements. Virchows Archiv A Pathological Anatomy and Histology 398: 19–31

1663. Horoupian D S 1980 Large mitochondria in a pituitary adenoma with hyperprolactinemia. Cancer 46: 537–542

1664. Horvath E, Kovacs K 1974 Misplaced exocytosis. Distinct ultrastructural feature in some pituitary adenomas. Archives of Pathology 97: 221–224

1665. Horvath E, Kovacs K 1978 Morphogenesis and significance of fibrous bodies in human pituitary adenomas. Virchows Archiv B Cell Pathology 27: 69–78

1666. Horvath E, Kovacs K 1980 Pathology of the pituitary gland. In: Ezrin C, Horvath E, Kaufman B, Kovacs K, Weiss M H (eds) Pituitary diseases. CRC Press, Boca Raton, Florida, p 1–83

1667. Horvath E, Kovacs K 1982 Gonadotroph cell adenomas of the human pituitary. Laboratory Investigation 46: 37A

1668. Horvath E, Kovacs K, Killinger D W, Smyth H S, Weiss M H, Ezrin C 1983 Mammosomatotroph cell adenoma of the human pituitary: a morphologic entity. Virchows Archiv A Pathological Anatomy and Histopathology 398: 277–289

1669. Horvath E, Kovacs K, Ryan N 1980 Null cell adenomas of the human adenohypophysis. Laboratory Investigation 42: 164A

1670. Horvath E, Kovacs K, Singer W, Ezrin C, Kerenyi N A 1977 Acidophil stem cell adenoma of the human pituitary. Archives of Pathology and Laboratory Medicine 101: 594–599

1671. Horvath E, Kovacs K, Singer W, Smyth H S, Killinger D W, Ezrin C, Weiss M H 1981 Acidophil stem cell adenoma of the human pituitary: clinicopathologic analysis of 15 cases. Cancer 47: 761–771

1672. Ilse G, Ryan N, Kovacs K, Ilse D 1980 Calcium deposition in human pituitary adenomas studied by histology, electron microscopy, electron diffraction and X-ray spectrometry. Experimental Pathology 18: 377–388

1673. Ishikawa H, Nogami H, Kamio M, Suzuki T 1983 Single secretory granules contain both GH and prolactin in pituitary mixed type of adenoma. Virchows Archiv A Pathological Anatomy and Histopathology 399: 221–226

1674. Kameya T, Tsumuraya M, Adachi I, Abe K, Ichikizaki K, Toya S, Demura R 1980 Ultrastructure, immunohistochemistry and hormone release of pituitary adenomas in relation to prolactin production. Virchows Archiv A Pathological Anatomy and Histology 387: 31–46

1675. Kepes J J 1978 Transitional cell tumor of the pituitary gland developing from a Rathke's cleft cyst. Cancer 41: 337–343

1676. Kovacs K 1977 Morphology of prolactin producing adenomas. Clinical Endocrinology 6, suppl: 71S–79S

1677. Kovacs K, Horvath E 1973 Pituitary 'chromophobe' adenoma composed of oncocytes. A light and electron microscopic study. Archives of Pathology 95: 235–239

1678. Kovacs K, Horvath E 1973 Vascular alterations in adenomas of human pituitary glands. An electron microscopic study. Angiologica 10: 299–309

1679. Kovacs K, Horvath E 1974 Amphophil adenoma of the human pituitary gland with masses of cytoplasmic microfilaments. Endokrinologie 63: 402–408

1680. Kovacs K, Horvath E, Corenblum B, Sirek A M, Penz G, Ezrin C 1975 Pituitary chromophobe adenomas consisting of prolactin cells. A histologic, immunocytological and electronic microscopic study. Virchows Archiv A Pathological Anatomy and Histology 366: 113–123

1681. Kovacs K, Horvath E, Ezrin C 1977 Pituitary adenomas. Pathology Annual 12, pt 2: 341–382

1682. Kovacs K, Horvath E, Ezrin C, Weiss M H 1982 Adenoma of the human pituitary producing growth hormone and thyrotropin. A histologic, immunocytologic and fine-structural study. Virchows Archiv A Pathological Anatomy and Histology 395: 59–68

1683. Kovacs K, Horvath E, Rewcastle N B, Ezrin C 1980 Gonadotroph cell adenoma of the pituitary in a woman with long standing hypogonadism. Archives of Gynecology 229: 57–65

1684. Kovacs K, Horvath E, Ryan N, Ezrin C 1980 Null cell adenoma of the human pituitary. Virchows Archiv A Pathological Anatomy and Histology 387: 165–174

1685. Kuromatsu C 1968 The fine structure of the human pituitary chromophobe adenoma with special reference to the classification of this tumor. Archivum Histologicum Japonicum 29: 41–61

1686. Kurosumi K, Shimizu T, Takeda F 1981 The pituitary gland. In: Johannessen J V (ed) Electron microscopy in human medicine, vol 10. Endocrine organs. McGraw-Hill, New York, pt 1, p 3–26

1687. Landolt A M, Hosbach H U 1974 Biological aspects of pituitary tumors as revealed by electron microscopy. Pathologica 66: 413–436

1688. Landolt A M, Oswald U W 1973 Histology and ultrastructure of an oncocytic adenoma of the human pituitary. Cancer 31: 1099–1105

1689. Landolt A M, Rothenbuhler V 1977 The size of growth hormone granules in pituitary adenomas producing acromegaly. Acta Endocrinologica 84: 461–469

1690. Landolt A M, Rothenbuhler V 1978 Extracellular growth hormone deposits in pituitary adenoma. Virchows Archiv A Pathological Anatomy and Histology 378: 55–65

1691. Lewis P D, Van Noorden S 1972 Pituitary abnormalities in acromegaly. Archives of Pathology 94: 119–126

1692. Lewis P D, Van Noorden S 1974 Nonfunctioning pituitary tumors: a light and electron microscopical study. Archives of Pathology 97: 178–182

1693. Liszczak T, Richardson E P Jr, Phillips J P, Jacobson S, Kornblith P L 1978 Morphological, biochemical, ultrastructural, tissue culture and clinical observations of typical and aggressive craniopharyngiomas. Acta Neuropathologica 43: 191–203

1694. Lloyd R V, Gikas P W, Chandler W F 1983 Prolactin and growth hormone-producing pituitary adenomas. An immunohistochemical and ultrastructural study. American Journal of Surgical Pathology 7: 251–260

1695. Martinez D, Barthe D 1982 Heterogeneous pituitary adenomas. A light microscopic, immunohistochemical and electron microscopic study. Virchows Archiv A Pathological Anatomy and Histology 394: 221–223

1696. Matsushima T, Fukui M, Ohta M, Yamakawa Y, Takaki T, Okano H 1980 Ciliated and goblet cells in craniopharyngioma. Light and electron microscopic studies at surgery and autopsy. Acta Neuropathologica 50: 199–205

1697. Mukai M 1983 Pituitary adenomas. Immunocytochemical study of 150 tumors with clinicopathologic correlation. Cancer 52: 648–653

1698. Pearl G S, Takei Y, Kurisaka M, Seyama S, Tindall G T 1981 Cystic prolactinoma. A variant of 'transitional cell tumor' of the pituitary. American Journal of Surgical Pathology 5: 85–90

1699. Poon M-C, Prchal J T, Murad T M, Galbraith J G 1979 Multiple myeloma masquerading as chromophobe adenoma. Cancer 43: 1513–1516

1700. Robert F, Hardy J 1975 Prolactin-secreting adenomas. A light and electron microscopical study. Archives of Pathology 99: 625–633

1701. Robert F, Pelletier G, Hardy J 1978 Pituitary adenomas in Cushing's disease. A histologic, ultrastructural and immunocytochemical study. Archives of Pathology and Laboratory Medicine 102: 448–455

1702. Roy S 1977 Ultrastructure of chromophobe adenoma of the human pituitary gland. Journal of Pathology 122: 219–223

1703. Roy S 1978 Cytoplasmic filamentous masses in chromophobe adenoma of the human pituitary gland. Journal of Pathology 125: 151–154

1704. Roy S 1978 Ultrastructure of oncocytic adenoma of the human pituitary gland. Acta Neuropathologica 41: 169–171

1705. Saeger W, Lüdecke D K 1982 Pituitary adenomas with hyperfunction of TSH. Frequency, histological classification, immunocytochemistry and ultrastructure. Virchows Archiv A Pathological Anatomy and Histology 394: 255–267

1706. Saeger W, Lüdecke D K 1983 Pituitary hyperplasia. Definition, light and electron microscopical structures and significance in surgical specimens. Virchows Archiv A Pathological Anatomy and Histopathology 399: 277–287

1707. Saeger W, Ruttmann E, Lüdecke D 1981 ACTH secreting pituitary adenoma in an infant of 18 months. Immuno-histochemical, electron-microscopic, and in-vitro studies. Pathology Research and Practice 173: 121–129

1708. Sandbank U, Borstein B, Najenson T 1974 Acidophilic adenoma of the pituitary with polyneuropathy. Journal of Neurology, Neurosurgery and Psychiatry 37: 324–329

1709. Scanarini M, Mingrino S 1980 Functional classification of pituitary adenomas. Acta Neurochirurgica 52: 195–202

1710. Schechter J 1973 Electron microscopic studies of human pituitary tumors. I. Chromophobic adenomas. American Journal of Anatomy 138: 371–385

1711. Schechter J 1973 Electron microscopic studies of human pituitary tumors. II. Acidophilic adenomas. American Journal of Anatomy 138: 387–399

1712. Schober R, Nelson D 1975 Fine structure and origin of amyloid deposits in pituitary adenoma. Archives of Pathology 99: 403–410

1713. Schochet S S, McCormick W F, Halmi N S 1972 Acidophil adenomas with intracytoplasmic filamentous aggregates. A light and electron microscopic study. Archives of Pathology 94: 16–22

1714. Shimizu T, Ishida Y, Takeda F 1978 Electron microscopy of human pituitary adenomas. Correlation of the secretory granules with the experimentally and clinically evaluated hormone synthesis function of the adenoma tissue. Neurologica Medico-Chirurgica 18: 107–117

1715. Stefaneanu L, Tasca C, Coculescu M 1981 A light and electron microscopical study of pituitary adenomas. Endocrinologie 19: 243–248

1716. Tomiyasu U, Hirano A, Zimmerman H M 1973 Fine structure of human pituitary adenoma. Archives of Pathology 95: 287–292

1717. Trouillas J, Girod C, Lhéritier M, Claustrat B, Dubois M P 1980 Morphological and biochemical relationships in 31 human pituitary adenomas with acromegaly. Virchows Archiv A Pathological Anatomy and Histology 389: 127–142

1718. Trouillas J, Girod C, Sassolas G, Claustrat B, Lhéritier M, Dubois M P, Goutelle A 1981 Human pituitary gonadotrophic adenoma: histological, immunocytochemical, and ultrastructural and hormonal studies in eight cases. Journal of Pathology 135: 315–336

1719. Vilches J, Lopez A, Martinez M C, Gomez J, Barbera J 1981 Scanning and transmission electron microscopy of a craniopharyngioma: X-ray microanalytical study of the intratumoral mineralized deposits. Ultrastructural Pathology 2: 343–356

## 42 TUMOURS OF THE THYROID GLAND

1720. Albores-Saavedra J, Altamirano-Dimas M, Alcorta-Anguizola B, Smith M 1971 Fine structure of human papillary thyroid carcinoma. Cancer 28: 763–774

1721. Asaadi A A 1981 Ultrastructure in C cell hyperplasia in asymptomatic patients with hypercalcitoninemia and a family history of medullary thyroid carcinoma. Human Pathology 12: 617–622

1722. Beaumont A, Ben Othman S, Fragu P 1981 The fine structure of papillary carcinoma of the thyroid. Histopathology 5: 377–388

1723. Braunstein H, Stephens C L, Gibson R L 1968 Secretory granules in medullary carcinoma of the thyroid: electron microscopic demonstration. Archives of Pathology 85: 306–313

1724. Burke J S, Butler J J, Fuller L M 1977 Malignant lymphomas of the thyroid. A clinical pathologic study of 35 patients including ultrastructural observations. Cancer 39: 1587–1602

1725. Bussolati G, Monga G 1979 Medullary carcinoma of the thyroid with atypical patterns. Cancer 44: 1769–1777

1726. Cameron R G, Seemayer T A, Wang N-S, Ahmed M N, Tabah E J 1975 Small cell malignant tumors of the thyroid. A light and electron microscopic study. Human Pathology 6: 731–740

1727. Carneiro F, Conçalves V, Sobrinho-Simoes M A 1980 Intranuclear cytoplasmic inclusions in thyroid papillary carcinomas. Journal of Submicroscopic Cytology 12: 137–143

1728. Cibull M L, Gray G F 1978 Ultrastructure of osteoclastoma-like giant cell tumor of thyroid. American Journal of Surgical Pathology 2: 401–405

1729. David R, Kim K M 1983 Dense-core matrical mitochondrial bodies in oncocytic adenoma of the thyroid. Archives of Pathology and Laboratory Medicine 107: 178–182

1730. Davis R I, Corson J M 1979 Renal metastases from well differentiated follicular thyroid carcinoma: a case report with light and electron microscopic findings. Cancer 43: 265–268

1731. Dayan A D, Woodhouse M A 1968 Amyloid and medullary carcinoma of the thyroid. Electron microscope observations on one case. Pathologia et Microbiologia 31: 93–96

1732. DeLellis R A, May L, Tashjian A H Jr, Wolfe H J 1978 C-cell granule heterogeneity in man. An ultrastructural immunocytochemical study. Laboratory Investigation 38: 263–269

1733. DeLellis R A, Nunnemacher G, Wolfe H J 1977 C-cell hyperplasia. An ultrastructural analysis. Laboratory Investigation 36: 237–248

1734. DeLellis R A, Wolfe H J 1981 The pathobiology of the human calcitonin (C)-cell: a review. Pathology Annual 16, pt 2: 25–52

1735. Deligdisch L, Subhani Z, Gordon R E 1980 Primary mucinous carcinoma of the thyroid gland: report of a case and ultrastructural study. Cancer 45: 2564–2567

1736. Dickersin G R, Vickery A L Jr, Smith S B 1980 Papillary carcinoma of the thyroid, oxyphil cell type, 'clear cell' variant. A light- and electron-microscopic study. American Journal of Surgical Pathology 4: 501–509

1737. Dralle H, Böcker W 1977 Immunohistochemical and electron microscope analysis of adenomas of the thyroid gland. I. A comparative investigation of hot and cold nodules. Virchows Archiv A Pathological Anatomy and Histology 374: 285–301

1738. Faria V, Vaz Saleiro J, Oliveira M C 1982 Atypical thyroid carcinoma: atypical follicular or atypical medullary carcinoma? Journal of Submicroscopic Cytology 13: 717–721

1739. Feldman P S, Horvath E, Kovacs K 1972 Ultrastructure of three Hürthle cell tumors of the thyroid. Cancer 30: 1279–1285

1740. Fernandez B J, Bedard Y C, Rosen I 1982 Mucus-producing medullary cell carcinoma of the thyroid gland. American Journal of Clinical Pathology 78: 536–540

1741. Fisher E R, Gregorio R, Shoemaker R, Horvat B, Hubay C 1974 The derivation of so-called giant cell and spindle cell undifferentiated thyroidal neoplasms. American Journal of Clinical Pathology 61: 680–689

1742. Fisher E R, Kim W S 1977 Primary clear cell thyroid carcinoma with squamous features. Cancer 39: 2497–2502

1743. Gaal J M, Horvath E, Kovacs K 1975 Ultrastructure of two cases of anaplastic giant cell tumor of the human thyroid gland. Cancer 35: 1273–1279

1744. Gonzalez-Licea A, Hartmann W H, Yardley J H 1968 Medullary carcinoma of the thyroid. Ultrastructural evidence of its origin from the parafollicular cell and its possible relation to carcinoid tumors. American Journal of Clinical Pathology 49: 512–520

1745. Gould V E, Gould N S, Benditt E P 1972 Ultrastructural aspects of papillary and sclerosing carcinomas of the thyroid. Cancer 29: 1613–1625

1746. Gould V E, Johannessen J V, Sobrinho-Simoes M 1981 The thyroid gland. In: Johannessen J V (ed) Electron microscopy in human medicine, vol 10. Endocrine organs. McGraw-Hill, New York, pt 2, p 29–107

1747. Graham H, Daniel J 1974 Ultrastructure of an anaplastic carcinoma of the thyroid. American Journal of Clinical Pathology 61: 690–696

1748. Hales M, Rosenau W, Okerlund M, Galante M 1982 Carcinoma of the thyroid with a mixed medullary and follicular pattern. Morphologic, immunohistochemical, and clinical laboratory studies. Cancer 50: 1352–1359

1749. Heimann P, Ljunggren J-G, Löwhagen T, Hjern B 1973 Oxyphilic adenoma of the human thyroid. A morphological and biochemical study. Cancer 31: 246–254

1750. Hofstädter F 1980 Electron microscopic investigations about the differentiation of thyroid carcinoma. Pathology Research and Practice 169: 304–322

1751. Huang S N, Goltzman D 1978 Electron and immunoelectron microscopic study of thyroidal medullary carcinoma. Cancer 41: 2226–2235

1752. Ibanez M L 1974 Medullary carcinoma of the thyroid. Pathology Annual 9: 263–290

1753. Jao W, Gould V E 1975 Ultrastructure of anaplastic (spindle and giant cell) carcinoma of the thyroid: Cancer 35: 1280–1292

1754. Johannessen J V, Gould V E, Jao W 1978 The fine structure of human thyroid cancer. Human Pathology 9: 385–400

1755. Johannessen J V, Sobrinho-Simoes M 1981 Papillary carcinoma of the human thyroid gland. An ultrastructural study with emphasis on scanning electron microscopy. Progress in Surgical Pathology 3: 111–128

1756. Johannessen J V, Sobrinho-Simoes M 1982 Follicular carcinoma of the human thyroid gland: an ultrastructural study with emphasis on scanning electron microscopy. Diagnostic Histopathology 5: 113–127

1757. Johannessen J V, Sobrinho-Simoes M 1982 The fine structure of follicular thyroid adenomas. American Journal of Clinical Pathology 78: 299–310

1758. Johannessen J V, Sobrinho-Simoes M 1983 Well differentiated thyroid tumors. Problems in diagnosis and understanding. Pathology Annual 18, pt 1: 255–285

1759. Johannessen J V, Sobrinho-Simões M, Finseth I, Pilström L 1982 Papillary carcinomas of the thyroid have pore-deficient nuclei. International Journal of Cancer 30: 409–411

1760. Johannessen J V, Sobrinho-Simões M, Finseth I, Pilström L 1983 Ultrastructural morphometry of thyroid neoplasms. American Journal of Clinical Pathology 79: 166–171

1761. Johannessen J V, Sobrinho-Simões M, Lindmo T, Tangen K O, Kaalhus O, Brennhovd I 1983 Anomalous papillary carcinoma of the thyroid. Cancer 51: 1462–1467

1762. Kakudo K, Spurlock B O, Miyauchi A, Kuma K, Shimaoka K, Matsuzuka F 1982 Unusual cytoplasmic inclusion bodies in medullary carcinoma of the thyroid gland. Acta Pathologica Japonica 32: 319–326

1763. Kalderon A E, Bogaars H A, Diamond I 1975 Immune complex deposition in thyroid carcinoma associated with chronic thyroiditis. Clinical Immunology and Immunopathology 4: 101–107

1764. Kameya T, Shimosato Y, Adachi I, Abe K, Kasai N, Kimura K, Baba K 1977 Immunohistochemical and ultrastructural analysis of medullary carcinoma in relation to hormone production. American Journal of Pathology 89: 555–574

1765. Kay S, Terz J J 1976 Ultrastructural observations on a follicular carcinoma of the thyroid gland. American Journal of Clinical Pathology 65: 328–336

1766. Lew W, Orell S R, Henderson D W 1984 Intranuclear vacuoles in nonpapillary carcinoma of thyroid: a report of three cases. Acta Cytologica 28: 581–586

1767. Löwhagen T, Sprenger E 1974 Cytologic presentation of thyroid tumors in aspiration biopsy smear. A review of 60 cases. Acta Cytologica 18: 192–197

1768. Luna M A, Mackay B, Hill C S, Hussey D H, Hickey R C 1980 The quarterly case: malignant small cell tumor of the thyroid. Ultrastructural Pathology 1: 265–270

1769. Lupulescu A P, Boyd C B 1972 Follicular adenomas. An ultrastructural and scanning electron microscopic study. Archives of Pathology 93: 492–502

1770. Marcus J N, Dise C A, Li Volsi V A 1982 Melanin production in a medullary thyroid carcinoma. Cancer 49: 2518–2526

1771. Marcus P B, Martin J H, Lieberman Z H 1979 Convoluted secretory material in thyroid follicular epithelial tumors. American Journal of Surgical Pathology 3: 279–281

1772. Martinelli G, Bazzocchi F, Govoni E, Santini D 1983 Anaplastic type of medullary thyroid carcinoma. An ultrastructural and immunohistochemical study. Virchows Archiv A Pathological Anatomy and Histopathology 400: 61–67

1773. Memoli V A, Johannessen J V, Warren W H, Blom P, Gould V E 1983 Ultrastructural and immunohistochemical heterogeneity of medullary thyroid carcinomas. Laboratory Investigation 48: 57A

1774. Meyer J S 1968 Fine structure of two amyloid forming medullary carcinomas of thyroid. Cancer 21: 406–425

1775. Mayer J S, Abdel Bari W 1968 Granules and thyrocalcitonin-like activity in medullary carcinoma of the thyroid gland. New England Journal of Medicine 278: 523–529

1776. Meyer J S, Hutton W E, Kenny A D 1973 Medullary carcinoma of thyroid gland. Subcellular distribution of calcitonin and relationship between granules and amyloid. Cancer 31: 433–441

1777. Newland J R, Mackay B, Hill C S Jr, Hickey R C 1981 Anaplastic thyroid carcinoma: an ultrastructural study of 10 cases. Ultrastructural Pathology 2: 121–129

1778. Normann T, Johannessen J V, Gautvik K M, Olsen B R, Brennhovd I O 1976 Medullary carcinoma of the thyroid. Diagnostic problems. Cancer 38: 366–377

1779. Olsen J L, Penney D P, Averill K A 1977 Fine structural studies of a human thyroid adenoma, with special reference to psammoma bodies. Human Pathology 8: 103–111

1780. Panke T W, Croxson M S, Parker J W, Carriere D P, Rosoff L Sr, Warner N E 1978 Triiodothyronine secreting toxic adenoma of the thyroid gland: light and electron microscopic characteristics. Cancer 41: 528–537

1781. Pontius K I, Hawk W A 1980 Loss of microsomal antigen in follicular and papillary carcinoma of the thyroid. An immunofluorescence and electron-microscopic study. American Journal of Clinical Pathology 74: 620–629

1782. Ruizvalesco R, Waisman J, Vanherle A J 1978 Cystic papillary carcinoma of the thyroid gland. Diagnosis by needle aspiration with transmission electron microscopy. Acta Cytologica 22: 38–42

1783. Saito R, Sharma K 1976 Fine structure of a diffuse undifferentiated small cell carcinoma of the thyroid. American Journal of Clinical Pathology 65: 623–630

1784. Satoh M, Yagawa K 1981 Electron microscopic study on mitochondria in Hürthle cell adenoma of thyroid. Acta Pathologica Japonica 31: 1079–1087

1785. Schürch W, Babai F, Boivin Y, Verdy M 1977 Light, electron microscopic and cytochemical studies on the morphogenesis of familial medullary thyroid carcinoma. Virchows Archiv A Pathological Anatomy and Histology 376: 29–46

1786. Shin W-Y, Aftalion B, Hotchkiss E, Schenkman R, Berkman J 1979 Ultrastructure of a primary fibrosarcoma of the human thyroid gland. Cancer 44: 584–591

1787. Sobrinho-Simoes M, Johannessen J V 1982 Surface features in human thyroid disorders. A scanning electron microscopic study of ninety five cases. Journal of Submicroscopic Cytology 14: 187–202

1788. Tasca C, Stefaneanu L 1980 Ultrastructural morphometry of the secretory granules in thyroid medullary carcinoma. Endocrinologie 18: 187–191

1789. Tateishi R, Takahashi Y, Naguchi A 1972 Histologic and ultracytochemical studies on thyroid medullary carcinoma. Diagnostic significance of argyrophil secretory granules. Cancer 30: 755–763

1790. Tonietti G, Baschieri L, Salabe G 1967 Papillary and microfollicular carcinoma of human thyroid. An ultrastructural study. Archives of Pathology 84: 601–614

1791. Valenta L J, Michel-Béchet M 1977 Electron microscopy of clear cell thyroid carcinoma. Archives of Pathology and Laboratory Medicine 101: 140–144

1792. Valenta L J, Michel-Béchet M 1977 Ultrastructure and biochemistry of thyroid carcinoma. Cancer 40: 284–300

1793. Valenta L J, Michel-Béchet M, Mattson J C, Singer F R 1977 Microfollicular thyroid carcinoma with amyloid rich stroma, resembling the medullary carcinoma of the thyroid (MCT). Cancer 39: 1573–1586

1794. Variakojis D, Getz M L, Paloyan E, Straus F H II 1975 Papillary clear cell carcinoma of the thyroid gland. Human Pathology 6: 385–390

1795. Vaz Saleiro J, Faria V, Oliveira M C 1981 Clear cell tumor of the thyroid gland. Journal of Submicroscopic Cytology 13: 75–77

1796. Weimann R, Vannineuse A, de Sloover C, Dor P 1978 Malignant lymphomas and undifferentiated small cell carcinoma of the thyroid: a clinicopathological review in the light of the Kiel classification for malignant lymphomas. Histopathology 2: 201–213

1797. Wolfe H J, DeLellis R A 1981 Familial medullary thyroid carcinoma and C cell hyperplasia. Clinics in Endocrinology and Metabolism 10: 351–365

## 43 TUMOURS OF THE PARATHYROID GLANDS

1798. Allen T B, Thorburn K M 1981 The oxyphil cell in abnormal parathyroid glands. A study of 114 cases. Archives of Pathology and Laboratory Medicine 105: 421–427

1799. Altenähr E 1981 The parathyroid glands. In: Johannessen J V (ed) Electron microscopy in human medicine, vol 10. Endocrine organs. McGraw-Hill, New York, pt 3, p 129–146

1800. Arnold B M, Kovacs K, Horvath E, Murray T M, Higgins H P 1974 Functioning oxyphil cell adenoma of the parathyroid gland: evidence for parathyroid secretory activity of oxyphil cells. Journal of Clinical Endocrinology and Metabolism 38: 458–462

1801. Bichel P, Thomsen O F, Askjaer S A, Nielsen H E 1980 Light and electron microscopic investigation of parathyroid carcinoma during dedifferentiation. Survey and study of a case. Virchows Archiv A Pathological Anatomy and Histology 386: 363–370

1802. Boquist L 1980 On the relationship between annulate lamellae and mitochondria in human parathyroid adenomas. Zeitschrift für Mikroskopisch-Anatomische Forschung 94: 241–249

1803. Capen C C, Roth S I 1973 Ultrastructural and functional relationships of normal and pathologic parathyroid cells. Pathobiology Annual 3: 129–175

1804. Castleman B, Roth S I 1978 Tumors of the parathyroid glands. Atlas of tumor pathology, 2nd series, fascicle 14. Armed Forces Institute of Pathology, Washington DC

1805. Chaudhry A P, Satchidanand S, Gaeta J F, Cerra F B, Nickerson P A 1979 A functional parathyroid gland adenoma of transitional oxyphil cells. A light and ultrastructural study. Pathology 11: 705–712

1806. Cinti S, Osculati F 1982 Ribosome-lamellae complex in the adenoma cells of the human parathyroid gland. Journal of Submicroscopic Cytology 14: 521–524

1807. Cinti S, Osculati F, Lo Casio V 1980 Submicroscopic aspects of the chief cells in a case of a parathyroid adenoma. Journal of Submicroscopic Cytology 12: 293–300

1808. Cinti S, Osculati F, Parravicini C 1982 RER-associated structure in parathyroid glands removed because of tertiary hyperparathyroidism. Ultrastructural Pathology 3: 263–268

1809. Dietel M, Altenähr E, Montz R, Hagemann J, Dorn G 1978 Correlation of electron microscopic and secretory response of human parathyroid adenomas with different calcium concentrations in organ culture. Virchows Archiv A Pathological Anatomy and Histology 378: 229–246

1810. Faccini J M 1970 Ultrastructure of parathyroid glands removed from patients with primary hyperparathyroidism: report of 40 cases, including 4 carcinomas. Journal of Pathology 102: 189–199

1811. Holck S, Pedersen N T 1981 Carcinoma of the parathyroid gland. A light and electron microscopic study. Acta Pathologica et Microbiologica Scandinavica. Section A Pathology 89: 297–302

1812. Kameya T, Tamaoki N, Watanabe Y, Tachikawa S, Wada T 1974 Light and electron microscopic observations on two cases of parathyroid adenoma. Calcified Tissue Research 15: 156

1813. Marshall R B, Roberts D K, Turner R A 1967 Adenomas of the human parathyroid. Light and electron microscopic study following selenium 75 methionine scan. Cancer 20: 512–524

1814. Murayama T, Kawabe K, Tagami M 1977 A case of parathyroid carcinoma concurred with hyperplasia: an electron microscopic study. Journal of Urology 118: 126–127

1815. Nilsson O 1977 Studies on the ultrastructure of the human parathyroid glands in various pathological conditions. Acta Pathologica et Microbiologica Scandinavica. Section A. Pathology, suppl: 1–88

1816. Ordonez N G, Ibanez M L, Mackay B, Samaan N A, Hickey R C 1982 Functioning oxyphil cell adenomas of parathyroid gland: immunoperoxidase evidence of hormonal activity in oxyphil cells. American Journal of Clinical Pathology 78: 681–689

1817. Philips J N, Wills E J, Joasoo A, Davies J S, Goldie J E, Ng A B 1983 Large parathyroid adenoma in a normocalcemic patient. Pathology 15: 491–496

1818. Roth S I, Capen C C 1974 Ultrastructural and functional correlations of the parathyroid gland. International Review of Experimental Pathology 13: 161–221

1819. Selzman H M, Fechner R E 1967 Oxyphil adenoma and primary hyperparathyroidism. Clinical and ultrastructural observations. Journal of the American Medical Association 199: 359–361

1820. Spagnoli L G, Viilaschi S, Oddi G, Cocchieri G 1980 Ultrastructural observations on two parathyroid adenomas. Tumori 66: 397–404

1821. Szakacs J E, Bryant M 1980 Ultrastructure of parathyroid adenomas. Annals of Clinical and Laboratory Science 10: 13–25

1822. Szilagyi G, Benedeczky I, Lapis K 1967 Multiple parathyroid adenoma. Clinical, histological and electron microscopical studies. Acta Medica Academiae Scientiarum Hungaricae 23: 125–138

1823. Urbanski S J, Horvath E, Gardiner G W, Kovacs K 1981 Parathyroid carcinoma containing Luse bodies. A case report, including electron microscopic study. Journal of Submicroscopic Cytology 13: 63–68

1824. Weymouth R J, Sheridan M N 1966 Fine structure of human parathyroid glands, normal and pathological. Acta Endocrinologica 53: 529–546

## 44 TUMOURS OF THE ADRENAL CORTEX AND MEDULLA

1825. Aiba M, Suzuki H, Kageyama K, Murai M, Tazaki H, Abe O, Saruta T 1981 Spironolactone bodies in aldosteronomas and in the attached adrenals. Enzyme histochemical study of 19 cases of primary aldosteronism and a case of aldosteronism due to bilateral diffuse hyperplasia of the zona glomerulosa. American Journal of Pathology 103: 404–410

1826. Akhtar M, Gosalbez T, Young I 1974 Ultrastructural study of androgen-producing adrenocortical adenoma. Cancer 34: 322–327

1827. Bahu R M, Battifora H, Shambaugh G III 1974 Functional black adenoma of the adrenal gland: light and electron microscopic study. Archives of Pathology 98: 139–142

1828. Beltran G, Leiderman E, Stuckey W J Jr, Ferrans V J, Mogabgab W J 1969 Metastatic ganglioneuroblastoma. Ultrastructural, histochemical, and virological studies in a case. Cancer 24: 552–559

1829. Blaschko H, Jerrome D W, Robb-Smith A H, Smith A D, Winkler H 1968 Biochemical and morphological studies on catecholamine storage in human phaeochromocytoma. Clinical Science 34: 453–465

1830. Brown W J, Barajas L, Waisman J, De Quattro V 1972 Ultrastructural and biochemical correlates of adrenal and extra-adrenal pheochromocytoma. Cancer 29: 744–759

1831. Caplan R H, Virata R L 1974 Functional black adenoma of the adrenal cortex. A rare cause of primary aldosteronism. American Journal of Clinical Pathology 62: 97–103

1832. Cervós-Navarro J, Bayer J M, Käser H 1973 Ultrastructural differentiation of pheochromocytoma. Virchows Archiv A Pathologische Anatomie 361: 51–69

1833. Cohn D, Jackson R V, Gordon R D 1983 Factors affecting the frequency of occurrence of spironolactone bodies in aldosteronomas and non-tumorous cortex. Pathology 15: 273–277

1834. Conde E, Lafarga M, Bureo E, Baro J, Garijo J, Recio M, Zubizaretta A 1982 Unusual ultrastructural findings in neuroblastoma. Cancer 50: 1115–1121

1835. Davis D A, Medlina N M 1970 Spironolactone (aldactone) bodies: concentric lamellar formations in the adrenal cortices of patients treated with spironolactone. American Journal of Clinical Pathology 54: 22–32

1836. Eto T, Kumamoto K, Kawasaki T, Omae T, Masaki Z, Yamamoto T 1979 Ultrastructural types of cell in adrenal cortical adenoma with primary aldosteronism. Journal of Pathology 128: 1–6

1837. Evans A E, Hummeler K 1973 The significance of primitive cells in marrow aspirates of children with neuroblastoma. Cancer 32: 906–912

1838. Garret R, Ames R P 1973 Black-pigmented adenoma of the adrenal gland. Report of three cases including electron microscopic study. Archives of Pathology 95: 349–353

1839. Gorgas K, Block P, Wuketich S 1976 Fine structure of a virilizing adrenocortical adenoma. Beiträge zur Pathologie 159: 371–397

1840. Hosoda S, Suzuki H, Oguri T, Ikuta K, Nagatsu T 1976 Adrenal pheochromocytoma with both benign and malignant components. Acta Pathologica Japonica 26: 519–531

1841. Huhtanieme I, Kahri A I, Pelkonen R, Salmenperla M, Sivula A, Vihko R 1978 Ultrastructural and steroidogenic characteristics of an androgen-producing adrenocortical tumour. Clinical Endocrinology 8: 305–314

1842. Iida Y, Nose O, Kai H, Okada A, Mori T, Lee P K, Kakudo K, Yanaihara N 1980 Watery diarrhea with a vasoactive intestinal peptide-producing ganglioneuroblastoma. Archives of Disease in Childhood 55: 929–936

1843. Jenis E H, Hertzog R W 1969 Effect of spironolactone on the zona glomerulosa of the adrenal gland. Light and electron microscopy. Archives of Pathology 88: 530–539

1844. Kano K, Sato S 1977 Fine structure of adrenal adenomata causing Cushing's syndrome. Virchows Archiv A Pathological Anatomy and Histology 374: 157–168

1845. Katenkamp D, Stiller D, Holzhausen H J 1983 Morphology of neuroblastoma. Light and electron microscopic studies as a contribution to diagnosis and differential diagnosis. Zentralblatt für allgemeine Pathologie und pathologische Anatomie 127: 207–218

1846. Koppersmith D L, Powers J M, Hennigar G R 1980 Angiomatoid neuroblastoma with cytoplasmic glycogen. A case report and histogenetic considerations. Cancer 45: 553–560

1847. Kovacs K, Horvath E, Delarue N C, Ladlaw J C 1974 Ultrastructural features of an aldosterone-secreting adrenocortical adenoma. Hormone Research 5: 47–56

1848. Kovacs K, Horvath E, Singer W 1973 Fine structure and morphogenesis of spironolactone bodies in the zona glomerulosa of the human adrenal cortex. Journal of Clinical Pathology 26: 949–957

1849. Kramer S A, Bradford W D, Anderson E E 1980 Bilateral adrenal neuroblastoma. Cancer 45: 2208–2212

1850. Lauper N T, Tyce G M, Sheps S G, Carney J A 1972 Pheochromocytoma: fine structural, biochemical and clinical observations. American Journal of Cardiology 30: 197–204

1851. Macadam R F 1970 Fine structure of a functional adrenal cortical adenoma. Cancer 26: 1300–1310

1852. Mackay B, Luna M A, Butler J J 1976 Adult neuroblastoma. Electron microscopic observations in nine cases. Cancer 37: 1334–1351

1853. Mackay B, Masse S R, King O Y, Butler J 1975 Diagnosis of neuroblastoma by electron microscopy of bone marrow aspirates. Pediatrics 56: 1045–1049

1854. Mazzocchi G, Robba C, Gottardo G, Meneghelli V, Nussdorfer G G 1982 Ultrastructure of aldosterone secreting adrenal adenomata. Journal of Submicroscopic Cytology 14: 179–185

1855. Meneghelli V, Bonanni G, Robba C, Ziliotto D, Mazzocchi G, Nussdorfer G G 1981 Observations on the fine structure of an adrenal adenoma provoking Cushing's syndrome. Journal of Submicroscopic Cytology 13: 69–74

1856. Misugi K, Misugi N, Newton W A Jr 1968 Fine structural study of neuroblastoma, ganglioneuroblastoma, and pheochromocytoma. Archives of Pathology 86: 160–170

1857. Mullins J D 1980 A pigmented differentiating neuroblastoma. A light and ultrastructural study. Cancer 46: 522–528

1858. O'Hare M J, Monaghan P, Neville A M 1979 The pathology of adrenocortical neoplasia: a correlated structural and functional approach to the diagnosis of malignant disease. Human Pathology 10: 137–153

1859. Osborn M, Altmannsberger M, Shaw G, Schauer A, Weber K 1982 Various sympathetic derived human tumors differ in neurofilament expression. Use in diagnosis of neuroblastoma, ganglioneuroblastoma and pheochromocytoma. Virchows Archiv B Cell Pathology 40: 141–156

1860. Powers J M, Balentine J D, Wisniewski H M, Terry R D 1976 Retroperitoneal ganglioneuroblastoma – kaleidoscope of neuronal degeneration: a light and electron microscopic study. Journal of Neuropathology and Experimental Neurology 35: 14–25

1861. Reidbord H, Fisher E R 1969 Aldosteronoma and nonfunctioning adrenal cortical adenoma: comparative ultrastructural study. Archives of Pathology 88: 155–161

1862. Robba C, Bonanni G, Meneghelli V, Ziliotto D, Mazzocchi G, Nussdorfer G G 1980 Ultrastructure of cortisol-secreting adrenal adenomata. Virchows Archiv B Cell Pathology 33: 245–255

1863. Romansky S G, Crocker D W, Shaw K N F 1978 Ultrastructural studies on neuroblastoma. Evaluation of cytodifferentiation and correlation of morphology and biochemical and survival data. Cancer 42: 2392–2398

1864. Rosenthal I M, Greenberg R, Goldstein R, Katham R, Cadkin L 1966 Catecholamine metabolism in a pheochromocytoma. Correlation with electron micrographs. American Journal of Diseases of Children 11: 389–395

1865. Sano T, Saito H, Inaba H, Hizawa K, Saito S, Yamanoi A, Mizunuma Y, Matsumura M, Yuasa M, Hiraishi K 1983 Immunoreactive somatostatin and vasoactive intestinal polypeptide in adrenal pheochromocytoma. An immunochemical and ultrastructural study. Cancer 52: 282–289

1866. Sasano N, Ojima M, Masuda T 1980 Endocrinologic pathology of functioning adrenocortical tumors. Pathology Annual 15, pt 2: 105–141

1867. Shimada H 1982 Transmission and scanning electron microscopic studies on the tumors of neuroblastoma group. Acta Pathologica Japonica 32: 415–426

1868. Shin W-Y, Groman G S, Berkman J I 1977 Pheochromocytoma with angiomatous features. A case report and ultrastructural study. Cancer 40: 275–283

1869. Shrago S S, Waisman J, Cooper P H 1975 Spironolactone bodies in an adrenal adenoma. Archives of Pathology 99: 416–420

1870. Silva E G, Mackay B, Samaan N A, Hickey R C 1982 Adrenocortical carcinomas: an ultrastructural study of 22 cases. Ultrastructural Pathology 3: 1–7

1871. Tannenbaum M 1970 Ultrastructual pathology of adrenal medullary tumors. Pathology Annual 5: 145–171

1872. Tannenbaum M 1973 Ultrastructural pathology of the adrenal cortex. Pathology Annual 8: 109–156

1873. Tannenbaum M 1981 The adrenal glands. In: Johannessen J V (ed) Electron microscopy in human medicine, vol 10. Endocrine organs. McGraw-Hill, New York, pt 4, p 149–186

1874. Taxy J B 1980 Electron microscopy in the diagnosis of neuroblastoma. Archives of Pathology and Laboratory Medicine 104: 355–360

1875. Triche T J, Askin F B 1983 Neuroblastoma and the differential diagnosis of small-, round- blue-cell tumors. Human Pathology 14: 569–595

1876. Triche T J, Ross W E 1978 Glycogen-containing neuroblastoma with clinical and histopathologic features of Ewing's sarcoma. Cancer 41: 1425–1432

1877. Vacher-Lavenu M C, Lellouch-Tubiana A, Louvel A, Daudet-Monsac M, Abelanet R 1982 Spironolactone bodies. A light and electron microscopic study of four cases of Conn's adenomas. Annales de Pathologie 2: 311–319

1878. Voorhess M L 1974 Neuroblastoma-pheochromocytoma: products and pathogenesis. Annals of the New York Academy of Science 230: 187–194

1879. Wrzolkowa T, Mrozowicz M, Lewinski A, Pryczkowski J 1975 Phaeochromocytoma: electron microscopic study on catecholamine storage. Pathologia Europaea 10: 179–191

1880. Yunis E J, Agostini R M Jr, Walpusk J A, Hubbard J D 1979 Glycogen in neuroblastomas. A light- and electron-microscopic study of 40 cases. American Journal of Surgical Pathology 3: 313–323

1881. Zwierzina W-D 1982 Ultrastructure of a steroid producing adrenal cortex tumor and another one without endocrine activity. Zentralblatt für allgemeine Pathologie und pathologische Anatomie 126: 269–276

## 45 EXTRA-ADRENAL PARAGANGLIOMAS

1882. Alpert L I, Bochetto J F Jr 1974 Carotid body tumor: ultrastructural observations. Cancer 34: 564–573

1883. Amemiya T, Kadoya M 1980 Paraganglioma in the orbit. Journal of Cancer Research and Clinical Oncology 96: 169–179

1884. Beltrami C A, Montironi R, Cinti S 1980 Gangliocytic paraganglioma of the duodenum: case report. Tumori 66: 637–641

1885. Binkley W, Vakili S T, Worth R 1982 Paraganglioma of the cauda equina. Case report. Journal of Neurosurgery 56: 275–279

1886. Buss D H, Marshall R B, Baird F G, Myers R T 1980 Paraganglioma of the thyroid gland. American Journal of Surgical Pathology 5: 589–593

1887. Cabello A, Ricoy J R 1983 Paraganglioma of the cauda equina. Cancer 52: 751–754

1888. Chaudhry A P, Haar J G, Koul A, Nickerson P A 1979 A nonfunctioning paraganglioma of vagus nerve. An ultrastructural study. Cancer 43: 1689–1701

1889. Crowell W T, Grizzle W E, Siegel A L 1982 Functional carotid paragangliomas. Biochemical, ultrastructural, and histochemical correlations with clinical symptoms. Archives of Pathology and Laboratory Medicine 106: 599–603

1890. Dhom G, Hohbach Ch 1980 Case 11: chemodectoma of the larynx. Ultrastructural Pathology 1: 133–139

1891. Fernandez B B, Hernandez F J, Staley C J 1975 Chemodectoma of the vagus nerve. Report of a case with ultrastructural study. Cancer 35: 263–269

1892. Glenner G G, Grimley P M 1974 Tumors of the extra-adrenal paraganglion system (including chemoreceptors). Atlas of tumor pathology, 2nd series, fascicle 9. Armed Forces Institute of Pathology, Washington DC, p 43–52

1893. Gonzalez-Angulo A, Feria-Valasco A, Corvera J, Elias E Y 1968 Ultrastructure of the glomus jugulare tumor. Archives of Otolaryngology 87: 12–21

1894. Grimley P M, Glenner G G 1967 Histology and ultrastructure of carotid body paragangliomas. Comparison with the normal gland. Cancer 20: 1473–1488

1895. Hordijk G J, Ruiter D J, Bosman F T, Mauw B J 1981 Chemodectoma (paraganglioma) of the larynx. Clinical Otolaryngology 6: 249–254

1896. Houroupian D S, Kerson L A, Saiontz H, Valsamis M 1974 Paraganglioma of cauda equina. Clinicopathologic and ultrastructural studies on an unusual case. Cancer 33: 1337–1348

1897. Hull M T, Roth L M, Glover J L, Walker P D 1982 Metastatic carotid body paraganglioma in von Hippel-Lindau disease. An electron microscopic study. Archives of Pathology and Laboratory Medicine 106: 235–239

1898. Justrabo E, Michiels R, Calmettes C, Cabanne F, Bastein H, Horiot J C, Guerrin J 1980 An uncommon apudoma: a functional chemodectoma of the larynx. Report of a case and review of the literature. Acta Oto-laryngologica 89: 135–143

1899. Kahn L B 1976 Vagal body tumor (nonchromaffin paraganglioma, chemodectoma, and carotid body-like tumor) with cervical node metastasis and familial association. Ultrastructural study and review. Cancer 38: 2367–2377

1900. Kepes J J, Zacharias D L 1971 Gangliocytic paragangliomas of the duodenum. A report of two cases with light and electron microscopic examination. Cancer 27: 61–70

1901. Lack E E, Cubilla A L, Woodruff J M 1979 Paragangliomas of the head and neck region. A pathologic study of tumors from 71 patients. Human Pathology 10: 191–218

1902. Lack E E, Stillinger R A, Calvin D B, Groves R M, Burnette D G 1979 Aortico-pulmonary paraganglioma. Report of a case with ultrastructural study and review of the literature. Cancer 43: 269–278

1903. Liew S-H, Leong A S-Y, Tang H M K 1981 Tracheal paraganglioma. A case report with review of the literature. Cancer 47: 1387–1393

1904. Llena J F, Wisoff H S, Hirano A 1982 Gangliocytic paraganglioma in cauda equina region, with biochemical and neuropathological studies. Case report. Journal of Neurosurgery 56: 280–282

1905. Nabarra B, Sonsino E, Andrianarison I 1977 Ultrastructure of a polysome-lamellae complex in a human paraganglioma. American Journal of Pathology 86: 523–532

1906. Olson J L, Salyer W R 1978 Mediastinal paragangliomas (aortic body tumor). A report of four cases and a review of the literature. Cancer 41: 2405–2412

1907. Reed R J, Daroca P J Jr, Harkin J C 1977 Gangliocytic paraganglioma. American Journal of Surgical Pathology 1: 207–216

1908. Rippey J J, Röhm G F, van den Heeuer C M, de Wit L J 1981 Paraganglioma of the orbit — an exercise in diagnosis. A case report. South African Medical Journal 60: 148–150

1909. Robertson D I, Cooney T P 1980 Malignant carotid body paraganglioma: light and electron microscopic study of the tumor and its metastases. Cancer 46: 2623–2633

1910. Schaefer S D, Blend B L, Denton J G 1980 Laryngeal paragangliomas: evaluation and treatment. American Journal of Otolaryngology 1: 451–455

1911. Schmitt H P, Wurster K, Bauer M, Parsch K 1982 Mixed chemodectoma-ganglioneuroma of the conus medullaris region. Acta Neuropathologica 57: 275–281

1912. Schuller D E, Lucas J G 1982 Nasopharyngeal paraganglioma. Report of a case and review of the literature. Archives of Otolaryngology 108: 667–670

1913. Soffer D, Pittaluga S, Caine Y, Feinsod M 1983 Paraganglioma of cauda equina. A report of a case and review of the literature. Cancer 51: 1907–1910

1914. Taxy J B 1983 Paraganglioma of the cauda equina. Report of a rare tumor. Cancer 51: 1904–1906

1915. Tischler A S, Dichter M A, Biales B, DeLellis R A, Wolfe H 1976 Neural properties of cultured human endocrine tumor cells of proposed neural crest origin. Science 192: 902–904

## 46  PINEAL TUMOURS

1916. Cravioto H, Dart D 1973 The ultrastructure of pinealoma: seminoma-like tumor of the pineal region. Journal of Neuropathology and Experimental Neurology 32: 552–565

1917. Markesbery W R, Brooks W H, Milsow L, Mortara R H 1976 Ultrastructural study of the pineal germinoma in vivo and in vitro. Cancer 37: 327–337

1918. Markesbery W R, Haugh R M, Young A B 1981 Ultrastructure of pineal parenchymal neoplasms. Acta Neuropathologica 55: 143–149

1919. Misugi K, Liss L, Bradel E J 1967 Electron microscopic study of an ectopic pinealoma. Acta Neuropathologica 9: 346–356

1920. Nielsen S L, Wilson C B 1974 Ultrastructure of a pineocytoma. Gynecologic Oncology 2: 205–220

1921. Papasozomenos S, Shapiro S 1981 Pineal astrocytoma: report of a case, confined to the epiphysis, with immuno-cytochemical and electron microscopic studies. Cancer 47: 99–103

1922. Ramsey H J 1965 Ultrastructure of a pineal tumor. Cancer 18: 1014–1025

1923. Vuia O 1980 Embryonic carcinosarcoma (mixed tumour) of the pineal gland. Neurochirurgia 23: 47–54

## 47  TUMOURS OF THE CENTRAL NERVOUS SYSTEM

1924. Arnold A, Burrows D 1976 Comparative studies of tumors of the central nervous system of man by scanning electron microscopy, phase microscopy, and light microscopy. Scanning Electron Microscopy 2: 25–30

1925. Arseni C, Nereantiu F 1977 Ultrastructural aspects of medulloblastoma. Neurologie et Psychiatrie 15: 207–210

1926. Azzarelli B, Richards D E, Anton A H, Roessman U 1977 Central neuroblastoma. Electron microscopic observations and catecholamine determinations. Journal of Neuropathology and Experimental Neurology 36: 384–397

1927. Baloyannis S 1981 The fine structure of the isomorphic oligodendroglioma. Anticancer Research 1: 243–248

1928. Bertel C, Gouranton J, Menault F, Chatel M 1981 The intranuclear filamentous inclusions of a human glioma. Their relation with nuclear bodies. European Journal of Cell Biology 25: 36–45

1929. Bhrany D, Murphy M G, Morenstein S, Silbert S W 1974 Diffuse periventricular and meningeal glioma. Acta Neuropathologica 30: 243–249

1930. Boesel C P, Suhan J P, Bradel E J 1978 Ultrastructure of primitive neuroectodermal neoplasms of the central nervous system. Cancer 42: 194–201

1931. Boesel C P, Suhan J P, Sayers M P 1978 Melanotic medulloblastoma. Report of a case with ultrastructural findings. Journal of Neuropathology and Experimental Neurology 37: 531–543

1932. Carter L P, Beggs J, Waggener J D 1972 Ultrastructure of three choroid plexus papillomas. Cancer 30: 1130–1136

1933. Cervós-Navarro J, Pehlivan N 1981 Ultrastructure of oligodendrogliomas. Acta Neuropathologica suppl 7: 91–93

1934. Chaudhry A P, Montes M, Cohn G A 1978 Ultrastructure of a cerebellar hemangioblastoma. Cancer 42: 1834–1850

1935. Collins V P, Brunk U T, Fredricksson B A, Westermark B 1979 The fine structure of growing human glia and glioma cells. Whole cell preparations. Acta Pathologica et Microbiologica Scandinavica. Section A. Pathology 87: 29–36

1936. Cravioto H 1975 Human and experimental reticulum cell sarcoma (microglioma) of the nervous system. Acta Neuropathologica suppl 6: 135–140

1937. De Armond S J, Eng L F, Rubinstein L J 1980 The application of glial fibrillary acidic (GFA) protein immunohistochemistry in neurooncology. A progress report. Pathology Research and Practice 168: 374–394

1938. Ebhardt G, Cervós-Navarro J 1981 The fine structure of cells in astrocytomas of various grades of malignancy. Acta Neuropathologica suppl 7: 88–90

1939. Ejeckam G, Norman M G, Ivan L P 1978 Case report and ultrastructural study of intracranial embryonal carcinoma. Canadian Journal of Neurological Sciences 5: 447–450

1940. Friede R L, Janzer R C, Roessmann U 1982 Infantile small cell gliomas. Acta Neuropathologica 57: 103–110

1941. Friedländer M 1982 Centrioles and centrospheres in giant cells of human gliomas. Journal of Submicroscopic Cytology 14: 401–406

1942. Fu Y-S, Chen A T L, Kay S, Young H F 1974 Is subependymoma (subependymal conglomerate astrocytoma) an astrocytoma or ependymoma? A comparative ultrastructural and tissue culture study. Cancer 34: 1992–2008

1943. Gambarelli D, Hassoun J, Choux M, Toga M 1982 Complex cerebral tumor with evidence of neural, glial and Schwann cell differentiation. A histologic, immunocytochemical and ultrastructural study. Cancer 49: 1420–1428

1944. Garcia J H, Lemmi H 1970 Ultrastructure of oligo-dendroglioma of the spinal cord. American Journal of Clinical Pathology 54: 757–765

1945. Garcia J H, Mena H 1979 The diagnosis of central nervous system disorders by transmission electron microscopy. In: Trump B F, Jones R T (eds) Diagnostic electron microscopy, vol 2. John Wiley & Sons, New York, ch 8, p 351–394

1946. Goldammer D, Goebel H H 1980 Dense core vesicles in the desmoplastic variant of cerebral neuroblastoma. Acta Neuropathologica 50: 81–83

1947. Gonatas N K, Martin J, Evangelista I 1967 The osmiophilic particles of astrocytes. Viruses, lipid droplets or products of secretion? Journal of Neuropathology and Experimental Neurology 26: 369–376

1948. Gonzalez-Campora R, Haynes L W, Weller R O 1978 Scanning electron microscopy of malignant gliomas. A comparative study of glioma cells in smear preparations and in tissue culture. Acta Neuropathologica 41: 217–221

1949. Hadfield M G, Silverberg S C 1972 Light and electron microscopy of giant cell glioblastoma. Cancer 30: 989–996

1950. Hassoun J, Gambarelli D, Grisoli F, Pellet W, Salamon G, Pellissier J F, Toga M 1982 Central neurocytoma. An electron-microscopic study of two cases. Acta Neuro-pathologica 56: 151–156

1951. Hassoun J, Gambarelli D, Pellissier J F, Henin D, Toga M 1981 Germinomas of the brain. Light and electron microscopic study. A report of seven cases. Acta Neuropathologica suppl 7: 105–108

1952. Hess J R 1978 Frequency of surface micro-projections and coated vesicles with increased malignancy in human astrocytic neoplasms. Acta Neuropathologica 44: 151–153

1953. Hirano A 1975 A comparison of the fine structure of malignant lymphoma and other neoplasms in the brain. Acta Neuropathologica suppl 6: 141–145

1954. Hirano A 1978 Some contributions of electron microscopy to the diagnosis of brain tumors. Acta Neuropathologica 43: 119–128

1955. Horvat B, Pena C, Fisher E R 1969 Primary reticulum cell sarcoma (microglioma) of brain: an electron microscopic study. Archives of Pathology 87: 609–616

1956. Hwang T L, Borit A 1982 Rosenthal fibres in glioblastoma multiforme. Acta Neuropathologica 57: 230–232

1957. Ishida Y 1975 Fine structure of primary reticulum cell sarcoma of the brain. Acta Neuropathologica suppl 6: 147–153

1958. Jellinger K, Radaskiewicz Th, Slowik F 1975 Primary malignant lymphomas of the central nervous system in man. Acta Neuropathologica suppl 6: 95–102

1959. Johnson P C 1975 Ultrastructural study of two central nervous system lymphomas. Acta Neuropathologica suppl 6: 155–160

1960. Kalyanaraman V P, Henderson J P 1982 Intramedullary ganglioneuroma of spinal cord: a clinicopathologic study. Human Pathology 13: 952–955

1961. Kawamura J, Garcia J H, Kamijyo Y 1973 Cerebellar hemangioblastoma: histogenesis of stroma cells. Cancer 31: 1528–1540

1962. Kawano N, Morii S, Yada K, Aida Y, Yagishita S, Ishihara Y 1982 Contiguous malignant astrocytoma and Wilms'-like tumor in the brain. Cancer 49: 2505–2512

1963. Koide O, Watanabe Y, Sato K 1980 A pathological survey of intracranial germinoma and pinealoma in Japan. Cancer 45: 2119–2130

1964. Koinov R 1967 Crystal bodies in the ultrastructure of multiform glioblastoma. Cancer 20: 1181–1185

1965. Kuhajda F P, Mendelsohn G, Taxy J B, Long D M 1981 Pleomorphic xanthoastrocytoma: report of a case with light and electron microscopy. Ultrastructural Pathology 2: 25–32

1966. Kumar P, Kumar S, Marsden H B, Lynch P G, Earnshaw E 1980 Weibel-Palade bodies in endothelial cells as a marker for angiogenesis in brain tumors. Cancer Research 40: 2010–2019

1967. Liu H M, McLone D G, Clark S 1977 Ependymomas of childhood. II. Electron-microscopic study. Childs Brain 3: 281–296

1968. Llena J F, Hirano A, Wisoff H S 1978 Fine structure of an unusual spongy variant of medulloblastoma. Acta Neuro-pathologica 44: 83–84

1969. Lynn J A, Panopio I T, Martin J H, Shaw M L, Race G J 1968 Ultrastructural evidence for astroglial histogenesis of the monstrocellular astrocytoma (so-called monstrocellular sarcoma of brain). Cancer 22: 356–366

1970. Lyser K M 1975 Human nervous system tumors. Observations by high voltage electron microscopy. Acta Neuropathologica 32: 313–324

1971. Markesbery W R, Challa V R 1979 Electron microscopic findings in primitive neuroectodermal tumors of the cerebrum. Cancer 44: 141–147

1972. Masucci E F, Ferrero A A, Kurtzke J F, Fox J L 1966 Glioblastoma multiforme involving the posterior fossa. Case report and review of literature. Diseases of the Nervous System 27: 47–51

1973. Masuzawa T, Shimabukuro H, Yoshimizu N, Sato F 1981 Ultrastructure of disseminated choroid plexus papilloma. Acta Neuropathologica 54: 321–324

1974. Mathews T, Moosy J 1974 Gliomas containing bone and cartilage. Journal of Neuropathology and Experimental Neurology 33: 456–471

1975. McComb R D, Burger P C 1983 Choroid plexus carcinoma. Report of a case with immunohistochemical and ultrastructural observations. Cancer 51: 470–475

1976. McLone D G 1980 Ultrastructure of the vasculature of central nervous system tumors of childhood. Childs Brain 6: 242–254

1977. Mena H, Garcia J H 1978 Primary brain sarcomas: light and electron microscopic features. Cancer 42: 1298–1307

1978. Milhorat T H, Davis D A, Hammock M K 1976 Choroid plexus papilloma. II. Ultrastructure and ultracytochemical localization of Na-K-ATPase. Childs Brain 2: 290–303

1979. Misugi K, Liss L 1970 Medulloblastoma with cross-striated muscle. A fine structural study. Cancer 25: 1279–1285

1980. Nakamura Y, Becker L E, Marks A 1983 S100 protein in human chordoma and in human and rabbit notochord. Archives of Pathology and Laboratory Medicine 107: 118–120

1981. Nakashima N, Goto K, Takeuchi J 1982 Papillary carcinoma of choroid plexus. Light and electron microscopic study. Virchows Archiv A Pathological Anatomy and Histology 395: 303–318

1982. Nakashima N, Goto K, Tsukidate K, Sobue M, Toida M, Takeuchi J 1983 Choroid plexus papilloma. Light and electron microscopic study. Virchows Archiv A Pathological Anatomy and Histopathology 400: 201–211

1983. Navas J J, Battifora H 1978 Choroid plexus papilloma: light and electron microscopic study of three cases. Acta Neuropathologica 44: 235–239

1984. Ojeda V J, Jacobsen P F, Papadimitriou J M 1980 Primary cerebral neuroblastoma. Case report with light microscopy, tissue culture and electron microscopy study. Pathology 12: 269–274

1985. Pearl G S, Mirra S S, Miles M L 1981 Intracerebral ganglioneuroblastoma with intracytoplasmic microtubular aggregates: case report and ultrastructural study. Ultrastructural Pathology 2: 337–342

1986. Pearl G S, Takei Y 1981 Cerebellar 'neuroblastoma': nosology as it relates to medulloblastoma. Cancer 47: 772–779

1987. Pearl G S, Takei Y, Stefanis G S, Hoffman J C 1981 Intraventricular neuroblastoma in a patient with von Hippel-Lindau's disease. Light and electron microscopic study. Acta Neuropathologica 53: 253–256

1988. Peters A, Palay S L, Webster H de F 1976 The fine structure of the nervous system: the neurons and supporting cells. W B Saunders Company, Philadelphia

1989. Polak M 1975 Microglioma and/or reticulosarcoma of the nervous system. Acta Neuropathologica suppl 6: 115–118

1990. Pollak A, Friede R L 1977 Fine structure of medulloepithelioma. Journal of Neuropathology and Experimental Neurology 36: 712–725

1991. Poon T P, Hirano A, Zimmerman H M 1979 Tumors. In: Johannessen J V (ed) Electron microscopy in human medicine, vol 6. Nervous system, sensory organs and respiratory tract. McGraw-Hill, New York, ch 3 p 85–134

1992. Pritchett P S, King T I 1978 Dysplastic gangliocytoma of the cerebellum: an ultrastructural study. Acta Neuropathologica 42: 1–5

1993. Prokopanow H, Gabryel P, Topilko A 1974 Light and electron microscopic observations on human ependymomas. Annals of the Medical Section of the Polish Academy of Sciences 19: 145–146

1994. Raimondi A J 1967 Correlation of structure and function in selected tumors of the human nervous system. Acta Neuropathologica 8: 149–162

1995. Rhodes R H, Davis R L, Kassel S H, Clague B H 1978 Primary cerebral neuroblastoma: a light and electron microscopic study. Acta Neuropathologica 41: 119–124

1996. Robertson I, Cook M G, Wilson D F, Henderson D W 1983 Malignant Schwannoma of cranial nerves. Pathology 15: 421–429

1997. Rubinstein L J 1982 Tumors of the central nervous system (supplement). Atlas of tumor pathology, 2nd series, fascicle 6. Armed Forces Institute of Pathology, Washington DC

1998. Rubinstein L J, Herman M M 1979 Recent advances in human neuro-oncology. Recent Advances in Neuropathology 1: 179–223

1999. Rubinstein L J, Herman M M, Hanbery J W 1974 The relationship between differentiating medulloblastoma and dedifferentiating diffuse cerebellar astrocytoma. Light, electron microscopic, tissue, and organ culture observations. Cancer 33: 675–690

2000. Russell D S, Rubinstein L J 1977 Pathology of tumours of the nervous system. 4th ed. Edward Arnold, London

2001. Schlote W 1982 Diagnostic electron microscopy in diseases of the nervous system. In: High resolution electron microscope EM10. Application in pathology. Zeiss, Oberkochen, p 3–30

2002. Schochet S S Jr, Peters B, O'Neal J, McCormick W F 1975 Intracranial esthesioneuroblastoma. A light and electron microscopic study. Acta Neuropathologica 31: 181–189

2003. Seyama S, Ohta M, Nishio S, Matsushima T, Kitamura K 1982 Cells constituting cerebellar hemangioblastomas. Ultrastructural study. Acta Pathologica Japonica 32: 399–413

2004. Sima A A 1980 Peroxisomes (microbodies) in human glial tumors. A cytochemical ultrastructural study. Acta Neuropathologica 51: 113–117

2005. Spence A M, Rubinstein L J 1975 Cerebellar capillary hemangioblastoma: its histogenesis studied by organ culture and electron microscopy. Cancer 35: 326–341

2006. Staley N A, Poleksy H F, Bensch K G 1967 Fine structural and biochemical studies on the malignant ganglioneuroma. Journal of Neuropathology and Experimental Neurology 26: 634–653

2007. Stern J B, Helwig E B 1981 Ultrastructure of subcutaneous sacrococcygeal myxopapillary ependymoma. Archives of Pathology and Laboratory Medicine 105: 524–526

2008. Stinson J C 1981 Unidentified intracellular structures in an astrocytoma. Ultrastructural Pathology 2: 397–400

2009. Szymás J, Gabryel P, Biczysko W 1980 Isomorphous and anaplastic (polymorphous) oligodendroglioma. Neurosurgical Review 3: 227–231

2010. Tani E 1976 Aggregated plasmalemmal vesicles and microvilli in human astrocytoma. Acta Neuropathologica 36: 125–135

2011. Tani E, Ikeda K, Kudo S, Yamagata S, Nishiura M 1974 Specialized intercellular junctions in human intracranial germinomas. Acta Neuropathologica 27: 139–151

2012. Tani E, Maeda Y, Natsume S, Ito Y 1977 Membrane structures of human oligodendroglioma. Acta Neuropathologica 38: 11–19

2013. Tani E, Nakano M, Itagaki T, Fukumori T 1978 Cell membrane structure of human giant-celled glioblastoma. Acta Neuropathologica 41: 61–65

2014. Tani E, Nishiura M, Higashi N 1973 Freeze-fracture studies of gap junctions of normal and neoplastic astrocytes. Acta Neuropathologica 26: 127–138

2015. Vraa-Jensen J 1974 Massive congenital intracranial teratoma. Acta Neuropathologica 30: 271–276

2016. Vuia O 1975 Primary cerebral reticulosis and plasma cell differentiation. Acta Neuropathologica suppl 6: 161–166

2017. Waggener J D, Beggs J L 1976 Vasculature of neural neoplasms. Advances in Neurology 15: 27–49

2018. Wakai S, Matsutani M, Mizutani H, Sano K 1979 Tight junctions in choroid plexus papillomas. Acta Neuropathologica 45: 159–160

2019. Wilson N, Rosen M 1974 Primary intracranial adenoid cystic carcinoma (cylindroma). An electron microscopic study. Virchows Archiv B Zellpathologie 16: 95–109

2020. Wolff M, Santiago H, Duby M M 1972 Delayed distant metastasis from a subcutaneous sacrococcygeal ependymoma. Case report, with tissue culture, ultrastructural observations, and review of the literature. Cancer 30: 1046–1067

2021. Wolfson W L, Brown J 1977 Disseminated choroid plexus papilloma. An ultrastructural study. Archives of Pathology and Laboratory Medicine 101: 366–368

2022. Yagishita S, Itoh Y, Chiba Y, Kuwana N 1982 Morphological investigations on cerebellar 'neuroblastoma' group. Acta Neuropathologica 56: 22–28

2023. Yagishita S, Itoh Y, Chiba Y, Yamashita T, Nakazima F, Kuwabara T 1980 Cerebellar neuroblastoma. A light and ultrastructural study. Acta Neuropathologica 50: 139–142

2024. Yagishita S, Itoh Y, Chiba Y, Yuda K 1978 Cerebral neuroblastoma. Virchows Archiv A Pathological Anatomy and Histology 381: 1–11

2025. Yokoyama M, Okada K, Tokue A, Takayasu H 1973 Ultrastructural and biochemical study of benign ganglioneuroma. Virchows Archiv A Pathologische Anatomie 361: 195–209

## 48 MENINGEAL TUMOURS

2026. Botticelli A R, Villani M, Angiari P, Peserico L 1983 Meningeal melanocytoma of Meckel's cave associated with ipsilateral Ota's nervus. Case report. Cancer 51: 2304–2310

2027. Budka H 1982 Hyaline inclusions (pseudopsammoma bodies) in meningiomas: immunocytochemical demonstration of epithel-like secretion of secretory component and immunoglobulins A and M. Acta Neuropathologica 56: 294–298

2028. Copeland D D, Bell S W, Shelburne J D 1978 Hemidesmosome-like intercellular specializations in human meningiomas. Cancer 41: 2242–2249

2029. Ermel A E 1974 Histogenesis of angiomatous areas in meningiomas. An electron microscope study. Pathologia Europaea 9: 217–231

2030. Font R L, Croxatto J O 1980 Intracellular inclusions in meningothelial meningioma. A histochemical and ultrastructural study. Journal of Neuropathology and Experimental Neurology 39: 575–583

2031. Goldman J E, Horoupian D S, Johnson A B 1980 Granulofilamentous inclusions in a meningioma. Cancer 46: 156–161

2032. Humeau C, Vic P, Sentein P, Vlahovitch B 1979 The fine structure of meningiomas: an attempted classification. Virchows Archiv A Pathological Anatomy and Histology 382: 201–216

2033. Kepes J J 1975 The fine structure of hyaline inclusions — pseudopsammona bodies, in meningiomas. Journal of Neuropathology and Experimental Neurology 34: 282–294

2034. Kepes J J 1982 Meningiomas: biology, pathology, and differential diagnosis. Masson Publishing USA, New York, ch 26, p 150–182

2035. Kubota T, Hirano A, Yamamoto S 1982 The fine structure of hyaline inclusions in meningioma. Journal of Neuropathology and Experimental Neurology 41: 81–86

2036. Lam R M Y, Malik G M, Chason J L 1981 Osteosarcoma of the meninges. Clinical, light, and ultrastructural observations of a case. American Journal of Surgical Pathology 5: 203–208

2037. Limas C, Tio F O 1972 Meningeal melanocytoma ('melanotic meningioma'). Its melanocytic origin as revealed by electron microscopy. Cancer 30: 1286–1294

2038. Michaud J, Gagné F 1983 Microcystic meningioma. Clinicopathologic report of eight cases. Archives of Pathology and Laboratory Medicine 107: 75–80

2039. Mirra S S, Miles M L 1982 Unusual pericytic proliferation in a meningotheliomatous meningioma. An ultrastructural study. American Journal of Surgical Pathology 6: 573–580

2040. Mirra S, Tindall S, Check I, Brynes R, Moore W 1983 Inflammatory meningiomas: an ultrastructural and immunologic study. Laboratory Investigation 48: 59A

2041. Nystrom S H 1965 A study on supratentorial meningiomas. With special reference to gross and fine structure. Acta Pathologica et Microbiologica Scandinavica. Section A. Pathology, suppl 176: 1–90

2042. Nystrom S H, Nyholm M 1966 The origin of the calcium deposits in psammoma bodies of human spinal meningiomas. Naturwissenschaften 53: 703–704

2043. Pena C E 1977 Meningioma and intracranial hemangiopericytoma. A comparative electron microscopic study. Acta Neuropathologica 39: 69–74

2044. Pena C E 1978 Ribosome submembranous density complex. A new specialized cell unit. Acta Neuropathologica 44: 249–250

2045. Pietruszka M, Salazar H, Pena C 1978 Malignant meningioma: ultrastructure and observations on histogenesis. Pathology 10: 169–173

2046. Popoff N A, Malinin T I, Rosomoff H L 1974 Fine structure of intracranial hemangiopericytoma and angiomatous meningioma. Cancer 34: 1187–1197

2047. Rozzoli H V, Randall J D, Smith D R 1978 Psammoma bodies in meningioma. Appearance by scanning electron microscopy. Virchows Archiv A Pathological Anatomy and Histology 380: 317–325

2048. Tani E, Ikeda K, Yamagata S, Nishiura M, Higashi N 1974 Specialized junctional complexes in human meningioma. Acta Neuropathologica 28: 305–315

2049. Tani E, Nishiura M, Higashi N 1974 Freeze-fracture studies of gap junctions in human meningioma. Acta Neuropathologica 30: 305–314

2050. Tedeschi F, Brizzi R, Lechi A, Trabattoni G, Ferrari C, Tagliavini F 1981 Meningiomas. A light and electron microscopy study. Acta Neuropathologica suppl 7: 122–125

2051. Virtanen I, Lehtonen E, Wartiovaara J 1976 Structure of psammoma bodies of a meningioma in scanning electron microscopy. Cancer 38: 824–829

## 49 TUMOURS OF PERIPHERAL NERVES

2052. Alvira M M, Mandybur T I, Menefee M G 1976 Light microscopic and ultrastructual observations of a metastasizing malignant epithelioid schwannoma. Cancer 38: 1977–1982

2053. Averback P 1978 Spheroidal filamentous inclusion body cells in von Recklinghausen's disease. Virchows Archiv A Pathological Anatomy and Histology 377: 363–368

2054. Bair E D, Woodside J R, Williams W L, Borden T A 1978 Perirenal malignant Schwannoma presenting as renal cell carcinoma. Urology 11: 510–512

2055. Chandra S, Jerva M J, Clemis J D 1975 Ultrastructural characteristics of human neurilemoma cell nuclei. Cancer Research 35: 2000–2006

2056. Chen K T K, Latorraca R, Fabich D, Padgug A, Hafez G R, Gilbert E F 1980 Malignant Schwannoma. A light microscopic and ultrastructural study. Cancer 45: 1585–1593

2057. Chitale A R, Dickersin G R 1983 Electron microscopy in the diagnosis of malignant Schwannomas. A report of six cases. Cancer 51: 1448–1461

2058. Conley F K, Herman M M 1973 Intracellular septate desmosome-like structures in a human acoustic Schwannoma in vitro. Journal of Neurocytology 2: 457–464

2059. Das L, Chang C–H, Cushing B, Jewell P 1982 Congenital primitive neuroectodermal tumor (neuroepithelioma) of the chest wall. Medical and Pediatric Oncology 10: 349–358

2060. Elder D E, Ainsworth A M, Goldman L I, Inoue K, Clark W H Jr 1981 Malignant melanocytic Schwannoma. Report of a case with some histologic features of desmoplastic melanoma. In: Ackerman A B (ed) Pathology of malignant melanoma. Masson Publishing USA, New York, p 251–261

2061. Erlandson R A, Woodruff J M 1982 Peripheral nerve sheath tumors: an electron microscopic study of 43 cases. Cancer 49: 273–287

2062. Factor S, Turi G, Biempica L 1976 Primary cardiac neurilemoma. Cancer 37: 883–890

2063. Fethiere W, Carter H W, Sturim H S 1974 Elephantiasis neuromatosa of the penis. Light and electron microscopical studies. Archives of Pathology 97: 326–330

2064. Finkel G, Lane B 1982 Granular cell variant of neurofibromatosis: ultrastructure of benign and malignant tumors. Human Pathology 13: 959–963

2065. Fisher E R, Vuzevski V D 1968 Cytogenesis of schwannoma, neurilemoma, neurofibroma, dermatofibroma and dermatofibrosarcoma as revealed by electron microscopy. American Journal of Clinical Pathology 49: 141–154

2066. Friedmann I, Cawthorne T, Bird E S 1965 Broad-banded striated bodies in the sensory epithelium of the human macula and in neurinoma. Nature 207: 171–174

2067. Gallager R L, Helwig E B 1980 Neurothekeoma — A benign cutaneous tumor of neural origin. American Journal of Clinical Pathology 74: 759–764

2068. Gibson A A, Hendrick E B, Conen P E 1966 Intracerebral schwannoma. Report of a case. Journal of Neurosurgery 24: 552–557

2069. Goldman F 1980 Intermetatarsal neuromas: light and electron microscopic observation. Journal of the American Podiatry Association 70: 265–278

2070. Greer R O Jr, James R 1981 Benign nerve sheath neoplasm: a light microscopic and ultrastructural evaluation with differential diagnostic guidelines. Journal of Oral Surgery 39: 951–953

2071. Gregorios J B, Chou S M, Bay J 1982 Melanotic schwannoma of the spinal cord. Neurosurgery 11: 57–60

2072. Herrera G A, Reimann E F, Salinas J A, Turbat E A 1982 Malignant Schwannomas presenting as malignant fibrous histiocytomas. Ultrastructural Pathology 3: 253–261

2073. Hwang W S, Benediktsson H 1982 Lamellar bodies in benign and malignant schwannomas. Acta Pathologica, Microbiologica et Immunologica Scandinavica. Section A. Pathology 90: 89–93

2074. Johnson D E, Kaesler K E, Mackay B M, Ayala A G 1975 Neurofibrosarcoma of spermatic cord. Urology 5: 680–683

2075. Junqueira L C, Montes G S, Kaupert D, Shigihara K M, Bolonhani T M, Krisztán R M 1981 Morphological and histochemical studies on the collagen in neurinomas, neurofibromas, and fibromas. Journal of Neuropathology and Experimental Neurology 40: 123–133

2076. Kasantikul V, Brown W J 1981 Ultrastructure of capillaries in acoustic neurilemmoma. Surgical Neurology 16: 30–35

2077. Kasantikul V, Brown W J, Cahan L D 1981 Intracerebral neurilemmoma. Journal of Neurology, Neurosurgery and Psychiatry 44: 1110–1115

2078. Kedar A, Glassman M, Voorhess M L, Fisher J, Allen J, Jenis E, Freeman A I 1981 Severe hypertension in a child with ganglioneuroblastoma. Cancer 47: 2077–2080

2079. Kemmann E, Conrad P, Chen C K, Nicastri A D 1977 Pelvic neurilemmoma. Report of a case, electron microscopic studies and review of the literature. Gynecologic Oncology 5: 387–395

2080. Kimura M, Kamata Y, Matsumoto K, Takaya H 1974 Electron microscopical study on the tumor of von Recklinghausen's neurofibromatosis. Acta Pathologica Japonica 24: 79–91

2081. Lallemand R C, Weller R O 1973 Intraneural neurofibromas involving the posterior interosseous nerve. Journal of Neurology, Neurosurgery and Psychiatry 36: 991–996

2082. Lassmann H, Gebhart W, Stockinger L 1975 The reaction of connective tissue fibers in the tumor of Recklinghausen's disease. Virchows Archiv B Cell Pathology 19: 167–177

2083. Lassmann H, Jurecka W, Lassmann G, Gebhart W, Matras H, Watzek G 1977 Different types of benign nerve sheath tumors. Light microscopy, electron microscopy and autoradiography. Virchows Archiv A Pathological Anatomy and Histology 375: 197–210

2084. Lazarus S S, Trombetta L D 1978 Ultrastructural identification of a benign perineurial cell tumor. Cancer 41: 1823–1829

2085. Ma C K, Raju U, Fine G, Lewis J W Jr 1981 Primary tracheal neurilemoma. Report of a case with ultrastructural examination. Archives of Pathology and Laboratory Medicine 105: 187–189

2086. Mandybur T I 1974 Melanotic nerve sheath tumors. Journal of Neurosurgery 41: 187–192

2087. Marcus P B, Couch W D, Martin J H 1981 Crystals in a gastric Schwannoma. Ultrastructural Pathology 2: 139–145

2088. Matakas F, Cervós-Navarro J 1969 Electron microscopic study of tissue alterations in type B neurinomas. Virchows Archiv A Pathologische Anatomie 347: 160–175

2089. Mennemayer R P, Hammar S P, Tytus J S, Hallman K O, Raisis J E, Bockus D 1979 Melanotic schwannoma. Clinical and ultrastructural studies of three cases with evidence of intracellular melanin synthesis. American Journal of Surgical Pathology 3: 3–10

2090. Mullins J D 1980 A pigmented differentiating neuroblastoma: a light and ultrastructural study. Cancer 46: 522–528

2091. Nakamura Y, Becker L E, Mancer K, Gillespie R 1982 Peripheral medulloepithelioma. Acta Neuropathologica 57: 137–142

2092. Neely J G, Armstrong D, Benson J, Neblett C 1981 'Onion bulb' formation associated with a solitary neoplasm of the eighth nerve sheath. American Journal of Otolaryngology 2: 307–313

2093. Pineda A 1964 Neurolemmomas: a correlative study with silver carbonate techniques and electron microscopy. Transactions of the American Neurological Association 89: 241–242

2094. Pineda A 1966 Electron microscopy of the lemmocyte in peripheral nerve tumors — neurolemmomas. Journal of Neurosurgery 25: 35–44

2095. Rao M S, Chaudhuri B, Scarpelli D G 1981 A transplantable human malignant Schwannoma. Journal of Pathology 135: 169–177

2096. Rootman J, Goldberg C, Robertson W 1982 Primary orbital schwannomas. British Journal of Ophthalmology 66: 194–204

2097. Sian C S, Ryan S F 1981 The ultrastructure of neurilemoma with emphasis on Antoni B tissue. Human Pathology 12: 145–160

2098. Smith T W, Bhawan J 1980 Tactile-like structures in neurofibromas. An ultrastructural study. Acta Neuropathologica 50: 233–236

2099. Stefansson K, Wollmann R, Jerkovic M 1982 S-100 protein in soft tissue tumors derived from Schwann cells and melanocytes. American Journal of Pathology 106: 261–268

2100. Taxy J B, Battifora H 1981 Epithelioid Schwannoma: diagnosis by electron microscopy. Ultrastructural Pathology 2: 19–24

2101. Taxy J B, Battifora H, Trujillo Y, Dorfman H D 1981 Electron microscopy in the diagnosis of malignant Schwannoma. Cancer 48: 1381–1391

2102. Tsuneyoshi M, Enjoji M 1979 Primary malignant peripheral nerve tumors (malignant schwannomas). A clinicopathologic and electron microscopic study. Acta Pathologica Japonica 29: 363–375

2103. Uri A K, Witzleben C L, Raney R B 1984 Electron microscopy of glandular Schwannoma. Cancer 53: 493–497

2104. Vuia O 1977 Morphologic aspects of the neurofibrosarcoma — neurogenic sarcoma. European Neurology 16: 1–10

2105. Warner T F C S, Louie R, Hafez G R, Chandler E 1983 Malignant nerve sheath tumor containing endocrine cells. American Journal of Surgical Pathology 7: 583–590

2106. Webb J N 1982 The ultra-structure of a melanotic Schwannoma of the skin. Journal of Pathology 137: 25–36

2107. Weiser G 1975 An electron microscope study of Pacinian neurofibroma. Virchows Archiv A Pathological Anatomy and Histology 366: 331–340

2108. Weiser G 1978 Neurofibroma and perineurial cell. Electron microscopic examinations of 9 neurofibromas. Virchows Archiv A Pathological Anatomy and Histology 379: 73–83

2109. Weiss S W, Langloss J M, Enzinger F M 1983 Value of S-100 protein in the diagnosis of soft tissue tumors with particular reference to benign and malignant Schwann cell tumors. Laboratory Investigation 49: 299–308

2110. Weller R O, Cervós-Navarro J 1977 Pathology of peripheral nerves. Butterworths, London, ch 6, p 144–207

2111. Woodruff J M, Chernik N L, Smith M C, Millett W B, Foote F W Jr 1973 Peripheral nerve tumors with rhabdomyosarcomatous differentiation (malignant 'Triton' tumors). Cancer 32: 426–439

2112. Woodruff J M, Godwin T A, Erlandson R A, Susin M, Martini N 1981 Cellular schwannoma. A variety of schwannoma sometimes mistaken for a malignant tumor. American Journal of Surgical Pathology 5: 733–744

## 50 GRANULAR CELL TUMOURS

2113. Bhawan J, Malhotra R, Naik D R 1983 Gaucher-like cells in a granular cell tumor. Human Pathology 14: 730–733

2114. Christ M L, Ozzello L 1971 Myogenous origin of a granular cell tumor of the urinary bladder. American Journal of Clinical Pathology 56: 736–749

2115. Fenoglio J J, McAllister H A Jr 1976 Granular cell tumors of the heart. Archives of Pathology and Laboratory Medicine 100: 276–278

2116. Garancis J C, Komorowski R A, Kuzma J F 1970 Granular cell myoblastoma. Cancer 25: 542–550

2117. Goldstein B G, Font R L, Alper M G 1982 Granular cell tumor of the orbit: a case report including electron microscopic observations. Annals of Ophthalmology 14: 231–232, 236–238

2118. Gonzalez-Almaraz G, De Buen S, Tsutsumi V 1975 Granular cell tumor (myoblastoma) of the orbit. American Journal of Ophthalmology 79: 606–612

2119. Kay S, Elzay R P, Willson M A 1971 Ultrastructural observations on a gingival granular cell tumor (congenital epulis). Cancer 27: 674–680

2120. Kindblom L-G, Olsson K-M 1981 Malignant granular cell tumor. A clinico-pathologic and ultrastructural study of a case. Pathology Research and Practice 172: 384–393

2121. Lack E E, Perez-Atayde A R, McGill T J, Vawter G F 1982 Gingival granular cell tumor of the newborn (congenital 'epulis'): ultrastructural observations relating to histogenesis. Human Pathology 13: 686–689

2122. Manara G C, De Panfilis G, Bacchi A B, Ferrari C, Tedeschi F, Brusati R, Scandroglio R, Allegra F 1981 Fine structure of granular cell tumor of Abrikossoff. Journal of Cutaneous Pathology 8: 277–282

2123. Markesbery W R, Duffy P E, Cowen D 1973 Granular cell tumors of the central nervous system. Journal of Neuropathology and Experimental Neurology 32: 92–109

2124. Morgan G 1976 Granular cell myoblastoma of the orbit. Report of a case. Archives of Ophthalmology 94: 2135–2142

2125. Moscovic E A, Azar H A 1967 Multiple granular cell tumors (myoblastomas). Case report with electron microscopic observations and review of the literature. Cancer 20: 2032–2047

2126. Pour P, Althoff J, Cardesa A 1973 Granular cells in tumors and in nontumorous tissue. Archives of Pathology 95: 135–138

2127. Reyes C V, Kathuria S, Molnar Z 1980 Granular cell tumor of the esophagus: a case report. Journal of Clinical Gastroenterology 2: 365–368

2128. Roberston A J, McIntosh W, Lamont P, Guthrie W 1981 Malignant granular cell tumour (myoblastoma) of the vulva: report of a case and review of the literature. Histopathology 5: 69–79

2129. Rode J, Dhillon A P, Papadacki L 1982 Immunohistochemical staining of granular cell tumour for neurone specific enolase: evidence in support of a neural origin. Diagnostic Histopathology 5: 205–211

2130. Schulster P L, Khan F A, Azueta V 1975 Asymptomatic pulmonary granular cell tumor presenting as a coin lesion. Chest 68: 256–258

2131. Sobel H J, Marquet E 1974 Granular cells and granular cell lesions. Pathology Annual 9: 43–79

2132. Sobel H J, Marquet E, Schwartz R 1973 Is schwannoma related to granular cell myoblastoma? Archives of Pathology 95: 396–401

2133. Takei Y, Mirra S S, Miles M L 1976 Eosinophilic granular cells in oligodendrogliomas. An ultrastructural study. Cancer 38: 1968–1976

2134. Usui M, Ishii S, Yamawaki S, Sasaki T, Minami A, Hizawa K 1977 Malignant granular cell tumor of the radial nerve. An autopsy observation with electron microscopic and tissue culture studies. Cancer 39: 1547–1555

2135. Whitten J B 1968 The fine structure of an intraoral granular-cell myoblastoma. Oral Surgery, Oral Medicine and Oral Pathology 26: 202–213

## 51 TUMOURS OF THE EYE

2136. Archer D B, Gardiner T A 1982 An ultrastructural study of carcinoid tumor of the iris. American Journal of Ophthalmology 94: 357–368

2137. Astarita R W, Minckler D, Taylor C R, Levine A, Lukes R J 1980 Orbital and adnexal lymphomas. A multiparameter approach. American Journal of Clinical Pathology 73: 615–621

2138. Bierring F, Egeberg J, Jensen O A 1967 A contribution to the ultrastructural study of retinoblastomas. Acta Ophthalmologica 45: 424–428

2139. Bunt A H, Tso M O 1981 Feulgen-positive deposits in retinoblastoma. Incidence, composition and ultrastructure. Archives of Ophthalmology 99: 144–150

2140. Cohen B H, Green W R, Iliff N T, Taxy J B, Schwab L T, de la Cruz Z 1980 Spindle cell carcinoma of the conjunctiva. Archives of Ophthalmology 98: 1809–1813

2141. Craft J L, Robinson N L, Roth N A, Albert D M 1978 Scanning electron microscopy of retinoblastoma. Experimental Eye Research 27: 519–531

2142. Dark A J, Streeten B W 1980 Preinvasive carcinoma of the cornea and conjunctiva. British Journal of Ophthalmology 64: 506–514

2143. Diaz-Flores L, Carreras B Jr, Caballero T, Martas S, Lopez-Marin I 1979 Retinoblastoma. An optic-ultrastructural correlation. Presence of dense-core vesicles. Morfología Normal y Patológica 3: 145–162

2144. Dickson D H, Ramsey M S, Tonus J G 1976 Synapse formation in retinoblastoma tumours. British Journal of Ophthalmology 60: 371–375

2145. Ehlers N, Jensen O A 1982 Juxtapapillary retinal hemangioblastoma (angiomatosis retinae) in an infant: light microscopical and ultrastructural examination. Ultrastructural Pathology 3: 325–333

2146. Font R L, Jakobiec F A 1979 The role of electron microscopy in ophthalmic pathology. In: Trump B F, Jones R T (eds) Diagnostic electron microscopy, vol 2, John Wiley & Sons, New York, ch 4, p 163–219

2147. Iwamoto T, Jakobiec F A 1982 A comparative ultrastructural study of the normal lacrimal gland and its epithelial tumors. Human Pathology 13: 236–262

2148. Iwamoto T, Witmer R, Landolt E 1967 Diktyoma: a clinical, histological and electron microscopical observation. Albrecht von Graefes Archiv für Klinische und Experimentelle Ophthalmologie 172: 293–316

2149. Jakobiec F A, Font R L 1979 Ocular and orbital tumors. In: Johannessen J V (ed) Electron microscopy in human medicine, vol 6. Nervous system, sensory organs and respiratory tract. McGraw-Hill, New York, ch 8, p 316–345

2150. Jakobiec F A, Font R L, Tso M O M, Zimmerman L E 1977 Mesectodermal leiomyoma of the ciliary body. A tumor of presumed neural crest origin. Cancer 39: 2102–2113

2151. Jakobiec F A, Iwamoto T, Knowles D M II 1982 Ocular adnexal lymphoid tumors. Correlative ultrastructural and immunologic marker studies. Archives of Ophthalmology 100: 84–98

2152. Jauregui H O, Klintworth G K 1976 Pigmented squamous cell carcinoma of cornea and conjunctiva. A light microscopic, histochemical, and ultrastructural study. Cancer 38: 778–788

2153. Knowles D M, Jakobiec F A, Potter G D, Jones I S 1976 Ophthalmic striated muscle neoplasms. Survey of Ophthalmology 21: 219–261

2154. Kroll A J, Ricker D P, Robb R M, Albert D M 1981 Vitreous hemorrhage complicating retinal astrocytic hamartoma. Survey of Ophthalmology 26: 31–38

2155. Moor Sunba M S, Rahi A H, Garner A, Alexander R A, Morgan G 1980 Tumours of the anterior uvea. III. Oxytalan fibres in the differential diagnosis of leiomyoma and malignant melanoma of the iris. British Journal of Ophthalmology 64: 867–874

2156. Offret H, Saraux H 1980 Adenoma of the iris pigment epithelium. Archives of Ophthalmology 98: 875–883

2157. Ohnishi Y 1977 The histogenesis of retinoblastoma. An electron microscopic analysis of rosette. Ophthalmologica 174: 129–136

2158. Radnot M 1975 Synaptic lamellae in retinoblastoma. American Journal of Ophthalmology 79: 393–404

2159. Radnot M 1978 Scanning electron microscopy of retinoblastoma. Journal of Pediatric Ophthalmology 15: 36–39

2160. Riddle P J, Font R L, Zimmerman L E 1982 Carcinoid tumors of the eye and orbit: a clinicopathologic study of 15 cases with histochemical and electron microscopic observations. Human Pathology 13: 459–469

2161. Smith P J, Ablett G A, Sheridan J W 1983 Histopathological and tissue culture studies of a melanizing cell line derived from a retinoblastoma. Pathology 15: 431–435

2162. Weigent C E, Staley N A 1976 Meibomian gland carcinoma: report of a case with electron microscopic findings. Human Pathology 7: 231–234

2163. Zimmerman L E, Font R L, Anderson S R 1972 Rhabdomyosarcomatous differentiation in malignant intraocular medulloepitheliomas. Cancer 30: 817–835

## 52 TUMOURS OF THE EAR

2164. Busuttil A 1981 Electron microscopy in otorhinolaryngological oncology. Clinical Otolaryngology 6: 377–378

2165. Gillanders D A, Worth A J, Honore L H 1974 Ceruminous adenoma of the middle ear. Canadian Journal of Otolaryngology 3: 194–201

2166. Inoue S, Tanaka K, Kannae S 1982 Primary carcinoid tumour of the ear. Virchows Archiv A Pathological Anatomy and Histology 396: 357–363

2167. Michael R G, Woodard B H, Shelburne J D, Bossen E H 1978 Ceruminous gland adenocarcinoma: a light and electron microscopic study. Cancer 41: 545–553

2168. Riches W G, Johnston W H 1982 Primary adenomatous neoplasms of the middle ear. Light and electron microscopic features of a group distinct from the ceruminomas. American Journal of Clinical Pathology 77: 153–161

2169. Wetli C V, Pardo V, Millard M, Gerston K 1972 Tumors of ceruminous glands. Cancer 29: 1169–1178

## 53 GENERAL ASPECTS OF MESENCHYMAL TUMOURS, AND MISCELLANEOUS TUMOURS

2170. Bearman R M, Noe J, Kempson R L 1975 Clear cell sarcoma with melanin pigment. Cancer 36: 977–984

2171. Berthold F, Kracht J, Lampert F, Millar T J, Müller T H, Reither M, Unsicker K 1982 Ultrastructural, biochemical, and cell-culture studies of a presumed extraskeletal Ewing's sarcoma with special reference to differential diagnosis from neuroblastoma. Journal of Cancer Research and Clinical Oncology 103: 293–304

2172. Bloustein P A, Silverberg S G, Waddell W R 1976 Epithelioid sarcoma. Case report with ultrastructural review, histogenetic discussion, and chemotherapeutic data. Cancer 38: 2390–2400

2173. Boudreaux D, Waisman J 1978 Clear cell sarcoma with melanogenesis. Cancer 41: 1387–1394

2174. Brooks J J 1982 Immunohistochemistry of soft tissue tumors. Progress and Prospects. Human Pathology 13: 969–974

2175. Chung E B, Enzinger F M 1978 Chondroma of soft parts. Cancer 41: 1414–1424

2176. Chung E B, Enzinger F M 1983 Malignant melanoma of soft parts. A reassessment of clear cell sarcoma. American Journal of Surgical Pathology 7: 405–413

2177. Cooney T P, Hwang W S, Robertson D I, Hoogstraten J 1982 Monophasic synovial sarcoma, epithelioid sarcoma and chordoid sarcoma: ultrastructural evidence for a common histogenesis, despite light microscopic diversity. Histopathology 6: 163–190

2178. Cozzutto C, Comelli A, Bandelloni R 1982 Ectomesenchymoma. Report of two cases. Virchows Archiv A Pathological Anatomy and Histology 398: 185–195

2179. d'Andiran G, Gabbiani G 1980 A metastasizing sarcoma of the pleura composed of myofibroblasts. Progress in Surgical Pathology 2: 31–40

2180. Dardick I, Ho S P E, McCaughey W T E 1981 Soft-tissue sarcoma of undetermined histogenesis. An ultrastructural study. Archives of Pathology and Laboratory Medicine 105: 214–217

2181. Dardick I, Lagacé R, Carlier M T, Jung R C 1983 Chordoid sarcoma (extraskeletal myxoid chondrosarcoma). A light and electron microscope study. Virchows Archiv A Pathological Anatomy and Histopathology 399: 61–78

2182. De Schryver-Kecskemeti K, Kraus F T, Engleman W, Lacy P E 1982 Alveolar soft-part sarcoma — a malignant angioreninoma. Histochemical, immunocytochemical, and electron-microscopic study of four cases. American Journal of Surgical Pathology 6: 5–18

2183. Denk H, Krepler R, Artlieb U, Gabbiani G, Rungger-Brändle E, Leoncini P, Franke W W 1983 Proteins of intermediate filaments. An immunohistochemical and biochemical approach to the classification of soft tissue tumors. American Journal of Pathology 110: 193–208

2184. Dickman P S, Liotta L A, Triche T J 1982 Ewing's sarcoma. Characterization in established cultures and evidence of its histogenesis. Laboratory Investigation 47: 375–382

2185. Dickman P S, Triche T J 1981 Ultrastructural comparison of Ewing's sarcoma of bone with diverse pediatric soft tissue sarcomas: diagnostic criteria for soft tissue sarcoma resembling Ewing's sarcoma. Laboratory Investigation 44: 15A

2186. Ekfors T O, Kalimo H, Rantakokko V, Latvala M, Parvinen M 1979 Alveolar soft part sarcoma. A report of two cases with some histochemical and ultrastructural observations. Cancer 43: 1672–1677

2187. Enzinger F M, Shiraki M 1972 Extraskeletal myxoid chondrosarcoma. An analysis of 34 cases. Human Pathology 3: 421–435

2188. Enzinger F M, Weiss S W 1983 Soft tissue tumors. C V Mosby Company, St. Louis

2189. Fisher E R, Horvat B 1972 The fibrocytic derivation of the so-called epithelioid sarcoma. Cancer 30: 1074–1081

2190. Fisher E R, Reidbord H 1971 Electron microscopic evidence suggesting the myogenous derivation of the so-called alveolar soft part sarcoma. Cancer 27: 150–159

2191. Font R L, Jurco S III, Zimmerman L E 1982 Alveolar soft-part sarcoma of the orbit: a clinicopathological analysis of seventeen cases and a review of the literature. Human Pathology 13: 569–579

2192. Frable W J, Kay S, Lawrence W, Schatzki P F 1973 Epithelioid sarcoma. An electron microscopic study. Archives of Pathology 95: 8–12

2193. Gabbiani G, Fu Y–S, Kaye G I, Lattes R, Majno G 1972 Epithelioid sarcoma. A light and electron microscopic study suggesting a synovial origin. Cancer 30: 486–499

2194. Gillespie J J, Roth L M, Wills E R, Einhorn L H, Willman J 1979 Extraskeletal Ewing's sarcoma. Histologic and ultrastructural observations in three cases. American Journal of Surgical Pathology 3: 99–108

2195. Gonzalez-Crussi F, Goldschmidt R A, Hsueh W, Trujillo Y P 1982 Infantile sarcoma with intracytoplasmic filamentous inclusions. Distinctive tumor of possible histiocytic origin. Cancer 49: 2365–2375

2196. Hajdu S I 1979 Pathology of soft tissue tumors. Lea & Febiger, Philadelphia

2197. Hashimoto K, Brownstein M H, Jakobiec F A 1974 Dermatofibrosarcoma protuberans. A tumor with perineural and endoneural cell features. Archives of Dermatology 110: 874–885

2198. Hoffman G J, Carter D 1973 Clear cell sarcoma of tendons and aponeuroses with melanin. Archives of Pathology 95: 22–25

2199. Kaye G I 1981 The futility of electron microscopy in determining the origin of poorly differentiated soft tissue tumors. Progress in Surgical Pathology 3: 171–179

2200. Kindblom L–G, Lodding P, Angervall L 1983 Clear-cell sarcoma of tendons and aponeuroses. An immunohistochemical and electron microscopic analysis indicating neural crest origin. Virchows Archiv A Pathological Anatomy and Histopathology 401: 109–128

2201. Klima M, Smith M, Spjut H J, Root E N 1975 Malignant mesenchymoma. Case report with electron microscopic study. Cancer 36: 1086–1094

2202. Kubo T 1969 Clear-cell sarcoma of patellar tendon studied by electron microscopy. Cancer 24: 948–953

2203. Lattes R 1982 Tumors of the soft tissues (revised). Atlas of tumor pathology, 2nd series, fascicle 1. Armed Forced Institute of Pathology, Washington D C

2204. Levine A M, Reddick R, Triche T 1978 Intracellular collagen fibrils in human sarcomas. Laboratory Investigation 39: 531–540

2205. Machinami R, Kikuchi F, Matsushita H 1982 Epithelioid sarcoma. Enzyme histochemical and ultrastructural study. Virchows Archiv A Pathological Anatomy and Histology 397: 109–120

2206. Mackay B 1977 Electron microscopy of soft tissue tumors. In: Management of primary bone and soft tissue tumors. Year Book Medical Publishers, Chicago, p 259–269

2207. Mahoney J P, Ballinger W E Jr, Alexander R W 1978 So-called extraskeletal Ewing's sarcoma. Report of a case with ultrastructural analysis. American Journal of Clinical Pathology 70: 926–931

2208. Mathew T 1982 Evidence supporting neural crest origin of an alveolar soft part sarcoma. An ultrastructural study. Cancer 50: 507–514

2209. Mehio A R, Ferenczy A 1978 Extraskeletal myxoid chondrosarcoma with chordoid features. Chordoid sarcoma. American Journal of Clinical Pathology 70: 700–705

2210. Miettinen M, Foidart J–M, Ekblom P 1983 Immunohistochemical demonstration of laminin, the major glycoprotein of basement membranes, as an aid in the diagnosis of soft tissue tumors. American Journal of Clinical Pathology 79: 306–311

2211. Miettinen M, Lehto V-P, Vartio T, Virtanen I 1982 Epithelioid sarcoma. Ultrastructural and immuno-histochemical features suggesting a synovial origin. Archives of Pathology and Laboratory Medicine 106: 620–623

2212. Mills S E, Fechner R E, Bruns D E, Bruns M E, Clurman B 1981 Intermediate filaments in epithelioid sarcoma: an ultrastructural and electrophoretic study. Laboratory Investigation 44: 44A

2213. Mills S E, Fechner R E, Bruns D E, Bruns M E, O'Hara M F 1981 Intermediate filaments in eosinophilic cells of epithelioid sarcoma. A light-microscopic, ultrastructural, and electrophoretic study. American Journal of Surgical Pathology 5: 195–202

2214. Mirra S S, Miles M L 1982 Subplasmalemmal linear density: a mesodermal feature and a diagnostic aid. Human Pathology 13: 365–380

2215. Mukai M, Iri H, Nakajima T, Hirose S, Torikata C, Kageyama M, Ueno N, Murakami K 1983 Alveolar soft-part sarcoma. A review on its histogenesis and further studies based on electron microscopy, immunohistochemistry, and biochemistry. American Journal of Surgical Pathology 7: 679–689

2216. Ozzello L, Hamels J 1976 The histiocytic nature of dermatofibrosarcoma protuberans. Tissue culture and electron microscopic study. American Journal of Clinical Pathology 65: 136–148

2217. Parker J B, Marcus P B, Martin J H 1980 Spinal melanotic clear cell sarcoma: a light and electron microscopic study. Cancer 46: 718–724

2218. Patchefsky A-S, Soriano R, Kostianovsky M 1977 Epithelioid sarcoma. Ultrastructural similarity to nodular synovitis. Cancer 39: 143–152

2219. Pontius K I, Sebek B A 1981 Extraskeletal Ewing's sarcoma arising in the nasal fossa. Light- and electron-microscopic observations. American Journal of Clinical Pathology 75: 410–415

2220. Rao U, Cheng A, Didolkar M S 1978 Extraosseous osteogenic sarcoma. Clinicopathological study of eight cases and review of the literature. Cancer 41: 1488–1496

2221. Reddick R L, Michelitch H, Triche T J 1979 Malignant soft tissue tumors (malignant fibrous histiocytoma, pleomorphic liposarcoma, and pleomorphic rhabdomyosarcoma): an ultrastructural study. Human Pathology 10: 327–343

2222. Schmidt D, Mackay B, Osborne B M, Jaffe N 1982 The quarterly case: recurring congenital lesion of the cheek. Malignant ectomesenchymoma. Ultrastructural Pathology 3: 85–90

2223. Schmidt D, Mackay B, Sinkovics J G 1981 Quarterly case: retroperitoneal tumor with vertebral metastasis in a 25-year-old female (alveolar soft part sarcoma). Ultrastructural Pathology 2: 383–388

2224. Simonati A, Vio M, Iannucci A M, Bricolo A, Rizzuto N 1981 Lumbar epidural Ewing sarcoma. Light and electron microscopic investigation. Journal of Neurology 225: 67–72

2225. Smith M T, Farinacci C J, Carpenter H A, Bannayan G A 1976 Extraskeletal myxoid chondrosarcoma. A clinicopathological study. Cancer 37: 821–827

2226. Sobel H J, Marquet E, Sobrinho-Simoes M, Johannessen J V 1981 Tumors and tumor-like conditions of soft tissues. In: Johannessen J V (ed) Electron microscopy in human medicine, vol 4. Soft tissues, bones and joints. McGraw-Hill, New York, p 143–256

2227. Steeper T A, Rosai J 1983 Aggressive angiomyxoma of the female pelvis and perineum. Report of nine cases of a distinctive type of gynecologic soft-tissue neoplasm. American Journal of Surgical Pathology 7: 463–475

2228. Sugarbaker P H, Auda S, Webber B L, Triche T J, Shapiro E, Cook W J 1981 Early distant metastases from epithelioid sarcoma of the hand. Cancer 48: 852–855

2229. Taxy J B, Battifora H 1980 The electron microscope in the study and diagnosis of soft tissue tumors. In: Trump B F, Jones R T (eds) Diagnostic electron microscopy, vol 3. John Wiley & Sons, New York, ch 3, p 97–174

2230. Trono D, Stalder J, Cox J N 1983 Extraskeletal myxoid chondrosarcoma. A case report with histochemical and ultrastructural features. Applied Pathology 1: 139–148

2231. Tsuneyoshi M, Enjoji M, Iwasaki H, Shinohara N 1981 Extraskeletal myxoid chondrosarcoma. A clinicopathologic and electron microscopic study. Acta Pathologica Japonica 31: 439–447

2232. Tsuneyoshi M, Enjoji M, Kubo T 1978 Clear cell sarcoma of tendons and aponeuroses: a comparative study of 13 cases with a provisional subgrouping into the melanotic and synovial types. Cancer 42: 243–252

2233. Tsuneyoshi M, Enjoji M, Shinohara N 1980 Epithelioid sarcoma. A light clinicopathologic and electron microscopic study. Acta Pathologica Japonica 30: 411–420

2234. Tsuneyoshi M, Hashimoto H, Enjoji M 1983 Myxoid malignant fibrous histiocytoma versus myxoid liposarcoma. A comparative ultrastructural study. Virchows Archiv A Pathological Anatomy and Histopathology 400: 187–199

2235. Unni K K, Soule E H 1975 Alveolar soft part sarcoma. An electron microscopic study. Mayo Clinic Proceedings 50: 591–598

2236. van Haelst U J G M 1980 General considerations on electron microscopy of tumors of soft tissues. Progress in Surgical Pathology 2: 225–257

2237. Waxman M, Vuletin J C, Saxe B I, Monteleone F A 1981 Extraskeletal osteosarcoma: light and electron microscopic study. Mount Sinai Journal of Medicine 48: 322–329

2238. Weiss S W 1976 Ultrastructure of the so-called 'chordoid sarcoma'. Evidence supporting cartilaginous differentiation. Cancer 37: 300–306

2239. Welsh R A, Bray D M III, Shipkey F H, Meyer A T 1972 Histogenesis of alveolar soft part sarcoma. Cancer 29: 191–204

2240. Wigger H J, Salazar G H, Blanc W A 1977 Extraskeletal Ewing sarcoma. An ultrastructural study. Archives of Pathology and Laboratory Medicine 101: 446–449

## 54 FIBROUS, FIBRO-ELASTIC AND FIBROHISTIOCYTIC TUMOURS

2241. Akhtar M, Miller R M 1977 Ultrastructure of elastofibroma. Cancer 40: 728–735

2242. Alguacil-Garcia A, Unni K K, Goellner J R 1977 Malignant giant cell tumor of soft parts. An ultrastructural study of four cases. Cancer 40: 244–253

2243. Allegra S R, Broderick P A 1973 Desmoid fibroblastoma. Intracellular collagenosynthesis in a peculiar fibroblastic tumor: light and ultrastructural study of a case. Human Pathology 4: 419–429

2244. Angervall L, Hagmar B, Kindblom L-G, Merck C 1981 Malignant giant cell tumor of soft tissues: a clinico-pathologic, cytologic, ultrastructural, angiographic and microangiographic study. Cancer 47: 736–747

2245. Battifora H, Hines J R 1971 Recurrent digital fibromas of childhood. An electron microscope study. Cancer 27: 1530–1536

2246. Benjamin E, Wells S, Fox H, Reeve N L, Knox F 1982 Malignant fibrous histiocytomas of salivary glands. Journal of Clinical Pathology 35: 946–953

2247. Benjamin S P, Mercer R D, Hawk W A 1977 Myofibroblastic contraction in spontaneous regression of multiple congenital mesenchymal hamartomas. Cancer 40: 2342-2352

2248. Bhawan J, Bacchetta C, Joris I, Majno G 1979 A myofibroblastic tumor. Infantile digital fibroma (recurrent digital fibrous tumor of childhood). American Journal of Pathology 94: 19-36

2249. Blitzer A, Lawson W, Biller H F 1977 Malignant fibrous histiocytoma of the head and neck. Laryngoscope 87: 1479-1499

2250. Burry A F, Kerr J F R, Pope J H 1970 Recurring digital fibrous tumour of childhood: an electron microscopic and virologic study. Pathology 2: 287-291

2251. Chen W, Chan C W, Mok C K 1982 Malignant fibrous histiocytoma of the mediastinum. Cancer 50: 797-800

2252. Chung E B, Enzinger F M 1975 Proliferative fasciitis. Cancer 36: 1450-1458

2253. Chung E B, Enzinger F M 1981 Infantile myofibromatosis. Cancer 48: 1807-1818

2254. Churg A M, Kahn L B 1977 Myofibroblasts and related cells in malignant fibrous and fibrohistiocytic tumors. Human Pathology 8: 205-218

2255. Cozzutto C, Bronzini E, Bandelloni R, Guarino M, De Bernardi B 1981 Malignant, monomorphic histiocytoma in children. Cancer 48: 2112-2120

2256. Cozzutto C, De Bernardi B, Guarino M, Comelli A, Soave F 1978 Retroperitoneal fibrohistiocytic tumors in children: report of five cases. Cancer 42: 1350-1363

2257. Craver J L, McDivitt R W 1981 Proliferative fasciitis. Ultrastructural study of two cases. Archives of Pathology and Laboratory Medicine 105: 542-545

2258. Crocker D J, Murad T M 1969 Ultrastructure of fibrosarcoma in a male breast. Cancer 23: 891-899

2259. Dahl I, Säve-Söderbergh J, Angervall L 1973 Fibrosarcoma in early infancy. Pathologia Europaea 8: 193-209

2260. Daroca P J Jr, Pulitzer D R, LoCicero J III 1982 Ossifying fasciitis. Archives of Pathology and Laboratory Medicine 106: 682-685

2261. Dupree W B, Weiss S W 1983 Pigmented dermatofibrosarcoma protuberans (Bednár tumor): a clinicopathologic, ultrastructural, and immunohistochemical study. Laboratory Investigation 48: 21A

2262. Enzinger F M 1977 Recent developments in the classification of soft tissue tumors. In: Management of primary bone and soft tissue tumors. Year Book Medical Publishers, Chicago, p 219-234

2263. Escalona-Zapata J, Fernandez E A, Escuin F L 1981 The fibroblastic nature of dermatofibrosarcoma protuberans. A tissue culture and ultrastructural study. Virchows Archiv A Pathological Anatomy and Histology 391: 165-175

2264. Farragiana T, Churg J, Strauss L, Voglino A 1981 Ultrastructural histochemistry of infantile digital fibromatosis. Ultrastructural Pathology 2: 241-247

2265. Feiner H, Kaye G I 1976 Ultrastructural evidence of myofibroblasts in circumscribed fibromatosis. Archives of Pathology and Laboratory Medicine 100: 265-268

2266. Fishbein M C, Ferrans V J, Roberts W C 1975 Endocardial papillary elastofibromas. Histologic, histochemical, and electron microscopical findings. Archives of Pathology 99: 335-341

2267. Fu Y-S, Gabbiani G, Kaye G I, Lattes R 1975 Malignant soft tissue tumors of probable histiocytic origin (malignant fibrous histiocytomas): general considerations and electron microscopic and tissue culture studies. Cancer 35: 176-198

2268. Gabbiani G, Majno G 1972 Dupuytren's contracture: fibroblast contraction? An ultrastructural study. American Journal of Pathology 66: 131-146

2269. Goellner J R, Soule E H 1980 Desmoid tumors. An ultrastructural study of eight cases. Human Pathology 11: 43-50

2270. Gokel J M, Hübner G 1977 Intracellular 'fibrous long spacing' collagen in morbus Dupuytren (Dupuytren's contracture). Beiträge zur Pathologie 161: 176-186

2271. Gokel J M, Hübner G 1977 Occurrence of myofibroblasts in the different phases of morbus Dupuytren (Dupuytren's contracture). Beiträge zur Pathologie 161: 166-175

2272. Gonzalez-Crussi F 1970 Ultrastructure of congenital fibrosarcoma. Cancer 26: 1289-1299

2273. Gonzalez-Crussi F, Wiederhold M D, Sotelo-Avila C 1980 Congenital fibrosarcoma. Presence of a histiocytic component. Cancer 46: 77-86

2274. Govoni E, Bazzocchi F, Pileri S, Martinelli G 1982 Primary malignant fibrous histiocytoma of the spleen: an ultrastructural study. Histopathology 6: 351-361

2275. Hardy T J, An T, Brown P W, Terz J J 1978 Postirradiation sarcoma (malignant fibrous histiocytoma) of axilla. Cancer 42: 118-124

2276. Harris M 1980 The ultrastructure of benign and malignant fibrous histiocytomas. Histopathology 4: 29-44

2277. Hoffman M A, Dickersin G R 1983 Malignant fibrous histiocytoma: an ultrastructural study of eleven cases. Human Pathology 14: 913-922

2278. Iwasaki H, Kikuchi M, Eimoto T, Enjoji M, Yoh S, Sakurai H 1983 Juvenile aponeurotic fibroma: an ultrastructural study. Ultrastructural Pathology 4: 75-83

2279. Iwasaki H, Kikuchi M, Mori R, Miyazono J, Enjoji M, Shinohara N, Matsuzaki A 1980 Infantile digital fibromatosis. Ultrastructural, histochemical and tissue culture observations. Cancer 46: 2238-2247

2280. Iwasaki H, Kikuchi M, Takii M, Enjoji M 1982 Benign and malignant fibrous histiocytomas of the soft tissues. Functional characterization of the cultured cells. Cancer 50: 520-530

2281. Jakobiec F A, Tannenbaum M 1974 The ultrastructure of orbital fibrosarcoma. American Journal of Ophthalmology 77: 899-917

2282. Järvi O H, Saxén A E, Hopsu-Havu V K, Wartiovaara J J, Vaissalo V T 1969 Elastofibroma — a degenerative pseudotumor. Cancer 23: 42-63

2283. Johnson W W, Coburn T P, Pratt C B, Smith J W, Kumar A P M, Dahlin D C 1978 Ultrastructure of malignant histiocytoma arising in the acromion. Human Pathology 9: 199-209

2284. Kay S 1978 Inflammatory fibrous histiocytoma (? xanthogranuloma). Report of two cases with ultrastructural observations in one. American Journal of Surgical Pathology 2: 313-319

2285. Kindblom L-G, Merck C, Angervall L 1979 The ultrastructure of myxofibrosarcoma. A study of 11 cases. Virchows Archiv A Pathological Anatomy and Histology 381: 121-139

2286. Kindblom L-G, Spicer S S 1982 Elastofibroma. A correlated light and electron microscopic study. Virchows Archiv A Pathological Anatomy and Histology 396: 127-140

2287. Kobayashi Y, Watanabe H, Suzuki H, Konno T, Yamamoto T Y 1981 Ultrastructural studies on congenital generalised fibromatosis regressed spontaneously. Tohoku Journal of Experimental Medicine 134: 431-445

2288. Lagacé R, Dalage C, Seemayer T A 1979 Myxoid variant of malignant fibrous histiocytoma: ultrastructural observations. Cancer 43: 526-534

2289. Leu H J, Makek M 1982 Angiomatoid malignant fibrous histiocytoma. Case report and electron microscopic findings. Virchows Archiv A Pathological Anatomy and Histology 395: 99-107

2290. Liew S–H, Haynes M 1981 Localized form of congenital generalized fibromatosis. A report of 3 cases with myofibroblasts. Pathology 13: 257–266

2291. Limacher J, Delage C, Lagacé R 1978 Malignant fibrous histiocytoma. Clinicopathologic and ultrastructural study of 12 cases. American Journal of Surgical Pathology 2: 265–274

2292. Madri J A, Dise C A, LiVolsi V A, Merino M J, Bibro M C 1981 Elastofibroma dorsi: an immunochemical study of collagen content. Human Pathology 12: 186–190

2293. McLay A L C, McGregor F M, Toner P G 1980 Langerhans granules in malignant fibrous histiocytoma. Journal of Submicroscopic Cytology 12: 145–148

2294. Meister P, Gokel J M, Romberger K 1979 Palmar fibromatosis — 'Dupuytren's contracture'. A comparison of light, electron and immuno-fluorescence microscopic findings. Pathology Research and Practice 164: 402–412

2295. Merino M J, LiVolsi V A 1980 Inflammatory malignant fibrous histiocytoma. American Journal of Clinical Pathology 73: 276–281

2296. Merkow L P, Frich J C Jr, Slifkin M, Kyreages C G, Pardo M 1971 Ultrastructure of a fibroxanthosarcoma (malignant fibroxanthoma). Cancer 28: 372–383

2297. Miller R, Kreutner A Jr, Kurtz S M 1980 Malignant inflammatory histiocytoma (inflammatory fibrous histiocytoma). Report of a patient with four lesions. Cancer 45: 179–187

2298. Mortimer G, Gibson A A M 1982 Recurring digital fibroma. Journal of Clinical Pathology 35: 849–854

2299. Navas-Palacios J J 1983 The fibromatoses. An ultrastructural study of 31 cases. Pathology Research and Practice 176: 158–175

2300. Okeda R, Mochizuki T, Terao E, Matsutani M 1980 The origin of intracranial fibrosarcoma. Acta Neuropathologica 52: 223–230

2301. Osamura R Y, Watanabe K, Yoneyama K, Hayashi T 1978 Malignant fibrous histiocytoma of the renal capsule. Light and electron microscopic study of a rare tumor. Virchows Archiv A Pathological Anatomy and Histology 380: 327–334

2302. Paulsen S M, Egeblad K 1983 Sarcoma of the pulmonary artery. A light and electron microscopic study. Journal of Submicroscopic Cytology 15: 811–821

2303. Ramos C V, Gillespie W, Narconis R J 1978 Elastofibroma. A pseudotumor of myofibroblasts. Archives of Pathology and Laboratory Medicine 102: 538–540

2304. Rodu B, Weathers D R, Campbell W G Jr 1981 Aggressive fibromatosis involving the paramandibular soft tissues. A study with the aid of electron microscopy. Oral Surgery, Oral Medicine, Oral Pathology 52: 395–403

2305. Roessner A, Immenkamp M, Weidner A, Hobik H P, Grundmann E 1981 Benign fibrous histiocytoma of bone. Light- and electron-microscopic observations. Journal of Cancer Research and Clinical Oncology 101: 191–202

2306. Rosenberg H S, Stenback W A, Spjut H J 1978 The fibromatoses of infancy and childhood. Perspectives in Pediatric Pathology 4: 269–348

2307. Shah A A, Churg A, Sbarbaro J A, Sheppard J M, Lamberti J 1978 Malignant fibrous histiocytoma of the heart presenting as an atrial myxoma. Cancer 42: 2466–2471

2308. Shin W Y, Abramson A L 1976 The value of electron microscopy in the diagnosis of fibrosarcoma of the larynx. Transactions American Academy of Ophthalmology and Otolaryngology 82: 582–587

2309. Smith P S, Pieterse A S, McClure J 1982 Fibroma of tendon sheath. Journal of Clinical Pathology 35: 842–848

2310. Stiller D, Katenkamp D 1975 Cellular features in desmoid fibromatosis and well differentiated fibrosarcomas: an electron microscopic study. Virchows Archiv A Pathological Anatomy and Histology 369: 155–164

2311. Sun C–C J, Toker C, Breitenecker R 1982 An ultrastructural study of angiomatoid fibrous histiocytoma. Cancer 49: 2103–2111

2312. Taxy J B, Battifora H 1977 Malignant fibrous histiocytoma. An electron microscopic study. Cancer 40: 254–267

2313. Tralka T S, Yee C, Triche T J, Costa J, Dienes H P 1982 Unusual intranuclear inclusions in malignant fibrous histiocytoma: presence in primary tumor, metastases, and xenografts. Ultrastructural Pathology 3: 161–167

2314. Tsuneyoshi M, Enjoji M 1980 Postirradiation sarcoma (malignant fibrous histiocytoma) following breast carcinoma: an ultrastructural study of a case. Cancer 45: 1419–1423

2315. Tsuneyoshi M, Enjoji M, Shinohara N 1981 Malignant fibrous histiocytoma. An electron microscopic study of 17 cases. Virchows Archiv A Pathological Anatomy and Histology 392: 135–145

2316. Turi G K, Albala A, Fenoglio J J Jr 1980 Cardiac fibromatosis: an ultrastructural study. Human Pathology 11: 577–580

2317. Van Haelst U J G M, de Haas van Dorsser A H 1976 Giant cell tumor of soft parts. An ultrastructural study. Virchows Archiv A Pathological Anatomy and Histology 371: 199–217

2318. Vasudev K S, Harris M 1978 A sarcoma of myofibroblasts. An ultrastructural study. Archives of Pathology and Laboratory Medicine 102: 185–188

2319. Verity M A, Ebert J T, Hepler R S 1977 Atypical fibrous histiocytoma of the orbit: an electron microscopic study. Ophthalmologica 175: 73–79

2320. Waisman J, Smith D W 1968 Fine structure of an elastofibroma. Cancer 22: 671–677

2321. Wang N–S, Knaack J 1982 Fibromatosis hyalinica multiplex juvenilis. Ultrastructural Pathology 3: 153–160

2322. Wigger H J, Mitsudo S M 1976 Fibrous histiocytoma simulating congenital fibromatosis: a light, electron microscopic and tissue culture study. Virchows Archiv A Pathological Anatomy and Histology 370: 255–266

2323. Williamson J C, Johnson J D, Lamm D L, Tio F 1980 Malignant fibrous histiocytoma of the spermatic cord. Journal of Urology 123: 785–788

2324. Winkelmann R K, Sams W M Jr 1969 Elastofibroma. Report of a case with special histochemical and electron-microscopic studies. Cancer 23: 406–415

2325. Woyke S, Domagala W, Olszewski W 1970 Ultrastructure of a fibromatosis hyalinica multiplex juvenilis. Cancer 26: 1157–1168

2326. Yoshida H, Matsui K, Hashimoto K, Yumoto T, Mihara M 1982 Dermatofibrosarcoma protuberans and its tissue culture study — ultrastructural, enzyme histochemical and immunological study. Acta Pathologica Japonica 32: 83–91

2327. Zardawi I M, Earley M J 1982 Inclusion body fibromatosis. Journal of Pathology 137: 99–107

## 55 LIPOMA, HIBERNOMA AND LIPOSARCOMA

2328. Alba Greco M, Garcia R L, Vuletin J C 1980 Benign lipoblastomastosis. Ultrastructure and histogenesis. Cancer 45: 511–515

2329. Allen P W 1981 Tumors and proliferations of adipose tissue. A clinicopathologic approach. Masson Publishing USA, New York

2330. Battifora H, Nunez-Alonso C 1980 Myxoid liposarcoma: study of ten cases. Ultrastructural Pathology 1: 157–169

2331. Bolen J W, Thorning D 1980 Benign lipoblastoma and myxoid liposarcoma: a comparative light- and electron-microscopic study. American Journal of Surgical Pathology 4: 163–174

2332. Bolen J W, Thorning D 1981 Spindle-cell lipoma. A clinical, light- and electron-microscopical study. American Journal of Surgical Pathology 5: 435–441

2333. Dardick I 1978 Hibernoma: a possible model of brown fat adipogenesis. Human Pathology 9: 321–329

2334. Desai U, Ramos C V, Taylor H B 1978 Ultrastructural observations in pleomorphic liposarcoma. Cancer 42: 1284–1290

2335. Enzinger F M, Harvey D A 1975 Spindle cell lipoma. Cancer 36: 1852–1859

2336. Flenker H 1976 Myxoid liposarcoma. Light and electron microscopic investigation. Virchows Archiv A Pathological Anatomy and Histology 371: 171–176

2337. Fu Y S, Parker F G, Kaye G I, Lattes R 1980 Ultrastructure of benign and malignant adipose tissue tumors. Pathology Annual 15, pt 1: 67–89

2338. Gaffney E F, Hargreaves H K, Semple E, Vellios F 1983 Hibernoma: distinctive light and electron microscopic studies and relationship to brown adipose tissue. Human Pathology 14: 677–687

2339. Guevara M E, Machinami R, Higaki S 1981 Crystalline inclusion in myxoid liposarcoma. Acta Pathologica Japonica 31: 689–694

2340. Kim Y H, Reiner L 1982 Ultrastructure of lipoma. Cancer 50: 102–106

2341. Kindblom L G, Angervall L, Fassina A S 1982 Atypical lipoma. Acta Pathologica, Microbiologica, et Immunologica Scandinavica. Section A. Pathology 90: 27–36

2342. Kindblom L-G, Säve-Söderbergh J 1979 The ultrastructure of liposarcoma. A study of 10 cases. Acta Pathologica et Microbiologica Scandinavica. Section A. Pathology 87: 109–121

2343. Lagacé R, Jacob S, Seemayer T A 1979 Myxoid liposarcoma. An electronmicroscopic study: biological and histogenetic considerations. Virchows Archiv A Pathological Anatomy and Histology 384: 159–172

2344. Lazarus S S, Trombetta L D 1981 Ultrastructural and histochemical identification of sclerosing liposarcoma. Histopathology 5: 223–235

2345. Levine G D 1972 Hibernoma. An electron microscopic study. Human Pathology 3: 351–359

2346. Sadeghi E M, Sauk J J Jr 1982 Liposarcoma of the oral cavity. Clinical, tissue culture, and ultrastructure study of a case. Journal of Oral Pathology 11: 263–275

2347. Seemayer T A, Knaack J, Wang N-S, Ahmed M N 1975 On the ultrastructure of hibernoma. Cancer 36: 1785–1793

2348. Wetzel W, Alexander R 1979 Myxoid liposarcoma. An ultrastructural study of two cases. American Journal of Clinical Pathology 72: 521–528

### 56 SMOOTH MUSCLE TUMOURS

2349. Almagro U A, Schulte W J, Norback D H, Turcotte J K 1981 Glomus tumor of the stomach. Histologic and ultrastructural features. American Journal of Clinical Pathology 75: 415–419

2350. Angervall L, Berlin O, Kindblom L-G, Stener B 1980 Primary leiomyosarcoma of bone. A study of five cases. Cancer 46: 1270–1279

2351. Bloustein P A 1978 Hepatic leiomyosarcoma: ultrastructural study and review of the differential diagnosis. Human Pathology 9: 713–715

2352. Böcker W, Strecker H 1975 Electron microscopy of uterine leiomyosarcomas. Virchows Archiv A Pathological Anatomy and Histology 367: 59–71

2353. Bures J C, Barnes L, Mercer D 1981 A comparative study of smooth muscle tumors utilizing light and electron microscopy, immunocytochemical staining and enzymatic assay. Cancer 48: 2420–2426

2354. Burkhardt A, Otto H F, Kaukel E 1981 Multiple pulmonary (hamartomatous?) leiomyomas. Light and electron microscopic study. Virchows Archiv A Pathological Anatomy and Histology 391: 133–141

2355. Chang V, Aikawa M, Druet R 1977 Uterine leiomyoblastoma. Ultrastructural and cytological studies. Cancer 39: 1563–1569

2356. Chen K T, Kuo T T, Hoffmann K D 1981 Leiomyosarcoma of the breast: a case of long survival and late hepatic metastasis. Cancer 47: 1883–1886

2357. Cornog J L Jr 1974 Gastric leiomyoblastoma. A clinical and ultrastructural study. Cancer 34: 711–719

2358. Darby A J, Papadaki L, Beilby J O 1975 An unusual leiomyosarcoma of the uterus containing osteoclast-like giant cells. Cancer 36: 495–504

2359. di Sant'Agnese P A, de Masy Jensen K L 1983 Thick (myosin) filaments in a glomus tumor. American Journal of Clinical Pathology 79: 130–134

2360. Ferenczy A, Richart R M, Okagaki T 1971 A comparative ultrastructural study of leiomyosarcoma, cellular leiomyoma, and leiomyoma of the uterus. Cancer 28: 1004–1018

2361. Gabella G 1981 Structure of smooth muscles. In Bülbring E, Brading A F, Jones A W, Tomita T (eds) Smooth muscle: an assessment of current knowledge. Edward Arnold, London, ch 1, p 1–46

2362. Gould V E, Patel N S, Dardi L E, Memoli V A 1982 The quarterly case: painful lytic lesion of the left femur in an adult male (leiomyosarcoma). Ultrastructural Pathology 3: 301–307

2363. Hayata T, Sato E 1977 Primary leiomyosarcoma arising in the trunk of pulmonary artery: a case report and review of literature. Acta Pathologica Japonica 27: 137–144

2364. Henrichs K J, Wenisch H J C, Hofmann W, Klein F 1979 Leiomyosarcoma of the pulmonary artery. A light and electron-microscopical study. Virchows Archiv A Pathological Anatomy and Histology 383: 207–216

2365. Hernandez F J 1978 Leiomyosarcoma of male breast originating in the nipple. American Journal of Surgical Pathology 2: 299–304

2366. Hernandez F J, Stanley T M, Ranganath K A, Rubinstein A I 1979 Primary leiomyosarcoma of the aorta. American Journal of Surgical Pathology 3: 251–256

2367. Herrera G A, Miles P A, Greenberg H, Reimann B E F, Weisman I M 1983 The origin of the pseudoglandular spaces in metastatic smooth muscle neoplasm of uterine origin. Report of a case with ultrastructure and review of previous cases studied by electron microscopy. Chest 83: 270–274

2368. Jakobiec F A, Howard G M, Rosen M, Wolff M 1975 Leiomyoma and leiomyosarcoma of the orbit. American Journal of Ophthalmology 80: 1028–1042

2369. Jakobiec F A, Jones I S, Tannenbaum M 1973 Leiomyoma: an unusual tumour of the orbit. British Journal of Ophthalmology 57: 825–831

2370. Jakobiec F A, Witschel H, Zimmerman L E 1976 Choroidal leiomyoma of vascular origin. American Journal of Ophthalmology 82: 205–212

2371. Jernstrom P, Gowdy R A 1975 Leiomyosarcoma of the long saphenous vein. American Journal of Clinical Pathology 63: 25–31

2372. Johnson S, Rundell M, Platt W 1978 Leiomyosarcoma of the scrotum: a case report with electron microscopy. Cancer 41: 1830–1835

2373. Katenkamp D, Stiller D 1980 Unusual leiomyoma of vulva with fibroma-like pattern and pseudoelastin production. Virchows Archiv A Pathological Anatomy and Histology 388: 361–368

2374. Kawai T, Suzuki M, Mukai M, Hiroshima K, Shinmei M 1983 Primary leiomyosarcoma of bone. An immuno-histological and ultrastructural study. Archives of Pathology and Laboratory Medicine 107: 433–437

2375. King M E, Dickersin G R, Scully R E 1982 Myxoid leiomyosarcoma of the uterus. A report of six cases. American Journal of Surgical Pathology 6: 589–598

2376. Kuo T-T, London S N, Dinh T V 1980 Endometriosis occurring in leiomyomatosis peritonealis disseminata. Ultrastructural study and histogenetic consideration. American Journal of Surgical Pathology 4: 197–204

2377. Mackay B, Legha S S, Pickler G M 1981 Quarterly case: coin lesion of the lung in a 19-year-old male. Ultrastructural Pathology 2: 289–294

2378. Mair W G P, Tomé F M S 1972 Atlas of the ultrastructure of diseased human muscle. Churchill Livingstone, Edinburgh

2379. Marchevsky A M, Kaneko M 1983 Subcutaneous leiomyosarcoma with lymphomatous elements: histogenetic implications of an unusual sarcoma. Human Pathology 13: 86–88

2380. Mechlin D C, Hamasaki C K, Moore J R, Davis W E, Templer J 1980 Leiomyoma of the maxilla — report of a case. Laryngoscope 90: 1230–1233

2381. Miettinen M, Lehto V-P, Virtanen I 1983 Glomus tumor cells: evaluation of smooth muscle and endothelial cell properties. Virchows Archiv B Cell Pathology Including Molecular Pathology 43: 139–149

2382. Morales A R, Fine G, Pardo V, Horn R C Jr 1975 The ultrastructure of smooth muscle tumors with a consideration of the possible relationship of glomangiomas, hemangio-pericytomas, and cardiac myxomas. Pathology Annual 10: 65–92

2383. Murao T 1982 A comparative electron microscopic study of leiomyosarcoma and leiomyoma of the duodenum. Acta Pathologica Japonica 32: 621–632

2384. Nevalainen T J 1978 Ultrastructure of gastric leiomyo-sarcoma. Virchows Archiv A Pathological Anatomy and Histology 379: 25–33

2385. Nistal M, Paniagua R, Picazo M L, Cermeno de Giles F, Ramos Guerreira J L 1980 Granular changes in vascular leiomyosarcoma. Virchows Archiv A Pathological Anatomy and Histology 386: 239–248

2386. O'Brien S E, Shier K H 1974 Leiomyoblastoma of the stomach. Canadian Journal of Surgery 17: 105–110

2387. Overgaard J, Frederiksen P, Helmig O, Jensen O M 1977 Primary leiomyosarcoma of bone. Cancer 39: 1664–1671

2388. Pieslor P C, Orenstein J M, Hogan D L, Breslow A 1979 Ultrastructure of myofibroblasts and decidualized cells in leiomyomatosis peritonealis disseminata. American Journal of Clinical Pathology 72: 875–882

2389. Pritchett P S, Fu Y-S, Kay S 1975 Unusual ultrastructural features of leiomyosarcoma of the lung. American Journal of Clinical Pathology 63: 901–908

2390. Roth J A, Carter H, Costabile D 1978 An unusual multifocal leiomyosarcoma of the stomach: a light and electron microscopic study. Human Pathology 9: 345–351

2391. Seifert H W 1981 Ultrastructural investigation on cutaneous angioleiomyoma. Archives of Dermatological Research 271: 91–99

2392. Seo I S, Warner T F C S, Glant M D 1980 Retroperitoneal leiomyosarcoma: a light and electron microscopic study. Histopathology 4: 53–62

2393. Shamsuddin A K, Reyes F, Harvey J W, Toker C 1980 Primary leiomyosarcoma of bone. Human Pathology 11: 581–583

2394. Silverman J F, Kay S 1976 Multiple pulmonary leiomyomatous hamartomas. Report of a case with ultrastructure examination. Cancer 38: 1199–1204

2395. Small J V, Sobieszek A 1980 The contractile apparatus of smooth muscle. In: Bourne G H, Danielli J F (eds) International review of cytology, vol 64. Academic Press, New York, p 241–306

2396. Starr G F 1974 Pathologic features of smooth muscle tumors. Journal of the American Medical Association 229: 1219–1220

2397. Sun C C, Zelman J, Toker C 1980 Familial cutaneous leiomyomata: a case report with electron microscopic study. Mount Sinai Journal of Medicine 47: 40–44

2398. Tajima Y, Weather D R, Neville B W, Benoit P W, Pedley D M 1981 Glomus tumor (glomangioma) of the tongue. A light and electron microscopic study. Oral Surgery 52: 288–293

2399. Tobon H, Murphy A I, Salazar H 1973 Primary leiomyosarcoma of the vagina. Light and electron microscopic observations. Cancer 32: 450–457

2400. Tsuneyoshi M, Enjoji M 1982 Glomus tumor. A clinicopathologic and electron microscopic study. Cancer 50. 1601–1607

2401. Wang N S, Seemayer T A, Ahmed M N, Morin J 1974 Pulmonary leiomyosarcoma associated with an arteriovenous fistula. Archives of Pathology 98: 100–105

2402. Wang T-Y, Erlandson R A, Marcove R C, Huvos A G 1980 Primary leiomyosarcoma of bone. Archives of Pathology and Laboratory Medicine 104: 100–104

2403. Weiss R A, Mackay B 1981 Malignant smooth muscle tumors of the gastrointestinal tract: an ultrastructural study of 20 cases. Ultrastructural Pathology 2: 231–240

2404. Wolff M, Silva F, Kaye G 1979 Pulmonary metastases (with admixed epithelial elements) from smooth muscle neoplasms. Report of nine cases, including three males. American Journal of Surgical Pathology 3: 325–342

## 57 STRIATED MUSCLE TUMOURS

2405. Albrechsten R, Ebbeson F, Vangpedersen S 1974 Extra-cardiac rhabdomyoma. Light and electron microscopic studies of two cases in the mandibular area, with a review of previous reports. Acta Otolaryngologica 78: 458–464

2406. Altmannsberger M, Osborn M, Treuner J, Hölscher A, Weber K, Schauer A 1982 Diagnosis of human childhood rhabdomyosarcoma by antibodies to desmin, the structural protein of muscle specific intermediate filaments. Virchows Archiv B Cell Pathology 39: 203–215

2407. Bale P M, Parsons R E, Stevens M M 1983 Diagnosis and behavior of juvenile rhabdomyosarcoma. Human Pathology 14: 596–611

2408. Battifora H A, Eisenstein R, Schild J A 1969 Rhabdomyoma of the larynx. Ultrastructural study and comparison with granular cell tumors (myoblastomas). Cancer 23: 183–190

2409. Bleisch V R, Kraus F T 1980 Polypoid sarcoma of the pulmonary trunk: analysis of the literature and report of a case with leptomeric organelles and ultrastructural features of rhabdomyosarcoma. Cancer 46: 314–324

2410. Bundtzen J La V, Norback D H 1982 The ultrastructure of poorly differentiated rhabdomyosarcomas: a case report and literature review. Human Pathology 13: 301–313

2411. Churg A, Ringus J 1978 Ultrastructural observations on the histogenesis of alveolar rhabdomyosarcoma. Cancer 41: 1355–1361

2412. Cori G, Faraggiana T, Grandi C, Nardi F 1977 The diagnostic usefulness of electron microscopy investigation of orbital embryonal rhabdomyosarcomas. Tumori 63: 205–213

2413. Cornog J L Jr, Gonatas N K 1967 Ultrastructure of rhabdomyoma. Journal of Ultrastructure Research 20: 433–450

2414. Crist W M, Edwards R H, Pereira F 1978 Rhabdomyosarcoma diagnosed by electron microscopy in a child with acute lymphocytic leukemia. Journal of Pediatrics 93: 893–894

2415. Czernobilsky B, Cornog J L Jr, Enterline H T 1968 Rhabdomyoma: report of a case with ultrastructural and histochemical studies. American Journal of Clinical Pathology 49: 782–789

2416. Dehner L P, Enzinger F M, Font R L 1972 Fetal rhabdomyoma. An analysis of nine cases. Cancer 30: 160–166

2417. Fenoglio J J Jr, Diana D J, Bowen T E, McAllister H A Jr, Ferrans V J 1977 Ultrastructure of a cardiac rhabdomyoma. Human Pathology 8: 700–706

2418. Fenoglio J J Jr, McAllister H A Jr, Ferrans V J 1976 Cardiac rhabdomyoma: a clinicopathologic and electron-microscopic study. American Journal of Cardiology 38: 241–251

2419. Franzini-Armstrong C, Peachey L D 1981 Striated muscle — contractile and control mechanisms. Journal of Cell Biology 91: 166s–186s

2420. Freeman A I, Johnson W W 1968 A comparative study of childhood rhabdomyosarcoma and virus-induced rhabdomyosarcoma in mice. Cancer Research 28: 1490–1500

2421. Gonzalez-Crussi F, Black-Schaffer S 1979 Rhabdomyosarcoma of infancy and childhood. Problems of morphologic classification. American Journal of Surgical Pathology 3: 157–171

2422. Gould J H, Bossen E H 1976 Benign vaginal rhabdomyoma. A light and electron microscopic study. Cancer 37: 2283–2294

2423. Hanrinck E, Moulaert A J, Rohmer J, Brom A G 1974 Cardiac rhabdomyoma in infancy. Acta Paediatrica Scandinavica 63: 283–286

2424. Hański W, Hagel E 1976 Histological and ultrastructural studies of a case of rhabdomyoma polyposum vaginae. Annals of the Medical Section of the Polish Academy of Sciences 21: 47–48

2425. Henderson D W, Raven J L, Pollard J A, Walters M N-I 1976 Bone marrow metastases in disseminated alveolar rhabdomyosarcoma: case report with ultrastructural study and review. Pathology 8: 329–341

2426. Hildebrand H F, Krivosic I, Grandier-Vazeille X, Tetaert D, Biserte G 1980 Perineal rhabdomyosarcoma in a newborn child: pathological and biochemical studies with emphasis on contractile proteins. Journal of Clinical Pathology 33: 823–829

2427. Horvat B L, Caines M, Fisher E R 1970 The ultrastructure of rhabdomyosarcoma. American Journal of Clinical Pathology 53: 555–564

2428. Hosoda S, Suzuki H, Kawabe Y, Watanabe Y, Isojima G 1971 Embryonal rhabdomyosarcoma of the middle ear. Cancer 27: 943–947

2429. Kahn H J, Yeger H, Kassim O, Jorgensen A O, MacLennan D H, Baumal R, Smith C R, Phillips M J 1983 Immunohistochemical and electron microscopic assessment of childhood rhabdomyosarcoma. Increased frequency of diagnosis over routine methods. Cancer 51: 1897–1903

2430. Kanegaonkar G, McDougall J, Grant H R 1981 Rhabdomyosarcoma of the maxillary antrum in an adult. A case report with ultrastructural observations. Journal of Laryngology and Otology 95: 863–872

2431. Kay S, Gerszten E, Dennison S M 1969 Light and electron microscopic study of a rhabdomyoma arising in the floor of the mouth. Cancer 23: 708–716

2432. Konrad E A, Meister P, Hübner G 1981 Typing of extracardiac rhabdomyoma. Pathologe 3: 45–50

2433. Konrad E A, Meister P, Hübner G 1982 Extracardiac rhabdomyoma. Report of different types with light microscopic and ultrastructural studies. Cancer 49: 898–907

2434. Lack E E, Perez-Atayde A R, Shuster S R 1981 Botryoid rhabdomyosarcoma of the biliary tract. Report of five cases with ultrastructural observations and literature review. American Journal of Surgical Pathology 5: 643–652

2435. Lehtonen E, Asikainen U, Badley R A 1982 Rhabdomyoma. Ultrastructural features and distribution of desmin, muscle type of intermediate filament protein. Acta Pathologica Microbiologica et Immunologica Scandinavica. Section A. Pathology 90: 125–129

2436. Leone P G, Taylor H B 1973 Ultrastructure of a benign polypoid rhabdomyoma of the vagina. Cancer 31: 1414–1417

2437. Masuzawa T, Shimabukuro H, Kamashita S, Sato F 1982 The ultrastructure of primary cerebral rhabdomyosarcoma. Acta Neuropathologica 56: 307–310

2438. Mierau G W, Favara B E 1980 Rhabdomyosarcoma in children: ultrastructural study of 31 cases. Cancer 46: 2035–2040

2439. Miller R, Kurtz S M, Powers J M 1978 Mediastinal rhabdomyoma. Cancer 42: 1983–1988

2440. Morales A R, Fine G, Horn R C Jr 1972 Rhabdomyosarcoma: an ultrastructural appraisal. Pathology Annual 7: 81–106

2441. Papadimitriou J M, Mastaglia F L 1982 Ultrastructural changes in human muscle fibres in disease. Journal of Submicroscopic Cytology 14: 525–551

2442. Prince F P 1981 Ultrastructural aspects of myogenesis found in neoplasms. Acta Neuropathologica 54: 315–320

2443. Riehle R A Jr, Venkatachalam H 1982 Electron microscopy in diagnosis of adult paratesticular rhabdomyosarcoma. Urology 19: 658–661

2444. Roy S, Bhatia R, Nauda N R 1980 Primary rhabdomyosarcoma of the cerebellum. Journal of Pathology 132: 235–241

2445. Sarkar K, Tolnai G, McKay D E 1973 Embryonal rhabdomyosarcoma of the prostate. An ultrastructural study. Cancer 31: 442–448

2446. Scrivner D, Meyer J S 1980 Multifocal recurrent adult rhabdomyoma. Cancer 46: 790–795

2447. Shin K H, Whitehead V M 1980 Rhabdomyosarcoma of the brain. Canadian Journal of Surgery 23: 576–578

2448. Silseth C, Veress B, Bergström B 1982 A case of adult rhabdomyoma in the tonsillar region. A light and electron microscopic study. Acta Pathologica Microbiologica et Immunologica Scandinavica. Section A. Pathology 90: 1–4

2449. Silverman J F, Kay S, Chang C H 1978 Ultrastructural comparison between skeletal muscle and cardiac rhabdomyomas. Cancer 42: 189–193

2450. Silverman J F, Kay S, McCue C M, Lower R R, Brough A J, Chang C H 1976 Rhabdomyoma of the heart. Ultrastructural study of three cases. Laboratory Investigation 35: 596–606

2451. Simha M, Doctor V, Dalal S, Manghani D K, Dastur D K 1982 Postauricular fetal rhabdomyoma: light and electron microscopic study. Human Pathology 13: 673–677

2452. Smith M T, Armbrustmacher V W, Violett T W 1981 Diffuse meningeal rhabdomyosarcoma. Cancer 47: 2081–2086

2453. Sulser H 1978 The rhabdomyosarcoma with regard to age, sex, localization, pathological anatomy, and prognosis. Virchows Archiv A Pathological Anatomy and Histology 379: 35–71

2454. Trillo A A, Holleman I L, White J T 1978 Presence of satellite cells in a cardiac rhabdomyoma. Histopathology 2: 215–223

2455. Ueda K, Gruppo R, Unger F, Martin L, Bove K 1977 Rhabdomyosarcoma of lung arising in congenital cystic adenomatoid malformation. Cancer 40: 383–388

2456. Vartio T, Nickels J, Höckerstedt K, Scheinin T M 1980 Rhabdomyosarcoma of the oesophagus. Light and electron microscopic study of a rare tumor. Virchows Archiv A Pathological Anatomy and Histology 386: 357–361

2457. Warner T F, Kelly M 1974 Unusual ultrastructural features in alveolar rhabdomyosarcoma. Irish Journal of Medical Science 143: 220–226

2458. Yagishita S, Itoh Y, Chiba Y, Fujino H 1979 Primary rhabdomyosarcoma of the cerebrum. An ultrastructural study. Acta Neuropathologica 45: 111–115

## 58  MYXOMAS

2459. Bell D A, Alba Greco M 1981 Cardiac myxoma with chondroid features: a light and electron microscopic study. Human Pathology 12: 370–374

2460. Coltart D J, Billingham M E, Popp R L, Caves P K, Harrison D C, Stinson E B 1975 Left atrial myxoma. Diagnosis, treatment and cytological observations. Journal of the American Medical Association 234: 950–953

2461. Feldman P S 1979 A comparative study including ultrastructure of intramuscular myxoma and myxoid liposarcoma. Cancer 43: 512–525

2462. Feldman P S, Horvath E, Kovacs K 1977 An ultrastructural study of seven cardiac myxomas. Cancer 40: 2216–2232

2463. Ferrans V J 1980 Cardiac tumors. In: Johannessen J V (ed) Electron microscopy in human medicine, vol 5. Cardiovascular system, lymphoreticular and hematopoietic system. McGraw-Hill, New York, pt 1, ch 9, p 68–74

2464. Ferrans V J, Roberts W C 1973 Structural features of cardiac myxomas. Histology, histochemistry, and electron microscopy. Human Pathology 4: 111–146

2465. Hasleton P S, Simpson W, Craig R D 1978 Myxoma of the mandible: a fibroblastic tumor. Oral Surgery, Oral Medicine and Oral Pathology 46: 396–406

2466. Kelly M, Bhagwat A G 1972 Ultrastructural features of a recurrent endothelial myxoma of the left atrium. Archives of Pathology 93: 219–226

2467. Matsuyama K, Oneda G 1967 Histogenesis of primary myxoma of the heart: a case report. Gann 58: 435–440

2468. Morales A, Fine G, Castro A, Nadji M 1981 Cardiac myxoma (endocardioma). An immunocytochemical assessment of histogenesis. Human Pathology 12: 896–899

2469. Seo I S, Warner T F C S, Colyer R A, Winkler R F 1980 Metastasizing atrial myxoma. American Journal of Surgical Pathology 4: 391–399

2470. Wold L E, Lie J T 1981 Scanning electron microscopy of intracardiac myxoma. Mayo Clinic Proceedings 56: 198–200

## 59  VASOFORMATIVE TUMOURS

2471. Alvarez-Fernandez E, Salinero-Paniagua E 1981 Vascular tumors of the mammary gland. A histochemical and ultrastructural study. Virchows Archiv A Pathological Anatomy and Histology 391: 31–37

2472. Andrioli G C, Scanarini M, Iob I 1979 Intrinsic haematopoietic activity of cerebellar haemangioblastomas. Ultrastructural study of three cases. Neurochirurgia 22: 24–28

2473. Balázs M, Dénes J, Lukács V F 1978 Fine structure of multiple neonatal haemangioendothelioma of the liver. Virchows Archiv A Pathological Anatomy and Histology 379: 157–168

2474. Battifora H 1973 Hemangiopericytoma: ultrastructural study of five cases. Cancer 31: 1418–1432

2475. Bednár B 1980 Solid dendritic cell angiosarcoma: reinterpretation of extraskeletal sarcoma resembling Ewing's sarcoma. Journal of Pathology 130: 217–222

2476. Braun-Falco O, Schmoeckel C, Hübner G 1976 The histogenesis of Kaposi sarcoma. A histochemical and electronmicroscopical study. Virchows Archiv A Pathological Anatomy and Histology 369: 215–227

2477. Cancilla P A, Zimmerman H M 1965 The fine structure of a cerebellar haemangioblastoma. Journal of Neuropathology and Experimental Neurology 24: 621–628

2478. Carstens P H B 1981 The Weibel-Palade body in the diagnosis of endothelial tumors. Ultrastructural Pathology 2: 315–325

2479. Chaudhuri B, Ronan S G, Manaligod J R 1980 Angiosarcoma arising in a plexiform neurofibroma. A case report. Cancer 46: 605–610

2480. Dabska M 1969 Malignant endovascular papillary angioendothelioma of the skin in childhood. Clinicopathologic study of 6 cases. Cancer 24: 503–510

2481. Dixon A Y, McGregor D H, Lee S H 1981 Angiolipomas: an ultrastructural and clinicopathological study. Human Pathology 12: 739–747

2482. Echevarria R A, Arean V M, Galindo L 1978 Hepatic tumors of long duration with eventual metastases. Two cases of leiomyosarcomatosis possibly arising from hamartomas of liver. American Journal of Clinical Pathology 69: 624–631

2483. Eckstein R P, Wills E J, Segelov J N 1981 Haemangioblastoma of the optic nerve. Case report with study by light and electron microscopy. Pathology 13: 357–364

2484. Eimoto T 1977 Ultrastructure of an infantile hemangiopericytoma. Cancer 40: 2162–2170

2485. Feldman P S, Shneidman D, Kaplan C 1978 Ultrastructure of infantile hemangioendothelioma of the liver. Cancer 42: 521–527

2486. Friendly D S, Font R L, Milhorat T H 1982 Hemangioendothelioma of frontal bone. American Journal of Ophthalmology 93: 482–490

2487. Fulling K H, Gersell D J 1983 Neoplastic angioendotheliomatosis. Histologic, immunohistochemical, and ultrastructural findings in two cases. Cancer 51: 1107–1118

2488. Gindhart T D, Tucker W Y, Choy S H 1979 Cavernous hemangioma of the superior mediastinum. Report of a case with electron microscopy and computerized tomography. American Journal of Surgical Pathology 3: 353–361

2489. Govoni E, Pileri S, Bazzocchi F, Severi B, Martinelli G 1981 Postmastectomy angiosarcoma: ultrastructural study of a case. Tumori 67: 79–86

2490. Hahn M J, Dawson R, Esterly J A, Joseph D J 1973 Hemangiopericytoma. An ultrastructural study. Cancer 31: 255–261

2491. Hargreaves H K, Scully R E, Richie J P 1982 Benign hemangioendothelioma of the testis: case report with electron microscopic documentation and review of the literature. American Journal of Clinical Pathology 77: 637–642

2492. Harrison A C, Kahn L B 1978 Myogenic cells in Kaposi's sarcoma: an ultrastructural study. Journal of Pathology 124: 157–160

2493. Kaul B K, Sinhal G D, Rastogi B L 1974 Hemangiosarcoma in children: two case reports. American Surgeon 40: 643–646

2494. Kimura S 1981 Ultrastructure of so-called angioblastoma of the skin before and after soft X-ray therapy. Journal of Dermatology 8: 235–243

2495. Kindblom L–G, Ullman A 1983 Malignant hemangiopericytoma with admixed glandular structures in breast and lung metastases. A light and electron microscopic and histochemical study of a case. Applied Pathology 1: 50–59

2496. Kojimahara M, Yamazaki K, Ooneda G 1981 Ultrastructural study of hemangiomas. 1. Capillary hemangioma of the skin. Acta Pathologica Japonica 31: 105–115

2497. Kreutner A Jr, Smith R M, Trefny F A 1978 Intravascular papillary endothelial hyperplasia. Light and electron microscopic observations of a case. Cancer 42: 2304–2310

2498. Llombart-Bosch A, Peydro-Olaya A, Pellin A 1982 Ultrastructure of vascular neoplasms. A transmission and scanning electron microscopical study based upon 42 cases. Pathology Research and Practice 174: 1–41

2499. Llombart-Bosch A, Peydro-Olaya A, Paris-Romeu F 1981 Fine structure of a malignant hemangioendothelioma of the esophagus. Virchows Archiv A Pathological Anatomy and Histology 391: 107–115

2500. McNutt N S, Fletcher V, Conant M A 1983 Early lesions of Kaposi's sarcoma in homosexual men. An ultrastructural comparison with other vascular proliferations in skin. American Journal of Pathology 111: 62–77

2501. Meade J B, Whitwell F, Bickford B J, Waddington J K 1974 Primary haemangiopericytoma of lung. Thorax 29: 1–15

2502. Millstein D I, Tang C–K, Campbell E W Jr 1981 Angiosarcoma developing in a patient with neurofibromatosis (von Recklinghausen's disease). Cancer 47: 950–954

2503. Murad T M, von Haam E, Murthy M S N 1968 Ultrastructure of a hemangiopericytoma and a glomus tumor. Cancer 22: 1239–1249

2504. Nagao K, Matsuzaki O, Shigematsu H, Kaneko T, Katoh T, Kitamura T 1980 Histopathologic studies of benign infantile hemangioendothelioma of the parotid gland. Cancer 46: 2250–2256

2505. Newland R C, Maxwell L E, Constance T J, Fox R M 1978 Malignant haemangiopericytoma: case report and ultrastructural study. Pathology 10: 277–283

2506. Nunnery E W, Kahn L B, Reddick R L, Lipper S 1981 Hemangiopericytoma: a light microscopic and ultrastructural study. Cancer 47: 906–914

2507. Ongkasuwan C, Taylor J E, Tang C K, Prempree T 1982 Angiosarcomas of the uterus and ovary: clinicopathologic report. Cancer 49: 1469–1475

2508. Ordónez N G, Bracken R B, Stroehlein K B 1982 Hemangiopericytoma of kidney. Urology 20: 191–195

2509. Otsuki Y, Kobayashi S, Hayashi T, Omori M 1973 Angiosarcoma of the heart: report of a case and review of the literature. Acta Pathologica Japonica 23: 407–413

2510. Pasyk K A, Grabb W C, Cherry G W 1982 Cellular haemangioma. Light and electron microscopic studies of two cases. Virchows Archiv A Pathological Anatomy and Histology 396: 103–126

2511. Paullada J J, Lisci-Garmilla A, Gonzales-Angulo A, Jurado-Mendoza J, Quijano-Narezo M, Gomez-Peralta L, Doria-Medina M 1968 Hemangiopericytoma associated with hypoglycemia. Metabolic and electron microscopic studies of a case. American Journal of Medicine 44: 990–999

2512. Petito C K, Gottlieb G J, Dougherty J H, Petito F A 1978 Neoplastic angioendotheliosis: ultrastructural study and review of the literature. Annals of Neurology 3: 393–399

2513. Pollard S M, Millward-Sadler G H 1974 Malignant haemangioendothelioma involving the liver. Journal of Clinical Pathology 27: 214–221

2514. Ramsey H J 1966 Fine structure of hemangiopericytoma and hemangioendothelioma. Cancer 19: 2005–2018

2515. Reyes J W, Shinozuka H, Garry P, Putong P B 1977 A light and electron microscopic study of a hemangiopericytoma of the prostate with local extension. Cancer 40: 1122–1126

2516. Rosai J, Sumner H W, Kostianovsky M, Perez-Mesa C 1976 Angiosarcoma of the skin. A clinicopathologic and fine structural study. Human Pathology 7: 83–109

2517. Rossi N P, Kioschos J M, Aschenbrener C A, Ehrenhaft J L 1976 Primary angiosarcoma of the heart. Cancer 37: 891–896

2518. Scott P W, Silvers D N, Helwig E B 1975 Proliferating angioendotheliomatosis. Archives of Pathology 99: 323–326

2519. Silverberg S G, Kay S, Koss L G 1971 Post-mastectomy lymphangiosarcoma: ultrastructural observations. Cancer 27: 100–108

2520. Steiner G C, Dorfman H D 1972 Ultrastructure of hemangioendothelial sarcoma of bone. Cancer 29: 122–135

2521. Sun C C, Tang C K, Hill J L 1980 Mesenteric lymphangioma. A case report with transmission and scanning electron microscopic studies. Archives of Pathology and Laboratory Medicine 104: 316–318

2522. Tani E, Ikeda K, Kudo S, Yamagaia S, Higashi N 1974 Fenestrated vessels in human haemangioblastoma. Journal of Neurosurgery 40: 696–705

2523. Tavassoli F A, Weiss S 1981 Hemangiopericytoma of the breast. American Journal of Surgical Pathology 5: 745–752

2524. Taxy J B, Gray S R 1979 Cellular angiomas of infancy. An ultrastructural study of two cases. Cancer 43: 2322–2331

2525. Ulbright T M, Santa Cruz D J 1980 Intravenous pyogenic granuloma. Case report with ultrastructural findings. Cancer 45: 1646–1652

2526. Venkatachalam M A, Greally J G 1969 Fine structure of glomus tumor: similarity of glomus cells to smooth muscle. Cancer 23: 1176–1184

2527. Volmer J, Pickartz H, Jautzke G 1980 Vascular tumors in the region of the breast. Virchows Archiv A Pathological Anatomy and Histology 385: 201–214

2528. Vuia O 1978 Malignant haemangioblastoma: haemangiosarcoma of the meninges. Neurochirurgia 21: 164–172

2529. Waldo E D, Vuletin J C, Kaye G I 1977 The ultrastructure of vascular tumors: additional observations and a review of the literature. Pathology Annual 12, pt 2: 279–308

2530. Weiss S W, Enzinger F M 1982 Epithelioid hemangioendothelioma. A vascular tumor often mistaken for a carcinoma. Cancer 50. 970–981

2531. Wick M R, Scheithauer B W, Okazaki H, Thomas J E 1982 Cerebral angioendotheliomatosis. Archives of Pathology and Laboratory Medicine 106: 342–346

2532. Wynne-Roberts C, Anderson C, Turano A M, Baron M 1977 Synovial haemangioma of the knee: light and electron microscopic findings. Journal of Pathology 123: 247–255

2533. Yang H–Y, Wasielewski J F, Lee W, Lee E, Paik Y K 1981 Angiosarcoma of the heart: ultrastructural study. Cancer 47: 72–80

## 60 SYNOVIAL AND TENDON SHEATH TUMOURS

2534. Allred C D, Gondos B 1982 Ultrastructure of synovial chondromatosis. Archives of Pathology and Laboratory Medicine 106: 688–690

2535. Carstens H B 1978 Giant cell tumors of tendon sheath. An electron microscopical study of 11 cases. Archives of Pathology and Laboratory Medicine 102: 99–103

2536. Chimenti S, Calvieri S, Ribuffo M 1982 Synovial sarcoma of the foot. Journal of Dermatologic Surgery and Oncology 8: 882–886

2537. Corson J M, Weiss L M, Banks-Schlegal S P, Pinkus G S 1983 Keratin proteins in synovial sarcoma. American Journal of Surgical Pathology 7: 107–109

2538. Dardick I, O'Brien P K, Jeans M T, Massiah K A 1982 Synovial sarcoma arising in an anatomical bursa. Virchows Archiv A Pathological Anatomy and Histology 397: 93–101

2539. Dische F E, Darby A J, Howard E R 1978 Malignant synovioma: electron microscopical findings in three patients and review of the literature. Journal of Pathology 124: 149–155

2540. Dryll A, Lansamann J, Peltier A P, Ryckewaert A 1980 Cellular junctions in normal and inflammatory human synovial membrane revealed by tannic acid and freeze fracture. Virchows Archiv A Pathological Anatomy and Histology 386: 293–302

2541. Edwards J C W, Sedgwick A D, Willoughby D A 1981 The formation of a structure with the features of synovial lining by subcutaneous injection of air: an *in vivo* tissue culture system. Journal of Pathology 134: 147–156

2542. Ekfors T O, Rantakokko V 1979 Clear cell sarcoma of tendons and aponeuroses: malignant melanoma of soft tissues? Report of four cases. Pathology Research and Practice 165: 422–428

2543. Ferlito A, Gale N, Hvala A, Masera A 1981 Synovial sarcoma of the soft palate in a child: a light and electron microscopic study. Journal of Laryngology and Otology 95: 197–204

2544. Fernandez B B, Hernandez F J 1976 Poorly differentiated synovial sarcoma. A light and electron microscopic study. Archives of Pathology and Laboratory Medicine 100: 221–223

2545. Gabbiani G, Kaye G I, Lattes R, Majno G 1971 Synovial sarcoma. Electron microscopic study of a typical case. Cancer 28: 1031–1039

2546. Ghadially F N 1980 Overview article: the articular territory of the reticuloendothelial system. Ultrastructural Pathology 1: 249–264

2547. Golomb H M, Gorny J, Powell W, Graff P, Ultmann J E 1975 Cervical synovial sarcoma at the bifurcation of the carotid artery. Cancer 35: 483–489

2548. Graabaek P M 1982 Ultrastructural evidence for two distinct types of synoviocytes in rat synovial membrane. Journal of Ultrastructure Research 78: 321–339

2549. Kahn L B 1973 Malignant giant cell tumor of the tendon sheath. Ultrastructural study and review of the literature. Archives of Pathology 95: 203–208

2550. Katenkamp D, Stiller D 1980 Synovial sarcoma of the abdominal wall. Light microscopic, histochemical and electron microscopic investigations. Virchows Archiv A Pathological Anatomy and Histology 388: 349–360

2551. Klein W, Huth F 1974 The ultrastructure of malignant synovioma. Beiträge zur Pathologie 153: 194–202

2552. Krall R A, Kostianovsky M, Patchefsky A S 1981 Synovial sarcoma. A clinical, pathological, and ultrastructural study of 26 cases supporting the recognition of a monophasic variant. American Journal of Surgical Pathology 5: 137–151

2553. Kubo T 1974 A note on fine structure of synovial sarcoma. Acta Pathologica Japonica 24: 163–168

2554. Mickelson M R, Brown G A, Maynard J A, Cooper R R, Bonfiglio M 1980 Synovial sarcoma. An electron microscopic study of monophasic and biphasic forms. Cancer 45: 2109–2118

2555. Miettinen M, Lehto V-P, Virtanen I 1982 Keratin in the epithelial-like cells of classical biphasic synovial sarcoma. Virchows Archiv B Cell Pathology 40: 157–161

2556. Nunez-Alonso C, Gashti E N, Christ M L 1979 Maxillofacial synovial sarcoma. Light- and electron-microscopic study of two cases. American Journal of Surgical Pathology 2: 23–30

2557. Roth J A, Enzinger F M, Tannenbaum M 1975 Synovial sarcoma of the neck: a followup study of 24 cases. Cancer 35: 1243–1253

2558. Sajjad S M, Mackay B 1982 Hyaline inclusions in a synovial sarcoma following intra-arterial chemotherapy. Ultra-structural Pathology 3: 313–318

2559. Schmidt D, Mackay B 1982 Ultrastructure of human tendon sheath and synovium: implications for tumor histogenesis. Ultrastructural Pathology 3: 269–283

## 61  TUMOURS OF BONE

2560. Aho A J, Aho H J 1982 Ultrastructure of human osteosarcoma. Malignant transformation of a multipotential connective tissue cell. Pathology Research and Practice 174: 53–67

2561. Aho H J, Aho A J, Einola S 1982 Aneurysmal bone cyst, a study of ultrastructure and malignant transformation. Virchows Archiv A Pathological Anatomy and Histology 395: 169–179

2562. Angervall L, Kindblom L-G 1980 Clear-cell chondro-sarcoma. A light- and electron-microscopic study of two cases. Virchows Archiv A Pathological Anatomy and Histology 389: 27–41

2563. Aparisi T 1978 Giant cell tumor of bone. Electron microscopic and histochemical investigations. Acta Orthopaedica Scandinavica suppl 173: 1–38

2564. Aparisi T, Arborgh B, Ericsson J L 1977 Giant cell tumor of bone: detailed fine structural analysis of different cell components. Virchows Archiv A Pathological Anatomy and Histology 376: 273–298

2565. Aparisi T, Arborgh B, Ericsson J L 1977 Giant cell tumor of bone: fine structural localization of acid phosphatase. Virchows Archiv A Pathological Anatomy and Histology 376: 299–308

2566. Aparisi T, Arborgh B, Ericsson J L 1978 Giant cell tumor of bone. Fine structural localization of alkaline phosphatase. Virchows Archiv A Pathological Anatomy and Histology 378: 287–295

2567. Aparisi T, Arborgh B, Ericsson J L 1979 Giant cell tumor of bone. Variations of patterns of appearance of different cell types. Virchows Archiv A Pathological Anatomy and Histology 381: 159–178

2568. Aparisi T, Arborgh B, Ericsson J L, Glothlin G, Nilsonne U 1978 Contribution to the knowledge of the fine structure of chondrosarcoma of bone. With a note on the localization of alkaline phosphatase and ATPase. Acta Pathologica et Microbiologica Scandinavica. Section A. Pathology 86: 157–167

2569. Apte N K 1965 Fibrosarcoma of the temporal bone. Journal of Laryngology and Otology 79: 1101–1104

2570. Ayala A G, Mackay B 1977 Ewing's sarcoma: an ultrastructural study. In: Management of primary bone and soft tissue tumors. Year Book Medical Publishers, Chicago, p 179–185

2571. Bender B L, Barnes L, Yunis E J 1980 Intraosseous 'chordoid' sarcoma, chondroblastic or lipoblastic origin? Virchows Archiv A Pathological Anatomy and Histology 387: 241–249

2572. Bertoni F, Picci P, Bacchini P, Capanna R, Innao V, Bacci G, Campanacci M 1983 Mesenchymal chondrosarcoma of bone and soft tissues. Cancer 52: 533–541

2573. Carbone A, Clemente C, Lombardi L 1977 The aid of electron microscopy in the diagnosis of osteosarcoma of the bone: case report. Tumori 63: 549–557

2574. Damjanov I, Maenza R M, Snyder G G III, Ruiz J W, Toomey J M 1978 Juvenile ossifying fibroma: an ultrastructural study. Cancer 42: 2668–2674

2575. Erlandson R A, Huvos A G 1974 Chondrosarcoma: a light and electron microscopic study. Cancer 34: 1642–1652

2576. Faraggiana T, Sender B, Glicksman P 1981 Light- and electron-microscopic study of clear cell chondrosarcoma. American Journal of Clinical Pathology 75: 117–121

2577. Ferguson R J, Yunis E J 1978 The ultrastructure of human osteosarcoma: a study of nine cases. Clinical Orthopaedics and Related Research 131: 234–246

2578. Friedman B, Gold H 1968 Ultrastructure of Ewing's sarcoma of bone. Cancer 22: 307–322

2579. Fu Y-S, Kay S 1974 A comparative ultrastructural study of mesenchymal chondrosarcoma and myxoid chondrosarcoma. Cancer 33: 1531–1542

2580. Garbe L R, Monges G M, Pellegrin E M, Payan H L 1981 Ultrastructural study of osteosarcomas. Human Pathology 12: 891–896

2581. Ghadially F N, Lalonde J M, Yong N K 1980 Amianthoid fibres in a chondrosarcoma. Journal of Pathology 130: 147–151

2582. Ghadially F N, Mehta P N 1970 Ultrastructure of osteogenic sarcoma. Cancer 25: 1457–1467

2583. Ghandur-Mnaymneh L, Zych G, Mnaymneh W 1982 Primary malignant fibrous histiocytoma of bone: report of six cases with ultrastructural study and analysis of the literature. Cancer 49: 698–707

2584. Grundmann E, Hobik H P, Immenkamp M, Roessner A 1979 Histodiagnostic remarks on bone tumors, a review of 3026 cases registered in 'Knochengeschwulstregister Westfalen'. Pathology Research and Practice 166: 5–24

2585. Grundmann E, Roessner A, Immenkamp M 1981 Tumor cell types in osteosarcoma as revealed by electron microscopy: implications for histogenesis and subclassification. Virchows Archiv B Cell Pathology 36: 257–273

2586. Hanaoka H, Friedman B, Mack R P 1970 Ultrastructure and histogenesis of giant-cell tumor of bone. Cancer 25: 1408–1425

2587. Herrera G A, Reimann B E, Scully T J, Difiore R J 1982 Nonossifying fibroma. Electron microscopic examination of two cases supporting a histiocytic rather than a fibroblastic reaction. Clinical Orthopaedics and Related Research 167: 269–276

2588. Hou-Jensen K, Priori E, Dmochowski L 1972 Studies on ultrastructure of Ewing's sarcoma of bone. Cancer 29: 280–286

2589. Huvos A G, Marcove R C, Erlandson R A, Miké V 1972 Chondroblastoma of bone. A clinicopathologic and electron microscopic study. Cancer 29: 760–771

2590. Ide F, Kusuhara S, Onuma H, Miyake T, Umemura S 1982 Xanthic variant of non-ossifying fibroma (so-called xanthofibroma) of the mandible. An ultrastructural study. Acta Pathologica Japonica 32: 135–142

2591. Inada O, Yumoto T, Furuse K, Tanaka T 1976 Ultrastructural features of malignant fibrous histiocytoma of bone. Acta Pathologica Japonica 26: 491–501

2592. Kadin M E, Bensch K G 1971 On the origin of Ewing's tumor. Cancer 27: 257–273

2593. Kahn L B 1976 Chondrosarcoma with dedifferentiated foci. A comparative and ultrastructural study. Cancer 37: 1365–1375

2594. Katenkamp D, Stiller D 1981 Malignant fibrous histiocytoma of bone. Light microscopic and electron microscopic examination of four cases. Virchows Archiv A Pathological Anatomy and Histology 391: 323–335

2595. Katenkamp D, Stiller D, Waldmann G 1978 Ultrastructural cytology of human osteosarcoma cells. Virchows Archiv A Pathological Anatomy and Histology 381: 49–61

2596. Kay S 1971 Ultrastructure of an osteoid type of osteogenic sarcoma. Cancer 28: 437–445

2597. Kay S, Schatzki P F 1972 Ultrastructural observations of a chordoma arising in the clivus. Human Pathology 3: 403–413

2598. Kempson R L 1966 Ossifying fibroma of the long bones. A light and electron microscopic study. Archives of Pathology 82: 218–233

2599. Knapp R H, Wick M R, Scheithauer B W, Unni K K 1982 Adamantinoma of bone. An electron microscopic and immunohistochemical study. Virchows Archiv A Pathological Anatomy and Histology 398: 75–86

2600. Lagacé R, Bouchard H-Ls, Delage C, Seemayer T A 1979 Desmoplastic fibroma of bone. An ultrastructural study. American Journal of Surgical Pathology 3: 423–430

2601. Le Charpentier Y, Forest M, Postel M, Tomeno B, Abelanet R 1979 Clear-cell chondrosarcoma. A report of five cases including ultrastructural study. Cancer 44: 622–629

2602. Lee W R, Laurie J, Townsend A L 1975 Fine structure of a radiation-induced osteogenic sarcoma. Cancer 36: 1414–1425

2603. Levine G D, Bensch K G 1972 Chondroblastoma — the nature of the basic cell. A study by means of histochemistry, tissue culture, electron microscopy and autoradiography. Cancer 29: 1546–1562

2604. Llombart Bosch A, Peydro Olaya A, Lopez Fernandez A 1974 Non-ossifying fibroma of bone. A histochemical and ultrastructural characterisation. Virchows Archiv A Pathological Anatomy and Histology 362: 13–21

2605. Llombart-Bosch A, Blache R, Peydro-Olaya A 1982 Round cell sarcomas of bone and their differential diagnosis (with particular emphasis on Ewing's sarcoma and reticulosarcoma). A study of 233 tumors with optical and electron microscopic techniques. Pathology Annual 17, pt 2: 113–115

2606. Llombart-Bosch A, Blache R, Peydro-Olaya A 1978 Ultrastructural study of 28 cases of Ewing's sarcoma: typical and atypical forms. Cancer 41: 1362–1373

2607. Llombart-Bosch A, Ortuno-Pacheco G 1978 Ultrastructural findings supporting the angioblastic nature of the so-called adamantinoma of the tibia. Histopathology 2: 189–200

2608. Llombart-Bosch A, Peydro-Olaya A 1983 Scanning and transmission electron microscopy of Ewing's sarcoma of bone (typical and atypical variants). An analysis of nine cases. Virchows Archiv A Pathological Anatomy and Histopathology 398: 329–346

2609. Llombart-Bosch A, Peydro-Olaya A, Gomar F 1980 Ultrastructure of one Ewing's sarcoma of bone with endothelial character and a comparative review of the vessels in 27 cases of typical Ewing's sarcoma. Pathology Research and Practice 167: 71–87

2610. Lorenzo J C, Dorfman H D 1980 Giant-cell reparative granuloma of short tubular bones of the hands and feet. American Journal of Surgical Pathology 5: 551–563

2611. Mahoney J P, Alexander R W 1978 Ewing's sarcoma. A light- and electron-microscopic study of 21 cases. American Journal of Surgical Pathology 2: 283–298

2612. Makek M, Leu H J 1982 Malignant fibrous histiocytoma arising in a recurrent chordoma. Case report and electron microscopic findings. Virchows Archiv A Pathological Anatomy and Histology 397: 241–250

2613. Marquart K-H 1981 Intracisternal crystalline arrays of coated parallel tubules in cells of a human osteosarcoma. Virchows Archiv A Pathological Anatomy and Histology 391: 309–313

2614. Martínez-Tello F J, Navas-Palacios J J 1982 The ultrastructure of conventional, parosteal, and periosteal osteosarcomas. Cancer 50: 949–961

2615. Martínez-Tello F J, Navas-Palacios J J 1982 Ultrastructural study of conventional chondrosarcomas and myxoid- and mesenchymal-chondrosarcomas. Virchows Archiv A Pathological Anatomy and Histology 396: 197–211

2616. Martínez-Tello F J, Navas-Palacios J J, Calvo-Asensio M, Loizaga-Iriondo J M 1981 Malignant fibrous histiocytoma of bone. A clinico-pathological and electronmicroscopical study. Pathology Research and Practice 173: 141–158

2617. Meister P, Konrad E, Hübner G 1979 Malignant tumor of humerus with features of 'adamantinoma' and Ewing's sarcoma. Pathology Research and Practice 166: 112–122

2618. Murad T M, Murthy M S N 1970 Ultrastructure of a chordoma. Cancer 25: 1204–1215

2619. Nakayama I, Tsuda N, Muta H, Fujii H, Tsuji K, Matsuo T, Takahara O 1975 Fine structural comparison of Ewing's sarcoma with neuroblastoma. Acta Pathologica Japonica 25: 251–268

2620. Newland R C, Harrison M A, Wright R G 1975 Fibroxanthosarcoma of bone. Pathology 7: 203–208

2621. Pardo-Mindan F J, Guillen F J, Villas C, Vazquez J J 1981 A comparative ultrastructural study of chondrosarcoma, chordoid sarcoma, and chordoma. Cancer 47: 2611–2619

2622. Pieterse A S, Smith P S, McClure J 1982 Adamantinoma of long bones: clinical, pathological and ultrastructural features. Journal of Clinical Pathology 35: 780–786

2623. Povýsil C, Matejovský Z 1977 Ultrastructure of Ewing's tumour. Virchows Archiv A Pathological Anatomy and Histology 374: 303–316

2624. Povýsil C, Matejovský Z 1979 Ultrastructure of benign chondroblastoma. Pathology Research and Practice 166: 80–89

2625. Povýsil C, Matejovský Z 1981 Ultrastructure of adamantinoma of long bones. Virchows Archiv A Pathological Anatomy and Histology 393: 233–244

2626. Reddick R L, Michelitch H J, Levine A M, Triche T J 1980 Osteogenic sarcoma. A study of the ultrastructure. Cancer 45: 64–71

2627. Reddick R L, Popovsky M A, Fantone J C III, Michelitch H J 1980 Parosteal osteogenic sarcoma. Ultrastructural observations in three cases. Human Pathology 11: 373–380

2628. Reinholt F P, Engfeldt B, Hjerpe A, Jansson K 1982 Stereological studies on the epiphyseal growth plate with special reference to the distribution of matrix vesicles. Journal of Ultrastructure Research 80: 270–279

2629. Ringus J C, Riddell R H 1981 Small cell osteosarcoma: ultrastructural description and differentiation from atypical Ewing's sarcoma. Laboratory Investigation 44: 55A

2630. Robertson D I, Hogg G R 1980 Chordoid sarcoma. Ultrastructural evidence supporting a synovial origin. Cancer 45: 520–527

2631. Roessner A, Grundmann E 1982 Electron microscopy in bone tumor diagnosis. Current Topics in Pathology 71: 153–198

2632. Roessner A, Hobik H P, Grundmann E 1979 Malignant fibrous histiocytoma of bone and osteosarcoma. A comparative light and electron microscopic study. Pathology Research and Practice 164: 385–401

2633. Roessner A, Immenkamp M, Weidner A, Hobik H P, Grundmann E 1981 Benign fibrous histiocytoma of bone. Light- and electron-microscopic observations. Journal of Cancer Research and Clinical Oncology 101: 191–202

2634. Roessner A, Voss B, Rauterberg J, Immenkamp M, Grundmann E 1982 Biologic characterisation of human bone tumors. I. Ewing's sarcoma. A comparative electron and immunofluorescence microscopic study. Journal of Cancer Research and Clinical Oncology 104: 171–180

2635. Rosai J 1969 Adamantinoma of the tibia: electron microscopic evidence of its epithelial origin. American Journal of Clinical Pathology 51: 786–792

2636. Schajowicz F, Cabrini R L, Simes R J, Klein-Szanto A J 1974 Ultrastructure of chondrosarcoma. Clinical Orthopaedics and Related Research 100: 378–386

2637. Schmidt D, Mackay B, Ayala A G 1982 Ewing's sarcoma with neuroblastoma-like features. Ultrastructural Pathology 3: 143–151

2638. Sela I, Bab I A, Muhlrad A, Stein H 1981 Extracellular matrix vesicles in human osteogenic neoplasms: an ultrastructural and enzymatic study. Cancer 48: 1602 1610

2639. Sela J, Bab I A 1979 The realtionship between extracellular matrix vesicles and calcospherites in primary mineralization of neoplastic bone tissue. TEM and SEM studies on osteosarcoma. Virchows Archiv A Pathological Anatomy and Histology 382: 1–9

2640. Shapiro F 1981 Malignant fibrous histiocytoma of bone: an ultrastructural study. Ultrastructural Pathology 2: 33–42

2641. Shapiro F 1983 Ultrastructural observations on osteosarcoma tissue: a study of 10 cases. Ultrastructural Pathology 4: 151–161

2642. Spjut H J, Dorfman H D, Fechner R E, Ackerman L V 1971 Tumors of bone and cartilage. Atlas of tumor pathology, 2nd series, fascicle 5. Armed Forces Institute of Pathology, Washington, D C, p 216–229

2643. Steiner G C 1974 Fibrous cortical defect and nonossifying fibroma of bone. A study of the ultrastructure. Archives of Pathology 97: 205–210

2644. Steiner G C 1976 Ultrastructure of osteoid osteoma. Human Pathology 7: 309–325

2645. Steiner G C 1977 Ultrastructure of osteoblastoma. Cancer 39: 2127–2136

2646. Steiner G C 1979 Ultrastructure of benign cartilaginous tumors of intraosseous origin. Human Pathology 10: 71–86

2647. Steiner G C 1981 Tumors and tumor-like conditions of bone and joints. In: Johannessen J V (Ed) Electron microscopy in human medicine, vol 4. Soft tissues, bones and joints. McGraw-Hill, New York, p 54–140

2648. Steiner G C, Ghosh L, Dorfman H D 1972 Ultrastructure of giant cell tumors of bone. Human Pathology 3: 569–586

2649. Steiner G C, Mirra J M, Bullough P G 1973 Mesenchymal chondrosarcoma. A study of the ultrastructure. Cancer 32: 926–939

2650. Szakacs J E, Carta M, Szakacs M R 1974 Ewing's sarcoma, extraskeletal and of bone. Case report with ultrastructural analysis. Annals of Clinical and Laboratory Science 4: 306–322

2651. Terashima K, Suda A, Imai Y, Watanabe Y, Kasajima T, Matsuda M, Dobashi M 1981 Malignant fibrous histiocytoma of bone associated with focal hemangiopericytomatous pattern. Acta Pathologica Japonica 31: 1063–1078

2652. Toremalm N G, Lindstrom C, Malm L 1976 Chondromyxoid fibroma of the pterygo-palatine space. Journal of Laryngology and Otology 90: 971–978

2653. Tornberg D N, Rice R W, Johnston A D 1973 The ultrastructure of chondromyxoid fibroma. Its biologic and diagnostic implications. Clinical Orthopaedics and Related Research 95: 295–299

2654. Ushigome S, Takakuwa T, Shinagawa T, Kishida H, Yamazaki M 1982 Chondromyxoid fibroma of bone. An electron microscopic observation. Acta Pathologica Japonica 32: 113–122

2655. Valderrama E, Kahn L B, Lipper S, Marc J 1983 Chondroid chordoma. Electron-microscopic study of two cases. American Journal of Surgical Pathology 7: 625–632

2656. Van Haelst U J, de Haas van Dorsser A H 1975 A perplexing malignant bone tumor. Highly malignant so-called adamantinoma or non-typical Ewing's sarcoma. Virchows Archiv A Pathological Anatomy and Histology 365: 63–74

2657. Vuletin J C 1977 Myofibroblasts in parosteal osteogenic sarcoma. Archives of Pathology and Laboratory Medicine 101: 272

2658. Wetzel W J, Reuhl K R 1980 Microtubular aggregates in the rough endoplasmic reticulum of a myxoid chondrosarcoma. Ultrastructural Pathology 1: 519–525

2659. Williams A H, Schwinn C P, Parker J W 1976 The ultrastructure of osteosarcoma. A review of twenty cases. Cancer 37: 1293–1301

2660. Willis R A 1967 Pathology of tumours, 4th edn. Butterworths, London, ch 43 & 55, p 702–703 & 857–885

2661. Yoneyama T, Winter W G, Milsow L 1977 Tibial adamantinoma: its histogenesis from ultrastructural studies. Cancer 40: 1138–1142

## 62 THYMIC TUMOURS

2662. Baud M, Stamenkovic I, Kapanci Y 1981 Malignant thymomas: clinicopathologic study of 13 cases. Progress in Surgical Pathology 3: 129–146

2663. Bloodworth J M B Jr, Hiratsuka H, Hickey R C, Wu J 1975 Ultrastructure of the human thymus, thymic tumors, and myasthenia gravis. Pathology Annual 10: 329–391

2664. Chalk S, Donald K J 1977 Carcinoid tumour of the thymus. A case report including discussion of the morphological diagnosis and the cell of origin. Virchows Archiv A Pathological Anatomy and Histology 377: 91–96

2665. Cossman J, Deegan M J, Schnitzer B 1978 Thymoma: an immunologic and electron microscopic study. Cancer 41: 2183–2191

2666. Fetissof F, Boivin F, Jobard P 1982 Microfilamentous carcinoid of the thymus: correlation of ultrastructural study with Grimelius stain. Ultrastructural Pathology 3: 9–15

2667. Kay S, Willson M A 1970 Ultrastructural studies of an ACTH-secreting thymic tumor. Cancer 26: 445–452

2668. Lemos L B, Hamoudi A B 1978 Malignant thymic tumor in an infant (malignant histiocytoma). Archives of Pathology and Laboratory Medicine 102: 84–89

2669. Levine G D 1973 Primary thymic seminoma — a neoplasm ultrastructurally similar to testicular seminoma and distinct from epithelial thymoma. Cancer 31: 729–741

2670. Levine G D, Bearman R M 1980 The thymus. In: Johannessen J V (ed) Electron microscopy in human medicine, vol 5. Cardiovascular system, lymphoreticular and hematopoietic system. McGraw-Hill, New York, pt 4, p 216–254

2671. Levine G D, Polliack A 1975 The T-cell nature of the lymphocytes in two human epithelial thymomas: a comparative immunologic, scanning and transmission electron microscopic study. Clinical Immunology and Immunopathology 4: 199–208

2672. Levine G D, Rosai J 1976 A spindle cell variant of thymic carcinoid tumor. A clinical, histologic, and fine structural study with emphasis on its distinction from spindle cell thymoma. Archives of Pathology and Laboratory Medicine 100: 293–300

2673. Levine G D, Rosai J 1978 Thymic hyperplasia and neoplasia: a review of current concepts. Human Pathology 9: 495–515

2674. Levine G, Bensch K G 1972 Epithelial nature of spindle cell thymoma. An ultrastructural study. Cancer 30: 500–511

2675. Llombart-Bosch A 1975 Epithelio-reticular cell thymoma with lymphocytic emperipolesis. An ultrastructural study. Cancer 36: 1794–1803

2676. Otto H F 1978 Investigations on the ultrastructure of lympho-epithelial thymomas with special reference to 'emperipolesis'. Virchows Archiv A Pathological Anatomy and Histology 379: 335–349

2677. Pak H Y, Yokota S B, Friedberg H A 1982 Thymoma diagnosed by transthoracic fine needle aspiration. Acta Cytologica 26: 210–216

2678. Pascoe H R, Miner M S 1976 An ultrastructural study of nine thymomas. Cancer 37: 317–326

2679. Pedraza M A 1977 Thymoma immunological and ultrastructural characterization. Cancer 39: 1455–1461

2680. Rao U, Takita H 1977 Carcinoid tumour of possible thymic origin: case report. Thorax 32: 771–776

2681. Reddick R L, Jennette J C 1983 Immunologic and ultrastructural characterization of the small cell population in malignant thymoma. Human Pathology 14: 337–380

2682. Rosai J, Higa E, Davie J 1972 Mediastinal endocrine neoplasm in patients with multiple endocrine adenomatosis. A previously unrecognized association. Cancer 29: 1075–1083

2683. Rosai J, Levine G D 1976 Tumors of the thymus. Atlas of tumor pathology, 2nd series, fascicle 13. Armed Forces Institute of Pathology, Washington DC, p 108–130

2684. Rosai J, Levine G, Weber W R, Higa E 1976 Carcinoid tumors and oat cell carcinomas of the thymus. Pathology Annual 11: 201–226

2685. Sajjad S M, Lukeman J M, Llamas L, Fernandez T 1982 Needle biopsy diagnosis of thymoma. A case report. Acta Cytologica 26: 503–506

2686. Seemayer T A, Jerry T M, Shapiro L, Sullivan A K 1976 Spindle cell epithelial thymoma: fine structural and tumor lymphocyte observations. American Journal of Clinical Pathology 65: 612–622

2687. Snover D C, Levine G D, Rosai J 1982 Thymic carcinoma. Five distinctive histological variants. American Journal of Surgical Pathology 6: 451–470

2688. Swinborne-Sheldrake K, Gray G F Jr, Glick A D 1983 Primary epithelial neoplasms of the thymus with emphasis on differential diagnosis and the usefulness of electron microscopy. Laboratory Investigation 48: 83A

2689. Tanaka T, Tanaka S, Kimura H, Ito J 1974 Mediastinal tumor of thymic origin and related to carcinoid tumor. Acta Pathologica Japonica 24: 413–426

2690. Toker C 1968 Thymoma: an ultrastructural study. Cancer 21: 1157–1163

2691. Watanabe H 1966 A pathological study of thymomas. Acta Pathologica Japonica 16: 323–358

2692. Wick M R, Scheithauer B W 1982 Oat-cell carcinoma of the thymus. Cancer 49: 1652–1657

2693. Wick M R, Scheithauer B W, Weiland L H, Bernatz P E 1982 Primary thymic carcinomas. American Journal of Surgical Pathology 6: 613–630

2694. Wolfe J T III, Wick M R, Banks P M, Scheithauer B W 1983 Clear cell carcinoma of the thymus. Mayo Clinic Proceedings 58: 365–370

## 63 MALIGNANT LYMPHOMAS — GENERAL ASPECTS

2695. Dantchev D 1978 Scanning electron microscopy morphology of mononuclear phagocytes in normal subjects and in patients with lymphoid and monocytoid neoplasias. Recent Results in Cancer Research 64: 94–107

2696. Ewing E P Jr, Spira T J, Chandler F W, Callaway C S, Brynes R K, Chan W C 1983 Unusual cytoplasmic body in lymphoid cells of homosexual men with unexplained lymphadenopathy. A preliminary report. New England Journal of Medicine 308: 819–822

2697. Hansen J A, Good R A 1974 Malignant disease of the lymphoid system in immunological perspective. Human Pathology 5: 567–599

2698. Ioachim H L 1980 The pathological lymph node. In: Johannessen J V (ed) Electron microscopy in human medicine, vol 5. Cardiovascular system, lymphoreticular and hematopoietic system. McGraw-Hill, New York, pt 6, ch 32, p 421–470

2699. Ioachim H L 1980 The pathological spleen. In: Johannessen J V (ed) Electron microscopy in human medicine, vol 5. Cardiovascular system, lymphoreticular and hematopoietic system. McGraw-Hill, New York, pt 6, ch 34, p 477–496

2700. Kadin M E, Berard C W, Nanba K, Wakasa H 1983 Lymphoproliferative diseases in Japan and western countries: proceedings of the United States–Japan seminar, September 6 and 7, 1982, in Seattle, Washington. Human Pathology 14: 745–772

2701. Kjeldsberg C R, Kim H 1981 Polykaryocytes resembling Warthin-Finkeldey giant cells in reactive and neoplastic lymphoid disorders. Human Pathology 12: 267–272

2702. Mollo F, Monga G, Coda R, Palestro G 1975 Ultrastructural features of human lymphomas. Acta Neuropathologica suppl 6: 17–20

2703. Mori Y, Lennert K 1969 Electron microscopic atlas of lymph node cytology and pathology. Springer-Verlag, Berlin

2704. Peiper S C, Kahn L B 1982 Ultrastructural comparison of Hodgkin's and non-Hodgkin's lymphomas. Histopathology 6: 93–109

2705. Polliack A 1978 Surface morphology of lymphoreticular cells: review of data obtained from scanning electron microscopy. Recent Results in Cancer Research 64: 66–93

2706. Rilke F, Giardini R, Lombardi L, Pilotti S, Clemente C 1980 Malignant lymphomas — histopathological diagnoses and their conceptual bases. Progress in Surgical Pathology 2: 145–185

## 64 NON-HODGKIN'S LYMPHOMAS

2707. Abe M, Takahashi K, Mori N, Kojima M 1982 'Waldenström's macroglobulinemia' terminating in immuno-blastic sarcoma. A case report. Cancer 49: 2580–2586

2708. Agudelo C A, Schumacher H R, Glick J H, Molina J 1981 Non-Hodgkin's lymphoma in systemic lupus erythematosus: report of 4 cases with ultrastructural studies in 2. Journal of Rheumatology 8: 69–78

2709. Al-Irhayim B 1981 Functional studies of lymph nodes infiltrated by non-Hodgkin's lymphoma. Diagnostic Histopathology 4: 137–148

2710. Aliaga A, Bombi J A, Barbera E, Fortea J M 1980 Woringer-Kolopp disease. Dermatologica 160: 45–56

2711. Ansell J, Bhawan J, Cohen S, Sullivan J, Sherman D 1982 Histiocytic lymphoma and malignant angioendo-theliomatosis. One disease or two? Cancer 50: 1506–1512

2712. Azar H A, Jaffe E S, Berard C W, Callihan T R, Braylan R R, Cossman J, Triche T J 1980 Diffuse large cell lymphomas (reticulum cell sarcomas, histiocytic lymphomas). Correlation of morphological features with functional markers. Cancer 46: 1428–1441

2713. Bedetti C D, Ollapally E 1983 Malignant lymphoma with a high content of epithelioid histocytes (so-called Lennert's lymphoma). Immunocytochemical and ultrastructural observations. Virchows Archiv A Pathological Anatomy and Histopathology 399: 255–264

2714. Bellomi A, Gamoletti R 1981 Malignant histiocytic tumour presenting as a primary uterine neoplasm: a cytochemical and electron microscopy study. Journal of Pathology 134: 233–241

2715. Belpomme D, Dantchev D, Karima A M, LeLarge N, Joseph R, Caillou B, Lafleur M, Mathé G 1976 Search for correlations between immunological criteria used to classify lymphoid leukemias and non-Hodgkin's hematosarcomas, with special reference to scanning electron microscopy and T and B membrane markers. Recent Results in Cancer Research 56: 131–143

2716. Bockman D E, Wu L Y, Lawton A R, Cooper M D 1974 Altered fine structure of B lymphocytes correlated with defective terminal differentiation. American Journal of Anatomy 140: 551–567

2717. Braun-Falco O, Schmoeckel C, Wolff H H 1977 The ultrastructure of mycosis fungoides, of Sézary's syndrome, and of Woringer-Kolopp's disease — Pagetoid reticulosis. Bulletin du Cancer 64: 191–208

2718. Braylan R C, Jaffe E S, Berard C W 1975 Malignant lymphomas: current classification and new observations. Pathology Annual 10: 213–270

2719. Breathnach S M, McKee P H, Smith N P 1982 Hypopigmented mycosis fungoides: report of five cases with ultrastructural observations. British Journal of Dermatology 106: 643–649

2720. Brehmer-Andersson E 1976 Mycosis fungoides and its relation to Sézary's syndrome, lymphomatoid papulosis, and primary cutaneous Hodgkin's disease. Acta Dermato-Venereologica 56, suppl 75: 1–42

2721. Broder S, Edelson R L, Lutzner M A, Nelson D L, MacDermott R P 1976 Sézary syndrome: malignant proliferation of helper T cells. Journal of Clinical Investigation 58: 1297–1306

2722. Broome J D, Zucker-Franklin D, Weiner M S, Bianco C, Nussenzweig V 1973 Leukemic cells with membrane properties of thymus derived (T) lymphocytes in a case of Sézary's syndrome: morphologic and immunologic studies. Clinical Immunology and Immunopathology 1: 319–329

2723. Brownlee T R, Murad T M 1970 Ultrastructure of mycosis fungoides. Cancer 26: 686–698

2724. Brunning R D, Maldonado J E 1980 Sézary's syndrome. In: Johannessen J V (ed) Electron microscopy in human medicine, vol 5. Cardiovascular system, lymphoreticular and hematopoietic system. McGraw-Hill, New York, pt 5, ch 28, p 377–378

2725. Buss D H, Marshall R B, Holleman I L Jr, Myers R T 1980 Malignant lymphoma of the thyroid gland with plasma cell differentiation (plasmacytoma). Cancer 46: 2671–2675

2726. Caorsi I, Figuerola C D, Rodríguez E M 1982 Morphologic and morphometric study of the two main cell lineages involved in mycosis fungoides: the lymphoid cells and the Langerhans cells. Ultrastructural Pathology 3: 119–136

2727. Carr I 1975 Ultrastructure of malignant reticulum and Reed-Sternberg cells. Lancet i: 926

2728. Catovsky D, Greaves M F, Rose M, Galton D A G, Goolden A W G, McCluskey D R, White J M, Lampert I, Bourikas G, Ireland R, Brownell A I, Bridges J M, Blattner W A, Gallo R C 1982 Adult T-cell lymphoma-leukaemia in blacks from the West Indies. Lancet i: 639–643

2729. Chu A C, Morgan E W, MacDonald D M 1980 Ultrastructural identification of T lymphocytes in tissue sections of mycosis fungoides. Journal of Investigative Dermatology 74: 17–20

2730. Chu A C, Morgan E W, MacDonald D M 1982 An ultrastructural study of the mononuclear cell infiltrate of mycosis fungoides and poikiloderma atrophicans vasculare. Clinical and Experimental Dermatology 7: 11–19

2731. Chu H, Foucar K, Barlogie B, Middleman E 1982 Tubular complexes of endoplasmic reticulum in lymphoblastic lymphoma: case report. Cancer 49: 1629–1635

2732. de Vries E, van Leeuwen A W F M, van de Putte L B A, Lafeber G J M, Maijer C L M 1977 Atypical T-cells in rheumatoid synovial membranes. Virchows Archiv B Cell Pathology 24: 19–26

2733. Domagala W, Emeson E E, Greenwald E, Koss L G 1977 A scanning electron microscopic and immunologic study of B cell lymphosarcoma cells in cerebrospinal fluid. Cancer 40: 715–720

2734. Edelson R L, Kirkpatrick C H, Shevach E M, Schein P S, Smith R W, Green I, Lutzner M 1974 Preferential cutaneous infiltration by neoplastic thymus-derived lymphocytes. Morphologic and functional studies. Annals of Internal Medicine 80: 685–692

2735. Edelson R L, Lutzner M A, Kirkpatrick C H, Shevach E M, Green I 1974 Morphologic and functional properties of the atypical T lymphocytes of the Sézary syndrome. Mayo Clinic Proceedings 49: 558–566

2736. Eimoto T, Mitsui T, Kikuchi M 1981 Ultrastructure of adult T-cell leukaemia/lymphoma. Virchows Archiv B Cell Pathology 38: 189–208

2737. Feltkamp C A, van Heerde P, Feltkamp-Vroom T M, Koudstaal J 1981 A malignant tumor arising from interdigitating cells: light microscopical, ultrastructural, immuno- and enzyme-histochemical characteristics. Virchows Archiv A Pathological Anatomy and Histology 393: 183–192

2738. Feremans W W, Neve P, Caudron M 1978 IgM-lambda cytoplasmic crystals in three cases of immunocytoma: a clinical, cytochemial, and ultrastructural study. Journal of Clinical Pathology 31: 250–258

2739. Fisher E R, Horvat B L, Wechsler H L 1972 Ultrastructural features of mycosis fungoides. American Journal of Clinical Pathology 58: 99–110

2740. Flaxman B A, Zelazny G, Van Scott E J 1971 Nonspecificity of characteristic cells in mycosis fungoides. Archives of Dermatology 104: 141–147

2741. Gillespie J J 1978 The ultrastructural diagnosis of diffuse large-cell ('histiocytic') lymphoma. Fine structural study of 30 cases. American Journal of Surgical Pathology 2: 9–20

2742. Gisser S D, Young I 1978 Mycosis fungoides-like cells. Their presence in a case of pityriasic dermatitis with a comment on their significance as an indicator of primary T-cell dyscrasia. American Journal of Surgical Pathology 2: 97–101

2743. Glick A D, Leech J H, Waldron J A, Flexner J M, Horn R G, Collins R D 1975 Malignant lymphomas of follicular center cell origin in man. II. Ultrastructural and cytochemical studies. Journal of the National Cancer Institute 54: 23–36

2744. Golomb H M, Braylan R, Reese C, Variakojis D, Brynes R K, Yachnin S 1975 The Sézary syndrome cell: surface ultrastructural characteristics. Acta Haematologica 54: 106–114

2745. Habeshaw J A, Stuart A E 1975 Cell receptor studies on seven cases of diffuse histiocytic malignant lymphoma (reticulum cell sarcoma). Journal of Clinical Pathology 28: 289–297

2746. Harris M, Eyden B, Read G 1981 Signet ring cell lymphoma: a rare variant of follicular lymphoma. Journal of Clinical Pathology 34: 884–891

2747. Hauch T W, Shelbourne J D, Cohen H J, Mason D, Kremer W B 1975 Meningeal mycosis fungoides: clinical and cellular characteristics. Annals of Internal Medicine 82: 499–505

2748. Henry K 1975 Electron microscopy in the non-Hodgkins lymphomata. British Journal of Cancer 31, suppl 2: 73–93

2749. Henry K, Bennett M H, Farrer-Brown G 1978 Classification of the non-Hodgkin's lymphomas. Advances in Histopathology 10: 275–302

2750. Henry K, Bennett M H, Farrer-Brown G 1978 Morphological classification of non-Hodgkins lymphomas. Recent Results in Cancer Research 64: 38–56

2751. Holden C A, Morgan E W, MacDonald D M 1982 A technique for immunoultrastructural identification of T6-positive Langerhans cells and indeterminate cells in mycosis fungoides. Journal of Investigative Dermatology 79: 382–384

2752. Iossifides I, Mackay B, Butler J J 1980 Signet ring cell lymphoma. Ultrastructural Pathology 1: 511–517

2753. Isaacson P, Wright D H, Jones D B 1983 Malignant lymphomas of true histiocytic (monocyte/macrophage) origin. Cancer 51: 80–91

2754. Jimbow K, Chiba M, Horikoshi T 1982 Electron microscopic identification of Langerhans cells in the dermal infiltrates of mycosis fungoides. Journal of Investigative Dermatology 78: 102–107

2755. Jimbow K, Katoh M, Nishio C, Jimbow M 1981 Characterisation of surface markers and cytoplasmic organelles in benign and malignant lymphoid lesions of the skin. Journal of Cutaneous Pathology 8: 283–298

2756. Kaiserling E 1978 Ultrastructure of non-Hodgkin's lymphomas. In: Lennert K Malignant lymphomas other than Hodgkin's disease. Histology. Cytology. Ultrastructure. Immunology. Springer-Verlag, Berlin, pt 5, p 471–528

2757. Kaiserling E, Stein H, Lennert K 1973 IgM-producing malignant lymphomas without macroglobulinemia. Morphological and immunochemical findings. Virchows Archiv B Zellpathologie 14: 1–18

2758. Katayama I, Ceccacci L, Valu A F, Horne E O 1977 Histiocytic lymphoma with sclerosis arising from a nodular lymphoma with a special stromal reaction. An ultrastructural study. Cancer 40: 2203–2208

2759. Katayama I, Uehara H, Gleser R A, Weintraub L 1974 The value of electron microscopy in the diagnosis of Burkitt's lymphoma. American Journal of Clinical Pathology 61: 540–548

2760. Kim H, Dorfman R F, Rappaport H 1978 Signet ring cell lymphoma. A rare morphologic and functional expression of nodular (follicular) lymphoma. American Journal of Surgical Pathology 2: 119–132

2761. Kojima M, Imai Y, Mori N 1973 A concept of follicular lymphoma. A proposal for the existence of a neoplasm originating from the germinal centre. Gann 15: 195–207

2762. Laitio M T, Nevalainen T J 1975 Ultrastructure of primary lymphosarcoma of testis. Zeitschrift für Krebsforschung und Klinische Onkologie 84: 189–192

2763. Lennert K 1973 Follicular lymphoma. A tumor of the germinal centers. Gann 15: 217–231

2764. Leong A S-Y, Sage R E, Kinnear G C, Forbes I J 1980 Preferential epidermotropism in adult T-cell leukemia-lymphoma. American Journal of Surgical Pathology 4: 421–430

2765. Levine G D, Dorfman R F 1975 Nodular lymphoma: an ultrastructural study of its relationship to germinal centers and a correlation of light and electron microscopic findings. Cancer 35: 148–164

2766. Lutzner M A, Jordan H W 1968 The ultrastructure of an abnormal cell in Sézary's syndrome. Blood 31: 719–726

2767. Lutzner M, Edelson R, Schein P, Green I, Kirkpatrick C, Ahmed A 1975 Cutaneous T-cell lymphomas: the Sézary syndrome, mycosis fungoides, and related disorders. Annals of Internal Medicine 83: 534–552

2768. Mann R B, Jaffe E S, Braylan R C, Eggleston J C, Ransom L, Kaizer H, Berard C W 1975 Immunologic and morphologic studies of T-cell lymphoma. American Journal of Medicine 58: 307–313

2769. Matz L R, Papadimitriou J M, Carroll J R, Barr A L, Dawkins R L, Jackson J M, Herrmann R P, Armstrong B K 1977 Angioimmunoblastic lymphadenopathy with dysproteinemia. Cancer 40: 2152–2160

2770. McKenna R W, Bloomfield C D, Brunning R D 1975 Nodular lymphoma: bone marrow and blood manifestations. Cancer 36: 428–440

2771. McKenna R W, Brunning R D 1975 Reed-Sternberg-like cells in nodular lymphoma involving the bone marrow. American Journal of Clinical Pathology 63: 779–785

2772. McNutt N S, Crain W R 1981 Quantitative electron microscopic comparison of lymphocyte nuclear contours in mycosis fungoides and in benign infiltrates in skin. Cancer 47: 698–709

2773. McNutt N S, Heilbron D C, Crain W R 1981 Mycosis fungoides. Diagnostic criteria based on quantitative electron microscopy. Laboratory Investigation 44: 466–474

2774. Meyer C J L M, van Leeuwen A W F M, van der Loo E M, van de Putte L B A, van Vloten W A 1977 Cerebriform (Sézary like) mononuclear cells in healthy individuals: a morphologically distinct population of T cells. Relationship with mycosis fungoides and Sézary's syndrome. Virchows Archiv B Cell Pathology 25: 95–104

2775. Michel R P, Case B W, Moinuddin M 1979 Immunoblastic lymphosarcoma: a light, immunofluorescence and electron microscopic study. Cancer 43: 224–236

2776. Morris J A, Bird C C 1979 Ultrastructural and immunohistological study of immunoblastic sarcoma developing in child with immunoblastic lymphadenopathy. Cancer 44: 171–182

2777. Navas Palacios J J, Valdes M D, Montalban Pallares M A, Gomez de Salazar M D, Marcilla A G 1981 Lymphoblastic lymphoma/leukemia of T-cell origin: ultrastructural cytochemical, and immunological features of ten cases. Cancer 48: 1982–1991

2778. Neiman R S, Dervan P, Haudenschild C, Jaffe R 1978 Angioimmunoblastic lymphadenopathy. An ultrastructural and immunologic study with review of the literature. Cancer 41: 507–518

2779. Neiman R S, Sullivan A L, Jaffe R 1979 Malignant lymphoma simulating leukemic reticuloendotheliosis: a clinicopathologic study of ten cases. Cancer 43: 329–342

2780. O'Brien C, Lampert I A, Catovsky D 1983 The histopathology of adult T-cell lymphoma/leukaemia in blacks from the Caribbean. Histopathology 7: 349–364

2781. Ohno Y-I, Koya M, Yasuda N, Kanoh T, Uchino H, Fujii H 1982 Ultrastructure of vacuolated plasma cells in macroglobulinemia associated with production of mu-chain fragment. Cancer 49: 2489–2492

2782. Osborne B M, Mackay B, Butler J J, Ordonez N G 1983 Large cell lymphoma with microvillus-like projections: an ultrastructural study. American Journal of Clinical Pathology 79: 443–450

2783. Ough Y D, Miller W M, Leeb B, Holbrook D L, Klos J R 1983 Immunoblastic lymphoma with extracellular and intravascular immunoglobulin deposits: immuno-cytochemical and electron microscopic studies. Cancer 51: 623–630

2784. Padmalatha C, Warner T F C S, Hafez G R 1981 Pseudo-Gaucher cell in IgMk plasmacytoid lymphoma. American Journal of Surgical Pathology 5: 501–505

2785. Palutke M, Tabaczka P, Weise R W, Axelrod A, Palacas C, Margolis H, Khilanani P, Ratanatharathorn V, Piligian J, Pollard R, Husain M 1980 T-cell lymphomas of large cell type. A variety of malignant lymphomas: 'histiocytic' and mixed lymphocytic-'histiocytic'. Cancer 46: 87–101

2786. Pelc S, Fondu P, Otten J, Gompel C 1981 Immunoblastic sarcoma of the B-cell type in the CSF. Light- and electronmicroscopic study of the malignant cells and unusual macrophages. Acta Neuropathologica 55: 289–292

2787. Perez-Atayde A R, Chang Y C, Seiler M W 1982 Retroperitoneal lymphoma with ribosome-lamellae complexes, cytoplasmic projections and desmosome-like junctions: an ultrastructural study. Ultrastructural Pathology 3: 43–49

2788. Pileri S, Serra L, Govoni E, Martinelli G 1981 Signet ring cell lymphoma: a case report. Histopathology 5: 165–173

2789. Pinkus G S, Said J W, Hargreaves H 1979 Malignant lymphoma, T-cell type. A distinct morphologic variant with large multilobated nuclei, with a report of four cases. American Journal of Clinical Pathology 72: 540–550

2790. Polliack A, Djaldetti M 1978 Surface features of Sézary cells. A scanning electron microscopic study. Israel Journal of Medical Sciences 14: 1236–1241

2791. Polliack A, Djaldetti M, Reyes F, Biberfeld P, Daniel M T, Flandrin G 1977 Surface features of Sézary cells: a scanning electron microscopy study of 5 cases. Scandinavian Journal of Haematology 18: 207–213

2792. Rademakers L H P M, Peters J P J, van Unnik J A M 1983 Histiocytic and dendritic reticulum cells in follicular structures of follicular lymphoma and reactive hyperplasia. A quantitative electron microscopical analysis. Virchows Archiv B Cell Pathology 44: 85–98

2793. Reynes M, Diebold J 1977 Polysome lamellae complexes in a case of nodular pleomorphic lymphoblastosarcoma. Biomedicine Express 27: 55–57

2794. Robinowitz B N, Noguchi S, Roenigk H H 1976 Tumor cell characterization in mycosis fungoides. Cancer 37: 1747–1753

2795. Rosas-Uribe A, Variakojis D, Molnar Z, Rappaport H 1974 Mycosis fungoides: an ultrastructural study. Cancer 34: 634–645

2796. Rosas-Uribe A, Variakojis D, Rappaport H 1973 Proteinaceous precipitate in nodular (follicular) lymphomas. Cancer 31: 534–542

2797. Said J W, Hargreaves H K, Pinkus G S 1979 Non-Hodgkin's lymphomas: an ultrastructural study correlating morphology with immunologic cell type. Cancer 44: 504–528

2798. Said J W, Pinkus G S 1980 Immunoblastic sarcoma of the T cell type. An ultrastructural study of five cases. American Journal of Pathology 101: 515–525

2799. Schmitt D, Thivolet J 1980 Lymphocyte — epidermis interactions in malignant epidermotropic lymphomas. I. Ultrastructural aspects. Acta Dermato-Venereologica 60: 1–11

2800. Schneider G B, Katayama I 1978 Scanning electron microscopy of Burkitt's tumor cells: letter. American Journal of Clinical Pathology 69: 567–569

2801. Schnitzer B, Kass L 1973 Leukemic phase of reticulum cell sarcoma (histiocytic lymphoma). A clinicopathologic and ultrastructural study. Cancer 31: 547–559

2802. Schumacher H R, Rainey T, Davidson L, Simon D, Strong M, Creegan W J, Holloway M L, Stass S A 1978 American Burkitt's lymphoma, hand mirror variant. A detailed investigation of cytologic, ultrastructural, and immunologic features. American Journal of Clinical Pathology 70: 937–944

2803. Shaklai M, Mintz U, Pinkhas J, Pick A, Ben-Bassat M, Devries A 1974 Intestinal lymphoma with unusual sequence of serum IgA changes. American Journal of Digestive Diseases 19: 279–286

2804. Shigematsu T, Nagasaki T, Kikuchi M, Kishida K, Miyoshi M 1978 Scanning and transmission electronmicroscopy of leukemic lymphoma cells without T and B cell surface markers. Virchows Archiv B Cell Pathology 26: 225–232

2805. Souteyrand P, Thivolet J 1981 Mycosis fungoides and Sézary syndrome. Pathology Research and Practice 171: 240–261

2806. Spagnolo D V, Papadimitriou J M, Matz L R, Walters M N-I 1982 Nodular lymphomas with intracellular immunoglobulin inclusions: report of three cases and a review. Pathology 14: 415–427

2807. Stein H, Kaiserling E, Lennert K 1974 Evidence for B-cell origin of reticulum cell sarcoma. Virchows Archiv A Pathological Anatomy and Histology 364: 51–67

2808. Tan H K, Harrison M, Gralnick H R 1974 Nuclear topography in the abnormal cell of Sézary syndrome: observation by freeze etch electron microscopy. Journal of the National Cancer Institute 52: 1367–1371

2809. Tokunaga M, Hasui K, Sato E 1982 Ultrastructure of adult T-cell lymphoma. Gann 73: 748–757

2810. van Heerde P, Feltkamp C A, Feltkamp-Vroom T M, Koudstaal J, van Unnik J A 1980 Non-Hodgkin's lymphoma. Immunohistochemical and electronmicroscopic findings in relation to lightmicroscopy. A study of 74 cases. Cancer 46: 2210–2220

2811. van der Putte S C J, Toonstra J, Go D M D S, van Unnik J A M 1982 Mycosis fungoides. Demonstration of a variant simulating Hodgkin's disease. A report of a case with a cytomorphological analysis. Virchows Archiv B Cell Pathology 40: 231–247

2812. van der Putte S C J, Toonstra J, de Weger R A, van Unnik J A M 1982 Cutaneous T-cell lymphoma, multilobated type. Histopathology 6: 35–54

2813. van der Valk P, Hermans J, Brand R, Cornelisse C J, Spaander P J, Meijer C J 1982 Morphometric characterisation of diffuse large-cell (histiocytic) lymphomas. American Journal of Pathology 107: 327–335

2814. van der Valk P, te Velde J, Jansen J, Ruiter D J, Spaander P J, Cornelisse C J, Meijer C J L M 1981 Malignant lymphoma of true histiocytic origin: histiocytic sarcoma. A morphological, ultrastructural, immunological, cytochemical and clinical study of 10 cases. Virchows Archiv A Pathological Anatomy and Histology 391: 249–265

2815. Variakojis D, Rosas-Uribe A, Rappaport H 1974 Mycosis fungoides: pathologic findings in staging laparotomies. Cancer 33: 1589–1600

2816. Vernon S E, Voet R L 1983 Transformation of 'signet ring cell' lymphoma to typical nodular, poorly differentiated lymphocytic lymphoma: light microscopic, immunohisto-chemical and electron microscopic observations. Ultrastructural Pathology 4: 177–186

2817. Waldron J A, Leech J H, Glick A D, Flexner J M, Collins R D 1977 Malignant lymphoma of peripheral T-lymphocyte origin. Immunologic, pathologic, and clinical features in six patients. Cancer 40: 1604–1617

2818. Ward A M, Shortland J R, Darke C S 1971 Lymphosarcoma of the lung with monoclonal (IgM) gammopathy. A clinico-pathologic, histochemical, immunologic, and ultrastructural study. Cancer 27: 1009–1028

2819. Watanabe S, Shimosato Y, Shimoyama M, Minato K, Suzuki M, Abe M, Nagatani T 1980 Adult T cell lymphoma with hypergammaglobulinemia. Cancer 46: 2472–2483

2820. Willemze R, Ruiter D J, Van Vloten W A, Meijer C J 1982 Reticulum cell sarcomas (large cell lymphomas) presenting in the skin. High frequency of true histiocytic lymphoma. Cancer 50: 1367–1379

2821. Willemze R, Van Vloten W A, van der Loo E M, Meyer C J 1981 Primary lymphoblastic non-Hodgkin's lymphoma of the skin. British Journal of Dermatology 104: 333–338

2822. Zucker-Franklin D 1974 Properties of the Sézary lymphoid cell: an ultrastructural analysis. Mayo Clinic Proceedings 49: 567–574

2823. Zucker-Franklin D, Melton J W III, Quagliata F 1974 Ultrastructural, immunologic, and functional studies on Sézary cells: a neoplastic variant of thymus derived T lymphocytes. Proceedings of the National Academy of Sciences 71: 1877–1881

## 65 HODGKIN'S DISEASE

2824. Anagnostou D, Parker J W, Taylor C R, Tindle B H, Lukes R J 1977 Lacunar cells of nodular sclerosing Hodgkin's disease: an ultrastructural and immunohistologic study. Cancer 39: 1032–1043

2825. Archibald R B, Frenster J H 1973 Quantitative ultrastructural analysis of in vivo lymphocyte-Reed-Sternberg cell interactions in Hodgkin's disease. National Cancer Institute Monograph 36: 239–245

2826. Azar H A 1975 Significance of the Reed-Sternberg cell. Human Pathology 6: 479–484

2827. Bernau D, Feldmann G, Vorhauer W 1978 Hodgkin's disease: ultrastructural localization of intra-cytoplasmic immunoglobulins within malignant cells. British Journal of Haematology 40: 51–57

2828. Dorfman R F, Rice D F, Michell A D, Kempson R L, Levine G 1973 Ultrastructural studies of Hodgkin's disease. National Cancer Institute Monograph 36: 221–238

2829. Gladkowska-Dura M J, Dura W T, Johnson W W 1981 Light and immunoelectron microscopic study of Hodgkin's disease: evidence of immunoglobulin synthesis by tumor cells. Virchows Archiv B Cell Pathology 37: 109–124

2830. Glick A D, Leech J H, Flexner J M, Collins R D 1976 Ultrastructural study of Reed-Sternberg cells. Comparison with transformed lymphocytes and histiocytes. American Journal of Pathology 85: 195–208

2831. Halie M R, Splett-Romascano M, Nieweg H O 1974 Abnormal cells in the peripheral blood of patients with Hodgkin's disease. II. Ultrastructural studies. British Journal of Haematology 28: 323–328

2832. Hansmann M–L, Kaiserling E 1982 The lacunar cell and its relationship to interdigitating reticulum cells. Virchows Archiv B Cell Pathology 39: 323–332

2833. Harris N L, Dvorak A M, Smith J, Dvorak H F 1982 Fibrin deposits in Hodgkin's disease. American Journal of Pathology 108: 119–129

2834. Hayhoe F G, Burns G F, Cawley J C, Stewart J W 1978 Cytochemical, ultrastructural and immunological studies of circulating Reed-Sternberg cells. British Journal of Haematology 38: 485–490

2835. Ioachim H L 1975 New vistas in Hodgkin's disease. Pathology Annual 10: 419–459

2836. Kay M M 1975 Letter: Surface characteristics of Hodgkin's cells. Lancet ii: 459–460

2837. Kay M M 1976 Hodgkin's disease: a war between T-lymphocytes and transformed macrophages? Recent Results in Cancer Research 56: 111–121

2838. Kay M M, Kadin M 1975 Letter: Surface characteristics of Hodgkin's cells. Lancet i: 748–749

2839. Mikata A, Oishi T, Kagayama K 1973 Ultrastructure of Hodgkin's cell. A preliminary report. Gann 15: 287–291

2840. Parmley R T, Spicer S S, Morgan S K, Grush O C 1976 Hodgkin's disease and myelomonocytic leukemia. An ultrastructural and immunocytochemical study. Cancer 38: 1188–1198

2841. Parmley R T, Spicer S S, Pratt-Thomas H R, Morgan S K, Othersen H B 1975 Microorganism-like structures in Hodgkin disease. Electron microscopical demonstration. Archives of Pathology 99: 259–266

2842. Parmley R T, Spicer S S, Wright N J 1975 The ultrastructural identification of tissue basophils and mast cells in Hodgkin's disease. Laboratory Investigation 32: 469–475

2843. Peckman M J, Cooper E H 1973 Cell proliferation in Hodgkin's disease. National Cancer Institute Monograph 36: 179–189

2844. Peiper S C, Kahn L B, Ross D W, Reddick R L 1980 Ultrastructural organisation of the Reed-Sternberg cell: its resemblance to cells of the monocyte-macrophage system. Blood Cells 6: 515–523

2845. Poppema S, Elema J D, Halie M R 1978 The significance of intracytoplasmic proteins in Reed-Sternberg cells. Cancer 42: 1793–1803

2846. Schnitzer B, Mead M L 1975 Letter: Surface characteristics of Hodgkin's lymphoma cells. Lancet i: 223

2847. Seemayer T A, Lagacé R, Schürch W 1980 On the pathogenesis of sclerosis and nodularity in nodular sclerosing Hodgkin's disease. Virchows Archiv A Pathological Anatomy and Histology 385: 283–291

2848. Stiller D, Katenkamp D 1978 Intercellular substances in Hodgkin's lymphomas. Ultrastructural investigations. Virchows Archiv A Pathological Anatomy and Histology 380: 81–90

2849. Zucker-Franklin D, Schinella R 1981 Nature of the giant cell in Hodgkin's disease. Ultrastructural Pathology 2: 81–83

## 66 LEUKAEMIAS – GENERAL ASPECTS

2850. Anderson D R 1966 Ultrastructure of normal and leukemic leukocytes in human peripheral blood. Journal of Ultrastructure Research suppl 9: 1–42

2851. Azar H A 1979 The hematopoietic system. In: Trump B F, Jones R T (eds) Diagnostic electron microscopy, vol 2. John Wiley & Sons, New York, ch 3, p 47–161

2852. Beard M E, Fairley G H 1974 Acute leukemia in adults. Seminars in Hematology 11: 5–24

2853. Bessis M 1973 Cytologic diagnosis of leukaemias by electron microscopy. Recent Results in Cancer Research 43: 63–70

2854. Bessis M 1973 Living blood cells and their ultrastructure. Springer-Verlag, Berlin, p 555–672

2855. Breton-Gorius J, Gourdin M F, Reyes F 1981 Ultrastructure of the leukemic cell. In: Catovsky D (ed) The leukemic cell, Churchill Livingstone, Edinburgh, p 87–128

2856. Breton-Gorius J, Reyes F, Duhamel G, Najman A, Gorin N C 1978 Megakaryoblastic acute leukemia: identification by the ultrastructural demonstration of platelet peroxidase. Blood 51: 45–60

2857. Brunning R D, Maldonado J E 1980 Leukemias. In: Johannessen J V (ed) Electron microscopy in human medicine, vol 5. Cardiovascular system, lymphoreticular and hematopoietic system. McGraw-Hill, New York, pt 5, ch 25, p 279–353

2858. Brunning R D, Parkin J 1975 Ribosome-lamella complexes in neoplastic hematopoietic cells. American Journal of Pathology 79: 565–578

2859. Butler A E, Vardiman J W, Golomb H M 1982 Ultrastructural characterization of de novo and secondary leukaemias. Virchows Archiv B Cell Pathology 39: 239–257

2860. Cawley J C, Hayhoe F G J 1973 Ultrastructure of haemic cells. A cytological atlas of normal and leukaemic blood and bone marrow. W.B. Saunders Company, London

2861. Conforti A, Medolago-Albani L, Alessio L 1976 Ultrastructural changes in human leukaemic cell nuclei. Virchows Archiv B Cell Pathology 22: 143–149

2862. Coppola A, O'Connor J 1977 Ultrastructure of unusual cytoplasmic inclusions in a case of myeloproliferative disorder. Cancer 40: 2111–2115

2863. Dvorak A M, Monahan R A, Dickersin G R 1981 Diagnostic electron microscopy. I. Hematology: differential diagnosis of acute lymphoblastic and acute myeloblastic leukemia. Use of ultrastructural peroxidase cytochemistry and routine electron microscopic technology. Pathology Annual 16, pt 1: 101–137

2864. Frisch B, Lewis S M, Catovsky D 1978 Ultrastructural study of normal and leukaemic leucocyte processes. Biomedicine 28: 264–270

2865. Glick A D 1976 Acute leukemia: electron microscopic diagnosis. Seminars in Oncology 3: 229–241

2866. Glick A D, Paniker K, Flexner J M, Graber S E, Collins R D 1980 Acute leukemia of adults. Ultrastructural, cytochemical and histologic observations in 100 cases. American Journal of Clinical Pathology 73: 459–470

2867. Golomb R M, Reese C 1976 Surface ultrastructural and marker characteristics of leukemic cells. Scanning Electron Microscopy 2: 41–48

2868. Jacknow G, Muehleck S, Parkin J, Arthur D, McKenna R, Brunning R 1983 Morphologic, ultrastructural and cytogenetic features of acute megakaryoblastic leukemia. Laboratory Investigation 48: 40A

2869. Jansson S E, Gripenberg J, Vuopio P, Teerenhovi L, Andersson L C 1980 Classification of acute leukaemia by light and electron microscope cytochemisty. Scandinavian Journal of Haematology 25: 412–416

2870. Komiyama A, Ogawa M, Eurenius K, Spicer S S 1976 Unusual cytoplasmic inclusions in blast cells in acute leukemia. Archives of Pathology and Laboratory Medicine 100: 590–594

2871. Marie J P, Perrot J Y, Boucheix C, Zittoun J, Martyre M C, Kayibanda M, Rosenfeld C, Mishal Z, Zittoun R 1982 Determination of ultrastructural peroxidases and immunologic membrane markers in the diagnosis of acute leukemias. Blood 59: 270–276

2872. Marini M, Baguara G P, Biagini G, Baccarani M, Rosito P 1982 TdT-positive and TdT-negative human leukemic cells: specific density and morphology. Advances in Experimental Medicine and Biology 145: 357–370

2873. Polliack A 1977 Surface morphology of leukaemic cells. Application of scanning electron microscopy to the study of human leukaemias. Israel Journal of Medical Sciences 13: 701–709

2874. Polliack A 1982 The contribution of scanning electron microscopy in haematology: its role in defining leucocyte and erythrocyte disorders. Journal of Microscopy 123: 177–187

2875. Polliack A, Gamliel H, Ben Bassat H, Gurfel D, Leizerawitz R, Minowada J 1983 Surface morphology and membrane phenotype of cultured human leukemia-lymphoma cells. A scanning electron microscopic study of 36 cell lines. Cancer 51: 72–79

2876. Polliack A, Prokocimer M, Or R, Korkesh A, Leizerowitz R, Ben-Bassat H, Gamliel H 1981 Use of multiparameter studies and scanning electron microscopy in the interpretation and attempted correlation of surface morphology with cell type in 135 cases of human leukemias. Cancer Research 41: 1171–1179

2877. Rosen N R, DiFino S, Nelson D A 1979 Acute leukemia with unusual cytoplasmic inclusions. A cytochemical and ultrastructural study. Cancer 43: 2405–2409

2878. Schumacher H R, Szekely I E, Park S A, Rao U N, Fisher D R, Patel S B 1979 Acute leukemic cells. Qualitative and quantitative electron microscopy. American Journal of Pathology 73: 27–46

2879. Sébahoun G, Bayle J, Muratore R, Carcassonne Y 1979 Ribosome lamella complex in neoplastic cells of a Sézary's syndrome. Journal of Clinical Pathology 32: 1041–1044

2880. Topitko A, Radwańska U 1981 Present and future application of the electron microscopy in acute leukemias. Zentralblatt für allgemeine Pathologie und pathologische Anatomie 125: 460–472

2881. Youness E, Trujillo J M, Ahearn M J, McCredie K B, Cork A 1980 Acute unclassified leukemia: a clinicopathologic study with diagnostic implications of electron microscopy. American Journal of Hematology 9: 79–88

2882. Zafar M N, O'Brien M, Catovsky D 1982 Similarities in mitochondrial ultrastructure of leukemic cells and ethidium-bromide-treated normal cells. Journal of Ultrastructure Research 81: 133–138

2883. Zucker-Franklin D, Greaves M F, Grossi C E, Marmont A M 1981 Atlas of blood cells. Function and pathology, vols 1 and 2, Lea & Febiger, Philadelphia

## 67  LYMPHOCYTIC LEUKAEMIAS

2884. Boesen A M 1983 Stereological analysis of the ultrastructure of isolated human T and non-T lymphoid cells. III. Studies in chronic lymphoid leukaemias, hairy cell leukemia and some malignant lymphomas. Virchows Archiv B Cell Pathology Including Molecular Pathology 43: 165–178

2885. Brunning R D, Parkin J 1975 Ultrastructural studies of parallel tubular arrays in human lymphocytes. American Journal of Pathology 78: 59–70

2886. Brynes R K, Hamburg A, Reese C, Golomb H M 1975 Letter: Surface ultrastructural changes of lymphoid cells in chronic lymphocytic leukaemia. Lancet i: 687–688

2887. Capron F, Perrot J Y, Boucheix L, Reynes M, Tricottet V, Bernadou A, Diebold J 1982 Lysosomal localisation of parallel tubular arrays in chronic lymphocytic leukaemia of T cell origin: an ultrastructural study. Journal of Clinical Pathology 35: 167–171

2888. Catovsky D 1975 Letter: T-cell origin of acid phosphatase-positive lymphoblasts. Lancet ii: 327–328

2889. Catovsky D, Goldman J M, Okos A, Frisch B, Galton D A 1974 T lymphoblastic leukaemia: a distinct variant of acute leukaemia. British Medical Journal 2: 643–646

2890. Cawley J C, Emmines J, Goldstone A H, Hamblin T, Hough D, Smith J L 1975 Distinctive cytoplasmic inclusions in chronic lymphocytic leukaemia. European Journal of Cancer 11: 91–92

2891. Cawley J C, Smith J, Goldstone A H, Emmines J, Hamblin J, Hough D 1976 IgA and IgM cytoplasmic inclusions in a series of chronic lymphocytic leukaemia. Clinical and Experimental Immunology 23: 78–82

2892. Costello C, Catovsky D, O'Brien M 1981 Cytoplasmic inclusions in a case of prolymphocytic leukemia. American Journal of Clinical Pathology 76: 499–501

2893. Costello C, Catovsky D, O'Brien M, Galton D A 1980 Prolymphocytic leukaemia: an ultrastructural study of 22 cases. British Journal of Haematology 44: 389–394

2894. Costello C, Catovsky D, O'Brien M, Morilla R, Varadi S 1980 Chronic T-cell leukemias. I. Morphology, cytochemistry and ultrastructure. Leukemia Research 4: 463–476

2895. de Harven E 1975 Scanning electron microscopy of leukaemic and lymphoma cells. British Journal of Cancer 32: 278

2896. Djaldetti M, Landau M, Mandel E M, Har-Zaav L, Lewinski U 1974 Electron microscopic study of lymphosarcoma cell leukaemia. Blut 29: 210–215

2897. Enno A, Catovsky D, O'Brien M, Cherchi M, Kumaran T O, Galton A 1979 Prolymphocytoid transformation of chronic lymphocytic leukaemia. British Journal of Haematology 41: 9–18

2898. Fischer K, Cohnen G, Szaniawski W, Brittinger G 1977 Scanning electron microscopic study of leukemic human B lymphocytes. Acta Haematologica 57: 247–256

2899. Galton D A, Goldman J M, Wiltshaw E, Catovsky D, Henry K 1974 Prolymphocytic leukaemia. British Journal of Haematology 27: 7–23

2900. Gamliel H, Polliack A 1981 Positive identification of human leukaemic cells with scanning immuno-electron microscopy, using antibody coated polystyrene (latex) beads as markers. Scandinavian Journal of Haematology 26: 297–305

2901. Guglielmi P, Preud'Homme J L, Gourdin M F, Reyes F, Daniel M T 1982 Unusual intracytoplasmic immuno-globulin inclusions in chronic lymphocytic leukaemia. British Journal of Haematology 50: 123–134

2902. Guseo A 1975 Electron microscopy of lymphocytic leukaemia cells in the cerebrospinal fluid. Acta Neuropathologica suppl 6: 199–203

2903. Haemmerli G, Felix H, Sträuli P 1978 Dynamic morphology of human lymphoid leukaemias. Recent Results in Cancer Research 64: 113–117

2904. Huhn D, Thiel E, Rodt H, Schlimok G, Theml H, Rieber P 1983 Subtypes of T-cell chronic lymphocytic leukemia. Cancer 51: 1434–1447

2905. James V, Jupe D M, Proctor J 1980 Stereological studies on chronic lymphocytic leukaemia and hairy cell leukaemia. Scandinavian Journal of Haematology 24: 263–269

2906. Kjeldsberg C R, Bearman R M, Rappaport H 1980 Prolymphocytic leukemia. An ultrastructural study. American Journal of Clinical Pathology 73: 150–159

2907. Lambertenghi-Deliliers G, Zanon P, Boldini L, Nava M T, Pozzoli E 1980 Ultrastructural aspects of lymphocytes in B- and T-chronic lymphocytic leukaemia. Journal of Submicroscopic Cytology 12: 665–671

2908. Lin P S, Tsai S, Wallach D F, Ehrhart C 1975 Visualization of surface topography of human lymphoid cells by scanning electron microscopy. Bibliotheca Haematologica 40: 263–269

2909. Litovitz T L, Lutzner M A 1974 Quantitative measurements of blood lymphocytes from patients with chronic lymphocytic leukemia and the Sézary syndrome. Journal of the National Cancer Institute 53: 75–77

2910. Mathé G, Belpomme D, Dantchev D, Pouillart P, Jasmin C, Misset J L, Musset M, Amiel J L, Schlumberger J R, Schwarzenberg L, Hayat M, Devassal F, Lafleur M 1974 Immunoblastic acute lymphoid leukaemia. Biomedicine 20: 333–340

2911. McCann S R, Whelan A, Greally J 1978 Intracellular lambda light chain inclusions in chronic lymphocytic leukaemia. British Journal of Haematology 38: 367–371

2912. McKenna R W, Parkin J, Brunning R D 1979 Morphologic and ultrastructural characteristics of T-cell acute lymphoblastic leukemia. Cancer 44: 1290–1297

2913. Minerbrook M, Schulman P, Budman D R, Teichberg S, Vinciguerra V, Kardon N, Degnan T J 1982 Burkitt's leukemia: a re-evaluation. Cancer 49. 1444–1448

2914. Mirra S S, Miles M L, Jacobs J 1981 The coexistence of ribosome-lamella complex and annulate lamellae in chronic lymphocytic leukemia. Ultrastructural Pathology 2: 249–256

2915. Muller-Hermelink U, Muller-Hermelink H K 1977 Scanning electron microscopic investigations of acute leukaemia. Virchows Archiv B Cell Pathology 23: 227–236

2916. Paintrand M, Dantchev D, Mathé G 1973 Electron microscopic aspects of cells in the four subvarieties of acute lymphoid leukaemia. Recent Results in Cancer Research 43: 71–75

2917. Perera D J, Pegrum G D 1974 The lymphocyte in chronic lymphatic leukaemia. Lancet i: 1207–1209

2918. Peterson L C, Bloomfield C D, Sundberg R D, Gajl-Peczalska K J, Brunning R D 1975 Morphology of chronic lymphocytic leukemia and its relationship to survival. American Journal of Medicine 59: 316–324

2919. Polliack A, Froimovici M, Pozzoli E, Lambertenghi-Deliliers G 1976 Acute lymphoblastic leukaemia: a study of 25 cases by scanning electron microscopy. Blut 33: 359–366

2920. Polliack A, Siegal F P, Clarkson B D, Fu S M, Winchester R J, Lampen N, Siegal M, de Harven E 1975 A scanning electron microscopy and immunological study of 84 cases of lymphocytic leukaemia and related lymphoproliferative disorders. Scandinavian Journal of Haematology 15: 359–376

2921. Ralfkiaer E, Hou-Jensen K, Geisler C, Plesner T, Henschel A, Hansen M M 1982 Cytoplasmic inclusions in lymphocytes of chronic lymphocytic leukaemia. A report of 10 cases. Virchows Archiv A Pathological Anatomy and Histology 395: 227–236

2922. Reiffers J, Darmendrail V, Larrue J, Villenave I, Bernard P, Boisseau M, Broustet A 1981 Ultrastructural cytochemical prospective study of adult acute lymphoblastic leukemia: detection of peroxidase activity in patients failing to respond to treatment. Cancer 48: 927–931

2923. Rilke F, Pilotti S, Carbone A, Lombardi L 1978 Morphology of lymphatic cells and of their derived tumours. Journal of Clinical Pathology 31: 1009–1056

2924. Rozman C, Montserrat E, Feliu E, Woessner S 1980 Lymphocyte size and survival of patients with chronic lymphocytic leukaemia (B-type). Scandinavian Journal of Haematology 24: 315–320

2925. Said J W, Pinkus G S 1981 Immunologic characterization and ultrastructural correlations for 125 cases of B- and T-cell leukemias: studies of chronic and acute lymphocytic, prolymphocytic, lymphosarcoma cell and hairy cell leukemia, Sézary's syndrome and other lymphoid leukemias. Cancer 48: 2630–2642

2926. Schmalzl F, Huhn D, Abbrederis K, Braunsteiner H 1974 Acute lymphocytic leukaemia. Cytochemistry and ultrastructure. Blut 29: 87–95

2927. Schumacher H R, Mangel T K, Davis K D 1970 The lymphocyte of chronic lymphatic leukaemia. I. Electron microscopy — onset. Cancer 26: 895–903

2928. Schumacher H R, Szekely I E, Fisher D R 1975 Leukemic mitochondria. III. Acute lymphoblastic leukemia. American Journal of Pathology 78: 49–58

2929. Schumacher H R, Szekely I E, Park S A, Fisher D R 1973 Ultrastructural studies on the acute leukaemic lymphoblast. Blut 27: 369–406

2930. Schumaker H R, Thomas W J, Creegan W J, Pitts L L 1980 Infectious mononucleosis and acute lymphoblastic leukemia — hand mirror cells: a qualitative and quantitative ultrastructural study. American Journal of Hematology 9: 67–77

2931. Schweitzer M, Melief C J, Ploem J E 1973 Chronic lymphocytic leukaemia in 5 siblings. Scandinavian Journal of Haematology 11: 97–105

2932. Shah-Reddy I, Mirchandani I, Bishop C R 1981 Hand mirror cell leukemia — immunologic and ultrastructural studies. Cancer 47: 715–719

2933. Shamoto M 1983 Langerhans cells increase in the dermal lesions of adult T cell leukaemia in Japan. Journal of Clinical Pathology 36: 307–311

2934. Shamoto M, Murakami S, Zenke T 1981 Adult T-cell leukemia in Japan: an ultrastructural study. Cancer 47: 1804–1811

2935. Sharp J W, Stass S A, Creegan W J, Pitts L L, Schumacher H R 1979 Acute lymphoblastic leukemia, hand-mirror variant. A detailed ultrastructural study. American Journal of Clinical Pathology 72: 551–558

2936. Stass S A, Perlin E, Jaffe E S, Simon D R, Creegan W J, Robinson J J, Holloway M L, Schumacher H R 1978 Acute lymphoblastic leukemia, hand mirror cell variant. A detailed cytological and ultrastructural study with an analysis of the immunologic surface markers. American Journal of Hematology 4: 67–77

2937. Stathopoulos G, Papmichail M, Sheldon P, Catovsky D, Davies A J, Holborow E J, Wiltshaw E 1974 Immunological studies in a case of T-cell leukaemia. Journal of Clinical Pathology 27: 851–859

2938. Taylor H G, Butler W M, Rhoads J, Karcher D S, Detrick-Hooks B 1982 Prolymphocytic leukemia: treatment with combination chemotherapy to include doxorubicin. Cancer 49: 1524–1529

2939. Tricot G, Broeckaert-Van Orshoven A, Van Hoof A, Verwilghen R L 1982 Sudan Black B positivity in acute lymphoblastic leukaemia. British Journal of Haematology 51: 615–621

2940. Trubowitz S, Sobel H, Davis S 1980 Null cell (non-T, non-B) acute lymphoblastic leukemia terminating as malignant histiocytosis. American Journal of Clinical Pathology 73: 725–730

2941. Tsukada M, Hanamura K, Eguchi M, Komiyama A, Akabane T 1976 Scanning electron microscopic study of peripheral blood lymphocytes, thymic cells and acute lymphoblastic leukemic cells in children. Acta Haematologica Japonica 39: 43–52

2942. Weber A F 1974 Nuclear pockets in blood leukocytes, a morphological marker of possible early diagnostic value for lymphocytic leukaemia. Schweizerische Medizinische Wochenschrift 104: 284–286

2943. Woessner S, Rozman C 1976 Ribosome lamellae complex in chronic lymphatic leukaemia. Blut 33: 23–28

## 68 GRANULOCYTIC LEUKAEMIAS

2944. Ackerman G A 1975 Ultrastructural histochemical alteration of the plasma membrane in chronic myelocytic leukemia. Blood 46: 869–881

2945. Arnal-Moureal F M, Alvarez Fernandez J C, Sanchez Varela J M, Marini Diaz M 1981 Meningeal granulocytic sarcoma without evidence of leukemia. Light and ultrastructural study of one case. Virchows Archiv A Pathological Anatomy and Histology 392: 111–118

2946. Bain B, Catovsky D, O'Brien M, Spiers A S, Richards G H 1977 Megakaryoblastic transformation of chronic granulocytic leukaemia. An electron microscopy and cytochemical study. Journal of Clinical Pathology 30: 235–242

2947. Breton Gorius J, Houssay D 1973 Auer bodies in acute promyelocytic leukemia. Demonstration of their fine structure and peroxidase localization. Laboratory Investigation 28: 135–141

2948. Catovsky D, O'Brien M, Cherchi M, Benavides I 1978 Ultrastructural, cytochemical and surface marker analysis of cells during blast crisis of chronic granulocytic leukaemia. Bolletino dell' Istituto Sieroterapico Milanese 57: 344–354

2949. Chesney T M, Brown P, Neely C, Bell A 1980 A new cytoplasmic crystalline inclusion in myeloblastic leukemia (M2) morphologically distinct from the Auer rod. Laboratory Investigation 42: 105–106A

2950. Dittman W A, Kramer R J, Bainton D F 1980 Electron microscopic and peroxidase cytochemical analysis of pink pseudo-Chediak-Higashi granules in acute myelogenous leukemia. Cancer Research 40: 4473–4481

2951. Foa R, Oscier D G, Hillyard C J, Incarbone E, McIntyre I, Goldman J M 1982 Production of immunoreactive calcitonin by myeloid leukaemia cells. British Journal of Haematology 50: 215–223

2952. Freeman J A 1966 Origin of Auer bodies. Blood 27: 499–510

2953. Gralnick H R, Tan H K 1974 Acute promyelocytic leukemia. A model for understanding the role of the malignant cell in hemostasis. Human Pathology 5: 661–673

2954. Haider Y S, Phillips T M, Schumacher H R 1982 Acute myeloid leukemia with hand-mirror cells. Archives of Pathology and Laboratory Medicine 106: 271–274

2955. Holton C P, Johnson W W 1968 Chronic myelocytic leukemia in infant siblings. Journal of Pediatrics 72: 377–383

2956. Ito S, Hattori A 1974 Study on the fibrillar formation surrounding the nuclear bridge in some types of leukaemic cells. Scandinavian Journal of Haematology 12: 321–328

2957. Kondo K, Yoshitake J, Takemura K 1966 The fine structure of Auer bodies. Journal of Electron Microscopy 15: 237–248

2958. Ligorsky R D, Axelrod A R, Mandell G H, Palutke M, Prasad A S 1977 Acute myelomonocytic leukemia in a patient with macroglobulinemia and malignant lymphoma. Cancer 39: 1156–1162

2959. McKenna R W, Parkin J L, Foucar K, Brunning R D 1981 Ultrastructural characteristics of therapy-related acute nonlymphocytic leukemia: evidence for a panmyelosis. Cancer 48: 725–737

2960. McKenna R W, Parkin J, Bloomfield C D, Sundberg R D, Brunning R D 1982 Acute promyelocytic leukaemia: a study of 39 cases with identification of a hyperbasophilic microgranular variant. British Journal of Haematology 50: 201–214

2961. Mintz U, Djaldetti M, Rozenszajn L, Pinkhas J, de Vries A 1973 Giant lysosome-like structures in promyelocytic leukemia. Ultrastructural and cytochemical observations. Biomedicine Express 19: 426–430

2962. O'Donnell J R, Tansey P, Chung P, Burnett A K, Thomson J, McDonald G A 1982 Acute myelomonocytic leukaemia presenting as xanthomatous skin eruption. Journal of Clinical Pathology 35: 1200–1203

2963. Parkin J L, Brunning R D 1978 Unusual configurations of endoplasmic reticulum in cells of acute promyelocytic leukemia. Journal of the National Cancer Institute 61: 341–348

2964. Parkin J L, Brunning R D 1980 Tubular complexes of endoplasmic reticulum in myeloblasts of acute myelogenous leukemia. Ultrastructural Pathology 1: 55–65

2965. Parkin J L, McKenna R W, Brunning R D 1982 Philadelphia chromosome-positive blastic leukaemia: ultrastructural and ultracytochemical evidence of basophil and mast cell differentiation. British Journal of Haematology 52: 663–677

2966. Polliack A, McKenzie S, Gee T, Lampen N, de Harven E, Clarkson B D 1975 A scanning electron microscopic study of 34 cases of acute granulocytic, myelomonocytic, monoblastic and histiocytic leukemia. American Journal of Medicine 59: 308–315

2967. Rasore-Quartino A 1976 Acute promyelocytic leukaemia in children. An ultrastructural study. Pathologica 68: 539–545

2968. Schumacher H R, Szekely I E, Patel S B, Fisher D R 1974 Leukemic mitochondria. I. Acute myeloblastic leukemia. American Journal of Pathology 74: 71–82

2969. Shamoto M 1981 Emperipolesis of hematopoietic cells in myelocytic leukemia. Electron microscope and phase contract microscopic studies. Virchows Archiv B Cell Pathology 35: 283–290

2970. Shaw M T, Bottomley R H, Grozea P N, Nordquist R E 1975 Heterogeneity of morphological, cytochemical and cytogenetic features in the blastic phase of chronic granulocytic leukemia. Cancer 35: 199–207

2971. Skinnider L F, Card R T, Padmanabh S 1977 Chronic myelomonocytic leukemia. An ultrastructural study by transmission and scanning electron microscopy. American Journal of Clinical Pathology 67: 339–346

2972. Skinnider L F, Ghadially F N 1975 Ultrastructure of acute myeloid leukemia arising in multiple myeloma. Human Pathology 6: 379–384

2973. Smith W B, Ablin A, Goodman J R, Brecher G 1973 Atypical megakaryocytes in preleukemic phase of acute myeloid leukemia. Blood 42: 535–540

2974. Spremolla G, Gori Z, Bottone E 1976 Electron microscopy and cytochemistry of the bone marrow in acute promyelocytic leukaemia. Haematologica 61: 202–218

2975. Thiele J, Ballard A-Ch, Georgii A, Vykoupil K F 1977 Chronic megakaryocytic-granulocytic myelosis. I. Megakaryocytes and thrombocytes. Virchows Archiv A Pathological Anatomy and Histology 373: 191–211

2976. Thiele J, Ballard A-Ch, Georgii A, Vykoupil K F 1977 Chronic megakaryocytic-granulocytic myelosis — an electron microscopic study including freeze fracture. II. Granulocytes, erythrocytes, plasma cells and myeloid stroma. Virchows Archiv A Pathological Anatomy and Histology 375: 129–146

2977. Thiele J, Georgii A, Vykoupil K F 1976 Ultrastructure of chronic megakaryocytic granulocytic myelosis. Blut 32: 433–438

2978. Thiele J, Vykoupil K F, Georgii A 1980 Myeloid dysplasia (MD): a hematological disorder preceding acute and chronic myeloid leukemia. A morphological study on sequential core biopsies of the bone marrow in 27 patients. Virchows Archiv A Pathological Anatomy and Histology 389: 343–367

2979. Thiele J, Vykoupil K F, Georgii A 1980 Ultrastructure of blastic crisis in osteomyelofibrosis. A report of 2 cases with some unusual features. Virchows Archiv A Pathological Anatomy and Histology 389: 287–305

2980. Ullyot J L, Bainton D F 1975 Azurophil and specific granules of blood neutrophils in chronic myelogenous leukemia. An ultrastructural and cytochemical analysis. Blood 45: 469–482

2981. Valdivieso M, Rodriguez V, Drewinko B, Body G P, Ahearn M J, McCredie K, Freireich E J 1975 Clinical and morphological correlations in acute promyelocytic leukemia. Medical and Pediatric Oncology 1: 37–50

2982. Wada J 1980 Ultrastructural peroxidase cytochemistry of leukemic cells. I. Classification of acute myelogenous leukemia. Keio Journal of Medicine 29: 163–174

2983. Wada J 1980 Ultrastructural peroxidase cytochemistry of leukemic cells. II. Blast crisis of chronic myelogenous leukemia. Keio Journal of Medicine 29: 175–183

2984. Weiselberg L, Teichberg S, Vinciguerra V, Schulman P, Budman D, Degnan T 1981 Electron microscope cytochemical analysis of chronic myelocytic leukemia. A case report. Cancer 47: 533–536

2985. White J G 1967 Fine structural demonstration of acid phosphatase activity in Auer bodies. Blood 29, suppl: 667–682

2986. Wilson P D, Rustin G J, Smith G P, Peters T J 1981 Electron microscopic cytochemical localisation of nucleoside phosphatases in normal and chronic granulocytic leukemic human neutrophils. Histochemistry 13: 73–84

2987. Wolf D J, Fialk M A, Mouradian J, Gottfried E L, Pasmantier M W 1980 Unusual intracytoplasmic inclusions in acute myeloblastic leukemia. American Journal of Hematology 9: 413–420

2988. Wulfhekel U, Düllmann J, Bartels H, Hausmann K 1975 On the ultrastructure and cytochemistry of eosinophil-myelomonocytic leukemias. Virchows Archiv A Pathological Anatomy and Histology 365: 289–308

## 69 MONOCYTIC LEUKAEMIA AND ERYTHROLEUKAEMIA

2989. Begin L R, Osborne B M, Mackay B 1981 Monocytic leukemia with cutaneous involvement: ultrastructural observations on unusual cytoplasmic complexes. Ultrastructural Pathology 2: 11–18

2990. Burg G, Schmoeckel C, Braun-Falco O, Wolff H H 1978 Monocytic leukemia. Clinically appearing as malignant reticulosis of the skin. Archives of Dermatology 114: 418–420

2991. Catovsky D, O'Brien M 1981 Lysosomal granules in leukemic monocytes and their relation to maturation stages. Haematologie und Bluttransfusion 27: 167–173

2992. Dantchev D, Belpomme D 1977 Critical study of the mononuclear leukocyte morphology based on scanning electron microscopy in normal subjects and in patients with lymphoid or monocytoid proliferative disorders. Comparison with the T, B or null cell membrane phenotypes. Biomedicine 26: 202–222

2993. Feremans W W, Menu R, Hupin J, Bieva C J, Caudron M 1980 Acute promonocytic leukaemia with ribosome-lamella complexes and elevated muramidase activity in serum and urine. A clinical, morphological, cytochemical and immunochemical study. Acta Clinica Belgica 35: 212–221

2994. Glick A D, Horn R G 1974 Identification of promonocytes and monocytoid precursors in acute leukaemia of adults: ultrastructural and cytochemical observations. British Journal of Haematology 26: 395–403

2995. Huhn D, Schmalzl F 1974 Electron microscopic and cytochemic findings in Di-Guglielmo's syndrome and in other forms of leukaemia. Haematologie und Bluttransfusion 14: 36–49

2996. McKenna R W, Bloomfield C D, Dick F, Nesbit M E, Brunning R D 1975 Acute monoblastic leukemia: diagnosis and treatment of ten cases. Blood 46: 481–494

2997. O'Brien M, Catovsky D, Costello C 1980 Ultrastructural cytochemistry of leukaemic cells: characterisation of the early small granules of monoblasts. British Journal of Haematology 45: 201–208

2998. Parker A C, Dewar A E, Wilson C D, Young S, Stuart A E 1978 Surface membrane characteristics of cells from human acute monocytic leukaemia. Scandinavian Journal of Haematology 20: 467–478

2999. Rodgers G M, Carrera C J, Ries C A, Bainton D F 1982 Blastic transformation of a well differentiated monocytic leukemia: changes in cytochemical and cell surface markers. Leukemia Research 6: 613–622

3000. Schiffer C A, Sanel F T, Stechmiller B K, Wiernik P H 1975 Functional and morphologic characteristics of the leukemic cells of a patient with acute monocytic leukemia. Correlation with clinical features. Blood 46: 17–26

3001. Schumacher H R, Szekely I E, Park S A 1973 Monoblast of acute monoblastic leukemia. Cancer 31: 209–220

3002. Shaw M T, Nordquist R E 1975 'Pure' monocytic or histiomonocytic leukemia. A revised concept. Cancer 35: 208–214

3003. Strauss D J, Mertelsmann R, Koziner B, McKenzie S, de Harven E, Arlin Z A, Kempin S, Broxmeyer H, Moore M A, Menendez-Botet C J, Gee T S, Clarkson B D 1980 The acute monocytic leukemias: multidisciplinary studies in 45 patients. Medicine 59: 409–425

3004. Tsukada M, Saitoh H, Hara T, Komiyama A, Akabane T 1981 Electron microscopy of E-rosette-forming leukemic monocytes in a child with acute monocytic leukemia. Cancer 47: 1800–1803

## 70 HAIRY CELL LEUKAEMIA

3005. Alptuna E, Anteunis A, Krulik M, Astesano A, Robineaux R, Debray J 1978 Hairy cell leukemia. A clinical, immunological and ultrastructural study. New data for the origin of the hairy cell. Virchows Archiv B Cell Pathology 28: 135–149

3006. Bartl R, Frisch B, Hill W, Burkhardt R, Sommerfeld W, Sund M 1983 Bone marrow histology in hairy cell leukemia. Identification of subtypes and their prognostic significance. American Journal of Clinical Pathology 79: 531–545

3007. Braylan R C, Jaffe E S, Triche T J, Nanba K, Fowlkes B J, Metzger H, Frank M M, Dolan M S, Yee C L, Green I, Berard C W 1978 Structural and functional properties of the hairy cells of leukemic reticuloendotheliosis. Cancer 41: 210–227

3008. Brunning R D, Maldonado J E 1980 Hairy cell leukemia. In: Johannessen J V (ed) Electron microscopy in human medicine, vol 5. Cardiovascular system, lymphoreticular and hematopoietic system. McGraw-Hill, New York, pt 5, ch 27, p 374–376

3009. Burke J S, Mackay B, Rappaport H 1976 Hairy cell leukemia (leukemic reticuloendotheliosis). II. Ultrastructure of the spleen. Cancer 37: 2267–2274

3010. Burns C P, Hoak J C 1973 Freeze etching, scanning and thin section electron microscopic studies of the hairy leukocytes in leukemic reticuloendotheliosis. Journal of the National Cancer Institute 51: 743–750

3011. Catovsky D 1977 Hairy cell leukaemia and prolymphocytic leukaemia. Clinics in Haematology 6: 245–268

3012. Catovsky D, Frisch B, Okos A, Van Noorden S 1975 Letter: Scanning electron microscopy and the nature of the hairy cell. Lancet i: 462–463

3013. Catovsky D, Pettit J E, Galton D A, Spiers A S, Harrison C V 1974 Leukaemic reticuloendotheliosis — hairy cell leukaemia. A distinct clinico-pathological entity. British Journal of Haematology 26: 9–27

3014. Cawley J C, Burns G F, Hayhoe F G J 1980 Hairy cell leukaemia. Recent Results in Cancer Research, vol 72. Springer-Verlag, Berlin

3015. Daniel M T, Flandrin G 1974 Fine structure of abnormal cells in hairy cell (tricholeukocytic) leukemia with special reference to their in vitro phagocytic capacity. Laboratory Investigation 30: 1–8

3016. Debusscher L, Bernheim J L, Collard-Ronge E, Govaerts A, Hooghe R, Lejeune F J, Zeicher M, Stryckmans P A 1975 Hairy cell leukemia. Functional, immunologic, kinetic and ultrastructural characterization. Blood 46: 495–507

3017. Deegan M J, Cossman J, Chosney B T, Schnitzer B 1976 Hairy cell leukemia. An immunologic and ultrastructural study. Cancer 38: 1952–1961

3018. Espinouse D, Touraine J L, Schmitt D, Revol L 1980 Specific anti-hairy cell and anti-B cell antisera: characterisation of surface antigens and origin of hairy cells. Clinical and Experimental Immunology 39: 756–767

3019. Ghadially F N, Skinnider L F 1972 Ultrastructure of hairy cell leukemia. Cancer 29: 444–452

3020. Golde D W, Stevens R H, Quan S G, Saxon A 1977 Immunoglobulin synthesis in hairy cell leukaemia. British Journal of Haematology 35: 359–365

3021. Golomb H M, Braylan R, Polliack A 1975 Hairy cell leukaemia — leukaemic reticuloendotheliosis. A scanning electron microscopic study of eight cases. British Journal of Haematology 29: 455–460

3022. Golomb H M, Ganapathy R 1976 Letter: Hairy cells of leukaemic reticuloendotheliosis. Lancet ii: 39

3023. Golomb H M, Simon D 1977 Hairy cell leukaemia: letter. Lancet i: 372–373

3024. Golomb H M, Vardiman J, Sweet D L Jr, Simon D, Variakojis D 1978 Hairy cell leukaemia: evidence of the existence of a spectrum of functional characteristics. British Journal of Haematology 38: 161–170

3025. Haak H L, De Man J C, Hijmans W, Speck B 1974 Further evidence of the lymphocytic nature of leukaemic reticuloendotheliosis — hairy cell leukaemia. British Journal of Haematology 27: 31–38

3026. Haegert D G, Cawley J C, Collins R D, Flemans R J, Smith J L 1974 Leukaemic reticuloendotheliosis: a morphological and immunological study of four cases. Journal of Clinical Pathology 27: 967–972

3027. Hammar S P, Bockus D, Remington F, Hallman K, Huff J W, Ragen P A, Rudolph R H, Einstein A B, Bell J 1982 Autologous red blood cell and platelet engulfment in hairy cell leukemia. Ultrastructural Pathology 3: 243–252

3028. Hooper W C, Buss D H, Parker C L 1980 Leukemic reticuloendotheliosis (hairy cell leukemia): a review of the evidence concerning the immunology and origin of the cell. Leukemia Research 4: 489–503

3029. Hsu S-M, Yang K, Jaffe E S 1983 Hairy cell leukemia: a B cell neoplasm with a unique antigenic phenotype. American Journal of Clinical Pathology 80: 421–428

3030. Katayama I, Finkel H E 1974 Leukemic reticuloendotheliosis. A clinicopathologic study with review of the literature. American Journal of Medicine 57: 115–126

3031. Katayama I, Li C Y, Yam L T 1972 Ultrastructural characteristics of the 'hairy cells' of leukemic reticuloendotheliosis. American Journal of Pathology 67: 361–370

3032. Katayama I, Nagy G K, Balogh K Jr 1973 Light microscopic identification of the ribosome lamella complex in hairy cells of leukemic reticuloendotheliosis. Cancer 32: 843–846

3033. Katayama I, Pechet L 1975 Letter: Hairy cells. Lancet i: 976–977

3034. Katayama I, Schneider G B 1975 Letter: Cell surface structure in hairy cell leukaemia. Lancet i: 920–921

3035. Katayama I, Schneider G B 1977 Further ultrastructural characterization of hairy cells of leukemic reticuloendotheliosis. American Journal of Pathology 86: 163–182

3036. King G W, Hurtubise P E, Sagone A L Jr, Lobuglio A F, Metz E N 1975 Leukemic reticuloendotheliosis. A study of the origin of the malignant cell. American Journal of Medicine 59: 411–416

3037. Matre R, Talstad I, Haugen A 1977 Surface markers in non-phagocytic hairy cell leukaemia. Acta Pathologica et Microbiologica Scandinavica. Section C. Immunology 85: 406–412

3038. Palutke M, Tabaczka P, Mirchandani I, Goldfarb S 1981 Lymphocytic lymphoma simulating hairy cell leukemia: a consideration of reliable and unreliable diagnostic features. Cancer 48: 2047–2055

3039. Palutke M, Weise R W, Tabaczka P, Varadachair C, Axelrod A 1978 Hairy cells and macrophages: a comparative study. Laboratory Investigation 39: 267–280

3040. Pilon V, Davey F R, Gordon G B, Jones D B 1982 Splenic alterations in hairy-cell leukaemia: II. An electron microscopic study. Cancer 49: 1617–1623

3041. Roath S, Newell D G 1975 Letter: Cell surface characteristics in hairy cell leukaemia. Lancet i: 283–284

3042. Rosenszajn L A, Gutman A, Radnay J, David E B, Shoham D 1976 A study of the nature of hairy cells, with emphasis on enzymatic markers. American Journal of Pathology 66: 432–441

3043. Rosner M C, Golomb H M 1980 Ribosome-lamella complex in hairy cell leukemia. Ultrastructure and distribution. Laboratory Investigation 42: 236–247

3044. Rosner M C, Golomb H M 1982 Phagocytic capacity of hairy cells from seventeen patients. Virchows Archiv B Cell Pathology 40: 327–337

3045. Schnitzer B, Hammack W J 1975 Letter: The hairy cell. Human Pathology 6: 262–263

3046. Schnitzer B, Kass L 1974 Hairy cell leukemia. A clinicopathologic and ultrastructural study. American Journal of Clinical Pathology 61: 176–187

3047. Schnitzer B, Mead M L 1975 Letter: Nature of the hairy cell. Lancet i: 805

3048. Sutherland J C, Middleton E B, Banfield W G, Lee C W 1980 Lamella-particle complexes in the human placenta. Pathology Research and Practice 169: 323–329

3049. Vykoupil K F, Thiele J, Georgii A 1976 Hairy cell leukemia: bone marrow findings in 24 patients. Virchows Archiv A Pathological Anatomy and Histology 370: 273–289

## 71 HISTIOCYTOSES

3050. Basset F, Corrin B, Spencer H, Lacronique J, Roth C, Soler P, Battesti J-P, Georges R, Chrétien J 1978 Pulmonary histiocytosis X. American Review of Respiratory Disease 118: 811–820

3051. Basset F, Escaig J, LeCrom M 1972 A cytoplasmic membranous complex in histiocytosis X. Cancer 29: 1380–1386

3052. Cline M J, Golde D W 1973 A review and reevaluation of the histiocytic disorders. American Journal of Medicine 55: 49–60

3053. Corrin B, Basset F 1979 A review of histiocytosis X with particular reference to eosinophilic granuloma of the lung. Investigative & Cell Pathology 2: 137–146

3054. David R, Buchner A 1980 Langerhans' cells in a pleomorphic adenoma of submandibular salivary gland. Journal of Pathology 131: 127–135

3055. Divertie M B, Cassan S M, Brown A L Jr 1975 Application of ultrastructural morphometry to lung biopsy specimens in pulmonary histiocytosis X. Thorax 30: 326–332

3056. El-Labban N G 1982 The nature of Langerhans cell granules: an ultrastructural study. Histopathology 6: 317–325

3057. Flynn K J, Dehner L P, Gajl-Peezalska K J, Dahl M V, Ramsay N, Wang N 1982 Regressing atypical histiocytosis: a cutaneous proliferation of atypical neoplastic histiocytes with unexpectedly indolent biologic behavior. Cancer 49: 959–970

3058. Glick A D, Bennett B, Collins R D 1980 Neoplasms of the mononuclear phagocyte system: criteria for diagnosis. Investigative & Cell Pathology 3: 259–279

3059. Gold J, L'Heureux P, Dehner L P 1977 Ultrastructure in the differential diagnosis of pulmonary histiocytosis and pneumocystosis. Archives of Pathology and Laboratory Medicine 101: 243–247

3060. Griffin J D, Ellman L, Long J C, Dvorak A M 1978 Development of a histiocytic medullary reticulosis-like syndrome during the course of acute lymphocytic leukemia. American Journal of Medicine 64: 851–858

3061. Hashimoto K, Griffin D, Kohsbaki M 1982 Self-healing reticulohistiocytosis: a clinical, histologic, and ultrastructural study of the fourth case in the literature. Cancer 49: 331–337

3062. Henderson D W, Sage R E 1972 Malignant histiocytosis with eosinophilia. Cancer 32: 1421–1428

3063. Heustis D G, Bull B S, Handley G G 1977 Ultrastructure of the spleen in malignant histiocytosis. Archives of Pathology and Laboratory Medicine 101: 239–242

3064. Ho F C S, Todd D 1978 Malignant histiocytosis. Report of five Chinese patients. Cancer 42: 2450–2460

3065. Huhn D, Meister P 1978 Malignant histiocytosis: morphologic and cytochemical findings. Cancer 42: 1341–1349

3066. Ide F, Sano R, Shimura H, Kusama K, Umemura S 1981 An ultrastructural and immunohistochemical study on mandibular lesion of Letterer-Siewe disease. Journal of Oral Pathology 10: 386–397

3067. Imamura M, Muraya K 1971 Lymph node ultrastructure in Hand-Schüller-Christian disease. Cancer 27: 956–964

3068. Imamura M, Sakamoto S, Hanazono H 1971 Malignant histiocytosis: a case of generalized histiocytosis with infiltration of Langerhans' granule-containing histiocytes. Cancer 28: 467–475

3069. Kim H, Pangalis G A, Payne B C, Kadin M E, Rappaport H 1982 Ultrastructural identification of neoplastic histiocytes-monocytes. An application of a newly developed cytochemical technique. American Journal of Pathology 106: 204–223

3070. Lampert I A, Catovsky D, Bergier N 1978 Malignant histiocytosis: a clinico-pathological study of 12 cases. British Journal of Haematology 40: 65–77

3071. Lombardi L, Carbone A, Pilotti S, Rilke F 1978 Malignant histiocytosis: a histological and ultrastructural study of lymph nodes in six cases. Histopathology 2: 315–328

3072. Mierau G W, Favara B E, Brenman J M 1982 Electron microscopy in histiocytosis X. Ultrastructural Pathology 3: 137–142

3073. Morales A R, Fine G, Horn R C Jr, Watson J H L 1969 Langerhans cells in a localized lesion of the eosinophilic granuloma type. Laboratory Investigation 20: 412–423

3074. Newton W A Jr, Hamoudi A B 1973 Histiocytosis: a histologic classification with clinical correlation. Perspectives in Pediatric Pathology 1: 251–283

3075. Nezelof C 1979 Histiocytosis X: a histological and histogenetic study. Perspectives in Pediatric Pathology 5: 153–178

3076. Nezelof C, Basset F, Rousseau M F 1973 Histiocytosis X: histogenetic arguments for a Langerhans' cell origin. Biomedicine 18: 365–371

3077. Nezelof C, Jaubert F 1978 Histiocytic and/or reticulum cell neoplasias. Recent Results in Cancer Research 6: 118–125

3078. Rausch E, Kaiserling E, Goos M 1977 Langerhans cells and interdigitating reticulum cells in the thymus-dependent region in human dermatopathic lymphadenitis. Virchows Archiv B Cell Pathology 25: 327–343

3079. Rausch P G, Herion J C, Carney C N, Weinstein P 1979 Malignant histiocytosis. A cytochemical and electron microscopic study of an unusual case. Cancer 44: 2158–2164

3080. Risdall R J, Sibley R K, McKenna R W, Brunning R D, Dehner L P 1980 Malignant histiocytosis. A light- and electron-microscopic and histochemical study. American Journal of Surgical Pathology 4: 439–450

3081. Ritter R A Jr 1966 Histiocytosis X. A case report with electron microscopic observations. Cancer 19: 1155–1164

3082. Rodriguez E M, Caorsi J 1978 A second look at the ultrastructure of the Langerhans cell of the human epidermis. Journal of Ultrastructure Research 65: 279–295

3083. Rousseau-Merck M F, Barbey S, Jaubert F, Bach M A, Chatenoud L, Nezelof C 1983 Reactivity of histiocytosis X cells with monoclonal antibodies. Pathology Research and Practice 177: 8–12

3084. Sagebiel R W, Reed T H 1968 Serial reconstruction of the characteristic granule of the Langerhans cell. Journal of Cell Biology 36: 595–602

3085. Sajjad S M, Luna M A 1982 Primary pulmonary histiocytosis X in two patients with Hodgkin's disease. Thorax 37: 110–113

3086. Shamoto M 1970 Langerhans cell granule in Letterer-Siwe disease. An electron microscopic study. Cancer 26: 1102–1108

3087. Shelley W B, Juhlin L 1978 The Langerhans cell: its origin, nature, and function. Acta Dermatovener, suppl 79: 7–22

3088. Skinnider L F, Ghadially F N 1977 Ultrastructure of cell surface abnormalities in neoplastic histiocytes. British Journal of Cancer 35: 657–667

3089. Smith M, McCormack L J, Van Ordstrand H S, Mercer R D 1974 Primary pulmonary histiocytosis X. Chest 65: 176–180

3090. Vernon M L, Fountain L, Krebs H M, Horta-Barbosa L, Fuccillo D A, Sever J L 1973 Birbeck granules (Langerhans' cell granules) in human lymph nodes. American Journal of Clinical Pathology 60: 771–779

3091. Vilpo J A, Klemi P, Lassila O, Fraki J, Sahni T T 1980 Cytological and functional characterisation of three cases of malignant histiocytosis. Cancer 46: 1795–1801

3092. Vogel J M, Vogel P 1972 Idiopathic histiocytosis: a discussion of eosinophilic granuloma, the Hand-Schüller-Christian syndrome and the Letterer-Siwe syndrome. Seminars in Hematology 9: 349–369

3093. Williams J W, Dorfman R F 1979 Lymphadenopathy as the initial manifestation of histiocytosis X. American Journal of Surgical Pathology 3: 405–421

## 72 PLASMACYTOMA/MYELOMATOSIS AND PLASMA CELL LEUKAEMIA

3094. Arkin C F, Federman M, Gerson B 1981 Paranuclear microfilaments in multiple myeloma associated with the presence of free light chains. Annals of Clinical and Laboratory Science 11: 506–510

3095. Asselah F, Crow J, Slavin G, Sowter G, Sheldon C, Asselah H 1982 Solitary plasmacytoma of the intestine. Histopathology 6: 631–645

3096. Azar H A 1973 Amyloidosis and plasma cell disorders. In: Azar H A, Potter M (eds) Multiple myeloma and related disorders, vol 1. Harper & Row, Hagerstown, ch 7, p 328–403

3097. Azar H A 1973 The myeloma cell. In: Azar H A, Potter M (eds) Multiple myeloma and related disorders, vol 1. Harper & Row, Hagerstown, ch 2, p 86–152

3098. Bartoloni C, Flamini G, Gentiloni N, Russo M A, Barone C, Gambassi G, Terranova T 1980 Immunochemical and ultrastructural study of multiple myeloma with a heavy chain protein in the serum. Journal of Clinical Pathology 33: 936–945

3099. Bassan H, Gutmann H, Djaldetti M 1981 Ultrastructural characteristics of the plasma cells of a patient with non secretory myeloma and plasma cell leukemia. Acta Haematologica 66: 129–133

3100. Bernier G M, Duca V D Jr, Brereton R, Graham R C Jr 1975 Multiple myeloma with intramedullary masses of M component. Blood 46: 931–935

3101. Blom J 1977 The ultrastructure of macrophages found in contact with plasma cells in the bone marrow of patients with multiple myeloma. Acta Pathologica et Microbiologica Scandinavica. Section A. Pathology 85: 335–344

3102. Blom J, Hansen O P, Mansa B 1980 The ultrastructure of bone marrow plasma cells obtained from patients with multiple myeloma during the clinical course of the disease. Acta Pathologica et Microbiologica Scandinavica. Section A. Pathology 88: 25–39

3103. Booth J B, Cheesman A D, Vincenti N H 1973 Extramedullary plasmacytomata of the upper respiratory tract. Annals of Otology, Rhinology and Laryngology 82: 709–715

3104. Brunning R D, Maldonado J E 1980 Plasma cell dyscrasias. In: Johannessen J V (ed) Electron microscopy in human medicine, vol 5. Cardiovascular system, lymphoreticular and hematopoietic system. McGraw-Hill, New York, pt 5, ch 26, p 354–373

3105. Cleary B, Binder R A, Kales A N, Veltri B J 1978 Simultaneous presentation of acute myelomonocytic leukemia and multiple myeloma. Cancer 41: 1381–1386

3106. Curtis S K, Propp R, Cowden R R, Tartaglia A P 1975 Ultrastructure of a human malignant IgA-producing plasmacytoma. Experimental and Molecular Pathology 22: 386–399

3107. Djaldetti M 1982 Mitochondrial abnormalities in the cells of myeloma patients. Acta Haematologica 68: 241–248

3108. Djaldetti M, Fishman P 1977 Scanning and transmission electron microscopy study on the plasma cells of a patient with multiple myeloma. Acta Haematologica 58: 173–180

3109. Djaldetti M, Lewinski U H 1978 Origin of intranuclear inclusions in myeloma cells. Scandinavian Journal of Haematology 20: 200–205

3110. El-Labban N G 1979 New findings of a lamina densa in relation to plasma cells. Histopathology 3: 287–294

3111. Ferrer-Roca O 1982 Primary gastric plasmacytoma with massive intracytoplasmic crystalline inclusions. A case report. Cancer 50: 755–759

3112. Foucar K, Raber M, Foucar E, Barlogie B, Sandler C M, Alexanian R 1982 Anaplastic myeloma with massive extramedullary involvement. Report of two cases. Cancer 51: 166–174

3113. Franklin R M, Kenyon K R, Green W R, Saral R, Humphrey R 1982 Epibulbar IgA plasmacytoma occurring in multiple myeloma. Archives of Ophthalmology 100: 451–456

3114. Graham R C Jr, Bernier G M 1975 Bone marrow in multiple myeloma: correlation of plasma cell ultrastructure and clinical state. Medicine (Baltimore) 54: 225–243

3115. Kalderon A E, Bogaars H A, Diamond I, Cummings F J, Kaplan S R, Calabresi P 1977 Ultrastructure of myeloma cells in a case with crystalcryoglubinemia. Cancer 39: 1475–1481

3116. Kitani T, Yonezawa T, Imanaka T, Hiraoka A, Nasu T 1982 Ultrastructural analysis of membrane-bound polysomes in human myeloma cells. Blut 44: 51–63

3117. Klain B, Lewinski U, Shabtai F, Freidin N, Djaldetti M 1977 Transmission and scanning electron microscopy study on plasma cell leukemia. Blut 35: 11–19

3118. Lazarus H M, Kellermeyer R W, Aikawa M, Herzig R H 1980 Multiple myeloma in young men. Clinical course and electron microscopic studies of bone marrow plasma cells. Cancer 46: 1397–1400

3119. Maldonado J E, Bayrd E D, Brown A L Jr 1965 The flaming cell in multiple myeloma. A light and electron microscopy study. American Journal of Clinical Pathology 44: 605–612

3120. Maldonado J E, Brown A L Jr, Bayrd E D, Pease G L 1966 Ultrastructure of the myeloma cell. Cancer 19: 1613–1627

3121. Maldonado J E, Kyle R A, Brown A L Jr, Bayrd E D 1966 Intermediate cell types and mixed cell proliferation in multiple myeloma. Electron microscopic observations. Blood 27: 212–226

3122. Maldonado J E, Brown A L Jr, Bayrd E D, Pease G L 1966 Cytoplasmic and intranuclear electron dense bodies in the myeloma cell. Archives of Pathology 81: 484–500

3123. Mancilla-Jimenez R, Tavassoli F A 1976 Solitary meningeal plasmacytoma. Report of a case with electron microscopic and immunohistologic observations. Cancer 38: 798–806

3124. Polliack A, Gamliel H, Froimovici M, Laskov R 1978 Myeloma cells: surface morphology as seen by scanning and transmission electron microscopy. Israel Journal of Medical Sciences 14: 1252–1258

3125. Polliack A, Leiserowitz R, Korkesh A, Matzner Y, Prokocimer M, Gamliel H 1981 Plasma cell leukemia and myeloma: a scanning electron-microscopic study of cell surface features in six cases. American Journal of Clinical Pathology 75: 834–838

3126. Polliack A, Nilsson K, Laskov R, Biberfeld P 1978 Characteristic surface morphology of human and murine myeloma cells. A scanning and transmission electron microscopic study. British Journal of Haematology 39: 25–32

3127. Renau-Piqueras J, Wetter O, Miragall F, Miguel A, Hertenstein Ch, Cervera J, Brandhorst D 1982 Extramedullary multiple myeloma. A qualitative and quantitative electron microscopic study. Virchows Archiv B Cell Pathology 40: 171–190

3128. Ricci A Jr, Monahan R A, Paradise C, Robinson S, Dvorak A M 1982 Unusual inclusions in plasmacytoid cells. Their occurrence in a patient with Waldenström's macroglobulinemia. Archives of Pathology and Laboratory Medicine 106: 452–457

3129. Rygaard-Olsen C, Boedker A, Emus H C, Olsen H A R 1982 Extramedullary plasmacytoma of the small intestine. A case report studied with electron microscopy and immunoperoxidase technique. Cancer 50: 573–576

3130. Sanchez J A, Rahman S, Strauss R A, Kaye G I 1977 Multiple myeloma masquerading as a pituitary tumor. Archives of Pathology and Laboratory Medicine 101: 55–56

3131. Schweers C A, Shaw M T, Nordquist R E, Rose D D, Kell T 1976 Solitary cecal plasmacytoma. Electron microscopic, immunologic, and cytochemical studies. Cancer 37: 2220–2223

3132. Shaw M T, Twele T W, Nordquist R E 1974 Plasma cell leukemia: detailed studies and response to therapy. Cancer 33: 619–625

3133. Smetana K, Lane M, Busch H 1966 Studies on nucleoli of leukemic agranulocytes and plasmacytes in multiple myeloma. Experimental and Molecular Pathology 5: 236–244

3134. Soffer D, Siegal T 1982 Solitary dural plasmacytoma with conspicuous cytoplasmic inclusions. Cancer 49: 2500–2504

3135. Stavem P, Froland S S, Haugen H F, Lislerud A 1976 Nonsecretory myelomatosis without intracellular immuno-globulin. Immunofluorescent and ultramicroscopic studies. Scandinavian Journal of Haematology 17: 89–95

3136. Stavem P, Hovig T, Froland S, Skrede S 1974 Immunoglobulin-containing intranuclear inclusions in plasma cells in a case of IgG myeloma. Scandinavian Journal of Haematology 13: 266–275

3137. Tavassoli M, Baughan M 1973 Virus-like particles in human myeloma without paraproteinemia. Archives of Pathology 96: 347–349

3138. Turesson I 1975 Nucleolar size in benign and malignant plasma cell proliferation. Acta Medica Scandinavica 197: 7–14

3139. Veloso F T, Saleiro J V, Oliveira A O, de Freitas A F 1983 Atypical plasma cells in alpha-chain disease. Cancer 52: 79–82

3140. Vital C, Vallat J M, Deminiere C, Loubet A, Leboutet M J 1982 Peripheral nerve damage during multiple myeloma and Waldenström's macroglobulinemia. An ultrastructural and immunopathologic study. Cancer 50: 1491–1497

3141. Weiss S, Lewinski U H, Pick A J, Gafter U, Djaldetti M 1978 Ultrastructural features of the plasma cells in non-secretory myeloma. Blut 36: 149–157

3142. Yasuda N, Kanoh T, Vchino H 1980 J chain synthesis in human myeloma cells: light and electron microscopic studies. Clinical and Experimental Immunology 40: 573–580

3143. Yonezawa T, Kitani T, Tamaki T, Kanayama Y, Hiraoka A, Tarui S 1982 Immunoglobulin production and secretion in Bence Jones protein myeloma and 'nonsecretory' myeloma. Ultrastructural and immunofluorescence study. Blut 45: 121–129

## 73 SUPPLEMENTARY REFERENCES

3144. Baden H P 1984 The keratinocyte has become the subject of intensive investigation. Journal of Investigative Dermatology 82: 305–307

3145. Capella C, Polak J M, Buffa R, Tapia F J, Heitz Ph, Usellini L, Bloom S R, Solcia E 1983 Morphologic patterns and diagnostic criteria of VIP-producing endocrine tumors. A histologic, histochemical, ultrastructural, and biochemical study of 32 cases. Cancer 52: 1860–1874

3146. Chase D R, Enzinger F M, Weiss S W, Langloss J M 1984 Keratin in epithelioid sarcoma. An immunohistochemical study. American Journal of Surgical Pathology 8: 435–441

3147. Edelman G M 1984 Cell-adhesion molecules: a molecular basis for animal form. Scientific American 250: 80–91

3148. Erlandson R A 1984 Diagnostic immunohistochemistry of human tumors. An interim evaluation. American Journal of Surgical Pathology 8: 615–624

3149. Payne C M, Nagle R B 1983 An ultrastructural study of intranuclear rodlets in a malignant extracranial neuroepithelial neoplasm. Ultrastructural Pathology 5: 1–13

3150. Yum M, Goheen M, Mandelbaum I 1984 Intracytoplasmic lumina in metastatic melanoma cells. Archives of Pathology and Laboratory Medicine 108: 183–184

# Index